WILLIAM OSLER

A Life in Medicine

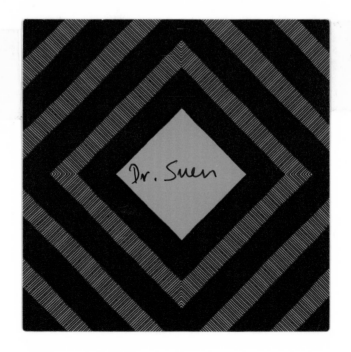

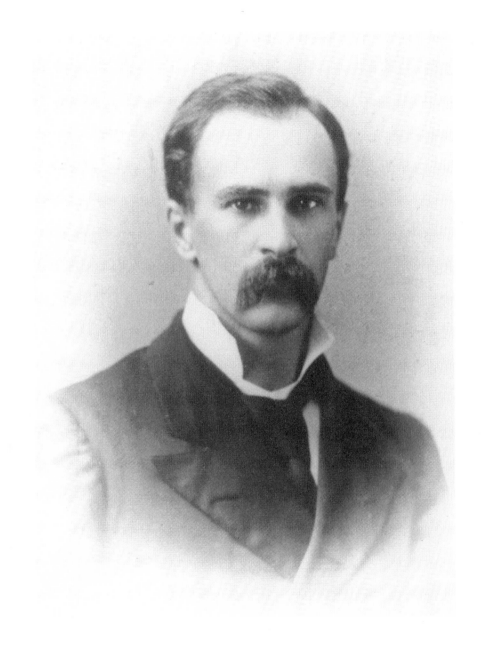

William Osler

WILLIAM OSLER
A Life in Medicine

MICHAEL BLISS

UNIVERSITY OF TORONTO PRESS
Toronto

Printed in Canada

Reprinted 2000

ISBN 0-8020-4349-6

Printed on acid-free paper

Canadian Cataloguing in Publication Data

Bliss, Michael, 1941–
William Osler : a life in medicine

Includes bibliographical references and index.
ISBN 0-8020-4349-6

1. Osler, William, Sir, 1849–1919.   2. Physicians – Biography.   I. Title.

R464.O8B54 1999   610′.92   C99-930825-4

University of Toronto Press acknowledges the financial assistance to its
publishing program of the Canada Council for the Arts and
the Ontario Arts Council.

We acknowledge the financial support of the Government of Canada
through the Book Publishing Industry Development Program (BPIDP)
for our publishing activities.
Canadä

To the memory of

Quartus Bliss, MD, Physician and Surgeon, 1903–1956

James Quartus Bliss, BSc, MD, PhD, Physiologist, 1930–1969

Contents

Illustrations follow pages 210 and 434

Preface: On Doing an Osler Autopsy

W as William Osler the greatest doctor in the history of the world? The idea was seriously advanced after his death in England, at Oxford, in 1919.

That would be a tough competition. Most of Osler's admirers were content to claim that he had merely been their era's most famous, most beloved, and most influential physician. These were no mean accolades either. Would any contemporary of Osler's – writer, artist, politician, scientist – have done so well in all three categories, and without anyone dissenting?

In seventy years from his birth in the backwoods of Canada, Osler had practiced, written about, and taught medicine at McGill University in Montreal, the University of Pennsylvania in Philadelphia, Johns Hopkins Hospital and University in Baltimore, and as Regius Professor of Medicine at Oxford. He had been a brilliant, innovative teacher, adored by his students, especially the young men and women who fanned out from Johns Hopkins as leaders in the new era of North American dominance of medicine.

Osler had literally written the book on his subject. *The Principles and Practice of Medicine*, issued in 1892, was the first great textbook of modern medicine. It dominated its market, had huge sales, went through many editions, and also proved to be the last text in which a single author dared to write on the whole range of the body's internal ills. In hundreds of other articles and monographs, Osler reported on the characteristics, diagnosis, and treatment of an amazing variety of diseases, syndromes, and cases – from staples, such as typhoid fever and syphilis, to all manner of exotic conditions, several of which came to bear his name.

What exactly did he discover? Very little – though when you map the frontiers of medicine in that era, you often find that Osler's were among the pioneers' tracks. But we are not asking the right question. Osler was an observer and scholar of the natural history of disease, a teacher of the natural history of illness, and a working doctor. He was not an experimental scientist, in the business of making discoveries. He honored and used the discoverers' breakthroughs, knowing that medicine must rest on science. As a clinical physician he went on from there, trying to heal and teaching the science and art of healing. The medical scientists and their discoveries could assist and supplement and arm, but they could never replace the doctor seeing patients. Osler's revolutionary impact as a teacher was to have medical students learn doctoring by working at the bedside.

When his students and colleagues were sick, Osler was usually their doctor. In his private practice he also saw poets, politicians, royalty, and nameless ordinary people with extraordinary conditions. He had a charismatic personality, as a physician and as a friend. His friends and the tribute they paid him seemed endless, both during his lifetime and for generations after his death. Osler had the best of two medical worlds, American and British, as patients and friends, and he never forgot his Canadian origins either. Everyone knew Osler, and almost everyone loved him. A few disciples literally worshiped him.

Much more than a physician, Osler was a literate, inspiring, humanist in science. His essays and addresses about the medical life, past, present, and future, were widely read and appreciated for their blending of scientific and literary knowledge with high idealism and sensible advice about getting on with the daily grind. In both his writings and his personal life, and through a prism of tragedy in the Great War, Osler seemed to embody the art of living. A friend said his story would be of interest to anyone who takes life seriously. William Welch, colleague and fellow medical giant, suggested that Osler's career had been a splendid match of character with situation, an 'almost perfect adaptation of his talents and temperament to the accidents and circumstances of his life.'[1]

In the last chapter I describe how those who had idolized Osler during his lifetime worked to ensure him immortality as a medical and inspirational role model. The fourteen-hundred-page, two-volume official biography, *The Life of Sir William Osler,* written by the great neurosurgeon Harvey Cushing, played a central role in the ongoing Osler mystique. For more than seventy years from its 1925 publication, Cushing's *Osler* was the authoritative, revered text, second in importance only to Osler's own inspirational and historical essays. The biography was acclaimed in its own right as a masterpiece and in the United States won a Pulitzer Prize. Would anyone ever supersede Cushing as a guide to Osler's life? Why would anyone want to try?

Later neurosurgeons, of course, were quick to improve on Cushing's surgical techniques. Even in its day, his Osler biography was a ponderous, repetitive narrative, which nonbelievers found difficult to approach and nearly impossible to finish. It seemed hagiographic. It was certainly uncritical. In time, it was dismissed for not addressing many of the questions historians were beginning to ask about Osler's life and his medical world.

The discovery of new primary sources further dated Cushing's pages. A large new corpus of writing about Osler gradually developed; some of it reflected high standards of scholarship and objectivity, and a few authors groped towards a revisionist view of the medical idol. Was William Osler's approach to medicine viable in the long run? Was his charisma real or contrived? Was he, like so many other historical figures, a captive of his generation's racial and gender biases? Was his reputation overblown, more hype than Hippocratic? Was he hypocritical in projecting an image of sanctity possibly not reflected in his personal life? By the 1980s anyone who tried to read Cushing or think about Osler knew how badly a new biography was needed.[2]

I became interested in Osler's life when I began to study medical history seriously after a first excursion into the subject which resulted in two books – *The Discovery of Insulin* (1982) and *Banting: A Biography* (1984) – and whetted my appetite. My Canadian connections first led me from insulin and Banting to Osler. But it was instantly clear that Osler had far outdistanced most of his countrymen, medical and lay, in a life of achievement and mobility, complexity, and, possibly, ongoing significance. It was also clear that writing a new Osler biography would be an exhausting job. The sources were vast and were scattered in archives in three countries. Much of Osler's work as a physician is technically difficult to understand and explain in context – and doubly so for a nonphysician. The Cushing biography, so packed with detail and the author's first-hand knowledge, awaited Osler explorers like a lush, hazardous, and tiresome jungle. What if the Osler territory turned out to be nothing more than a dense medical forest, impenetrable except to experts and acolytes? Publishers told me there was little interest in biographies of scientists, less in the lives of doctors. Daunted, I turned to more manageable topics and friendlier terrain.

Three books later, one of them a study of smallpox in Montreal during Osler's time, I reconsidered. I had a better sense of how to handle large bodies of sources, thanks in part to the wonderful capacities of the laptop computer; I was better prepared for some of the challenges involved in writing about medicine; and I had become familiar enough with Osler to be excited by the richness of his medical life and the splendor of his aspirations. His life and work, I realized, offered another way of reflecting on the human condition, of studying the meaning of life and death, the quest for salvation, and the forms of immortality.

Once I had decided that a new narration of Osler's life was apt to be interesting and illuminating, it did not particularly matter to me how he turned out as a human being. In my biography of Sir Frederick Banting, a co-discover of insulin, I had written frankly about a Canadian icon who was a mediocre scientist, a boor, and a chauvinist. At times Banting was best compared to a horse's ass, not always favorably. Nothing pleased me more than praise for the book's fairness from both those who loved and those who despised Banting. The ideal of objectivity is the *sine qua non* of historical scholarship.

These chapters are as fair-minded and objective a portrait of Osler as I can produce, using every tool of my trade. Immersing myself in the sources, expecting them to make possible a reasonable amount of icon bashing, I gradually found myself becoming struck by the power of the Osler image. Osler worship was more widespread than I had realized and was more heart-felt, less self-interested or promotional than I had anticipated. Osler shone partly by comparison with many of his colleagues, but it became clear to me that he was a man who would have stood out, did stand out, in any crowd – except that he had a habit of disappearing from crowds to find some children to play with. Nothing struck me more forcibly about the beauty of Osler's personality than the magic he could generate with little children. It shines in scores of his wonderfully whimsical, loving notes and in dozens of anecdotes and memoirs, many more than are recounted here. With children, Osler had Lewis Carroll's sensibilities without his peculiarities.

For some years Osler had minor tuberculous growths on his hands, known as 'cadaver wart,' which came from all his work with corpses. He had learned his trade as a pathologist, investigating the remains of the dead to find out what had gone wrong with them. All biography has to partake of what Joyce Carol Oates has labeled 'pathography,' and comparisons of historians to pathologists (and archives to morgues) are often apt. Rather to my surprise, this postmortem study of Osler has not found other significant warts or pathological conditions. His was a life that stands up almost too well to critical dissection, even microscopic scrutiny. In an age when biographers make their reputation by claiming to have discovered hidden internal derangements in their subjects, this project has been an unusual intellectual autopsy, at times something of a modern biographer's nightmare. Try as I might, I could not find a cause to justify the death of Osler's reputation. He lived a magnificent, epic, important, and more than slightly saintly life. For the most part, Osler 'revisionism' does not work. Even a splendidly Victorian sex scandal, celebrated in oral Osler history for years, appears to have been an invention.

The sources, and the life itself, proved far richer than I had anticipated, and they do lead in these pages to a great deal of new, revisionist views of Osler's friends, institutions, and medical world. The book has also been written in the context of the exploding and marvelously fruitful world of scholarship in medical history. But I have tried to make every paragraph intelligible to any reasonably literate reader, lay or medical, from high school student to molecular biologist, to tired general practitioner, to anyone with a taste for biography. From the outset I determined to tell the story of this life in one volume. Even brain surgery takes less time now than in Harvey Cushing's day.

William Osler's life illuminates his medical and cultural times in striking ways, and I hope it illuminates our times too. This book is about the coming of modern medicine, the training of doctors, the doctor-patient relationship, localism and holism in medical thought, role modeling, feminism, humanism, science and the humanities, Victorianism, the rise of the United States, the North Atlantic cultural triangle, the Great War, the decline of Christianity, our collapsing life expectancy, the religion of health care, the Anglican temperament, and much else. But the essence of any biography must be the attempt to recreate a human life, an effort that extends beyond intellectual pathology or social science. My aim has been to follow Walt Whitman, who happened to have been a patient of William Osler's, and who wrote that the poet 'drags the dead out of their coffins and stands them again on their feet ... He says to the past, Rise and walk before me that I may realize you.'[3] Osler, you will see, would have particularly appreciated that image.

For thanks and acknowledgments, please turn to page 557.

MICHAEL BLISS
SPRINGFIELD, PRINCE EDWARD ISLAND
SEPTEMBER 1998

WILLIAM OSLER
A Life in Medicine

We live forward, we understand backward.

WILLIAM JAMES

And I call to mankind, Be not curious about God
For I who am curious about each am not curious about God.

WALT WHITMAN

I call the effects of Nature the works of God.

SIR THOMAS BROWNE

What more delightful in literature than biography? And yet, how uncertain and
treacherous is the account which any man can give of another's life.

SIR WILLIAM OSLER

ONE

English Gentlemen with American Energy

William Osler was born in a parsonage in backwoods Canada on July 12, 1849. His parents had come out from England to serve the Anglican Church in an obscure corner of British North America. Their parish centered on the hamlet of Bond Head, Canada West, some forty miles north of the little city of Toronto. At the time of Osler's birth, Bond Head was still a frontier station on the edge of a savage wilderness. Thousands of miles across the Atlantic, Victorian Britain was approaching the height of its power, prestige, and cultural refinement.

Osler was of mainly Celtic descent. Many generations of his forebears had lived in Cornwall in southwestern England. The name Osler is derived from 'ostler,' a stableman at an inn, and has a common root with 'host' and 'hospitality.' The Canadian family pronounces the 'o' long as in 'host,' not short as in 'lost.'

Four older Oslers were particularly important in shaping a legacy for William. They were his grandfather, Edward Osler, of Falmouth, England; a physician-uncle, Edward Osler, of England and Wales; and, of course, his father and mother, the Reverend Featherstone Lake Osler and Ellen Free Pickton Osler. These relatives' ambitions and adventures, especially the parents' journey from genteel England to raw North America, set the stage for William's life and mission. As well, like most of us, he grew up to resemble and echo the people whose genes he bore.

Edward Osler, William's grandfather, born in 1758, had turned his back on his family's seafaring tradition to become a shopkeeper and shipowner in the ancient port city of Falmouth, on the southern Cornish coast. He became moderately prosperous and hoped his nine children, especially his four sons, would rise in the world. If not, they should at least maintain the family's degree of comfort and security. When the eldest son, Edward, decided to become a surgeon, a step up the ladder, the father was willing to bear considerable expense to help with his education.

Much of this book touches on the making of doctors. In England in the early 1800s the two ancient universities, Oxford and Cambridge, turned out only a handful of physicians, mostly from the upper classes. Most young Britons who wanted to study medicine or surgery served a local apprenticeship, then took courses at hospitals or privately run schools, usually in London, and finally wrote licensing examinations. Future-uncle Edward Osler took this route. He served an apprenticeship with a Falmouth surgeon, then sailed with his father to London to arrange for the rest of his training.

Medical education had become partially modern in the sense that students, then as now, began to know the body by studying bodies. They learned anatomy and pathology by working on cadavers, human preferably, other animals if necessary. Cutting up or dissecting dead bodies has always been a gruesome business for most lay people and would-be students to contemplate. But the ability to examine diseased, dying, and dead humans with at least outward detachment or calm was and is a *sine qua non* of practicing medicine.

On a June day in 1816, a year after the end of the Napoleonic Wars, the Edward Oslers, father and eighteen-year-old son, visited the well-known Blenheim Street anatomy 'school' run by Joshua Brookes. It was the only such London institution open in summer; other instructors were inhibited by the problem of corpses decomposing in the heat. When Brookes, once described by a colleague as 'the dirtiest professional person I've ever met with ... all and every part of him was dirt,' showed the Oslers his anatomical 'museum,' Edward senior recoiled in terror from the stench. He thought the odors themselves might poison him. The experience seemed to him like a descent into Hades.[1]

The son already had a medical student's apparent equanimity. He also had a lively pen and a gauche desire to shock the folk back in Falmouth. Perhaps also sublimating inner nausea, he described what it was like to work at Brookes's:

> On the second day of my attendance, I entered the dissecting room for the first time. The first object which met my view was the body of an old man stretched on a shutter in the court, the brain taken out, & the scalp hanging about his ears, whilst his straggling white locks were matted together by his blood. A hungry wolf was snarling at it, & straining to get at it as far as his chain would allow him. A tub full of human flesh was standing near it, some pieces of which I gave the eagles, who devoured it with avidity. On entering the room, the stink was most abominable. About 20 chaps were at work, carving limbs & bodies, in all stages of putrefaction, & of all colors; black, green, yellow, blue, while the pupils carved them apparently, with as much pleasure, as they would carve their dinner.[2]

The hometown readers were predictably disgusted. Reveling in their discomfort and enjoying indulging his 'scribbling propensity,' Edward supplied more graphic detail:

> We had a woman brought in three weeks ago, which was drowned in the Regents Canal. She is the fattest carcase I ever saw, so much so, that none of the pupils would take her. Her thigh is larger in circumference than my body. Three or four operations have been performed on her, & the fat is four inches deep in some places. Indeed, she is a ball of grease, & is now lying in the dissecting room untouched, except that one hip, shoulder, & breast, & her skull cap are taken off. She stinks most abominably, and when the sun shines hot, the yellow globules of melted fat run from her upon the floor, like fresh butter, and in the evening it congeals there like little saffron buns. I took a gentleman into the dissecting room last Monday, but he could not stand it a second, nor could I persuade him to enter it again ...
>
> I am now dissecting part of a female subject. Wonderful to relate, though 28 years of age her hymen was perfect. A handsome woman too. I gave it to Brookes at his request, to place among the rareties of his museum.[3]

Edward attended lectures at Brookes's school and at Guy's and St Thomas's hospitals, and he walked the wards of several hospitals to see cases. 'The ward smells worse than a dissecting room.' He was most interested in observing surgery. We are several decades before the advent of anesthesia:

> Mr. Travers castrated an Irishman this forenoon at St Thomas', who roared most lustily. He was to have performed the operation for Hydrocele [a scrotal cyst] on a poor devil of a taylor, but he being frightened I suppose at the terrible outcries of the Irishman, would not get upon the table. Mr. Travers endeavored to persuade him to undergo the operation, but in vain, & he accompanied his refusals with gesticulations, which gave such an effect to his pale, trembling, vacant, sartorial physiognomy, that the whole theatre was kept in a roar of laughter. Another patient was brought, & underwent the same operation without flinching, as might be expected ... The taylor ... slunk downstairs to his ward, amidst the laughter of the pupils, the hootings of the patients, who collected at the doors of the wards to see him pass, & the scolds of the nurses & sisters.[4]

British medical students no longer had to procure their own corpses for dissection. Graverobbing had become specialized: the recently dead were raised from their resting places and sold to the medical schools by professional bodysnatchers, nicknamed 'resurrection men.' The demand was very high, but so was resistance to the idea of mutilating the dead – widely feared as a kind of final, horrible assault on the person.[5] Families tried to forestall graverobbing with mortuaries and burglar-proof coffins, and sometimes with armed guards. Soon all the United Kingdom would be appalled to learn that some resurrectionists, notably William Burke and William Hare in Edinburgh, had bypassed the middleman, as it were, by murdering ('burking') the living to create bodies for dissection. In 1832 Parliament passed the Anatomy Act, based on French practice, making available the corpses of indigents for dissection. In other countries the search for teaching aids in medicine remained less regulated.

Edward Osler finished his training, became a licensed surgeon, and secured a promising position as resident surgeon to the Swansea Infirmary, one of the few hospitals in Wales. He hoped to fulfill his father's expectations and rise in Britain's layered society: 'I think I can climb a little way ... I cannot help thinking that I shall be somebody one day, if I live.'[6] He concentrated on ophthalmic, or eye surgery, a very early specialty.

Edward married and began to raise a family. But his young wife's health became precarious and she had to leave Swansea (which also was in decline). Edward resigned his position and indulged in an opportunity to go to sea as a medical officer and student of natural history. His wife died soon after his return, and he moved home to Falmouth. There he practiced little medicine, instead spending most of his time scribbling. He wrote poetry (not nearly as well as his contemporary in medical studies in London, John Keats), also natural history, many hymns, and theology, following in the tradition of his maternal relative Samuel Drew, a prolific author locally famous as 'the Cornish Metaphysician.'

Two of Edward's younger brothers were not having much success as Falmouth storekeepers. One of them, Sam, eventually became the family's black sheep, a drinker and womanizer. By the 1830s the septuagenarian father, Edward senior, was suffering from a bilious disorder. Edward junior prescribed regular purging; but the patient himself, 'after many experiments,' concluded that the best medicine for his condition was 'beef and good Port Wine.'[7] Edward *père* worried about his offspring's ability to sustain the family's 'respectability of station & character.' His boys' blasting of their good prospects disgusted him, and he was not pleased that young Edward appeared to be so contented to stay at home: 'I do sometimes grieve to think that after such an Education, no expense spared, he should have so mispent the best years of his life ... He is a peculiar character and I fear there is little prospect of his becoming independant of his Family ... I do like to see a Man more like a Man.'[8]

Edward *fils* finally left home again, marrying a second and eventually a third time. He became mainly a writer and an editor, based in Truro, Cornwall. He was deeply conservative in both religion and politics. He practiced a little medicine among the poor and became especially interested in the healing effect of anointing patients with olive and other oils, a practice dating from at least biblical times. Edward was a dreamy, impractical soul, far more interested in verses and books than in practicing physic. Once asked to treat a lady in a great house, he wandered into the library while waiting for his patient and became oblivious to time and the purpose of his visit.[9] But although Edward Osler never enjoyed the success his father hoped for, he was not in any way a disgrace. Given his brothers' problems and his sisters' apparent inability to make advantageous marriages, a doctor and a prolific author was a bit of an ornament in the Osler family. Some of his hymns are still sung in Anglican churches. His descendants touched the life of his nephew, William Osler, in many ways.

Edward Osler senior hoped that his fourth son, Featherstone Lake (William's father), born December 14, 1805, would do better than the others. An adventuresome lad who loved the sea, 'Fed' shipped aboard a relative's schooner at age fifteen, survived the vessel's dismasting in a terrible storm, and joined the Royal Navy as a cadet. 'He is a fine spirited lad & I have no doubt will fight his way through this rascally World as well as any person I know,' his first master wrote of him.[10]

As a naval officer in the late 1820s, young Featherstone survived other shipwrecks, as well as outbreaks of yellow fever and battles with privateers and slave traders. He served briefly on the late Horatio Nelson's ship, HMS *Victory*, spent several years on South American patrol, and saw much of the rest of the world. His father made it a habit to cultivate people in high places; as a result the family knew several families with influence in naval affairs who could be counted on to advance Featherstone's interest when it came to promotion. Edward senior hoped for the best: 'You are my fourth Son and I do yet hope to see one who will be my pride, who will be respectable on his own merits, conduct, and situation, independent or without his Father.'[11]

A shortish, full-faced man, whose hairline was already receding in his twenties, Featherstone did his work with calm competence and a strong sense of duty – and, like brother Edward, with an urge to write. His journals and letters are in straightforward pleasing prose, less cluttered than Edward's. They portray a sober career-oriented officer, who could be resplendent in full uniform with his cocked hat and sword, and enjoyed galloping across the Argentine pampas, flirting with the better class of young ladies in port, and always having fresh flowers in his cabin. An agreeable fellow, seldom reflective, secure in the belief that family friends and patrons would look after him in the influence-riddled world of the as yet unreformed navy.[12]

Featherstone's personal philosophy was cheerfully fatalist: '"What is to be will be, and all we can do will not prevent it" ... I found "it was folly to fret."'[13] His superiors were entirely satisfied with him. One of his captains reported that Featherstone was 'everything he could wish him to be as an Officer and a Man.'[14]

Having endured shipwreck and pestilence and encounters with cannibals and slavers, Featherstone came close to death in port in 1828 at the hands of naval surgeons. He was accidentally struck on the head with a crowbar and a few days later was diagnosed as having inflamed lungs. To draw off the inflammation, the doctors opened a vein and bled him, eventually draining away one hundred ounces (almost three liters). Literally exhausted or exsanguinated, Featherstone was taken to a naval hospital to die. 'There,' he remembered many years later, 'the nurse, to save herself the trouble of giving me the medicine, threw away all I should have taken, and after a month's illness, I so far recovered that I was able to rejoin my ship.' When a chest problem recurred, Featherstone told his father that 'low diet, plenty of exercise and drinking nothing but water will soon put me to right better than any doctor.'[15]

As his tour of duty expired in 1831, Featherstone wrote frankly to his father about his prospects: 'I could easily get a larger ship as I could make rather strong interests in the Petticoat way. Lady Northesk will do anything in her power and I can have Lady Grey's (sister in law of the Earl Grey) by asking thru' my very good friend Mr. Lake. Every thing that has yet been done for me has been done unasked by me and I shall ask nothing till I really want it. I think I am secure of the Admiral's interests should any thing occur on the station. So my prospects are not bad on the whole and if they will but continue I shall be well contented.'[16] Just as he was leaving

South America for home, he received an offer to join a ship on the outward passage that needed a replacement for a surgeon/naturalist who was departing in a huff. The historical might-have-beens if Featherstone Osler had taken the opportunity to join the *Beagle* as Charles Darwin's co-worker are incalculable.[17]

While at sea, Featherstone received many letters of advice from his godfather, the Reverend Edward Lake, after whom he had been named. Lake was a well-placed clergyman, a member of the evangelical wing of the Church of England, who took his duties as Featherstone's surrogate father with characteristic earnestness. He made it his business to advance his godson's prospects in the navy. At the same time, he urged upon Featherstone a far more important duty – to consider the prospect of his immortal soul. 'The longest life is short when compared with Eternity,' Lake warned.[18]

In Featherstone's final months at sea, he fretted about being 'the wanderer' in the family, thought more often about getting married, and began to have second thoughts about his lifelong nonchalance towards religion. He thought of Lake as his 'other father' and began to see in him something of what today we call a role model. 'Since corresponding with Mr. Lake,' Featherstone wrote to a sister, 'I have sometimes thought differently to what I did before, and would freely give up all my prospects to be like him. Should I ever be religious I think I should not be lukewarm.'[19]

Featherstone had to set a future course in 1832, a year of crisis in his country's life and in his own. Britain was experiencing economic and social turmoil as agitation for political reform shook the kingdom to its constitutional foundations and threatened to erupt in serious violence. At the same time, a ghastly new plague, Asiatic cholera, carried off tens of thousands of victims. Godfather Lake interpreted these public events as God's judgment upon sinners: 'Our poor native country is in a most alarming state – The general cry is for Reform, indeed the mistaken [view is] that this will be a remedy for every evil – riots are taking place throughout the land – and the burning of farmers [property] is vastly on the increase – Trade is in a dreadful state – and many of the working people are in a starving state – Added to all this the cholera has broken out – and we may expect it will spread – May the rod of God which is thus lifted up help us as a people to repentence and may He in mercy withhold the scourge. Alas sin abounds – it has increased.' Featherstone began attending prayer meetings and was soon convinced that the cholera epidemic was 'God's judgment on the Earth and well we deserve it.'[20]

To his dismay, Featherstone lost his power to influence the navy's judgment of his just deserts. He passed his final examinations to qualify as a permanent officer only to find that the advent of the Whigs to government in Britain had undermined his Tory patrons. England was awash in qualified naval officers. Those with pull got ships; those without, including Featherstone Osler, found themselves on the shelf. Now what was he to do with his life?

Featherstone's wrestling with fundamental questions led to something of a conversion experience late in 1832. He described it to one of his sisters:

> You feel distress of mind, you find that your heart is so deceitful that you cannot trust it, sometimes you feel a something like hope, and then again all is dark, and you think you must be a hypocrite that you are not sincere. You look all around for comfort but comfort is not to be found in the world whilst a 'still small voice' rather whispers 'the end of these things is death.' You try to look to Jesus but no answer appears given to your prayers and you are ready to say there is no hope for me – Are these anything like your feelings? They have been mine ... You are seeking a Saviour and every obstacle that Satan and your own evil heart can find in your way you will find ... but when the Holy Spirit visits the soul as a [baptism] of fire and the Soul feels its wretchedness and evil condition ... the heartfelt cry is uttered 'Lord save or I Perish.'[21]

The fact that his father was dying may have added to Featherstone's agony. It certainly contributed to his reflections on life after death, which would always be a vital element of his faith. 'The greatest consolation I have experienced under our late affliction,' he told his mother after Edward Osler's death,

> has been and is the hope that in a very little while we shall be where there is

no partings. I could not bear to think of the dear departed as dead but as living perhaps watching over us, soothing our wounded minds and whilst we are mourning he is inexpressably happy. Dearest Mother how thankful we ought to feel for the hope that we shall meet in Heaven an unbroken family. Our Father having provided for us on earth is now gone to Heaven to be the first to welcome us there – We have one tie less to the earth – one more serious warning to give earnest heed to make our calling and election sure.[22]

By 1833 Featherstone had decided to become a minister of the Church of England. He boned up on Greek and Latin privately and then enrolled at St Catharine's Hall, Cambridge, to take a degree prior to ordination. As a clergyman he would not only be living his faith but would have solved his career dilemma. After all the years wandering the seas, he looked forward to settling down as a country parson, working quietly and usefully in some beautiful corner of England; he might enjoy a comfortable living, as most successful Anglican clergymen did in that time, perhaps under the wing of a noble patron. He continued to have faith in the utility of being well connected: 'My prospects of advancement were very good, as I had friends of high power in the Church.'[23]

Featherstone had a strong constitution and was never afraid of hard work. He went to Cambridge in his late twenties as a man who had seen the world and opted for the unworldly. With his future clear before him, he concentrated on his studies so earnestly that he almost drove himself to a breakdown.

Ellen Free Pickton, the future Ellen Osler, was born near London on December 14, 1806, into a merchant family, which also was probably of Cornish origin. Her mother was not well and was sent into the country and ordered to take the 'cow-house vapours' by sitting in a farmyard inhaling the breath of cows as they were milked. The treatment did not help. Little Ellen was petite all her very long life, with a dark complexion, black hair, and black eyes that made her seem vaguely un-English (Canadians later wondered if she had Indian blood). She was first given to a servant for nursing and then adopted at age five by a childless aunt and uncle, the Brittons of Falmouth.

Like Featherstone, Ellen was a child of Regency England, growing up before the full impact of the Industrial Revolution, before the age of social reform, before the heyday of the doctrine of progress. She remembered seeing the bodies of criminals displayed in chains near the scene of their crimes; and she remembered the time when Captain Britton, one day on the highroad, took up a poor woman's offer to sell them her baby for a guinea. (The woman had second thoughts and reclaimed the infant that night.) During the celebrations in Falmouth after the Battle of Waterloo, Ellen wore a white sash with 'Peace and Plenty' emblazoned in gold lettering. Two years later, she and all her schoolmates dressed in black to mourn the 1817 death of Princess Charlotte. Men, too, wore black armbands, and even poor beggars displayed wisps of black crepe as England grieved the passing of a royal.

The Brittons were a shipowning, churchgoing family of moderate means. 'Little Pick' grew up to be fond of nature and the heavens, was educated in a boarding school for young ladies, and was known as a spirited girl, pretty, and sometimes quick-tongued, but religious and loyal to friends. In her teens she once ventured into the disreputable Fish Hill area of Falmouth late at night to bring news of the safe return of a missing ship to a worried mother. She spent many days helping nurse a dear friend who was suffering from the terrible skin disease, pemphigus. When the doctor said each day that he thought the girl was better, Ellen finally exclaimed, 'Oh, doctor, how many "betters" does it take to make a person well?' The patient died.

Ellen had many admirers among the young men who frequented the Britton household. Some of the Oslers thought she would be an ideal match for the seafaring Featherstone. 'I wish you would reserve yourself for my brother, who is coming home next week,' one of the Osler boys told Ellen, to her intense annoyance. But when Featherstone came home, he was attracted to her and won her over. They corresponded during his last voyage and became engaged about 1832. They were to be married after Featherstone completed his training for the ministry.[24]

Featherstone had always trusted his patrons. It was not their fault that control of naval patronage had changed hands. His friends' influence in the church seemed more secure, and it did not occur to the theolog that his plans could again be upset. He failed to reckon with his promoters' belief in Christianity's mission to spread the Gospel and save souls. Instead of holding the easy-going, latitudinarian views common enough in the Anglican Church at most times, Featherstone's friends had been caught up in an evangelical revival, which competed in intensity and many of its doctrines with Methodist, Quaker, and Baptist sects, and other forms of Dissent. The Anglican Evangelicals were in deep earnest, and when persuaded of the need to do their duty or follow the Lord's calling, would not be dissuaded by wordly considerations.

One Sunday at the end of his last college long vacation, Featherstone received a letter from the newly formed Upper Canada Clergy Society. It had been founded by the very group of aristocratic evangelicals to whom he looked for advancement. They were responding to word of a desperate shortage of ministers for the settlers in far-off Canada. Looking for men to send out in answer to the Canadian call, the society chose Featherstone as one whose travels around the world had presumably fitted him for overseas service. St Paul had always favored evangelists without attachments. The good folk asked Featherstone if it was not his duty to take up this work on their behalf.

By all accounts, especially his own, Featherstone was appalled at the prospect of going to Canada. The thought of going abroad had no appeal to Ellen or her friends either. Britain's North American colonies were not popular with the Falmouth people. They were cold, poor places to which you sailed at great peril. Special peril: a number of the autumn mail packets that had set out from Falmouth for Nova Scotia had never been heard from again. To 'go to Halifax' had become local slang for going to your death.[25]

'I put the letter in my mother's hands,' Featherstone remembered, 'and while tears streamed down her cheeks, she returned it with the remark, "If it is God's will, go, and God bless you." ... I felt I could not refuse the appeal ... duty had evidently called me and I could not refuse.' 'If I were still in the navy,' he reasoned to Ellen, 'and I were ordered east, west, north, or south,

in the service of my king, I could not refuse to go, and shall I be less obedi-
ent to the call to go abroad to serve my Heavenly King?'[26]

Featherstone Osler and Ellen Pickton were married on February 6, 1837.
In March the Archbishop of Canterbury ordained Featherstone a deacon
of the church under special provision 'for the cure of souls in His Majesty's
Foreign Possessions.' The pious couple sailed from Falmouth for Canada on
April 6 on the barque *Bragila*. 'The pain, I may say the anguish, of parting I
will not attempt to describe,' Featherstone wrote to a friend.[27] During the
voyage Ellen realized that she was pregnant.

The Oslers' seven-week crossing of the North Atlantic to the New World
in the spring of 1837 was relatively uneventful. Even so, Featherstone kept
a detailed journal and wrote long letters, whether or not he was in 'a writing humour': 'Inclination says "Put it by for another day," but resolution
replies "No, begin at once," and ... resolution shall have the mastery.'[28] The
ocean weather was unseasonably warm, there were the usual squalls and
gales and passing bouts of seasickness, but the newlyweds were not affected.
They had a good supply of fresh food, including oranges, and Featherstone
was so attentive to his pregnant bride that Ellen feared she might develop
idle habits. Featherstone led morning prayers and Sunday service for their
little party and the ship's company, 'striving ever to bear in mind,' he wrote,
'that I am a dying man speaking to dying men.' Christian joke: Why won't
fish off the Grand Banks take the salt pork bait offered from the *Bragila*?
Answer: The cod must be Jewish.[29]

Their first sight of land was the bleak, snow-swept coast of Newfoundland. Entering the St Lawrence River, they narrowly avoided being ship-
wrecked on Egg Island. The immense forest dominated the landscape as
they sailed upriver. A few solitary houses appeared, then a fur-trading post,
and occasional clearings where fire had ravaged the woods and 'the black,
scorched pine stumps seemed mourning the desolation which reigned on
every side.'[30]

Then Featherstone noticed the sunlight, the glittering snow, the birds and seals and beluga whales, and the farmhouses and fields of cultivated land by the great river, and his mood changed. He concluded that all na-ture was singing the praises of the Creator. The Ile d'Orléans, just below Quebec, was beautifully pastoral, and the passengers amused themselves by pointing out prototypes of the houses they might have in Upper Canada. Rounding Point Lévis, they marveled as Quebec City burst into view, high above the river, its tin roofs sparkling in the sun. At the Albion Hotel the Oslers found accommodation far better than Featherstone had expected: 'Everything is conducted as far as possible in the English style; fare good, waiters civil, and we have our own private room.'[31]

While her husband went to see the Anglican bishop of Quebec, Ellen looked carefully at their tiny square room in the Albion – at the sheets that had been slept in, the dirty pillow on the bed, the badly mended handle on the water jug. She sat down on the floor, laid her head in her arms on a chair, and wept. Moments later she said to herself, 'Come, this will never do,' and washed her face. When Featherstone returned she was perfectly composed. The next morning, when she looked out the window, her heart sank again at the sight of raw wood strewn everywhere in the hotel yard. 'I can't say I enjoy my solitude at the inn,' she wrote to a sister, 'but I bear it patiently as I can ... Beseech the Lord for me, my dear Lizzy, that I may be fitted for all there is before me to do and bear.'[32]

The bishop raised Featherstone to priest's orders and gave him details of his missionary posting. He was to take up residence in the townships of Tecumseth and West Gwillimbury, just north of Toronto, the Lake Ontario town that served as provincial capital of Upper Canada. During the Seven Years' War, which had ended in 1763, Great Britain had conquered the land known as New France or Canada or Quebec. In the following decade Britain's northern possessions – which also included Newfoundland, Nova Scotia, and the Hudson's Bay Company's vast fur-trading domain – had not joined in the American rebellion, thereby staying in the Empire as British North America. In 1791 the mother country had divided the old Province of Quebec into Upper and Lower Canada (corresponding roughly to today's Canadian provinces of Ontario and Quebec).

Lower Canada was dominated by its long-settled French and Roman

Catholic majority. Upper Canada, which contained millions of acres of fertile, forested land in the triangle formed by Lakes Ontario, Erie, and Huron, was in its pioneering, settlement phase. Tens of thousands of emigrants from Great Britain arrived in Upper Canada every year in the 1830s, swelling a population originally seeded from the south by United Empire Loyalist refugees and land-hungry Yankee frontiersmen. When their St Lawrence steamer reached Upper Canada, the Osler party congratulated themselves 'on being in our own country.' They had a pleasant spring voyage up Lake Ontario – their stops and rambles in the forest spoiled only by mosquitoes reveling in fresh Old Country blood – and disembarked in Toronto.[33]

It was only a few miles, less than an hour's drive today, from the church spires and semi-refined society taking shape in muddy Toronto to the backwoods townships where the Oslers were to live and preach. In 1837 the journey took two days by stage and then wagon, with the roads and probably the travelers' spirits deterioriating as they penetrated the dense, primeval forest. Ellen and Featherstone finally arrived at their obscure Canadian station on June 19, 1837. One day later, back in London, eighteen-year-old Victoria Hanover ascended to the throne of Great Britain and its empire.

'We are a wild people here, Sir,' frontier folk said to Featherstone as he visited among them. He was minister to about two thousand settlers scattered in townships covering some 240 square miles. A fair bit of land had been cleared in the twenty years or so since the first axmen attacked the northern bush. Hamlets and villages had sprung up along mud tracks through the pine and cedar forests. Still, tracts of wilderness and swamp were everywhere, bears and wolves and wildcats shared the woods with the handful of humans, and schools and churches were hardly to be found. Most of the region's settlers had come from northern Ireland and were poor, Protestant, and proud in about equal measure. 'The Devil I fear to say almost reigns triumphant,' was Featherstone's first impression of his Canadian charge. 'Drunkenness, blasphemy & several species of vice is common.'

The god-fearing among the settlers had managed, under the prodding of visiting missionaries, to begin work on Anglican churches, seven miles apart, at West Gwillimbury and Tecumseth. Featherstone was to be their first settled minister. He and Ellen found temporary, cramped rooms with a farmer near a crossroads settlement in the middle of the territory, 'one of the most wicked places in the world.'[34]

The wickedness in the eye of the clerical beholder was mostly drinking, swearing, and desecrating the sabbath with sports and hunting. Were there layers of meaning in a convert's plaintive cry, 'No one told me I was a sinner till Mr. Osler came here'? The man's sins might have included following after the itinerant Methodist preachers who supplied the main competition for the Church of England in Upper Canada. 'The Methodists here are very different from those I had intercourse with at home,' Featherstone wrote. 'They are very ignorant, imagine conversion consists in highly wrought feelings ... They agree in one thing, bitter hatred and abuse of the Church; the most unfounded lies are propagated of the church services and ministers, but God will defend His own.'[35]

Featherstone was further dismayed by the illiteracy and ignorance of his sinful flock. In 1838 one of his parishioners was accused of bewitching a horse and causing its death. 'I thought that absurdity had quite gone out of date, but on inquiry find that most of my poor ignorant people firmly believe in it.' They also believed in placing crossed tongs over babies lying in cradles to protect them from the devil. One of Featherstone's first projects was to found a lending library, 'the books to be of a religious tendency,' but it did not last. Ellen had better luck with sewing and reading classes to help the farm women improve their domestic life; and Featherstone founded Sunday schools at each of his churches.[36]

He preached morning, noon, and night, in homes, barns, and stables, often competing with barking dogs, clucking chickens, and crying children. He traveled everywhere on horseback, an Anglican version of the frontier 'circuit rider,' bringing the word and the sacraments to pioneers who had not seen a minister for months, sometimes years. They were like sheep waiting for a shepherd, Featherstone reflected. Their joy and tears and thanks at his coming compensated for the bone-chilling cold of the winter rides, the searing heat and clouds of mosquitoes in summer, the fear of beasts in the night. 'You'll not see me often over this road, good people,' he said to himself the first time he led his horse along miles of floating corduroy road through a dark wolf-haunted swamp to the Innisfil settlement. 'But when I reached Innisfil ... the people received me as an angel of light, and could not tell how to express their gratitude and joy at being visited by a clergyman of the Church of England ... They had formerly been visited by the Methodists, who had left them because they did not get money enough.'[37]

The hardships of the first year in Canada almost broke Featherstone. After three months of living with a farm family in two small rooms – with all their household goods in storage in a barn, their last Old Country gingerbread eaten by the farmer's dog – the Oslers had to move. All that could be found for them was an old shed in the woods, which had been used to keep livestock. Ellen remembered how horses would come and look in the window at them, 'as much as to say, "Why have you taken our stable and shut us out?"' 'It is scarcely possible to move a step without being over shoes in dung and dirt,' Featherstone wrote. 'Nothing has tended so much to dishearten me. Fatigue I do not mind, but to be all together in one room, no place to write or study in, and surrounded with filth, I find difficulty.'[38]

Ellen had to move to the nearest town, Newmarket, to be near help when giving birth. Her husband was there with her in early December 1837 when incredible news arrived of an insurrection in the colony. Rebels were said to be marching on Toronto to overthrow British rule. 'The people seemed panic-struck,' Featherstone wrote in his journal. The Anglican Church gave unqualified support to the state, and Osler rode late into the night, 'giving intelligence, stirring up the men, and quieting the women.' He buried the family valuables in case of a rebel attack on their hut and then galloped back to Newmarket to stand guard over the women, children, and dogs sheltering at a friend's house. Word came from the south that Toronto was in flames. Then new word: it was the rebels who had been routed and their tavern burnt. The only shot Newmarket heard during the barely serious Upper Canada Rebellion came when a guard fired at his shadow.[39]

Milk froze a yard from the stove. Snow drifted through chinks in the logs. No servants would stay in the bush during winter. Featherstone could hardly bear the loneliness. In the spring of 1838 the Oslers, now three with the birth of a son, had to surrender their shed to cattle and move to an even smaller outbuilding, which had only loose boards for a floor. Possibly, Ellen had to lay her baby in a manger. The only stable for Featherstone's horse was three-quarters of a mile distant. After a week of traveling and preaching, after riding fourteen miles or more to lead two Sunday services, and after taking the horse to the stable, the walk back through the forest was almost too much for him: 'Often I have been on the point of dropping with fatigue; it is, indeed, more than I can bear.'[40]

He threatened to leave if the people did not produce decent accommodation. He had to organize much of the construction himself, but in midsummer 1838 the Oslers moved into a new home near the center of their community. The formerly wicked crossroads hamlet had been named Bond Head in honor of the governor of Upper Canada, Sir Francis Bond Head (whose authoritarian rule has often been blamed for sparking the rebellion); it may well have been Featherstone who suggested the name.

The move came just in time, Featherstone judged:

> A more anxious year than the past one I never passed and but for the experience I obtained & the habits I acquired when at sea I could not possibly have remained here. During the last three months especially my duties have been almost too much for me. I have risen on the Sunday Mornings with a feeling of almost overpowering weariness, yet could not rest, for who was to take my duties? ... My poor horse is so worn down that I am compelled to give him a holiday for a little while – but my own health has been graciously spared ... I may almost say I never knew fatigue till I came to Canada.[41]

At the new Trinity Church in Bond Head, Ellen Osler became the effective superintendent of the best Sunday school in the area. She had proved a perfect mate, uncomplaining, utterly loyal, a pillar of faith and piety. 'During my sojourn in a strange land and shut out from all congenial society,'

she wrote home, 'I can truly say that the Lord hath been my helper, continually suiting his mercies to my necessities, and graciously fulfilling to me his promise "As thy day so shall thy strength be."' When her husband was discouraged, Ellen was his rock: 'We must my dearest Fed look on all these crosses as coming direct from God and submit with cheerfulness to what He sees is necessary for us.'[42]

Ellen's ability to quote scripture exceeded Featherstone's, and in the Sunday school she somehow inspired the children to want to memorize huge chunks of the Bible. 'The boys whilst ploughing would have their Testament open, fastened to their ploughs, ploughing and learning at the same time,' Featherstone marveled, 'girls doing the same with their spinning-wheels.' In 1840 Ellen also supervised the baking, including three hundred rhubarb pasties, and other preparations for a grand Sunday school picnic and prize giving, one of the first ever held in Canada, attended by some seven hundred children, teachers, and parents. The prizes would have been for attendance and Scripture knowledge.[43]

As leaders in the community, the Oslers were more than preachers, teachers, and givers of tracts and prizes. Featherstone baptized his people's children, married the young, and buried the dead. He made out wills and often lent small sums of money, interest-free. While intending to minister to souls, he also found himself treating, or appearing to treat, bodies. Early in his ministry he took some store-bought medicine to a man said to be on his deathbed, persuaded the poor fellow to repent of his sins, brought more medicine, and, when the man recovered, was acclaimed a powerful physician. Others soon sought the benefit of his healing power:

A poor woman stopped me to say that she had a sick infant in her arms which she wished me to see and prescribe for – she had been to the doctor but would not give the child the medicine till she had consulted me. Another came to me with a bad leg, another with his arm, two women came to have their teeth drawn &c. Tis of no use for me to plead ignorance. They shake their heads and say 'Oh you know very well Sir' so that I am obliged to think of something always taking care to give nothing but what I am sure will do no hurt should it do no good.

'Confidence and a few simple medicines often did wonders,' Featherstone
wrote about his healing role, 'my good wife attending to the women and
children.'[44] Once he was called out in bitter cold in the dead of night to see
a dying person:

> I found the girl apparently very sick, and as they were expecting her to die
> many women were busy making her shroud. I found on examination that
> there was no sign of death, but they had persuaded her she was going to die,
> and she believed it. I ordered them to stop making the shroud, told her
> parents that I saw no immediate danger, prescribed a few simple remedies,
> made the girl take some nourishment, and left, promising to return in the
> evening ... I found the girl up sitting by the fire, and in a few days she was
> quite well, and was known for a long time afterwards in the locality as the
> resurrection girl.[45]

Featherstone drew the line when a respectable parishioner came to him
and asked to be venesected, or bled, to relieve the congestions of winter, a
custom analogous to spring cleaning: 'I referred him to the doctor. The
poor I rejoice to assist in every way in my power, but if I continue to give
medicine to all, gratis, my practice will increase to an extent which will be
troublesome.'[46] He toyed with the idea of asking well-to-do patients to contribute to a fund for building local schools. When physicians came to the
community, many of Featherstone's people were not sure how far to trust
them, and they sought the minister's advice about whether they should
follow doctors' orders.

Church-starved settlers in the forests north and west of Tecumseth town-
ship begged Featherstone to visit them and lead services. He obliged as best
he could, riding into the wilderness season after season to preach, found
churches, launch Sunday schools, and perhaps offer 'confidence and a few
simple medicines.' He often returned exhausted, desperate for rest, not seeing how it would come this side of the grave. He pleaded with the bishop of
Toronto, John Strachan, to put more workers into the territory. When
Strachan could not supply any – the Church of England was never the
established or even the leading denomination in Upper Canada –

Featherstone decided to make his own men. He organized a little seminary-cum-apprenticeship program at the Bond Head–Tecumseth parsonage, training six men who eventually became ministers. One was a younger brother, Henry, who came out from England, took well to the frontier work, and became pastor of a new church at nearby Lloydtown, a settlement that had been a hellhole of rebellion. Featherstone was immensely proud of the churches and clergy he spawned.

He dreamed for a time of founding a theological college. His Cambridge degree and the good working library at his parsonage made him an unusually well-read clergyman by backwoods standards. He and Ellen intensely valued education and manners; these were essential attributes of gentlefolk, whether frequenting the haunts of the mighty or on arduous errands in the northern wilderness. Featherstone's strongest subject at Cambridge had been mathematics, however, and in matters theological and literary he does not seem to have been much of a scholar. He would have been better at navigating his way through forest clearings with a sextant than fulfilling John Strachan's ideal of ministers so cultivated that they could proclaim the Gospels in Greek from horseback.[47] Strachan encouraged some of his more like-minded colleagues in more settled areas to proceed with the training of future ministers.

In his backwoods townships Featherstone Osler preached an evangelical message in plain English: We are sinners who will be damned for eternity if we do not accept Christ as our Salvation; with Christ we gain eternal happiness. Featherstone kept his distance from the movement towards a more liturgical Anglo-Catholicism that had begun in the church during his college days. In Canada he became extremely suspicious of the High Church tendencies of his own bishop and many of his colleagues. The Tractarian, or Oxford Movement, in the Church of England might be 'the Devil's work,' he told Ellen.[48]

On the other hand, he was repelled by the emotionalism of those to whom he was theologically closest, the Methodists. Their revival or camp meetings unleashed animal feelings, mere passions, he thought: 'Let me direct your attentions to those who are led away by them. Are they not the weak-minded and females? Is it not the case as people become educated,

they see the absurdity of such proceedings, and know that they are the effects of overwrought feelings, like Popery ... It is only suited to a state of
ignorance and both [Methodism and Popery] are actuated by the same principles, appealing to the passions and feelings rather than reason.'[49]

Passionate about doing his duty to his 'poor sheep in the wilderness,'[50]
passionate about the need to save immortal souls, Featherstone Osler was
always a solid middle-of-the-road Anglican. True religion was rational and
helped rational people control their passions and elevate themselves. True
religion was neither Catholic nor Protestant but a bridge, the best of both.
The bridge-building, common-sense mind-set would be one of Featherstone's
most important legacies to his physician son.

Featherstone Osler was a shining success as a frontier parson. Bishop
Strachan occasionally had doubts about the Cornishman's 'morbid disposition' and perhaps about his tendency to grumble, but otherwise offered only
praise. He reported that Osler was 'a Treasure, indefatigable in his labors
and journeys, judicious in his arrangements, frank, kind, and conciliatory
in his manners.' Back home, Osler was spoken of as the best missionary that
ever went out to Canada. His sponsors urged him to stay in Upper Canada
after his first five-year term. Torn between worries about his health and a
sense of being hard done by, on the one hand, and the call of duty and love
of his flock on the other, Featherstone agreed to stay.[51]

Ellen had the first trip home, in the winter of 1840–1. She bore their third
child there and longed for Fed's company. He had his turn in early 1843,
when a chronic cough and an abscess on his backside from the years on
horseback forced a rest and change. The people of Tecumseth and West
Gwillimbury organized a cavalcade of 110 sleighs and buggies to see their
minister off; on his return they met him with a procession of sixty wagons.
In the motherland he had a flattering reception from leading churchmen and
aristocrats, paid his fee at Cambridge to get his master of arts degree, and went
on a preaching tour of Ireland to raise money for the Canadian mission.[52]

In his prime, Featherstone was incapable of inactivity. Back in Canada
he set about doubling the capacity of Trinity Church at Bond Head. It had
become his principal responsibility, as seven other ministers now serviced
the outlying portions of his old domain. The parsonage had been enlarged

into a spacious, rambling home on a hillside with a beautiful view. It had a huge garden, then a working farm attached to it. The larder was always particularly well stocked: 'I like to keep a good supply of eatables as persons are continually calling and my poor back settlement people I always wish to be kindly treated when they come on any account.' The Oslers entertained visitors as an everyday part of their lives.[53]

By the mid-1840s, about the time of his fortieth birthday, Featherstone was beginning to slow down. He could afford to rest in comfort, substitute a cushioned carriage seat for a saddle, and enjoy the laurels of a race well run. It was important to him to savor his accomplishments, for his journals and reminiscences disclose a nagging dissatisfaction with his lot in life. He could have had other careers at home, perhaps rising to high position in the navy or serving the church without the fatigue and obscurity he had met in Canada. He had no desire, he told a daughter, that a son of his should become 'a misunderstood poorly paid Backwoods parson.' Unlike brother Henry in Lloydtown, Featherstone always yearned to return to England.

England was 'home' to this family growing up in the Canadian forest. A British education and gentility were to be acquired as a matter of course; and as Edward Osler senior had indicated to his children, career achievement was very important. From far-off Canada even doctor-brother Edward's accomplishments, especially the hymns and books he had written, seemed impressive. 'God has given you talents and me strength of body to endure fatigue,' Featherstone once wrote to him from Canada. As Featherstone entered middle age, one of his priorities was to help his children make their way in the world.[54]

Ellen had been over thirty when she was married, and she and Featherstone thought they might not have children. After the first three babies arrived – Featherston (without an 'e') in 1838, Britton Bath in 1839, and Ellen Mary ('the little English girl') in 1841 – husband wrote wife: 'I do not wish to see you again my precious E with a very large stomach.' But they either did not know how to practice effective birth control or did not believe in it. 'Ellen has proved such a breeder,' Featherstone told his mother ten years later.[55] Edward was born in 1842, Edmund Boyd in 1845, and the twins Charlotte and Frank in 1847 when their mother was forty-one. At age forty-three she bore her eighth child, a boy, on July 12, 1849.

Featherstone had planned to name him Walter after an Old Country patron. But there was only one name for a boy born on the Twelfth of July in a community of Irish Protestants. In 1690 King William III had defeated the forces of Stuart Catholicism at the Battle of the Boyne, assuring continued Protestant ascendency in Ireland. The victory had been celebrated ever since on the 'Glorious Twelfth.' When Featherstone showed the baby to the members of the Orange Order parading to his rectory, it was declared that a new Prince of Orange, a new William, had come into the world. (It was not an uncommon name in the community: Featherstone baptized one William Banting, the son of an Irish Protestant farmer in the locality, the same day he christened William Osler.)

'Don't spoil them ... I think there is much truth in the proverb that children like horses ought to be broken in by the time they are three years old,' Featherstone wrote. Like many British parents in the mid-nineteenth century, Featherstone and Ellen assumed that their children, especially the boys, were willful animals whose passions had to be tamed. But not with lash or whip: the clergyman and his wife were loving, playful parents, and there is no evidence in any of the family records of authority being abused. That 'the Pater' or 'the Governor,' as the boys came to call him, had authority and expected to be listened to was unquestioned, but he may not have been the more strict of the parents. 'Never was there a greater mistake than the idea that he is a Tartar to the children,' a perceptive niece wrote of Featherstone, and then switched to equine imagery: 'Aunt holds the reins far tighter than he does, and she never checks without absolute need.'[56]

Ellen was as like-minded with Featherstone in parenting as religion. The idea of raising four children would at one time have 'quite startled me,' she had written during her fourth pregnancy. 'Now half a score will not surprise or trouble more than two. I learn a lesson from the wren and the dove: "Coo coo, says the dove, what shall I do? for I have got two! Twit, twit, said the wren, I have got ten and shall bring them up like gentlemen."'[57]

Baby eight was known as Willie, except that the Oslers were addicted to using nicknames. Ellen called him Benjamin after the child of Rachel and Jacob's old age. He was dark eyed and dark haired like his mother and had the same olive-hued complexion, perhaps a reflection of Celtic or Iberian genes. Featherstone was impressed by his eyes, calling him 'Little burnt-holes-in-a-blanket.'

Willie's memories of childhood were vague and skimpy. He could recall only about twenty specific events of his first nine years, he once noted, most of them associated with pranks and punishment, though nothing severe or scarring: 'Perhaps it is because my childhood was so happy that it is so free from memories ... A distinguished physician said to me once, "Osler you must have had a happy home as a boy – You are always happy."'[58]

Another calf in the herd, Willie was not singled out for special attention – except, of course, on his birthday, when to his delight and his siblings' chagrin the whole community seemed to be celebrating. He believed he had an accurate first memory of his mother tethering him to a tree in the yard near the pasture where the beef calves were kept, and leaving a pail of milk for his nourishment. As he was drinking from the pail, one of the calves butted him into it.[59]

He also told a story of encountering a bear in a raspberry patch, though no one could corroborate it, and Dr Osler was known to embellish a tale. But, yes, he really did chop off sister Charlotte's ('Chattie's') finger one day when he was five years old and she kept putting her hand in the way of his little hatchet. She had the scar to prove it, and the event even caused the older boys to take notice: 'Charlotte had the top of her finger chopped off the other day by Master William with an axe. It is healing as well as could be expected.'[60]

Willie dimly remembered the family tragedy of those years, the 1853 death of the ninth and last Osler child, two-year-old Emma Henrietta. He had a confused memory of his mother bringing the white-clad body into the house so the family could say good-bye, of the contrast between the pale face and a black stove, and of trips with his mother to Emma's grave. Many years later, when Ellen Osler was near death, she told her son, 'I shall soon join little Emma.'[61]

There would always be preachers finding their way to backwoods settlements, but getting schoolteachers and founding decent permanent schools was much more difficult. Public schooling was only beginning to take shape on the Canadian frontier in the 1840s and 1850s and, despite Featherstone's best efforts to get a school going, was erratic at best in the Bond Head area. After elementary education, the oldest Osler boys were sent to board and attend school in nearby communities. Barrie, a big town about twenty miles north of Bond Head, had a particularly good grammar school, which grounded its teaching in knowledge of classical languages and culture – but Featherstone doubted he could afford to send the whole flock there. Mainly for the sake of his younger children's education, he asked his bishop for a move.

In early 1857 the Oslers left Bond Head to take up life in Dundas, Canada West (as Upper Canada was now called). Dundas was a thriving town at the head of Lake Ontario and on the main railway line forty miles west of Toronto. Although the family and the parishioners felt separation pangs after nearly twenty years of Featherstone's ministry, it was good to return to more advanced conditions of civilization. Not that the young Osler colts, or 'Tecumseth cabbages' as the townies nicknamed them, had seriously run wild in the bush. For the most part, the Osler boys grew up strong and healthy and versatile, hard-working, well-mannered gentlemen, who could shoot and ride and chop wood and quote Scripture and bits of Greek or Latin, and knew the value of a bushel of wheat and a side of bacon. In Dundas they would have better housing, better schools, and more opportunities – including, the older boys realized, more opportunities to meet young ladies.

The grass is unkempt in the one surviving family photo of the Bond Head years. Little Willie looks sullen. But he and his brothers all have their jackets on, buttons done up, and their hair brushed. Willie, too, was learning to handle guns and horses and to love the outdoors even as family discipline was curbing his animal spirits. His most vivid memory of the bush years was of going into the woods to make maple sugar in the spring.[62]

The Osler family's introduction to the quicker pace of Dundas life gave them all pause. Just before they arrived, the collapse of a bridge there caused one of the worst train wrecks in nineteenth-century Canada. Come to civilization and count the corpses. The story that Willie had the croup, thereby saving the family from being on the fatal train, is not true. When the wreck occurred, Ellen was in Toronto with the little ones waiting for Featherstone to come from a funeral in Tecumseth.[63]

Dundas nestled in hilly country at the head of bays and a great swamp. It had about four thousand people, macadamized streets, plank sidewalks, gas lighting, schools and churches, and extremely handsome accommodation for the Anglican parson in a rambling brick house on a hill overlooking the town. The oldest boy, Featherston ('Fen'), was already away from home, learning the law as an articled student in Barrie. Brother Britton Bath ('Brick' or 'B.B.'), a jack-of-all-trades, soon decided also to enter the legal profession. Sister Ellen Mary ('Nellie'), whose health was not good, stayed at home, and the third boy, Edward, whose idle habits were causing serious concern to his father, had already been enrolled in the Barrie school before the move. The remaining 'shrimps' or 'juveniles,' as their parents called them, who had a smattering of formal learning, public and private, from Bond Head days, went to the local Dundas schools.

In the late 1850s and early 1860s Canon Featherstone Osler, as he had become, took charge of the parishes of Dundas and Ancaster. Sons Featherston and B.B. embarked on careers in the law that would take them to great eminence in the Canadian bench and bar. Edward struggled with the law; Edmund went to work in a bank; Frank did poorly in school; and of master Willie little is known. He apparently continued to be a happy, hearty boy, not particularly studious or in any way remarkable – at least none of his family bothers to remark on him in the letters that have survived. Dundas offered good primary schooling for the times, but with rigid masters and an old-fashioned curriculum. Osler recalled that John King, MA of Trinity College, Dublin, 'across his *tie*, as he called it ... birched into me small Latin and less Greek.'[64]

He was touched by war, if only vicariously. As a child, he recoiled in terror at hearing of the biblical Israelites' slaughter of thousands, sparing neither man nor beast, woman nor child. As a boy in the early 1860s, he experienced American Civil War fever, parading through Dundas with other lads behind a single-starred bonnie-blue flag, singing 'Maryland! My Maryland' ('Avenge the patriotic gore / That flecked the streets of Baltimore / And be the battle-queen of yore / Maryland! My Maryland!'). Canadians, like the British, tended to sympathize with the South in the great and bloody conflict. An escaped Confederate soldier was said to have interested the Dundas boys in drilling with a view to going off to fight the Yankees. Years later, Dr Osler told American friends that as a boy of thirteen in Canada he had mobilized and drilled a squad of Confederate volunteers.[65]

Willie comes back into focus in 1864, just before his fifteenth birthday, when he is expelled from the Dundas grammar school for shouting abuse at one of the masters through a keyhole. Canon Osler stood up for his boy, berating the school's trustees for a disgraceful decision, apparently chalking it up to their being Methodists. In later life William reminisced about other pranks he got up to in those years – filling a schoolroom with geese, removing desks to an inaccessible attic – and sister Charlotte remembered him coming home on horseback calling out, 'Chattie, I've got the sack!' In fact, the Dundas trustees agreed to reinstate him on a promise of good behavior.[66]

About this time, Osler gave one of his first public performances. As senior boy in the senior Sunday school class at church, he was asked to read at the service. He had no trouble with the prayers as written out in the Church of England's *Book of Common Prayer*, but when he came to the injunction to the familiar Lord's Prayer, 'Our Father, which art in Heaven, &c,' the young man trying so anxiously to be on his best behaviour could not remember the words to '&c.'[67]

The children were 'neither very good or very bad,' Featherstone had written his mother in 1851. He probably felt the same about his domestic flock a decade later. He had made clear to his boys, particularly the eldest, that he expected them to be industrious and dutiful, and then to make their own way in life: 'I wish to give each of you the best start in my power and then your future prosperity must under God depend upon yourselves.'[68] As he aged, slowing down a bit, perhaps burned out from the early years in

Canada, Featherstone tended to fade into the background of family life, an amiable, woolly country parson, some of whose parishioners nicknamed him Sneezer.

Ellen continued to sparkle with vitality for decades. It was probably his mother who dosed Willie every spring and fall with quinine to protect him from the malaria that still lurked in the nearby marshes. It was certainly Ellen who made a point of attending to the children's moral health, saturating them with Holy Scripture, and urging the young Osler men to think about their immortal souls while avoiding the temptations of the World, the Flesh, and the Devil.[69]

Despite or because of being raised in a parsonage, on Scripture, daily family prayers, and two or three church services a week, none of the Osler boys adopted their mother's or even their father's religious zeal. At their best, they combined their parents' other strengths, especially a capacity for sustained hard work. A comment Willie made about another physician – that he was 'singularly fortunate in his parents ... strong earnest souls, well endowed with graces of the head and of the heart' – was also true of him. At least four of the Osler offspring (Edward remained a gray sheep and Frank became a black one) were intensely hard-working, ambitious, and men of obvious good breeding who went on to remarkable attainment. An English aunt later marveled at the Osler brothers as 'fine specimens of men ... English gentlemen with American energy.'

The Osler women were not expected to have careers and did not. The men broke a popular stereotype about ministers' children. As a Toronto rhymester once put it,

> You have heard the remark in different Places
> That clergymans sons always turn out hard cases
> When you hear of the Oslers you'll have to admit
> Some clergymans sons have both virtue & wit.

Featherstone and Ellen's branch of the Falmouth Oslers became the highest achievers of their clan, in fact the highest-achieving family in nineteenth-century Canada.[70]

After his adventures at the Dundas school, Willie was enrolled in the Barrie grammar school, where older brothers had gone; he boarded in the residence run by the headmaster, the Reverend W.F. Checkley, another MA from Trinity College, Dublin. The training was heavily weighted towards the traditional rote learning of classical languages and literature. 'Hoping that you are on terms of love and friendship with your books,' his mother wrote, promising to send the family copy of Horace. Featherstone Osler's library ran mostly to theology. Willie had been exposed to the Bible while taking his mother's milk, but otherwise he had done little more than sample his father's travel books and some fiction – forbidden fiction if opened on a Sunday. He had yet to form much of a friendship with literature, let alone Latin and Greek: 'We loathed Xenophen and his ten thousand, Homer was an abomination, while Livy and Cicero were names and tasks. Ten years with really able Trinity College, Dublin and Oxford teachers left me with no more real knowledge of Greek and Latin than of Chinese.'[71]

A classmate from the Barrie days, Ned Milburn, remembered that he, Charley Locke, and Osler had a happy series of schoolboy scrapes – hooking out at night to go swimming, raiding Sheriff Smith's melon patch, stealing a judge's prize dahlias – which got them known as 'Barrie's Bad Boys.' A few of Osler's letters to Milburn, his earliest surviving correspondence, suggest a sixteen-year-old testing limits, probably with some exaggeration. In Dundas in the summer of 1865 he played cricket, tried and disliked the new game of baseball, shot ducks, had the use of a horse and a boat whenever he liked, and was 'only ... on one drunk ... that was on the 5th at the Sunday School picnic and had lots of fun with the girls.' In Barrie that fall there was sailing every evening, and hours spent sitting around having 'two or three good horns' in the parlor of Meeking's hotel: 'And Mr. Stuart gets at the piano and sings the dirtiest songs out of jail ... We do nothing but play shinny and Charlie [Locke] and I go down town and get into Jo Locke's room and smoke and eat bullzies.' Nothing serious in the way of vices, and Milburn claimed that Osler was the best student in the school. The letters may confirm a contemporary's report that Barrie students were 'rather precociously sophisticated in ways not becoming a boy, & not adding to his good repute even when he came to man's estate.'[72]

Whether or not he was happy or successful in Barrie, Willie was agreeable to his father's plan to switch him to a new school in the village of Weston, a few miles west of Toronto, for 1866. A school whose circular promised instruction in singing and dancing could not be all that bad. So in January, Willie began attending Trinity College School, billed as a Canadian equivalent of England's Eton or Rugby. His first reports on Trinity glowed with enthusiasm for a 'regular English school' with 'all the old English rules.'[73]

Late in 1866, two of Willie's English cousins arrived in Dundas. Jennette Osler and Marian Osler Bath were daughters of Uncle Edward Osler, the surgeon-writer, by his second marriage. The young women, both in their mid-twenties, were at loose ends after their father's death in 1863 and then Marian's early widowhood. Screwing up their courage, and bringing Marian's little son with them, they ventured to America to see the wing of the family with which they had been corresponding all their lives. The Canadian Oslers seemed to share their values more thoroughly than some of the ne'er-do-well relatives at home.

Little Jennette and plumpish Marian were well read, observant, and quick witted. During their Atlantic passage Jennette had a shipboard dalliance with young Oliver Wendell Holmes, whose father was the famous literary physician, author of *The Autocrat of the Breakfast Table*: 'Marian cruelly failed to appreciate him & dragged me away ... saying "Don't cultivate him 'Toddles,' he is only an American."' Traveling through New York and Boston, the sisters were a little shocked by assertive American women and American ways, but when they crossed the border at Niagara and reached Dundas, Canada West, they were suddenly on familiar ground: 'A stout kindly looking gentleman in clerical costume came forward & welcomed us to Canada, I should have known him, he is so very like Aunt Lizzie and his voice is like Papa's and is full of English tone ... We felt at home &

happy at once ... At the upper gate stood a dear little dark woman in a nice little cap tied under her chin and this was Aunt Ellen. They welcomed us most warmly, we felt at once as if we had known them for years; they are all dears.'[74]

The English cousins settled in like two new sisters in the Canadian family. They liked all the Dundas brood, and their admiration for the parents only increased with time. 'Uncle is very nice; a large hearted considerate liberal minded man, unselfish & truly good. The more you know him the more highly you learn to appreciate him,' Jennette wrote home. As for Aunt Ellen: 'She is one of the blessed of the earth. One does not know how to respect & love her enough; I verily believe she has not a single proud or selfish thought; she just lives to do good.'[75]

One day in October the cousins were taken to Weston to meet William, who starred in most of the events at Trinity College School's games day. 'Willie is the handsomest of the family except that he is not tall & graceful like Edmund & Ned. He is extremely dark; a very nice gentlemanly boy,' Jennette observed.[76] All fall and winter Jennette and Marian lived with the Dundas and Lloydtown families – lost some of their British reserve, learned to dance, helped with the church bazaars and teas and concerts and the Christmas celebrations (twenty-three sat down to dinner in Dundas, followed by singing, and charades) and seemed to fit in and be loved by all. Willie was particularly impressed by Jennette, who was interested in snakes and star gazing, a bit of a naturalist like her father.

Young Featherston Osler and his bride lived in Toronto. Brick and his wife had one of Dundas's finest homes, Staplehurst, not far from the rectory. There was endless coming and going between the families, with Staplehurst's croquet lawns one of the favorite gathering places for the young men and women. As spring came to Canada in May 1867, late again, the pace of parties, or 'shines,' picked up. A dozen of the young folk would have a late afternoon croquet match, followed by high tea. A few more would drop in, there would be dancing and singing, and at about eleven a round of cake and wine. A last big square, another song or two, and these children of England's empire builders would conclude the evening with the national anthem, 'God Save the Queen,' in full chorus, and singing the 'colonial' verse:

> Far from our Fatherland,
> Nobly we'll fall or stand
> By England's Queen;
> In town or forest free,
> Britons unconquered we,
> Sing with true loyalty,
> God Save the Queen

On July 1, 1867, the three leading provinces of British North America were to be amalgamated in a confederation named the Dominion of Canada. The Oslers' correspondence suggests that they paid no attention to the events leading to the birth of a new country. For them, and perhaps most British North Americans, the chief holiday of the season was Queen Victoria's birthday on May 24, the occasion for more picnicking, bonfires, fireworks, and anthems. As the older Britons partied and sang, seventeen-year-old Willie spent that weekend rambling in the Canadian countryside, becoming born again to a new world of natural splendor and beginning to develop the passion that would lead him to medicine.[77]

TWO

Learning to See: Student Years

When Willie Osler entered Trinity College School in Weston in 1866, he was a happy-go-lucky sixteen-year-old. He liked hunting, sports, and fights with the day boys and villagers. Smallish – he had probably reached his adult height of five foot, five and three-quarter inches – but wiry and fit, he was a good athlete, known for the strength and accuracy of his throwing arm: 'Last Friday I was coming up and the Roman Catholic school was standing about 80 yards from the road and I bet a boy I could throw and break a window. The other fellow threw and did not come near it ... Mine went through the window and struck one of the boys on the head, there was a terrible row about it but I went down to the old Priest and made it all right and put in the window.'[1]

Willie took to the English-style discipline (a prefect system and liberal caning by the masters) of the newly founded Trinity College School; he liked his schoolmates, found headmaster Badgely 'firstrate' and the singing lessons and theatricals 'such jolly fun.' His mother disapproved of such 'mummeries' as being too worldly.[2] In a less worldly vein, Willie took the instruction leading to his formal confirmation as a member of the Church of England. Then his rowdy side took over, and he got into fairly serious trouble as one of the ringleaders in a student war against an unpopular matron at the school. With the tacit consent of the masters, who had asked the lady to go, the boys barricaded her in her room, fumigated it with sulfur and molasses, smashed the windows, and threw sticks and snowballs at her. She had them arrested and charged with assault. They may have spent a night or two in jail. Big brother Featherston defended the scholars in county court. The magistrate fined each of them one dollar and costs.[3]

Brother Frank, two years older than Willie, was also in hot water that spring, having quit school, failed to find work, and gone into debt. So Ellen Osler had two wayward boys to worry about, and she did not mince her words to the younger:

> It was an unfortunate affair that of all you boys being brought into public notice in such a disreputable manner and although I do not think it was meant to be more than a mere school boy freak, such things often tell against a person long after, and I hear many say they think it will injure the reputation of the school ...
>
> Could you only know my dear boy how earnestly my heart longs to see you walking in the paths of holiness you would I think strive to do well but there is One who loves you with a love far stronger than mine who gave Himself to die for you. He is 'the Way, the Truth, and the Life' in Him and only in Him is true peace and happiness to be found.

A few weeks later Frank ran off to sea to be a sailor like his father. That led to more maternal pressure on Willie:

> I can never cease to pray for him [Frank]. Indeed my dear Willie it is what I constantly do for each and all of you, that God would grant you the Teaching of His Holy Spirit, to convince of Sin, of righteousness and of Eternal Judgment. God is your kind loving Father and we ought to love him. He is our Master and we are bound to serve him. Consecrate yourself my dear boy to His Service and all will be well with you for Time and Eternity.

Perhaps wracked by adolescent guilt – his parents had never before been so serious about the state of his soul – Willie announced that he planned to become a minister. Changing tacks, Ellen responded with wise skepticism:

My first impulse was to thank God that he had heard my prayer and inclined one of my six boys to make choice of that as his path in life. It is a
matter not to be decided on hastily any more than is any other profession –
take your time for consideration and above all search your heart for the
motives inducing your decision, for remember that God always judges of us
by our motives while man can only judge of our actions ... I am quite sure
that if you do seriously and in earnest desire to be fitted for the service of
God in His Church Papa will do all he can to help you forward by giving
you a liberal education and both of us will bid you Godspeed.[4]

Willie won most of the events at the school games in May 1866, cap-
ping the day with a close victory in a grueling steeplechase – which did
him in until he was pleasantly revived by girls mopping his brow and ex-
claiming, 'Poor Osler.' His letters show that he was starting to take his
studies seriously, though without obvious enthusiasm. He was working earnestly at letter writing ('I am a gnat stupid at letter writing – Nellie ... is
lecturing me about my letters') and was berating himself for writing so
briefly and badly. A family letter-writing gene was beginning to express
itself in Willie, complete with punctuation defect.[5]

He won the Chancellor's Prize for head student in the 1866 midsummer
examinations, but he was just turning seventeen and was thought too young
to move up to the Anglicans' Trinity College in Toronto. He was not too
young to stand on guard for Canada that spring, turning out for regular
drill as able-bodied men prepared to meet invaders from the United States
– a ragtag army of Irish nationalists, some of them Civil War veterans, who
hoped to liberate their country by seizing British North America. The
Fenians were easily repulsed. Osler saw no action.

He had another summer of shooting and sports and dalliances with girls
(his first love being one of his Lloydtown cousins, Mary Osler; sister Nellie
advised that the best way to advance his cause was to keep quiet about it
for two or three years). At summer's end, Willie returned to the Weston
school as head prefect. There were no pranks or scrapes that year, but neither did anyone remember Osler exercising intellectual or oratorical leadership: 'His work was always done, and well done; but it was "work," not a
flash of inspiration, that brought results. It was no uncommon thing to see

him during "prep," sitting with his fingers in his ears struggling with some problem, and oblivious of the distractions to which the rest of us had yielded.' As prefect, Willie kept the younger boys more or less orderly, sometimes having them fight out their disagreements, sometimes standing up for them against village toughs. He could use his fists. 'Once we played the villagers a football match ...,' a classmate remembered. 'One huge bully threw himself ferociously and quite unnecessarily upon a little chap who could hardly be said to have been actually in the scrim; but Osler, who was, catapulted out of the vortex, and with one blow on the big fellow's jaw sent him to the ground and thence to bed for a week.' With admiring sisters and English cousins watching, he maintained his running and jumping and throwing leadership at the autumn games day, only to be kicked in the shin at football soon afterwards and laid up for several weeks with a serious leg injury, probably osteomyelitis.[6]

During his forced immobility in the winter of 1866–7, Willie saw much more of Trinity College School's founder and warden, the Reverend William Arthur Johnson. About the same age as Featherstone Osler, Johnson was also a child of the British Empire. Born to an officer serving in India, he had learned a little medicine, done a little military service, tried farming in Upper Canada, and finally found a spiritual home as a priest in the Church of England. As pastor of the Weston church, Johnson had started the school in his home to teach his sons, then deferred to more scholarly masters when it developed into a preparatory school for Trinity College. Over the years, Johnson's ritualistic High Anglicanism – he was really an Anglo-Catholic – landed him in no end of trouble with parishioners and fellow churchmen, including loss of the school, which was taken away from him shortly after Osler left and was moved to the town of Port Hope, Ontario, where it still resides.

This was of little consequence to Osler. All that mattered was that Old Johnson, as the boys called him, was a man who loved nature and had a special way of looking at it – through a microscope.

Nature studies, especially 'natural history,' were hugely popular, virtually a craze, in nineteenth-century British North America and in the mother country itself. Britons, Canadians, and Americans too, loved to ramble outdoors, collect insects, butterflies, and fossils, classify flora and fauna, and count samples and species. 'The Victorians took for granted that a familiarity with natural science and a sensitivity to scenery formed part of the intellectual equipment of every educated person,' writes Carl Berger. Doing natural history was an agreeable hobby for some; for others it was a vital intellectual pursuit related to the quest to understand the mechanisms of life and creation.

A few exceptionally zealous naturalists made a particular specialty of penetrating deeper into the mysteries of nature with wonderful magnifying instruments. Microscopes had been developed in the seventeenth century, but the new worlds revealed through their primitive lenses were at first murky and obscure. By the second quarter of the nineteenth century, the development of achromatic compound lenses made the microscope a special tool with a status not unlike computers a hundred and fifty years later. As the instrument came down in price, ownership widened from an original elite of tinkerers and visionaries, and by the 1850s no serious science student could be without one. Still, microscopes were neither cheap nor commonplace, especially in frontier societies such as Canada West. Willie Osler almost certainly never saw one until he began helping Rev. Johnson with his nature studies.[7]

Johnson was a gourmand naturalist, interested in collecting, noting, and sketching everything. He gathered roots, feathers, flowers, bees' tongues, rabbits' tongues, leaves, seeds, sand, shells, rocks, fossils, eggs, animal organs, fleas, mosquito heads, parasites, algae ... and in the winter of 1866–7 he was particularly interested in studying teeth and bones. Often he exchanged specimens with his great friend, fellow microscopist, and decidedly kindred spirit, Dr James Bovell. Another imperial wanderer, born in the West Indies and educated in the mother country, Bovell taught at Trinity College and practiced medicine in Toronto. He, too, was immersed in natural history, along with many other interests.

As physician to Trinity College School, Bovell probably treated Osler's bad leg. But the main reason for his visits to Weston was to get together with Johnson to see what their microscopes could teach them. The immobilized Osler began to help prepare specimens for their study, apparently starting by grinding up a crocodile scale. He also remembered cleaning up the mess of specimens and stains left on Johnson's study table after the Saturday nature studies.[8]

When spring finally came in 1867, Johnson took some of the TCS students on field trips along the banks and marshes of the Humber River, which ran past Weston. While Willie's siblings and cousins in Dundas were enjoying their croquet and teas and dancing, Johnson was showing the boy a new world. The one person Willie felt he might tell about it was cousin Jennette. He wrote to her the day after the Queen's birthday, mentioning that he had a milk snake for her in a bottle of whisky and would look for more. His new enthusiasm spilled out:

> I have splendid times with Mr. Johnson out after specimens of all sorts. I wish you had been with us last Tuesday down at the Peat Swamp, there are such splendid flowers down there and the Moss is so nice and springy one would like to make a bed of it. We got the smallest and rarest variety of Ladies Slipper or Indian Moccasin plant. I would so like you to see them they are the most beautful of all Canadian wild flowers there are none about Dundas not being the right sort of soil for them to grow in.

More wondrously, Johnson had shown him what pond scum looked like under the microscope:

> And if you could only see the Algae, that green stuff that you see on ponds and stagnant water, it is so beautiful, the thousands upon thousands of small animals all alive and kicking that are in it. We got some dirty looking brown stuff that at this time covers all the stones of the river and we found that on every pin point there were one hundred of the small creatures, fancy what there would be on a square inch and on a square mile.

Suddenly self-conscious, Willie realized that this was not normal boy-to-girl or cousin-to-cousin talk: 'I suppose you will think this sort of thing rather dry so I will stop it and turn to something perhaps nicer. We are having such a splendid run of Cricket Matches this term.'[9]

A new young man began to emerge from the chrysalis of cricket and shooting and dreary recitations of Homer, Livy, and Cicero. In 'Father' Johnson, Osler had found a real teacher, the first of the three great mentors of his life. 'Imagine the delight of a boy of an inquisitive nature,' he recalled years later, 'to meet a man who cared nothing about words, but who knew about things – who knew the stars in their courses, and could tell us their names, whose delight was in the woods in springtime, who told us about the frogspawn and the caddice worms, and who read to us in the evenings Gilbert White [a popular naturalist] and Kingsley's "Glaucus" [*Glaucus: Or the Wonders of the Shore*], who showed us with the microscope the marvels in a drop of dirty pond water, and who on Saturday excursions up the river could talk of Trilobites and the Orthoceratites, and explain the formation of the earth's crust.'[10]

Osler had more health problems that summer of 1867 – 'conjestion of the lungs again,' according to Jennette – and had to postpone his matriculation examinations. His father, undoubtedly worrying that he might be prone to consumption (tuberculosis), considered sending him on a voyage for the fresh air, but nothing came of it. Father Johnson decided to come to Dundas to visit, causing Willie to revel, observed Nellie, 'in the thoughts of the hunts for "beasts" he will have.' The two nature lovers wandered through the sprawling Cootes Paradise marsh below the town. Along the wooden sides of a canal basin, a few feet below the surface, Johnson and Osler noticed extensive and mysterious gelatinous growths. They put samples under Johnson's lens. 'Judge of our delight,' Osler recalled, 'when we found the whole surface of the jelly was composed of a collection of tiny animals of surpassing beauty, each of which thrust out to our view in the zoophyte trough a crescent-shaped crown of tentacles.'[11]

Johnson's textbooks could not explain the growth pattern, but a new article in the *American Naturalist* happened to describe these freshwater polyzoa. Willie began what would be a decade-long study of them, supplementing his fascination with the diatoms, or algae, Johnson had first shown him along the banks of the Humber. As a young naturalist he became an intense observer, a careful classifier, a thorough searcher – both out-of-doors and in the scholarly literature Johnson introduced him to – and a skilled microscopist. We can imagine Johnson saying to him again and again, 'Look carefully Osler. Use your eyes, lad. What do you see? What exactly do you see?'

His lungs cleared and he was able to get on with his formal education. Osler entered the University of Trinity College in Toronto in the autumn of 1867, intending to engage in studies of the classics and divinity appropriate to entering the ministry. Trinity was a struggling sectarian institution, founded in 1851 by Bishop Strachan as an alternative to the 'godless' provincial University of Toronto. It had not flourished. Jennette Osler was disappointed in her visit to Trinity, finding it small and poor and with only forty-five students. Willie, who had won a scholarship, was one of only four entering scholars that year. The college building was bleak and cold, and was barred at ground level to prevent the students from skipping out after curfew. Osler's courses in his first year included Algebra, Euclid, Greek, the Catechism, Trigonometry, Latin Prose, Roman History, and Classics.[12]

He did not have an interest to lose in these subjects. None of his teachers had interested him in classical literature. He hated mathematics. His interest in the church was more a matter of convenience than commitment. At Trinity his reading suddenly blossomed, but not in the intended direction. He was obsessed with natural history: 'Early in my college life I kicked over the traces and exchanged the classics with "divvers" [divinity] as represented by Pearson, Browne and Hooker, for Hunter, Lyell and Huxley.' When not reading in his spare time, he visited Bovell to work on slides for the microscope and bring in algae and other pond creatures.[13]

James Bovell taught at both Trinity College and the Toronto School of Medicine, the latter a fairly typical North American 'proprietary' medical school. Owned and run by a group of physicians in a building rented from the University of Toronto, the Toronto school offered courses leading to qualification as a physician and surgeon. The teachers were paid from the students' fees. Neither the university nor Trinity College had been able to maintain faculties of medicine. There was a rival school in Toronto affiliated with the Methodists' Victoria University. One of Osler's schoolfriends,

Arthur Jukes Johnson, a son of the Reverend W.A., was studying at the Toronto School of Medicine and often did natural history with Osler and Bovell on Saturdays. Bovell frequently invited Osler to come over to the school of medicine and sit in on his lectures, and soon Osler was at the TSM every afternoon. Johnson Jr urged him to think about switching to medicine.[14]

During Christmas vacation Willie read Charles Lyell's *Principles of Geology*. The family member who was most likely to share his new interests, cousin Jennette, was back home in England, and he wrote to her asking how he could obtain her father's monograph on molluscs. 'The boy is more cracy [sic] about Natural Science than ever,' sister Nellie told Jennette.

By the spring of 1868, Nellie was becoming seriously concerned that Willie was throwing away his scholarship and losing his interest in entering the ministry, for the sake of natural history and what was then called 'natural theology' (taught at Trinity by Bovell). Contrary to legend, Osler's parents, or at least his father, did not seem to mind. 'Entering the Ministry is of his own free choice. Papa would prefer his becoming almost any thing except a misunderstood poorly paid Backwoods parson,' Nellie explained to Jennette. 'No, my objections were that Willie was neglecting the works that from choice & his own will he chose to take up & instead of reading for his Scholarship & honours, wasted his time over intricate Theological controversy.'[15]

The 'controversy' was the great nineteenth-century dispute about the relationship between the world of biblical revelation and the world the naturalists revealed. It had been simmering for decades when the 1859 publication of Darwin's *Origin of Species* brought matters to a boil. The 1860s were, as Osler remembered, 'a decade of mental tumult.' Thomas Henry Huxley and other nonbelievers insisted that the fact of evolution through natural selection undercut the biblical notion of creation and many other items of Christian faith. Was it possible to believe in the truths of evolution and nature and also believe the Bible was true? Was it possible to have a scientific outlook and remain a Christian?

The controversy raged hotly at Trinity College in colonial Canada, and Osler's mentor, Bovell, was in the thick of it. Years before, in the tradition

of the classic synthesizer William Paley, Bovell had written a long and
dreary book, *Outlines of Natural Theology*, trying to show that there was no
contradiction between revealed religion and the divinity's natural handi-
work. Osler remembered listening to advanced students pepper Bovell with
questions on natural history, evolution and metaphysics generally:

> On Providence, Foreknowledge, Will and Fate,
> Fixed Fate, Freewill, Foreknowledge absolute.

He sat in on disputations about Genesis and geology. 'It seems hardly credible,' he reminisced many years later, 'but I heard a long debate on Philip
Henry Gosse's ... "Omphalos, an Attempt to untie the Geological Knot."
A dear old parson, Canon Reade, stoutly maintained·the possibility of the
truth of Gosse's view that the strata and the fossils [and Adam's omphalos,
or navel] had been created by the Almighty to test our faith!'[16]

Osler the student appears to have listened and read, rather than spoken
or argued. He was an observer rather than a participant. If he underwent
personal 'mental tumult,' he camouflaged it then and for most of the rest of
his life. Early in his reading he hit upon a near-perfect personal guide to
living with, if not resolving, these issues. In the winter of 1868, under
Johnson's influence, he purchased his first copy of Sir Thomas Browne's
Religio Medici.

Browne was a seventeenth-century naturalist and physician in Norwich,
England. As a young man he wrote a private meditation on his religious
beliefs and their implications for his understanding of nature. Upon publication in 1642, *Religio Medici* (pronounced in English with a soft 'g' and
rhyming with 'shed a sigh') became an instant classic; it had been widely
translated and republished dozens of times before Osler first looked into its
pages. He found in them a stylistically beautiful, intellectually complex,
profoundly tolerant, and, for him, richly satisfying argument that anticipated most of Paley, Bovell, and the other nineteenth-century apologists'
arguments for the reconciliation of Christianity and human reason.

Browne insisted on being a follower of both revealed religion and nature: 'There are two Books from whence I collect my Divinity; besides that

written one of God, another of His servant Nature, that universal and publick Manuscript, that lies expans'd unto the Eyes of all ... I call the effects of Nature the works of God.' Where there appeared to be contradictions between the great books, Browne adroitly ducked – denying, taking refuge in seeing through a glass darkly, or just giving up: 'There are a bundle of curiosities, not only in Philosophy, but in Divinity, proposed and discussed by men of most supposed abilities, which indeed are not worthy our vacant hours, much less our serious Studies.'[17]

Aphoristic and elusive, the *Religio* requires and repays rereading. During his life Osler came to use it virtually as a surrogate Bible. Eventually he knew the *Religio* and Browne's other writings almost as well as his parents knew their Old and New Testaments; but his first copy is not widely marked or well thumbed. I suspect that after realizing that Browne had all the answers he needed, at least to avoid coming down firmly on one side or having to discuss matters further – Willy spent his vacant hours in 1868 hunting for more specimens to study under the microscope. He was too busy at that period of his life to spend much time becoming a learned Brunonian.

That spring he made his first observations of beasts within beasts when he saw in a piece of human muscle the *Trichinella spiralis* entozoa that had killed its host, a man in New York State. Thus Osler met parasites, a form of life most commonly studied by dissecting the dead.

His mentors still hoped he would enter the church. Johnson was both a naturalist and a priest, and Bovell, also a High Churchman, was himself thinking about becoming a priest. When Nellie Osler went to Bovell, as Willie's greatest friend, in the spring of 1868 to ask advice about her brother's future, Bovell told her emphatically not to dissuade Willie from entering the church. 'Underneath the surface' Nellie reported Bovell saying, 'his feelings were deep & sincere & the boy having varied talents, was never likely to strikingly excel in any one thing.' The one person who thought differently and apparently hoped Willie would not go into the ministry was cousin Jennette.[18] In any case, Nellie soon abdicated the solicitous sister role by eloping with a man the family did not like (whose early death doomed her to a life of piously helpful widowhood).

Willie had done well enough in his first year at Trinity to be awarded another scholarship. The competition may not have been very stiff. Early in his second year, he found himself in hot water with the provost of Trinity. This may have been because of his disinterest in his studies or because of a fetus he brought to the college from the dissecting room of the Toronto School of Medicine, which became the subject of many pranks and much ostentatious outrage by the divinity students. The provost held the sons of prominent churchmen to particularly high standards of decorum and performance, and apparently gave Osler a tongue lashing culminating in what a classmate remembered as his stock tantrum: 'Sir, you are persistently and essentially bad – you are a disgrace to yourself, to your family, to your college, to your church – and – and – you may go now sir.' Osler decided to go and study medicine. When he told James Bovell of his decision, he received immediate support. 'That's splendid,' Osler remembered Bovell saying. 'Come along with me.'[19]

Willie had decided to become a physician, a practitioner of physic, the art of healing through knowledge of nature. He would be entering one of the oldest professions, a brotherhood that in the Western world traced its lineage to ancient Greece. It had two Hellenic roots: the cult and temples of healing centered on the god Aesculapius, he of the snake-entwined staff; and the teachings of Hippocrates of Cos, reputed father of the oath Osler and most other young medical men would take before entering their practice.

Later in his life Osler celebrated ideas of medical lineage and collegiality, what he called the 'apostolic succession' that ran from the age of Hippocrates through Galen, Avicenna, and countless others who preserved the secrets of the art through unchanging centuries. New medical giants had emerged in the Renaissance – Paracelsus, the rebel against authority; Vesalius, the father of anatomy; Harvey, discoverer of the circulation of the blood – to begin to build recognizable foundations for modernity. Challenges were mounted to the Greco-Roman view of disease as an imbalance of the body's four fundamental ingredients, or humors. Thomas Sydenham and other skeptics insisted on observing and classifying disease carefully. Giovanni Morgagni emphasized the postmortem examination as a way of finding out what happened to the body in illness. John Hunter turned physicians back to the study of nature, insisting that they master knowledge of bodily parts in sickness and health.

New medical systematizers in the eighteenth century Enlightenment posited universal principles that seemed to control sickness and health. Perhaps the balance the body sought was between being too inflamed or excited on the one hand and being too low or depleted on the other. If disease was either stimulating ('sthenic') or weakening ('asthenic'), perhaps constitutional health could be restored by countermeasures, a therapeutic approach not greatly different from that of Greek times. The natural principle, or *vis medicatrix naturae*, it seemed, was to build strength by eating or drinking and to expel irritants by sweating, bleeding, vomiting, urinating, and defecating. Givers of physic could help restore nature's equilibrium through treatments that encouraged depletion or, less often, repletion. So doctors drew off blood, prescribed compounds that promoted sweating, blistering, vomiting, et cetera, ordered changes in diet, and occasionally gave a tonic or other stimulant. Featherstone Osler, we saw, was depleted in a major way in the 1820s by the draining off of one hundred ounces of his blood in the hope of reducing inflammation.

The passion to find out what was happening to diseased bodies in an age of growing scientific inquiry led to an emphasis on literally looking inside the dead – necropsy or autopsy. What Osler came to call medicine's 'great awakening' in the early nineteenth century was driven by pathologists' cutting open corpses in 'dead houses,' probing the mysteries of morbid anatomy to see how disease and death left their marks. Clinician pathologists, especially those working in the great hospitals of Paris, related the postmortem condition of organs and tissues to the symptoms of illness they had cataloged in life and began to assemble descriptions of specific diseases, such as tuberculosis, typhus, and typhoid fever. Often specific lesions could be located, suggesting that disease had a local impact or site, rather than being some vague impairment of the whole system. Disease seemed to attack selectively, specifically. You could describe its effect on the organs and tissues of the body; you could test remedies to see if they treated these effects.

Doctors had learned to bring all their senses into play in observing living patients. They not only listened to patients' complaints but looked carefully at their bodies. They learned to feel the bodies, palpating for signs of disease. They took the pulse. They tapped or percussed the chest and back, feeling vibrations and listening to internal echoes. They looked at urine and stool for bleeding and other signs. The sugary taste of urine might confirm a diagnosis of diabetes.

By the mid-nineteenth century technology was extending doctors' sensitivity. A few had put ear to chest or abdomen to try to listen to the body. Now the introduction of the stethoscope revealed a world of sounds made by the pumping heart, by air in the lungs, by blood coursing through arteries. Thermometers made it possible to measure body temperature. Gadgets with lenses and mirrors enabled doctors to see into the eye, down the throat, eventually into all the body's orifices. Physicians no longer just questioned and looked at their patients. They examined them, deducing from the outside what was happening on the inside.[20]

The microscope revealed amazing new worlds to medical investigators as surely as it did to other students of nature. The very structure of living things seemed to be laid bare; they all consisted of masses of tiny distinct globules, or cells. How the cells worked, in sickness and health, would take generations to explore. The publication of Rudolf Virchow's *Cellular Pathology* in 1858, a year before Darwin on the origin of species, was one of the great milestones in nineteenth-century scientific medicine. The sense of windows opening on the nature of life itself would not be repeated until the discovery of the structure of DNA a century later.

The enemies of life, the very causes of disease, also seemed to be appearing in the lenses of those studying human cells and tissue, the early histologists. Minute creatures, or animalcules, lived on and in animal matter, just as they lived on and in ponds and the wooden sides of the Desjardins Canal. Did some of them prey on the system, causing disease? William Osler entered medicine just as an age-old theory that many illnesss were

caused by infection from minute germs was finally being given scientific
verification. The study of these micro-organisms, microbiology, would be a
frontier of science for the rest of the century and beyond. In France, Louis
Pasteur began publishing his fascinating research on the role of microbes
in fermentation and putrefaction in the late 1850s. We saw Osler observe
the deadly trichinosis parasite, one of the first of the animalcules to have
been identified, while still a student at Trinity College.

All of these medical and scientific developments were disappointing in
one crucial way. It was now possible to separate fevers into typhoid and
typhus, suggest that consumption was a consequence of the creation of
tubercules in the lungs, and show that a symptom complex involving gas-
trointestinal upset and severe muscle pain was due to a parasite in food. It
was also possible to show, both from pathological investigation and from
statistical studies of cases, that many traditional treatments had no impact
on these diseases. They fell into disfavor; the reaction against bloodletting
and many other depletion therapies was particularly marked. What was
not possible was to find alternative therapies that would actually work to
cure disease. Virtually the sole exception was the discovery of the effectiveness of an extract of cinchona bark, quinine, in cases of malaria. It
happened that malaria was particularly hard to distinguish from other fevers, so, as in the Osler family, you dosed up on it as a general tonic – and
many doctors thought it worked against several kinds of fever.

The powerlessness of doctors to cure disease was a not-so-hidden secret
of the Victorian age. Making too much of that shortcoming is an all-too-
common failure of our era's historical judgment and imagination.

Ministering to the sick involves much more than curing. Without
curing disease, it was still possible to reduce pain, increase feelings
of well-being, and, above all, prevent the onset of many sicknesses. It was
possible, for example, to safeguard people from one of the most deadly
and loathsome of all scourges, smallpox, through the vaccination procedure developed by the careful observations of an English country doctor,
Edward Jenner, in the 1790s. No one was quite sure how that prophylac-
tic measure worked, nor were they yet sure which diseases could be stopped
through sanitary measures and which through isolation or quarantine,

but by the 1860s there was no doubt at all that epidemics of cholera, typhus, diphtheria, and yellow fever could be contained and reduced, to the
immense benefit of humanity. In an age of discovery, progress, and prevention, it was unforgivable to surrender to the old fatalism and acqui-
esce to plagues being God's judgment on sinful humans. Possibly venereal
disease was a kind of consequence of sin, but to avoid being ravaged by
syphilis, which was almost as terrible as AIDS would become and far more
widespread, one had to be chaste or careful, not a churchgoer.

In 1867, the year before William Osler entered medicine, Britain's Joseph
Lister published a paper outlining techniques to stop the microbes that
Pasteur and others were writing about from causing putrefaction, or *sepsis*,
during surgery. Years earlier, Ignatz Semmelweis and Oliver Wendell Holmes
through observation had learned to preach a gospel of rigid sanitation in
childbirth, a practice that saved millions of lives. From the 1840s the terrible
pain of surgery (and ultimately childbirth) was alleviated by the use of
anesthetics. Setting broken limbs, excising surface growths from the body,
amputating, and doing cesarian sections were useful surgical functions about
to be made more bearable and safer in the era of anti- and asepsis. Soon
surgeons would be entering the body itself to attack disease.

People have always looked to physicians to relieve pain. By the 1860s
opium and one of its alkaloids, morphine, were in use as wonderfully effective albeit dangerous painkillers. Of course, the original mood-altering drug,
alcohol, had all sorts of medicinal uses all along the spectrum, from analge-
sic to stimulant to narcotic. There may no longer have been theoretic
justification for the use of traditional tonics, elixirs, and other sthenic compounds, but include enough alcohol and there was no doubt that people
felt good after taking them. Sometimes people felt better after being given
an emetic to make them vomit or a cathartic to move their bowels, or a
mustard plaster on their chest, even if there was no impact on the real
source of their sickness. Sometimes, if they believed enough in their doctors' power to help them, they felt better on bread or sugar pills or from just
being reassured of recovery.

Changes in diet could make fever patients feel better; changes in atmosphere could help consumptives. A doctor might help a patient by telling

her to stay in bed or by telling her to get out of bed. Anyone who has been sick knows that medical meteorology – the offering of a forecast or prognosis for an illness – is often comforting and almost always welcome, even when negative. Those who built hospitals where the desperately poor could find a bed and food, and emergency and palliative care were reducing suffering. The doctors, nurses, and lay trustees who cared about making hospitals cleaner and better institutions were helping reduce suffering. It was a great thing to learn how to treat the insane without having to chain and imprison them.

If you were a wise up-to-date physician, by the middle of the nineteenth century you realized that it might be better not to try to do too much. The Paris clinicians, the pathologists, the histologists, a still heterogenous collection of laboratory workers, and perhaps your own eyes were showing that many disease conditions cleared up on their own with time. Bodies often healed themselves, as Jacob Bigelow argued in his 1835 classic, *Discourse upon Self-Limited Diseases*. Many of the traditional remedies, especially the old extremes of bleeding and blistering, and lathering with mercury compounds were not only useless but positively harmful. A physician could help reduce suffering by practicing and by prescribing better medicine or by not prescribing any medicine at all. At the beginning of the 1860s, the famous Boston physician and writer Oliver Wendell Holmes (father of the Holmes with whom Jennette Osler had flirted) delivered an instantly notorious challenge to the old therapeutics: 'I firmly believe that if the whole materia medica, as now used, could be sunk to the bottom of the sea, it would be all the better for mankind, and all the worse for the fishes.' Holmes took care to except wine, opium, and specifics such as quinine.[21]

Medical intelligence seemed to be accumulating in unmanageable proportions. In the 1840s James Jackson said that there was more known about medicine than the mind of man could grasp.[22] Good physicians tried to keep up-to-date, clubbing together in medical societies to share knowledge, and subscribing to an ever-increasing flow of medical periodicals. The electric telegraph was the world's first communications internet. Within a few weeks of Virchow's latest pathological investigations being published in Germany, doctors in California could read about them in their local journals. And when a son finished his basic medical training at the local proprietary school, the up-to-date American medical father would help finance his trip to Europe to see at first hand the world's greatest practitioners of medical science and art.

Not that there was perfect agreement on the state of the art or the nature of science. Medical communities were always in flux. In Britain, for example, there had long been three quite distinct bodies of healers – physicians, surgeons, and apothecaries – each with its own college, traditions, licensing practices, and class identification. The best physicians were gentlemen, surgeons were craftsmen, druggists were in trade. The ferment of American society had thrown up almost as many medical sects and cults as it had religious ones. Depending on whatever medical 'system' they believed in, sectarian physicians could prescribe almost anything. The Thomsonites used only botanical remedies. Homeopaths diluted their doses almost to infinity. Hydropaths believed that water was the universal restorative. Eclectics prescribed a little bit of everything. So it went. Without licensing laws in most states, every man could be a doctor, any woman a midwife or concoctor of potions and possibly spells (some women could even be doctors: Elizabeth Blackwell had graduated in medicine from a New York college in 1849, the year of Osler's birth), and any clergyman could be a faith healer or part-time physician. The sick poor had to take whatever quasi-medical comfort they could get or afford. Sometimes it was not very much – though perhaps better than nothing. There was a market for cheap medicine everywhere, including in the more regulated countries of Europe.

In the conservative provinces of British North America, physicians were more apt to have to get a license, though in Osler's Ontario in the late 1860s a man could be a licensed sectarian, as though it were possible to be a member of a Methodist parish of the Anglican Church. Willie Osler would not have considered sectarian options. His family's position in the province's professional and religious establishment, their belief in education, his contacts with James Bovell, and his interest in scientific learning all dictated that he would enter the medical mainstream.

The first recourse was in Toronto. The prospect was not particularly exciting. From the 1830s Toronto had supported two and sometimes three rival schools of medicine, all of them proprietary, some at times affiliated with the University of Toronto, Trinity College, or the Methodists' Victoria University. The doctors who gave courses changed adherences almost seasonally, it seemed, and no one thought medical education was the better for it. None of the struggling schools had significant supporting facilities, such as libraries, pathological museums, or laboratories. Rented lecture rooms and maybe a dissecting room in the basement made up a medical school. Students paid their fees directly to the professors, listened to their lectures over a few short terms, did some dissecting, and saw a few live patients on the wards of the Toronto General Hospital.

Assuming that the hospital was open. In the summer of 1867 the trustees of the fifty-year-old, debt-ridden charitable institution decided they had had enough in their dealings with the provincial government and simply closed Toronto General. It reopened in the summer of 1868, just as Osler began his studies at the Toronto School of Medicine. The hospital took only twenty-five indigent patients at a time, and students from the competing medical schools could see only their own professors' cases.[23]

One of Osler's classmates, J. Beattie Crozier, torched the Toronto School of Medicine in his memoirs. The teachers in their professorial chairs, Crozier wrote, 'rayed out from these high and sunless peaks mere cold and darkness, without enthusiasm, humour, or human geniality.' Their lectures were given without cases or specimens, and were a compound of textbook material and quotations from authorities, 'the whole being flung at us pell-mell without word of guidance, and leaving us standing helpless, bewildered, and starved in the midst of what seemed a superabundance of wealth.' Scholarship students found they could learn faster from books at home and only appeared for the compulsory number of lectures. Others 'yawned away the time lying listlessly about the seats,' said Crozier: 'Particularly during the evening lectures we might be seen dozing and snoring on the floor of the open plateau above the level of the amphitheatre, so that a stranger entering by the upper door in the shaded light, might have stumbled over body after body of us as we lay strewn about like corpses on a battlefield.'[24]

The only legible lecture notes surviving from Osler's years at the Toronto School of Medicine (written in a small, crabbed hand, much like his father's) are from his course on materia medica, the substances of drugs, given by one of the city's older practitioners, E.A. Ogden. Ogden was of the old school. He discussed the strengths and weaknesses of cathartics ('Castor oil & calomel may be given together, calomel on liver, castor oil in bowels below, you have in this way a more complete depletion of portal systems ... Rhubarb will relieve flatulence after eating. It is one of the best remedies you can administer after debilitated conditions of bowels, small doses of Rhubarb with bicarb of soda is very useful in cases of jaundice'), the strengths and weaknesses of the tonics ('cod liver oil – the darker the oil, the worse the taste ... It is the only remedy that exerts a marked influence over the tuberculous diathesis'), and the properties of the narcotics. Osler cared little for materia medica but stayed awake well enough to take his notes. He was so happy to have found his real calling in life that the only criticism he ever made of the Toronto medical school was that its building was 'dirty beyond belief.'[25]

Classmates remembered that he attended most of his lectures (there is no evidence that he had a scholarship) and spent the rest of his time in the dissecting room – where a good professor of anatomy helped make it a favorite subject – and at Bovell's microscope. Inside and outside the medical school he indulged his passion for examining the 'beasts' of the natural world. In Toronto's rivers and ponds, back in Dundas, and at Niagara, Barrie, and London, Ontario, he collected diatoms and polyzoa. He sat in on a course on natural history at the University of Toronto and regularly presented the professor, Rev. William Hincks, with specimens. A sunken barge near the mouth of the Humber proved a cornucopia of rare polyzoa.

Today's hardy Canadian boys sometimes shovel off their driveways and play basketball in the middle of winter. On Christmas Day 1868, Willie Osler went outdoors with his collecting bottles and stick to see what he could find. He could not find an unfrozen stream. Then he remembered a nearby spring that never froze. The barrel someone had put by it proved a naturalist's delight. He found so many interesting little creatures in his scrapings that he thought the tale worth telling. In the form of a letter to *Hardwicke's Science-Gossip*, he described his adventure for fellow naturalists in Great Britain, 'as it will give them some idea of what lovers of science meet with in this country.' Entitled 'Christmas and the Microscope' and prefaced with a Latin epigram (putting the hated classics training to use), it was his first publication.[26]

Pre-Christmas celebrations a year later proved fatal for two members of a Hamilton family. They died after eating an uncooked ham. In specimens from the victims and in the ham itself young Osler again saw the *Trichinella spiralis* parasite, enclosed in its cyst. Trichinosis was rare in Canada, so Osler must have been astonished a few months later when he was routinely dissecting the corpse of a German janitor from the hospital and found muscles riddled with encysted trichinae. Still a second-year medical student, he decided to make a special study of the parasite by inducing its growth in animals. In his first piece of research, he fed infected human flesh to rabbits, cats, and dogs, but without success. He saved his notes for future reference and began searching for other entozoa in animals and fish, becoming particularly interested in tapeworm in pike.

That spring he published a major paper in the *Canadian Naturalist* describing the 110 species of Canadian diatomaceae he had observed in his wanderings. Classmates noticed the appetite for hard work. Osler usually ate his lunch in the dissecting room so as not to waste time.[27] Nowhere in a lifetime of writing did he ever discuss the repugnance or other sensitivities some medical students have about cutting up humans; for him, dead bodies seem to have been instructive inanimate matter.

The medical students had no facilities for organized games, but they occasionally indulged in sporting fisticuffs, the challenge being to see if anyone could beat 'Long John' Standish, the school champion. Osler, to everyone's surprise, was at least able to land some punches. Medical students everywhere were notoriously rowdy, but nothing survives in the way of stories from Osler's years at Toronto School of Medicine. It was probably earlier, at Trinity, that he and Ned Milburn answered an American farmer's ad for a bride, enticed the man to Toronto, and met him at the station in drag. The farmer chose to woo the blond Milburn over the brunette Osler but never made a second visit.[28]

Osler still saw a lot of the Reverend W.A. Johnson – they were constantly on the trail of specimens together – and in 1868 and 1869 he spent time helping a local Dundas doctor, Holford Walker. He confused the medicine bottles, he later recalled, nearly killing Walker's best patient. Walker introduced Osler to two of the basic medical instruments, the laryngoscope and ophthalmoscope, and he had an exceptionally fine microscope. Another kindred spirit, who liked to work at Bovell's on specimens, was a young veterinary surgeon, Griffith Evans, who was stationed in Toronto with the Royal Artillery. Evans was fresh from taking a medical degree at Montreal's McGill University and was also a keen man for the microscope. 'Treat it gently, as you would a lady,' he told Osler.[29]

By far the dominant personality in Osler's life during his medical studies in Toronto was James Bovell. Osler worked with Bovell constantly the first year and lived in his house the second. In fact, his Toronto medical training was virtually an apprenticeship to a medical father-figure. Later, Osler occasionally doodled Bovell's name in notebooks and on papers. He always acknowledged Bovell as his second great mentor, Johnson being the first. Often they would all be immersed in microscopy at Bovell's on a Saturday morning, when a patient would show up and the pious doctor-scientist would curse the need to earn 'the damned guinea.'[30]

James Bovell had been a major figure in Toronto medicine and medical teaching for more than a generation. He was arguably the best-educated physician in Toronto, having trained at Guy's Hospital in London under several great names in British medicine, including three still associated with diseases: Bright, Hodgkin, and Addison. Bovell, recalled Osler, 'taught us to reverence his great masters' while also transmitting a fundamental belief in the unity of physiological and pathological processes. Bovell owned a rich and varied medical library, possibly the best in Toronto, in which Osler had free rein the year they lived together:

> That winter gave me a good first-hand acquaintance with the original works
> of many of the great masters. After fifty years the position in those rooms of

special books is fixed in my mind: Morton's 'Crania Americana,' Annesley's 'Diseases of India' with the fine plates, the three volumes of Bright, the big folios of Dana, the monographs of Agassiz. Dr Bovell had a passion for the great physician-naturalists, and it was difficult for him to give a lecture without a reference to John Hunter. The diet was too rich and varied, and contributed possibly to the development of my somewhat 'splintery' and illogical mind.

Osler would sit before a grate fire in Bovell's cluttered study on cold winter evenings, a blanket over his legs, another around his shoulders, reading and dreaming: 'I remember the awe and reverence inspired by the man who could write such wonderful books ... I used to wonder if I should ever be so fortunate as to see any of these great men.'[31]

Bovell also became for Osler a model of roles to avoid – a rather sad, sad-eyed case. Bovell could not focus his energies, he talked about everything but succeeded at doing little, and became notoriously absent-minded and negligent in the pursuit of his profession. He had to make most of his living from the practice of medicine, but he lost the addresses of patients he was supposed to see, and he gave away the income he was supposed to live on. Charitably, Osler spoke of Bovell as having had 'a quadrilateral mind, which he kept spinning like a teetotum.' He thought Bovell lacked self-discipline because he had been born into a life of ease, and that he was 'a typical example of a class' in falling far below his brilliant promise. There were strong elements of dreamy Anglo-Catholicism in the physician's drift towards a religious vocation. Bovell is remembered today in Canadian medical history for his attempts at transfusing milk into the arteries of cholera victims in the 1840s (having thought his microscope showed milk being converted into white blood corpuscles) and as one of Osler's mentors.[32]

Bovell's family returned to the West Indies in 1869. The Toronto School of Medicine was floundering in penury, paying its faculty very little, and in the summer of 1870 Bovell visited the West Indies and decided to stay. He and Osler had probably already talked over the desirability of Osler finding a better medical school. (Believing that India was far more promising than Canada, Bovell had encouraged the boy to dream of working in the Indian

Medical Service; Griffith Evans went on from Toronto to India.) If Osler was really going to be a physician rather than a microscopist, he would need to see patients – the patients Bovell did not have or was not interested in, the patients it was difficult to get access to in the Toronto General Hospital – a rich variety of patients like those Bovell had seen as a student at Guy's. Books were all very well, Bovell had taught Osler, but a man learned medicine on the wards of hospitals. He had marked for Osler a passage in Latham's *Clinical Medicine:* 'It is by your own eyes, and your ears and your own minds and ... your own hearts that you must observe and learn and profit.'[33]

When Osler learned that Bovell would not be returning to Toronto, he felt that he had 'lost a father and a friend.' He probably would have moved on anyway. His real father, Featherstone Osler, was a somewhat distant figure in his life in these years, but perhaps wise fathers know when to keep their distance, and certainly both father and son had their eye on Willie's advancement. 'Willie has gone to Montreal to McGill College where the hospital advantages are greater than at Toronto,' Featherstone wrote in October 1870. 'I wish to give him every advantage in my power though it is very expensive.'

James Bovell became a priest and served for ten years in dire poverty on the island of Nevis. He had given Osler his stethoscope but kept his microscope, and he studied nature to the end – 'anything to relieve this cruel monotony.' He died in 1880 at the age of sixty-three.[34]

Medical education at McGill was the best Canada had to offer. Montreal, Canada's largest city (population about 150,000) and its commercial metropolis, had become more than 50 per cent English-speaking in the century since the conquest of New France. Its Scots establishment had founded a university based on the solid principles in place at the University of Edinburgh in its golden age. McGill's Faculty of Medicine had high admission requirements by North American standards (James Bovell Johnson, son of one of Osler's mentors and namesake of the other, failed McGill's stiff entrance exam that autumn); the faculty had longer teaching sessions than most schools, required students to take its courses in sequence rather than in helter-skelter order, and required four years of training before graduation rather than the normal two or three. In his final two years, a medical student spent at least twelve months observing and working with medical and surgical cases in Montreal General Hospital and with obstetrics in the Lying-In Hospital. The medical school had a four-thousand-volume library, an anatomical and pathological museum, and a strong emphasis on dissection.

Few institutions anywhere in North America offered better facilities and hospital access or higher standards. McGill University's medical graduates were probably as well educated as its bachelors of arts. Harvard's medical school, while possibly the best in the United States, has been judged in those years to have been 'not much better than a diploma mill,' many of whose graduates were of doubtful literacy. In 1870 Harvard's president wrote: 'The ignorance and general incompetency of the average graduate of American Medical Schools, at the time when he receives the degree which turns him loose upon the community, is something horrible to contemplate.' McGill drew the majority of its 150 to 180 students from outside Quebec, many of them, like Osler, coming down from poorly serviced Ontario.[35]

By later standards, McGill's Faculty of Medicine was still primitive and its training grossly deficient. The two-storey brick building downtown on Côté Street, next to the Theatre Royal, housed a proprietary school that was only loosely affiliated with the university. Its staff were local practitioners, none of them trained as specialists, who passed on to their students what they had learned in practice and what they had picked up from textbooks. The students paid their fees, commonly twelve dollars a course,* directly to the professor. The 'late Dr Fenwick' was never on time, and

---

*Conversions of past to present monetary values are always inexact. At the end of the twentieth century, it took from twenty to forty American or Canadian dollars, depending on the situation, to do the work of one dollar in the last third of the nineteenth century. The effect of multiplying past values by thirty is sometimes noted in these pages (thus, each McGill course would cost about $360 in today's purchasing power, ignoring present disparities between the two countries' dollars), but usually I give past figures without comment. You will develop a feel for them on their own terms.

though considered the best surgeon in Montreal, he used no antiseptic methods until the late 1870s. William Fraser, Professor of the Institutes [fundamentals] of Medicine, taught physiology from an out-of-date textbook, used a blackboard as his only apparatus, and was nicknamed 'Old Commoonicate' for one of his pronunciational peculiarities. William Wright, Professor of Materia Medica, was another physician-clergyman, as long-winded about inconsequentials as Bovell at his fuzziest. Unlike Bovell, none of the professors at McGill used a microscope in his teaching. The medical building had no laboratory. The students copied and passed on lecture notes from year to year to year. The best performances they saw were next door at the theater.[36]

The Montreal General Hospital's building on Dorchester Street accommodated a hundred and fifty patients and very many rats, the latter sometimes bold enough to attack the former and to snatch their food. Some of the nurses, tough old birds who reminded the students of Dickens's Sairey Gamp, were adept at snatching the alcoholic stimulants liberally prescribed for the patients.[37] Fenwick and the other surgeons operated in blood-stained old frock coats (it was like donning painting clothes) on blood-stained wooden operating tables, washing their hands but nothing else. Medical and surgical patients were jumbled together in the same wards, Osler recalled, which was not wholly inappropriate because 'the physic of the men who were really surgeons was better than the surgery of the men who were really physicians, which is the best that can be said.' Francis Shepherd, a contemporary and later colleague of Osler's at McGill, remembered Dr William Fraser's nonphysic, nonsurgical approach to emptying one of the hospital beds:

> Old Nurse Sheehan ... reported to Dr Fraser that she thought a sailor in a certain bed was malingering, so he called for some brown paper, which he soaked in alcohol, and then ordered the man's abdomen to be exposed. On this he put the paper and then suddenly pulled a match out of his pocket, struck it, and applied it to the paper. In a few seconds there was a blaze, a yell from the man, who jumped out of the bed and rushed out of the ward ... The paper burned a large hole in the bedclothes.[38]

Osler began his McGill student life by giving a paper on his studies of
the diatoms to the Montreal Natural History Society. Through the winter
of 1870–1 he continued to study entozoa, dissecting a lynx, a cat, a rat, and
more fish. He took particularly detailed lecture notes in his course on 'The
Practice of Medicine,' given by Dr Palmer Howard, the most scholarly and
scientific of his professors, as well as the best teacher. Howard, himself a
McGill man who had done postgraduate work in Europe, seemed thoroughly up-to-date on such matters as the changing classifications of fevers,
the debate on the germ theory, diseases that were self-limiting, those that
called for heroic interventions (he still favored bloodletting in extreme
cases), and all other medical matters. Howard often brought pathological
specimens to class and, though not officially a teacher of clinical medicine,
was often followed around the hospital wards by students. Osler got to
know him right away: two weeks after he arrived in Montreal he had provided Howard with some microscopic slides of diseased kidney that Howard
used in a talk to the local Medico-Chirurgical Society.[39]

Osler did his required hospital service as a 'dresser' for surgeons and
'clerk' for physicians. These student positions were common in British but
not American hospitals. The young men did more than observe their masters. Osler's case notes indicate that he took patients' histories, learned to
do examinations, and regularly checked patients' pulse and temperature.
'In serious cases,' he remembered, 'we very often at night took our share in
nursing.'[40]

He lived with a gang of fellow Ontario students at 48 St Urbain Street
but had a second home with his English cousins, Jennette and Marian,
who had now immigrated to Canada and lived in Montreal with Marian's
second husband, George Francis, and a rapidly growing brood of children.
'Willie shed the light of his face on us this evening ...' Jennette wrote his
mother in January 1871. 'I cannot tell you what a pleasure it is to us to
have the dear merry fellow coming in & out ... We hear his praises on all
sides & from those whose good opinion is hard to win & well worth having. Your Benjamin is pronounced "thoroughly reliable," "as good as he is
clever," "the most promising student of the year," and finally, from a learned
Professor slow in approbation "a splendid fellow!" Now little Mother, purr

over that; we did! Willie says nothing himself & does not put on airs at all. He took me to church last night.'[41]

Strangely, in the spring of 1871 Osler did not take the 'preliminary' examinations required of McGill students after their third year. Despite clearly being a third-year student, he must not have felt or was not deemed well enough prepared for them. He never thought that he had great natural abilities, and he later told students of his despondency at first attempting to learn elementary anatomy. Just possibly he took the McGill exams and failed, but it is inconceivable that such an irony would never have been mentioned in a lifetime of reminiscing and advice giving. The set of preliminary exams he apparently did take that April were those held by the renascent Faculty of Medicine of the University of Trinity College in Toronto. It was being revived after a hiatus of fifteen years, and the first act of the newly appointed staff was to set examinations to sort out prospective students, many of whom would have studied at the Toronto School of Medicine or other schools.[42]

Why Osler wrote these examinations, presumably opening a door for his return to Toronto, is unclear. He stayed in Montreal during the summer of 1871 and was seriously short of money – 'Drat the dimes. I wish we could get along without them' – which may have been a factor. He was also, he remembered, very worried about the McGill final examination and what he would do afterwards. As well, James Bovell may have been planning a return to Toronto from the West Indies, for Trinity announced that he was to be professor of pathology in the new school, and that might have influenced Osler. And this may have been the season when he experienced another embarrassment as a speaker. Buried in a draft reminiscence there is one reference to a time when he gave lectures on physiology before a Young Men's Christian Association. 'They were a failure, so I stopped,' and we know nothing more.[43]

Bovell did not go back to Toronto, and Osler had a good summer in Montreal. He spent most of it working and learning in the hospital as a clinical clerk. Montreal medicine had adopted a British practice of having interesting hospital cases written up by the clerks and published in a local journal. Osler's first medical publications, in the September 1871 *Canada*

Medical Journal, were reports on five cases seen by D.C. 'Mickey Mac' MacCallum – the excision of a breast tumor, a fissure of the anus, Ludwig's angina, suppurative nephritism, and death from pleuropneumonia with delirium tremens. Osler studied the excised tumor under the microscope and did a full postmortem on the 'old toper,' whom they had had to tie down in his fits of delirium. Even a lay reader of his reports senses his fascination with the cysts, cells, and unidentifiable 'bodies' he saw in these human tissues.[44]

His interest in postmortems led to a cementing of his bond with Palmer Howard, whose outpatient clinics Osler was attending. Howard had become interested in a controversy about the specificity of tuberculosis as a disease, and he wanted to see every lung lesion found at the hospital. Osler brought specimens to him, often late at night. Fancy the slender, dark-complexioned student with a bag of organs slipping through the dark streets of gaslit Montreal and knocking on his professor's door. Howard's enthusiasm was infectious and inspiring as they pored over the literature in the midnight hours, forming in Osler's words an 'almost filial' relationship. His admiration for Howard, the third of his teachers and surrogate fathers, was warm and boundless: 'Since those days I have seen many teachers, and I have had many colleagues, but I have never known one in whom were more happily combined a stern sense of duty with the mental freshness of youth.' Knowing Howard, he eventually wrote, was a liberal education in itself. But he never got around to writing a planned profile of his mentor as 'a Canadian Sydenham.'[45]

That summer Osler experienced an important intellectual epiphany. One night, as he fretted about his future the way young people do, he came across an aphorism of Thomas Carlyle's: 'Our grand business undoubtedly is, not to *see* what lies dimly at a distance, but to *do* what lies clearly at hand.' Osler thought about it, decided to get on with each day's work as best he could, and found the habit so comforting that it gradually became the basis for a practical philosophy. He also decided to stay at McGill and write his degree thesis on postmortem studies of diseased organs. He pestered Palmer Howard for information and literature, and one day Howard gave him Samuel Wilks's *Lectures on Morbid Anatomy.* 'From that time,' Osler recalled, 'everything was plain sailing.'[46]

In his final year of medicine Osler is nearly invisible. Only one letter survives: he is working hard, taking regular exercise, and on Sundays managing to cram in churchgoing, dinner at Professor Howard's, and attempts to learn 'Dutch' (i.e., German). He suspends his natural history studies. He probably attends though cannot be found on the program of the medical students' annual 'footing supper.' This event was slowly evolving from an evening of beer and loose women in the dissecting room into a formal function at a downtown restaurant. The October 1871 supper at the Queen's Chop House was formally reported to have been run on 'strictly temperance principles.' Frank Shepherd's memory was that on such outwardly dry occasions the students became rowdier and more inebriated than ever, their ginger ale tasting much like brandy. Osler later compared the dinners to Bacchanalian orgies. He also recalled that his roommates on St Urbain Street went through several gallons of whisky a week. At least one brilliant friend from student days, Dick Zimmerman, had a promising career blighted by alcoholism, memories of which became the basis for some of Osler's later cautionary tales.[47]

McGill classmates had few memories of Osler, who was somewhat of a loner as he dissected and examined organs for his graduation thesis and boned up for his exams. He took McGill's course in materia medica that year, which was unusual for a fourth-year student (perhaps Ogden's weak Toronto course explains his examination problem). He also took courses in clinical medicine and surgery and medical jurisprudence, and became known as a protégé of Howard's. 'He sat in the centre of the front tier of semi-circular seats and was the cynosure of all eyes at the weekly "Grind" where Palmer Howard, with whom he was a great favourite, drew him out,' one classmate said. 'He was irregular in his attendance at lectures and retiring in character.' The brother of another classmate said that some of the men 'had no great respect for him though none disliked him. One of his year told me that he was not practical, and might have been plucked if he had not written some sort of a freak essay that happened to please Howard.'[48]

The 'freak essay' was his thesis, a formal degree requirement that had become almost obsolete at McGill. Many students paid a certain old Montreal physician twenty-five dollars to write a thesis for them. Osler did his own thesis, a report on twenty postmortems, illustrated with thirty-three microscopic slides and specimens. He presented it as a display in the Côté Street amphitheater. Many years later he remembered that a spell of warm weather and inadequate preservatives had made the presentation 'impressive in more ways than one.' Osler's thesis was judged by faculty members, Fraser as well as Howard, to be 'greatly distinguished for originality and research' and was awarded a special book prize. The specimens were given to McGill's medical museum. The full text of the thesis has not survived, but in a fragment from its introduction Osler states his faith in the importance of pathology: 'To investigate the causes of death, to examine carefully the condition of organs, after such changes have gone on in them as to render existence impossible and to apply such Knowledge to the prevention and treatment of disease, is one of the highest objects of the Physician.'[49]

Osler was the only McGill student that year to take both his primary and degree examinations. He stood eighth in the former competition, third in the latter, and was awarded the degree of Doctor of Medicine and Master of Surgery (MD, CM). He was twenty-two years old. With their hands uplifted, the graduates recited after the college registrar a Latin modification of the Hippocratic oath:

I swear by Apollo the physician and Aesculapius and Health (Hygeia) and All-Heal (Panacea) and all the gods and goddesses, that, according to my ability and judgement, I will keep this oath and this stipulation – to reckon him who taught me this art equally dear to me as my parents, to share my substance with him, and relieve his necessities if required; to look upon his offspring in the same footing as my own brothers, and to teach them this art, if they shall wish to learn it, without fee or stipulation; and that by precept, lecture, and every other mode of instruction, I will impart a knowledge of the art to my own sons, and those of my teachers, and to disciples bound by a stipulation and oath according to the law of medicine, but to none others. I will follow that system of regimen which, according to my ability and judgement, I consider for the benefit of my patients, and abstain from whatever is deleterious and mischievous.

I will give no deadly medicine to anyone if asked, nor suggest any such counsel; and in like manner I will not give to a woman a pessary to produce abortion.

With purity and with holiness I will pass my life and practise my art.

I will not cut persons labouring under the stone, but will leave this to be done by men who are practitioners of this work.

Into whatever houses I enter, I will go into them for the benefit of the sick, and will abstain from every voluntary act of mischief and corruption, and, further, from the abduction of females or males, or freeman and slaves. Whatever, in connection with my professional practice, or not in connection with it, I see or hear, in the life of men, which ought not to be spoken of abroad, I will not divulge, as reckoning that all such should be kept secret.

While I continue to keep this oath unviolated, may it be granted to me to enjoy life and the practice of the art, respected by all men in all times! But should I trespass and violate this oath, may the reverse be my lot![50]

Now what would he do? Rev. W.A. Johnson kept in touch with his prize student and disciple all through his medical education, writing him long letters of church and naturalist gossip, passing on books and advice on Christian living, and perhaps vicariously expanding his own horizons as Osler grew and traveled. Johnson knew the Osler family well, parents as well as children, knew the glittering achievements of some of the boys and the shortcomings of all of them. A few years after Willie graduated from McGill, Johnson warned his medical student son, who had finally made it to McGill, that Dr Osler should not be seen as a model:

He is an *Osler*, & there is that in him unless I am much mistaken which you must never admire. I would like to write you a good deal on the Osler character, but am too poorly. One thing only I see worthy of your imitation, that is, its *Application*. There does not appear to be any talent about them; or any high principles of action. Simply great application, and, *probably* the motive is money making.[51]

The soupçon of truth in Johnson's sour judgment (which may have been influenced by the fact that Canon Osler was on a bishop's committee investigating Johnson's suspiciously Romish stewardship of his parish) was that Willie, like most of his family, understood the need to make a living. All his life he watched his accounts carefully, and eventually he lived very well. In youth he benefited from his father's careful handling of family finances. Then he was especially blessed by the skill at moneymaking of his older brother Edmund Boyd ('E.B.'), who had moved from banking into brokering and other forms of investment and was on his way to becoming a very rich man, ultimately a millionaire (when a million dollars was still a fabulous sum).

Deeply impressed by the potential he had shown in his thesis, Osler's professors wanted him to stay at McGill. Osler wanted to be a teacher there. He knew that medical teachers could not support themselves solely from student fees but would have to practice medicine. Practicing medicine was not his first priority. Talking over the situation with Palmer Howard, he concluded that he could maximize his professional income and minimize the time he spent at it by becoming a specialist. Ophthalmology, his Uncle Edward's first interest, had continued to develop as an early medical specialty, now firmly based on a magnifying instrument, the ophthalmoscope. No one was practicing ophthalmology in Montreal.

There were no opportunities for postgraduate training in ophthalmology or any other specialty in Canada, and virtually none in the United States. To complete his education Osler, like thousands of North American medical students before him, would have to go to Europe. He decided to study in London, dividing his time between ophthalmology and advanced work in 'physiology,' an umbrella term coming into vogue to describe studies of bodily function. There were no scholarships, fellowships, or loan programs to finance higher education in medicine. Brother Edmund was the angel who made Willie's postgraduate training feasible, advancing $1,000, the equivalent of some $30,000 today, to fund his time abroad.

In the late spring of 1872 Willie picked up a few dollars relieving the house doctor in the Hamilton, Ontario, hospital. An unusual problem developed when a case of smallpox was brought to the hospital. Smallpox was too contagious to be allowed on the wards. Its victims had to be specially isolated. But where? Osler drove the patient up to the mayor of Hamilton's home, a sure way of getting action. Special accommodation was arranged in a secluded house. Osler visited the patient twice a day until he died, and then did an autopsy on the spot, helped by the German housekeeper. In July he and Edmund crossed the Atlantic together and did some sightseeing in Ireland and Scotland before going their separate ways. 'Be frugal: pay as you go,' Osler warned himself in his account book as he settled in to work in London.[52]

He shared a room on Gower Street, near the University of London, with another Canadian, and enrolled in a course in 'Practical Physiology' offered by John Burdon Sanderson, the Professor of Practical Physiology and Histology. One of his first hospital visits was to Guy's, the famous hospital complex south of the Thames: 'I spent the afternoon in looking over the wards & museum, both of which are remarkably well filled, the chief difference between them was that in the former the specimens (if I may so call them) were in beds, while in the latter they were in bottles.' A callous, callow comment, softened a bit by the fact that use of pathological specimens in teaching was highly developed in London. During ward rounds, British clinicians might refer to museum specimens as familiarly and with almost the same individuality as to the patient in the next bed. In London Osler attended 'museum classes' devoted entirely to the study of diseased organs.[53]

His career plans began to unravel right away. Palmer Howard wrote that two McGill graduates and one British specialist were planning to set up in Montreal as ophthalmologists. The market would be glutted. It would be better, Howard advised, 'to cultivate the whole field of Medicine & Surgery.' He obviously did not think it was yet too much for one man's mind.

'As you may imagine I was not a little disappointed at the blighting of my prospects as an ophthalmic surgeon, but I accept the inevitable with a good grace,' Osler wrote in his draft reply to Howard. But here he was, doing mostly laboratory work with Sanderson, and

... I now have to look forward to a general practice and I confess to you it is not with the greatest amount of pleasure ... The upshot of all this is, that I want something definite stated as regards my future connection with McGill College and I have written the Dean to that effect. It simply will not pay me to go on here spending quite half my time working at a subject [physiology] which may eventually become popular with the students, but the fees from which in Canada will never alone repay either the outlay required to qualify myself or the time spent over it.

I am sorry to have to appear so mercenary, but the recollection of my old friend Dr Bovell, who tried to work at Physiology and Practice both and failed in both, is too green in my memory to allow me to take any other course. My ambition is in time to work up a good Laboratory in connection with the College, and if I get a favourable answer from [Dean] Campbell, with that object in view I will continue my Physiological studies after this winter, but if not, I must turn my attention more fully to those branches which will enable me to engage in a general practice most successfully.

I hope you will not think me impudent in thus laying my case before the Dean, but I feel it is too unsatisfactory not having anything definite to go upon.[54]

The McGill faculty conferred with the university's dynamic principal, Sir William Dawson, a distinguished natural historian who had known Osler through his studies of diatoms. They decided to offer Osler a job teaching the botany course that was currently being given by Dawson to both arts and medical students. Osler might also give a half-year course in pathology, 'with the use of the microscope.' Possibly, at some future date, pathology could be hived off from the courses given by the professor of the institutes of medicine. Osler would, Dawson told him, have to develop 'special proficiency' in botany, preferably by studying in Germany.

Although Dawson hinted that a salaried chair might be established in the future, Dean Campbell added a harshly practical note:

Our chairs are not endowed, and the Professor depends upon his class fees for the remuneration, so that you must take your chance as all of us have done, and look chiefly to private practice for a *living* ...

The fact that we entertain such a high opinion of your acquirements and character, as to offer you the Chair of Botany, will give you, a comparative stranger in Montreal, a Great Advantage in commencing practice ... You should certainly devote the chief share of your attention to Medicine and Surgery. A young married couple might as reasonably expect to live upon love as a medical man to live upon science in this most practical country.

Sensing Osler's probable amazement at this unusual offer, Palmer Howard urged him to see it as a symbol of McGill's interest in him and to stay the course in cultivating an unusually good scientific training. Howard read the future remarkably accurately:

While it is quite plain that you must qualify yourself for the general practice of your profession, I am of opinion that you will be wise to cultivate those more scientific departments for which you have an aptitude & in which you have already done some work. It seems to me that two or three hours a day in a physiological laboratory need not prevent you from attending closely the wards of a general hospital & even pursuing your studies in morbid anatomy.

After you have finished your work in England, were I in your place I would go to Germany & work under some of the great histologists – Virchow or Rindfleish – in Berlin or Bonn or Vienna.

Your scientific education will be one of your best introductions to practice & will I have no doubt secure you a position as a teacher in a very short time in some one of the best Medical schools in this country. On that point I have no doubt ... In this rapidly growing country in which the Medical Schools are alive & enterprising, a man possessed of any scientific training beyond the average of his fellows is sure to make himself felt & more or less appreciated & the time must come when his services will be sought.[55]

Osler politely turned down McGill's offer. He knew next to nothing of botany and could not possibly learn enough to teach the subject intelligently: 'I would only make a fool of myself in accepting such a position.' But he appreciated the compliment of the offer and knew that it showed

McGill's regard for him. He also knew that his family would not understand his turning it down. The only relative he could confide in was Jennette in Montreal:

I would have made an ass of myself ... & that is not to my mind ... the Paternal as well as many others will think I was just as fitted to take Botany as anything else but I should feel like an imposter in a chair such as that.

I shall probably return to Montreal, but it will be as a private practitioner & – unless any further offer is made which I do not expect – not in connection with McGill. I do wish you would not build upon me for doing anything beyond my fellows. My abilities are but moderate and I can feel bitterly sometimes – that deficiencies in early education and want of thoroughness drag me back at every step. In addition to all of this I have my bread to earn: so that general medical studies demand the time which might be spent in acquiring – perhaps – a reputation.

One thing is certain, viz. cultivation of those scientific pursuits at the expense of paying [pursuits] is an injustice to oneself & – if he has one – his family.[56]

Amidst a busy social schedule in England – so many relatives and old family friends to be seen, so much sightseeing to be done – he tried to expand his general medical studies. Sanderson and other acquaintances introduced him at London's University College Hospital, where he observed a number of famous clinicians and surgeons – Erasmus Wilson, Tilbury Fox, Charlton Bastian, Sydney Ringer, Sir William Jenner, Sir Henry Thompson. He heard one of the surgeons tell students in a formal lecture that the art had all but reached its limit. He also attended Charles Murchison's clinics at St Thomas's Hospital and took a short course in embryology at the university's Brown Animal Sanitary Institution, a pioneering research institute dedicated to comparative medicine. He felt it was pretentious for Canadians to obtain British medical certification to get more letters after their names but went ahead and got his LRCP (licentiate of the Royal College of Physicians), for Howard had advised him that such qualifications carried utility back in Montreal. Certification from the Royal

Medical Society of Edinburgh would have been even more impressive with the Mac's and Mc's of Scots Canada.[57]

Most of Osler's London time was spent in Sanderson's laboratory, first taking Sanderson's physiology/pathology course ('I commenced as a green hand *ab initio*, in order that I might miss no little details') and then, at the suggestion of Sanderson, looking into certain reagents' effect on the white cells of the blood. Nothing came of that work other than his first scientific presentation in England, a paper read 'with many vasomoter accompaniments' to the Medical Microscopical Society.[58]

As Osler continued to examine samples of blood, often his own, in the microscope, he observed the presence of strange colorless granular masses, which were neither white nor red cells. Many others had seen these bodies in the thirty years since lenses had become clearer, but the literature was scanty, and Osler undertook a detailed study. 'An Account of Certain Organisms Occurring in the Liquor Saguinis' became his major piece of graduate research and significantly advanced knowledge of the characteristics of what others later named the blood 'platelets.' In his final paper he omitted an error he and a colleague, Edward Schäfer, had made in a preliminary publication in which they speculated that the platelets formed from or into other still-mysterious bodies, bacteria. While Osler was on the ground floor of platelet work, his research did not quite justify Palmer Howard's enthusiasm in labeling it 'a discovery of great interest' and issuing a public call for a friend of McGill's to endow a chair of physiological and pathological histology so that Osler could devote his time to the work 'and at the same time bring honour to himself and to Canada.'[59]

Most of Osler's letters to the Dundas family were later lost in a fire, but he wrote regularly and at length. His Canadian roommate and later colleague, Arthur Browne, was writing letters about the work in London for publication in the Canadian medical journals, inspiring Osler to draft an abortive attempt of his own. Browne shared his love of English literature with Osler, introducing him to Coleridge and Lamb to supplement a blooming passion for Shakespeare. During these years abroad, Osler was well on his way to becoming a compulsive writer and reader, infatuated with the written and printed word. Or most words – he always remembered reading the *Times* one October day in 1872 in a Tottenham Court Road teashop and being struck by a statement of John Ruskin's to the effect that no mind could resist for a year the dulling influence of the daily newspaper.[60]

Osler aimed higher. He came to know the great medical libraries of London, and his thesis book prize from McGill led to his being introduced to the bookselling brothers Nock, 'weird and desiccated specimens of humanity,' who kept an indescribably cluttered shop in Bloomsbury. Browne gave him a volume of Dr John Brown's *Horae Subsecivae* ('Spare Hours') essays, which he later recommended to all medical students as a guide to enlarging their cultural horizons. Brown's delightful, rambling, often historical and biographical meditations were designed, the author wrote, 'to give my vote for going back to the old manly intellectual and literary culture of the days of Sydenham, Arbuthnot, and Gregory; when a physician fed, enlarged and quickened his entire nature; when he lived in the world of letters as a free-holder, and reverenced the ancients, while, at the same time, he pushed on among his fellows, and lived in the present, believing that his profession and his patients need not suffer, though his *horae subsecivae* were devoted occasionally to miscellaneous thinking and reading.'[61]

Very little is known of the influence that Burdon Sanderson – a ubiquitous, towering figure in the early years of British experimental physiology and pathology – may have had on Osler. Although he had a somewhat absent-minded, forgettable personality (except on the memorable day in his lab when, intending to attack a sandwich, he is said to have bitten into one of his experimental frogs), Sanderson was extremely well connected. Through him and at the University Hospital, Osler was given an entrée into medical social circles which he happily cultivated: 'Last night I dined at Dr. Ringer's. Every thing was in grand style and the people very nice. Mrs. Ringer is like most Englishwomen very fresh looking, notwithstanding a number of bairns. Dr. Bird – a Red Republican – and myself had a long discussion on Canada & the States. Several others of the same "Kidney" were there.'[62]

Noticeably a bit of an outsider in student circles at Toronto and McGill, William worked hard to overcome his 'Osler reserve' and became unusually sociable – with fellow Canadian students, American students, and British physicians old and young. He formed friendships easily, and invariably attended to them. He made a particular point of meeting older, established figures. In this London season he attended a soirée of the Royal Society ('a very swell affair') where, among others, he met Charles Darwin. He thought of Darwin the day he did the Regent's Park zoo: – 'Not liking to do my nearest relatives in a careless manner I have determined to make a special afternoon at them. They say the new chimpanzee has made many converts to the Darwinian Theory, from its horrible likeness to some men.'[63]

He spent Christmas 1872 visiting the family of a classmate of his father's in Norfolk and might have been living a Trollope novel: 'Books Music and cats are the chief features in Witton vicarage. The former, I read, the second I listened to, and tried to understand, while the third I teased unmercifully. The girls are accomplished, good musicians &c but are lacking in looks which in spite of all else are very requisite.' At the county seat, Norwich, he inspected relics, not of a saint but of Sir Thomas Browne, whose coffin had been accidently opened some years earlier and whose skull was now on display in the local infirmary. A printed slip quoted Browne: 'To be knaved out of our graves, to have our skulls made drinking-bowls, and our bones turned into pipes, to delight and sport our enemies, are tragical abominations.'[64]

In October 1873 Osler left England for what North Americans were beginning to consider their medical meccas, Germany and Austria. In the second half of the century, leadership in both scientific and clinical medicine seemed to have passed to the German-speaking countries with their highly organized, research-oriented universities and hospitals, their outstanding scientists, their accessible postgraduate programs, and their devotion to scholarship as a way of life. American medical men, few of whom believed they could get a full education at home, had switched their preference from Paris to Vienna and other German centers. To spend as much time in Great Britain as Osler did was a bit unusual, though perhaps not for a colonial Canadian. As Osler knew before crossing the Atlantic, German, not English or French, had become the first language of advanced medicine.

On arrival in Berlin, Osler signed up for daily language lessons. He was alarmed at the cost of living in the German imperial capital, and by the stench of its open drains: 'Simply beastly ... London is sweetness itself by comparison. It reminds me of ... Montreal.' He had the usual adjustment problems – his courses started much later than he realized, and one of the professors to whom he had letters of introduction had just died, while another had left – but he got to know other visiting students and settled in happily: 'Dr. Sanderson gave me a very good letter to Professor Virchow, who received me very graciously, and told me to come to him whenever I wanted anything.'

Otherwise, Osler was just another foreign medical student (mistaken by Germans for a Frenchman more often than an American), taking notes in the tiered lecture theater at Berlin's huge hospital, the Charité Royal, as the masters examined and discussed their cases. Unlike British clinicians, each of whom had only a few dozen patients in the London hospitals, the German heads of service commanded scores of beds in the Charité – 'plentiful material,' as Osler put it in one of two Berlin letters he contributed to the *Canada Medical and Surgical Journal*. Of the two most prominent Berlin clinicians, Ludwig Traube and F.T. von Frerichs, the former went into his cases most fully 'and moreover possesses those necessary adjuncts to clinical teaching, a pleasant manner and a fluent style'; but Frerichs was the foreigners' favorite because he spoke so slowly that they could understand everything. The examinations of patients were not nearly as rigorous as those Murchison made by the bedside at St Thomas's, Osler noted. And it was one of Frerichs's student assistants, Osler remembered (perhaps apocryphally; surely this story is an old chestnut of medical education) who proved memorably casual:

'How is your patient this morning, Mr. Schmidt?'

'Very well indeed, very well; he is much better than yesterday.'

'Very well indeed; he died this morning; you will see what was the matter shortly.'

The medical superstar in Berlin was the great Virchow. Politician as well as pathologist, sanitarian, and man of many other parts, Rudolf Virchow was one of Germany's finest scientists of the nineteenth century. His medical specialty was Osler's greatest interest: 'It is the master mind of Virchow and the splendid Pathological Institute ... that specially attract foreign students to Berlin. This most remarkable man is yet in his prime ... comprehensive intellect and untiring energy ... Virchow himself performs a post-mortem on Monday morning making it with such care and minuteness that three or four hours may elapse before it is finished. The very first morning of my attendance he spent exactly half an hour in the description of the skull cap!' None of the other European teachers had anything like Virchow's impact on the young Canadian.[65]

American students preferred to take the plentiful courses available in Vienna, capital of the Austro-Hungarian Empire, whose vast general hospital, the Allgemeine Krankenhaus, offered a feast of interesting cases. Osler moved there at the beginning of 1874, found the place 'swarming' with fifty or sixty American students, and spent four months taking a wide variety of courses. He studied pediatrics with Hermann Wiederhoffer, skin diseases with Ferdinand Hebra ('*the* lecturer of the Vienna School'), general medicine with Heinrich von Bamberger ('a splendid diagnostician'), and ear diseases with Adam Politzer ('not that I am going to make a specialty of them, but I thought it well worth while, when an opportunity occurred, to make their acquaintance').

Like many North American students in Vienna, Osler was pleased to have a degree of access to obstetrical cases that was unthinkable at home for important reasons of patient privacy and modesty, though it led to American doctors graduating and even winning prizes in obstetrics without ever having seen a baby delivered. The students began by working with cadavers ('they have a fresh body about every second day, and any number of babies') and then graduated to the wards:

Every third day women come to be examined, to see whether their time is at hand. They are arranged on a series of beds, and the assistant takes a student to each case, and examines him on it. No matter how many students are present, all can have a 'finger in the pie,' and one feels sorry for the poor women, but Bandl says they don't mind. Operative cases occurring in the daytime are, if possible, delayed until the lecture hour, and then brought into the theatre. I begin next week to go on duty about every fifth or sixth day and hope to get three or four forceps cases before leaving.

Osler thought Vienna was 'infinitely below Berlin' in general medicine and pathology: 'After having seen Virchow, it is absolutely painful to attend post mortems here, they are performed in so slovenly a manner, and so little use is made of the material.' The Viennese founding father of pathology, Karl Rokitansky, taught only small select classes, which apparently did not include Osler; but the Canadian at least had the pleasure of observing the grand ceremonies on Rokitansky's seventieth birthday, including a huge torchlight parade of students, as medical Europe paid tribute to medical Vienna's brightest ornament.[66]

In the spring of 1874 Osler headed home via Paris and England. In later years he regretted the 'cobwebs in my pockets' that prevented him from buying anything but textbooks during that sojourn. Nor did he develop fluency in foreign languages: 'I made the great mistake both in Berlin & Vienna of living too much with the English-speaking students.' The German students, with their long hair, remarkable orderliness, dueling scars, and drinking societies were something of a mystery to him. 'If tobacco and beer have such a deteriorating effect on mind and body, as some of our advanced Tee-totallers affirm, we ought to see signs of it here.'[67]

For all his later regrets, he took home all the good effects, professional, personal, and cultural, that two years in Europe could have on any quick-witted North American eager to broaden his range of experience. He had seen art galleries, attended concerts, wandered in parks and by canals, read Shakespeare and George Eliot, made a host of friends, and been exposed to some of the best medical minds in the world. Whether it had happened in Europe (some said Sydney Ringer taught him the habit) or a bit earlier at home, exposure to tobacco had caused him to start smoking. He had continued to be a frequenter of churches everywhere he went – he was steeped in biblical lore and Christian culture – but had no particular interest in theology. After the frustrating go-round with McGill, he seems to have sublimated any long-term career worries into his day-at-a-time serenity. A single note of anxiety creeps into a letter from Berlin to sister Chattie: 'I am nearly a quarter of a century old and not on my own legs yet.'[68]

Any thoughts Osler may have had about how to take professional steps at home have not survived. Arriving late in the spring of 1874, he kicked around the Dundas-Hamilton area substituting for a local doctor, earning twenty-five dollars and a pair of boots.

Back at McGill, Dr Joseph Morley Drake, who had only recently been made Professor of the Institutes of Medicine, had developed heart trouble and could not carry on. He resigned his chair, and in July the McGill faculty decided to ask Dr Osler to join them as Lecturer in the Institutes of Medicine. 'Answer it at once,' Palmer Howard wrote Osler of the dean's invitation. 'Please present my congratulations to your father upon this gratifying recognition of your merits by the oldest medical school in Canada. All your friends here will be much pleased on your account.' Here was a magnificent opportunity for a young man to begin to stand on his own legs.[69]

THREE

The Baby Professor

'Silence, Gentlemen.'

This was the routine command to a room full of McGill medical students, taking a break from a long day of classes, to stop their singing, yelling, jostling, and settle in for another dreary hour of recitation from a gruff bewhiskered professor.

Their teacher of 'institutes,' Dr Osler, barely mustachioed, instead chose to stand and wait until the noise subsided of its own accord. He probably had no alternative at first. At twenty-five he was younger than some of the students. They called him 'the Baby Professor.' He was not a natural teacher. He had no flair for public speaking and little experience in it – some of it disastrous. He tended to talk quietly and was very nervous. Cousin Jennette proofread his lectures to improve their style. Cousin Marian helped him practice speaking out. 'My first appearance before the class filled me with a tremulous uneasiness and an overwhelming sense of embarrassment,' he recalled.

Even medical students are usually kind to novice lecturers, and Osler received polite attention. No one remembered him as a great speaker – at times he could be halting, almost stuttering – but the students soon realized he knew and believed in his material and was delivering it clearly and in good order. He had no problem with discipline, and his lectures were well attended. In any case, the Faculty of Medicine had moved from downtown Montreal to the McGill campus up on the mountain, and skipping out to the theater was no longer a possibility.

The hallway noise was a different matter. A number of the senior men, some of whom had known Osler as a fellow student, resented his having been elevated to such a high position. They made a habit of gathering in the corridor and disrupting his classes with loud chatter. After a few days, Osler posted a note on a bulletin board asking them to refrain. 'At the lecture hour the next morning,' a student remembered, 'the noise was even greater. After standing it for a while Osler opened the door, stepped into the corridor, pulled off his frock coat, and challenged the best man to step forward and fight it out with him. No one came forward, and peace and quiet reigned thereafter.'[1]

With or without fisticuffs, every teacher knows the ordeal of the first year. Osler had to produce a new lecture every day, about a hundred in total. His predecessor, J.M. Drake, offered to lend Osler his lectures to read to the students. Of course, Osler turned him down – though he had second thoughts after his first stock of ten or twelve lectures was used up and he had to work late into every night to have something to say to the students the next day: 'I reached January in an exhausted condition, but relief was at hand. One day the post brought a brand-new work on physiology by a well-known German professor, and it was remarkable with what rapidity my labours of the last half of the session were lightened. An extraordinary improvement in the lectures was noticed; the students benefited, and I gained rapidly in the facility with which I could translate from the German.' As well, his account book shows that in March he paid Drake the quite large sum of $64.50 'for Diagrams.'[2]

To cap the strenuous year, Osler's colleagues foisted on him the job of giving the farewell address to the graduating class. His first try at a form he would one day completely master was stilted and crammed with platitudinous advice to the young physicians to keep up their reading, plan to add to medical knowledge, make income a secondary consideration, speak no ill behind colleagues' backs, and consider becoming teetotalers. The talk had the merit of being relatively short, and it ended with an apt quotation.

Osler urged the McGill men to be, like one of Shakespeare's physicians, 'in what he did profess, well found.'[3]

At its end-of-term meeting the faculty concluded that Osler had been well found. Drake had decided to retire permanently, and Osler was promoted from lecturer to Professor of the Institutes of Medicine. Many years later, coming across Drake's heart in the McGill pathology museum, Osler remarked that its petering out was the key to his career.[4]

Professional men in Canada who netted $2,000–5,000 a year in the 1870s lived decently to comfortably. Osler's teaching brought him $1,129 in his first academic year, not much for even a fairly frugal bachelor. McGill had hired him because of his unusual promise as a medical scientist, but everyone, including Osler, knew he had to become a practicing physician to put bread on his table.

Where would the patients come from? He was an untried youngster, virtually an outsider, in a city bursting at its seams with doctors, more than a hundred and fifty of them, a ratio of about one per thousand Montrealers (many of whom were too poor to afford any doctor). His professorship in the fundamentals of medical science entailed neither clinical responsibility nor any access to patients in a hospital. About the best he could hope for would be referrals or consultations sent by senior colleagues. It would take a lot of patient visits, billed at the going rate of fifty cents or a dollar, to bring his income up to snuff.

With money advanced by his father, Osler had established himself in Montreal in August 1874, bought some office furniture, had a nameplate made, and launched himself in the practice of medicine. Practice was very slow – removing a speck from a cornea, a couple of office consultations, a couple of vaccinations against smallpox, treating the 'man on the SS Valetta.' Total income from patients in the first two months was about $9.75.[5]

In late October he met socially a visiting Englishman of about his own age named Austin Neville. On the evening of October 24, he was summoned to examine Neville, who had come down with a high fever, intense pains in his chest and back, and incessant vomiting. Neville thought it was a recurrence of a bilious condition.

The patient had a bad night, and next morning Osler found him still in pain with a strong reddening of the chest. He injected half a grain of morphine to try to give some relief. Osler saw Neville three more times that day. There was little improvement, with blue-black blotches starting to form on the chest and groin. When these had extended and multiplied the next morning, Osler called in Palmer Howard: 'My suspicions were confirmed and the diagnosis of smallpox made' – this despite Neville having the scars of an old vaccination. The doctors had Neville removed that evening, Saturday, to the smallpox ward of Montreal General.

Neville had a severe case of hemorrhagic, fulminating, or 'black' smallpox, the worst form of one of the world's worst diseases. He asked for an Anglican minister, who saw him several times. Osler spent Sunday morning with him and read him Scripture at his request. Neville vomited and passed blood, bled from his bowels, and began to lose coherence. His trunk turned plum purple, his face deep red, his eyelids black. 'The corneae appear sunk in dark red pits, giving to the patient a frightful appearance,' Osler noted.

Neville asked Osler to stay with him into the night. Around midnight he muttered some prayers 'and held out his hand, which I took,' recorded Osler, '& he said quite plainly "Oh thanks." These were the last words the poor fellow spoke.' He died about an hour later. Had the doctor done anything for him to deserve his thanks? 'As the son of a clergyman & knowing well what it is to be a "stranger in a strange land" I performed the last office of Christian friendship I could, & read the Commendatory Prayer at his departure.' Osler wrote Neville's parents a sensitive letter about their son's death, sparing them the details of the clinical record. Three weeks later, on November 20, he entered in his daybook a $24.50 payment of the account of the late Austin Neville. In a speech a few months later he quoted Sir Thomas Browne on the conundrums of a physician's fees: 'I desire rather to cure his infirmities than my own necessities; where I do him no good methinks it is scarce honest gain, though, I confess, 'tis but the unworthy salary of our well intended endeavours.'[6]

The irony was that smallpox really could be conquered by Jenner's wonderful discovery of vaccination. By Osler's day smallpox was rapidly being eliminated in the Western world. The case he had seen in Hamilton in 1872 was very rare for Ontario. Montreal, however, had a large French-Canadian population with a deep-seated aversion to vaccination. Through the 1870s the disease simmered and flared in the city, taking several hundred lives a year. The prevalence of smallpox, along with diphtheria, typhoid fever, and other infectious diseases, gave Canada's leading city a dark reputation as a nest of pestilence and unnecessary death. Most victims were French-Canadian children from the slums of the city. The unusual case of poor Neville was a reminder of the need for regular revaccination.

Late in 1874 Osler, who could claim considerable experience with the disease, obtained a position as physician to the smallpox ward at the Montreal General. The ward was separate from the main building, with a separate entrance, to try to prevent contagion. Doctors feared and hated smallpox almost as much as the general public did. Anyone who had been in contact with it became something of a pariah, as attendants had once been in leper colonies or would seem to be in the early days of AIDS. Being a smallpox doctor, a physician in the pesthouse, was to practice on the bottom rung of the medical ladder – not unlike a Christian missionary preaching in the northern wilderness.

Through most of 1875, Osler attended to smallpox patients, in hospital and in city hovels and brothels, seeing human suffering in one of its most ghastly, fetid forms. He treated eighty-one cases, including fourteen hemorrhagic ones, and did several postmortems, examining internal organs that had virtually dissolved in blood and pus. He observed his patients as carefully as he looked at specimens under a microscope, read up on the disease, and made his first real contribution to the literature of clinical medicine in a series of three articles discussing the initial rashes of smallpox, the hemorrhagic form, and one of its subforms.

In these papers Osler showed a facility for careful differentiation and description that became one of his hallmarks. Along with much else, he had learned that once this 'truly terrible disease' struck, there was little one could do other than learn more about it. In the hemorrhagic cases, he wrote: 'All the usual medicines indicated ... were tried, gallic-acid, ergot, turpentine, acetate of lead, &c., without the slightest benefit. Quinine was used in large doses, and in three cases I used the cold pack.' He tried 'all sorts of remedies' to stop victims being disfigured by smallpox scars, and found that none of them affected the lesions. He never forgot some of the women he saw caring for smallpox victims – in one instance an old-fashioned Dickensian nurse as good as any Osler ever saw later, in another a highbred French nun who came with him to the bedside when no one else could be found, and in another a slip of a teenaged prostitute who reminded him of St Theresa or De Quincey's Ann.[7]

Neither the smallpox work nor his interest in pathology helped Osler's private practice. He was working with the dying and the dead. He was examining highly contagious patients and disease-ridden corpses in an age before rubber gloves, masks, and gowns. Would he carry away the stink? the poisons? 'Willie went to a P[ost] M[ortem] this afternoon,' Jennette wrote during the Christmas season of 1875. 'We had to make him go through a course of hot water and carbolic soap before he was a pleasant neighbour at tea.' Osler thought he might have been responsible for infecting one of his recovering smallpox patients (a nine-year-old girl who was ready to leave hospital) with a fatal case of scarlet fever.[8]

Early in 1876, just as the work was winding down because of the opening of a new civic smallpox hospital, he came down with smallpox himself – something must have been wrong with his vaccination history – and had to be hospitalized. 'My attack was a wonderfully light one the pustules numbering sixteen, all told, and of these only two located themselves on my face; so that "my beauty has not been consumed away,"' he wrote, adding, 'You need not be afraid of this letter. I will disinfect it before sending.' He was not scarred. A few years later his mentor, the Reverend W.A. Johnson, died at Weston from an infection thought to have come from handling the body of a victim of the black smallpox which no one else would touch. [9]

The hospital paid Osler $600 for his smallpox service. He had spent most of it in advance, ordering fifteen Hartnack students' microscopes from Paris.

These were the essential apparatus for his first teaching innovation, an optional 'Practical Course' on microscopy and histology, based closely on what he had learned from Burdon Sanderson in London. Osler introduced it with a ringing manifesto about the need to keep up in the new age of practical medicine: 'Progress must be our watchword, and we must endeavour to keep pace with the old country institutions ... I may venture to congratulate McGill College as the first in this country to offer such a course.' Osler well knew the importance of microscopy for the advance of science, but he sold the course on the basis of its utility for studying bodily secretions, blood, food samples, et cetera, in general practice. It was not unusual for a professor to spend his own money on equipment. 'The rule has been that each lecturer from his fees shall provide his own teaching outfit,' he once noted.[10]

The faculty decided to hold a formal summer session in 1876, and Osler was appointed organizer. He repeated his histology course, giving it in the medical building's cloakroom, and following up a suggestion by a Harvard friend, Reginald Fitz, he added a new course of 'Practical Pathological Demonstrations' in the Montreal General Hospital's postmortem room. Osler and his students volunteered to do all the hospital's autopsies (previously done by the attending physicians, if they bothered), following Virchow's techniques. The course, which Osler claimed was the first of its kind in North America, was repeated on Saturdays the next winter. Working in a stove-heated old shack at the back of the hospital, Osler shared the pathological findings with the students and correlated the data with the clinical history, driving home the maxim that the postmortem was an essential part of the the history, the narrative, of any fatal case.[11]

He took the gospel of clinicopathology to the Medico-Chirurgical Society of Montreal, the local association of English-speaking doctors. In the summer of 1875 he gave his first presentation, a carefully worked-up paper, accompanied by specimens. A thirty-six-year-old Nova Scotian coal miner had died of smallpox. Osler had been astonished at the autopsy to find that the man had black lungs, saturated with carbon, and he had made a quick and quite pioneering study of the pathology of miner's lung, drawing on other specimens he found in the faculty's museum. He soon became the

Medico-Chirurgical Society's unofficial pathologist, showing syphilitic livers, perforated intestines, aneurysms, tumors, all manner of diseased organs. Within a few years the display of 'pathological specimens' had become a regular feature of Med-Chi meetings. Many of the members would have had only the haziest notion of the internal effects of the disease conditions they had been diagnosing for years; now they made a point of arriving on time to see what Osler would be showing. The young professor had effectively become pathologist for the whole city's medical community. [12]

As such, he was sometimes consulted by colleagues. A close friend remembered an occasion when a distinguished older surgeon asked Osler to examine a young adult's hand that he had amputed above the wrist for a supposedly malignant cancer. Osler realized the diagnosis was wrong. Rather than show up the old man, he submitted no report, forgoing a fee. When Osler told his friend about the case, years later, he said, 'No one but you and me ever knew of the unfortunate circumstance and we have both forgotten it.'[13]

On that occasion, he hid his light under a bushel. Normally, Osler acted on the biblical text he once advised should hang in all medical laboratories: 'Let your light so shine before men that they may see your good works.'[14] He was an eager joiner and subscriber, and as a researcher and publisher he mastered the knack of making the most of his material. An interesting case or specimen might be exploited for teaching purposes, first in the morgue, then in class. Then it would be presented at the Med-Chi, whose minutes would be published in one of the locally edited medical journals. Specially noteworthy cases, such as the study of miner's lung, were written up as separate articles and published in journals and then sometimes separately reprinted. Offprints were sent to friends, acquaintances, experts in the field. (Osler took an old-timer's advice to always stock up on offprints, and he ordered what amounted to more than a lifetime's supply of most of his works; they were still being given away, gratis, years after his death.) Later, Osler's cases might be agglomerated in lectures and papers on characteristics of diseases. Finally, the original pathological specimens would be preserved, labeled, and displayed in the faculty's museum.

A few of Osler's specimens have survived moves, breakage, fire, and neglect, and are still on view at McGill a hundred and twenty-five years after he first examined them. Those who wonder about the approximately thousand autopsies he and his students performed can find many of them in the 'Hospital Reports' sections of the journals, but more handily in *Montreal General Hospital: Pathological Report, for the Year Ending May 1st, 1877* (Montreal, 1878), by William Osler, MD. Osler proudly billed the volume as the first pathological report from a Canadian hospital, dedicated it to James Bovell, and supplied a quotation from Samuel Wilks on the title page: 'Pathology is the basis of all true instruction in Practical Medicine.' Two years later he arranged to have some of the hospital's clinicians publish their case studies along with his autopsies in another large volume of reports.

By all accounts Osler quickly became one of McGill's most popular professors. His lecturing style became more relaxed as he used illustrations and presented specimens in class and learned to speak from notes rather than read a text. Even so, two surviving sets of lecture notes from his basic 'institutes' course, mostly physiology, suggest that he was conventional for his day and unmemorable, though certainly clear and well organized. It was his special classes in pathology and histology that students found mesmerizing.

It has been said that great teaching cannot be reconstructed without film or tape. We will try anyway. Some of Osler's talks were published verbatim. Imagine the medical students clustering round Osler in the dead house, shivering a bit in the cold, perhaps smoking to cut the stench, as he discusses the specimens on the long wooden table. First, an aneurysm of the aorta:

> Notice, gentlemen the intima [inner lining]. You see it is uniformly coloured a brilliant red. Such colour is at once associated with active inflammation. I am sure that two-thirds of you would, if asked, tell me that the intima is here acutely inflamed; and a sad mistake you would make. For this colouration has nothing to do with inflammation – it is simply due to post-mortem staining, or imbibition of the blood-colouring matter.

Then certain pelvic organs from a different case:

Most of you saw the autopsy performed. We found extensive purulent peritonitis; about fifty ounces of thick, creamy pus filled the cavity; the coils of
intestines were deeply injected, matted together, and between them pockets of pus existed. On looking for the cause of this condition, no perforation
or ulceration could be found in the course of either small or large bowel.
But as we approached the sigmoid flexure of colon, we saw a projecting
mass lying between it and the psoas ... It was, in fact, an abscess in the left
broad ligament ... We found abscesses in both broad ligaments ... These
abscesses ... are by no means rare; and they often produce just this condition
... by perforating and discharging into the peritoneal cavity, when a general
peritonitis, of course ensues.

And other organs from a patient who had died of lung disease:

The liver in this case was fatty. This is of common occurrence in phthisis,
and needs no remark, but you had better examine the specimen sent round
carefully, as it is important to at once recognize this common condition ...

The appendix vermiformis shows an interesting condition in this case ...
These little faecal concretions often form in the appendix. They cause irri-
tation, and inflammation of the lining wall, and this may lead to ulceration
and perforation. Within a year, had this woman lived, she would have died
from peritonitis from this cause.[15]

Generations of physicians would use the adjectives 'infectious' and 'contagious' to describe Osler's enthusiasm, and they hardly found it work to
follow him on his journeys of medical detection. About this time, young
Arthur Conan Doyle was learning similar lessons from one of his great
teachers at Edinburgh, Joseph Bell, on whom he patterned Sherlock Holmes.
The students in the McGill classes were young Watsons; and the doctors
at the Med-Chi were old Watsons, listening to the elementary presentations.

Osler apparently never met or even referred to Conan Doyle. But he
and Holmes/Doyle/Bell had a common root, the 'method of Zadig,' as outlined in Voltaire's 1747 novelette, *Zadig or Destiny*. Zadig, a reasonable

man with an affinity for nature, reasons from apparently trivial details to give accurate descriptions of animals he has never seen. Joseph Bell considered Zadig's method the everyday foundation of medical teaching. In later years Osler, using the method to its fullest in diagnosis, had his students look up Voltaire's text.[16] Medical lore is rife, of course, with stories of cocky Zadigs being caught out. It was said that Joseph Bell's mentor in Edinburgh was once telling students a great deal about a child on the basis of his observations of its mother when the woman spoke up: 'Please sir, I am only his stepmother.' Another time, as he was saying, 'This I can tell, gentlemen, from the condition of the patient's teeth,' the patient asked if he would like to hand them around.

(There is only one recorded incident of Osler being involved in a medical murder mystery. In 1879 he assisted a colleague with the autopsy of a prominent Montrealer found dead in his sleigh. They reported perfect health in all the man's organs with the exception of the stomach, which they tied up carefully and left for the coroner with a Holmesian comment that the cause of death would probably be found there. Sure enough, large amounts of morphine were found in the stomach. The coroner's jury, however, reported death from natural causes, and it may have been that Osler and his colleague had bungled the case. They had not done anything to show that the poison had entered the system from the stomach and was the actual cause of death. The *Canada Medical and Surgical Journal* opined that autopsists skilled in medical jurisprudence would have done a better job.)[17]

Osler's relations with students were cemented after his appointment as faculty registrar in 1877. As their fee collector, counselor, and general factotum, he amazed the students by displaying another happy knack, the ability to remember names and faces. 'This was a new genus – a Registrar that knew his students by name at the second meeting.' The McGill University registrar at the time could not even remember the names of members of the faculty. More strikingly (if you were ever a green student away from home, you know the force of this), Dr Osler appeared to take a personal interest in the young men, their families, their work, mutual friends ... whatever seemed to strike a spark. One student who thought he must be specially privileged to have Osler's friendship found that practically everyone in the class also felt singled out. 'I never knew a man who possessed this capacity for intimacy with his students in any degree measuring up to that possessed of Osler,' he remembered. 'Once Osler shook his hand, the student had found a friend for life and he knew it.'[18]

Osler cast himself in the role of a faculty reformer. Along with his own teaching innovations, he was a moving spirit in having the thesis requirement abolished, examinations modernized, clinical training extended and reorganized, and a student medical society established. 'More than at any other time within the past fifty years the leading minds in the profession are occupied with the subject of medical education,' he told the students at the school's introductory lecture in 1877, 'and there is an almost universal feeling that in many quarters reform is needed.'[19] A few years before Osler's coming, the rejuvenation of the staff had begun with the appointment of twenty-seven-year-old George Ross as Professor of Clinical Medicine. Young Frank Shepherd of the class of '73, followed Osler's tracks to Europe and was hired in 1875 as a Demonstrator in Anatomy. In the same year, Thomas Roddick became Professor of Clinical Surgery at age twenty-nine; it was Roddick who, after several stints of training in Scotland, introduced antiseptic surgery to Montreal.

The young Canadians took the train south to see for themselves the results of an important reform agenda in the United States – President Charles W. Eliot's modernization, against much resistance, of Harvard's Faculty of Medicine. Osler had spent a week at Harvard in 1876; and he, Ross, and Shepherd visited again in 1877. The Boston medical school had become integrated with the university, had increased its yearly sessions to more than nine months, had caught up with McGill in holding an entrance examination and making its courses sequential, and had gone over to blind marking of written examinations. Osler pronounced it 'high time' the medical schools in the United States were 'being stirred up to some sense of the requirements and dignity of the profession they teach.' He noted (gently, in view of the professor being the great Oliver Wendell Holmes) that Harvard's approach to practical anatomy still fell short of British and Canadian standards, but that it had more than caught up in clinical teaching. He was dazzled by the facilities there – the well-equipped

laboratories in which chemistry and physiology were taught, and a postmortem room at the Massachusetts General Hospital which he judged to
be 'one of the most perfect in the world.' A major consequence of his investigation and pressure was McGill's decision to redo one of its lecture
rooms as a fully equipped physiological laboratory, designed by Osler. In
contrast to the bitter divisiveness of reform at Harvard and at the University of Pennsylvania, which was beginning to follow suit, the McGill changes
occurred without evident controversy.[20]

Another result of the Boston visits was Osler's developing friendship
with several of the Harvard professors. Wherever he went he made courtesy calls on the old pillars of the profession and got to know the young
movers. Both duties led him in Boston to the Bowditches, the aged Henry
Ingersoll Bowditch (who gave the reprint advice) and his physiologist
nephew, one of Harvard's key reformers, Henry Pickering Bowditch. Osler
got to know practically everyone else at medical Harvard and at the newly
reorganized Boston Medical Library. If he did not meet them on his first
visits, paths crossed at other medical gatherings or on the summer weeks in
1879 and 1883 that Osler spent at a Bostonian 'camp' in the Adirondacks
as a Bowditch guest.[21]

Osler had a second professorial appointment. The Montreal Veterinary
College had existed since 1866, the private enterprise of its principal, one
Duncan McEachran, an Edinburgh-trained veterinarian. McEachran had
arranged that his students would take some of their basic courses, including 'institutes,' at McGill. Osler not only inherited a handful of vet students, each paying the twelve-dollar fee per term, but he was appointed a
professor in the animal college. He listed himself there variously as Professor of Physiology, Professor of Physiology and Pathology, and Lecturer on
Helminthology. Over the years he gave special lectures, courses, and demonstrations at the Montreal Veterinary College, becoming the first serious
teacher of pathology at such an institution in North America (though also
following in the footsteps of James Bovell, who had lectured at the veteri-

nary school in Toronto). One historian of Osler's vet-school activities comments that he was bringing bedside teaching to the stables. In point of fact, as Osler was still without a hospital position, the stables were his only bedside.[22]

He was not merely moonlighting, for he had a serious interest in comparative anatomy and pathology. It had started with his student work on parasites and been reinforced by his understanding of Virchow on the basic unity of organisms and disease, and by his work with Burdon Sanderson at the Brown Animal Sanitory Institution in London. The germ theory and the rise of animal experimentation had made comparative medicine a leading field of interest – all the great bacteriologists and physiologists and most of the pathologists worked with animals.[23] Veterinary medicine was in itself a highly promising profession in an age when agriculture was North America's greatest industry. Osler was as keen to track down unusual cases in animals as in humans, and exhibited animal specimens both to the Medico-Chirurgical Society and the fledgling Montreal Veterinary Medical Association. In 1879–80 he served a term as president of the latter association; he never held office in the former.

He published in the veterinary journals. In 1877, for example, McEachran asked him to find out what was killing puppies at the Montreal Kennel Club. He found a new parasite in their bronchial tubes and named a new disease, verminous bronchitis. The parasite, a rare nematode, became known as *Filaroides osleri*, later *Oslerus osleri*.[24]

During an outbreak of what was known as 'pig typhoid' near Quebec City a few months later, the call again went out for Osler. He did a series of inoculation experiments and several postmortems, and concluded that the disease had no analogy to human typhoid fever and was probably not caused by bacteria. His paper 'On the Pathology of the So-Called Pig-Typhoid' was read to the Pathological Society of New York in January 1878, one of his first presentations outside Montreal. It was 'a good full meeting,' he wrote Jennette that night. 'A lot of swells and I got on as well as could be expected under circumstances. One thing was evident, nobody knew as much about it as we do, so the advantage was on our side ... The specimens and drawings were greatly admired and the mic. spcs. also. I went to see

Edwin Booth as Hamlet last night and enjoyed it very much, more I think than any play I have seen.'[25]

Osler was a busy young man by any standards, and in the rest of his life he never became significantly less busy. In his twenties, elaborating on the Carlylean maxim of taking one day at a time, he had already become unusually regular and disciplined in his habits. 'The secret of successful working lies in the systematic arrangement of what you have to do,' he told McGill students, advising them to make out a timetable rigidly allotting hours of study and recreation: 'I know of no better way to accomplish a large amount of work.' Osler soon became one of the breed of superproducers who accomplish in four hours what takes the rest of us sixteen, and who put in sixteen hours every day. He may have been influenced in his habits by Palmer Howard, the busiest practitioner in the city, who read medical articles in his carriage as he went from patient to patient. Osler became a notorious reader-traveller in vehicles. On foot he often ran the steep half mile up the mountain from the hospital to McGill.[26]

Edward Rogers, a student who lived with Osler in the late 1870s, remembered him as 'more regular and systematic than words can say; in fact, it was hardly necessary, living in the house with him, to have a timepiece of one's own. One could tell the time exactly from his movements from the hour of rising at seven-thirty until he turned out the light at eleven o'clock ... He always had a day's work laid out before the day began. Hours for meals, hours for recreation, hours for every duty were kept with absolute rigidity. He was always deliberate in every movement, never rushing, never hesitating.' Osler went to bed at 10 PM, Rogers remembered, and spent the next hour reading nonmedical classics. This became a legendary habit – an hour's worth of good reading a day – and it gave Osler a base of literary knowledge that was constantly expanding.[27]

We do not know whether he smoked as he read in bed. The spending on cigarettes, tobacco, and cigars listed in his accounts has been calculated as supporting the purchase of a hundred and fifty cigarettes, twelve ounces of tobacco, and three cigars a month.[28] Some of his smoking may have been during postmortems to counter the odors and, if Osler still followed older precautions, to create a healthy vapor to dissolve the poisons thought to be rising from the corpses.

After his first year in Montreal he drifted away from church attendance. The donations recorded in his accounts become fewer and fewer, then stop. Father Johnson, who visited Montreal from time to time before his death, thought that exposure to church divisions in England had eroded Osler's faith; but it is not clear that it had ever been very deep or personal, his only conversion having been to natural history and the microscope. In his student years, he had gravitated towards High Church services. As some Anglicans float higher in their beliefs, they drift into Roman Catholicism. For others, the faith just evaporates.

Neither Osler's practice nor his income rose substantially in the late 1870s, a time of considerable depression in Canada. His total annual earnings remained well below $2,000. While there is no doubt that he loved his pathological and histological investigations, he seems to have been regularly on the lookout for opportunities to treat patients. On Christmas Eve 1875, 'he was invited to a party at the Kenneth Campbells,' Jennette wrote. 'Marian would not hear of his refusing, for he was sure to meet nice people there & going into society is good for his practice ... Willie spent a pleasant evening & is invited there again for New Year's Eve.'[29]

He met other nice society people while serving for a month as hotel doctor in one of Montrealers' summer seaside resorts, Tadoussac on the lower St Lawrence. The arrangement was designed mainly to accommodate any summer medical needs of Canada's governor general. There were none. 'The only patient I have had was a poor French child with inf[lammation] of lungs following whooping cough – which is very prevalent among the natives.' He had time on his hands for trout fishing and a minor dalliance with a 'very agreeable' Boston girl, Edith Greenough. 'He is *very* handsome & the darkest man I ever saw,' she wrote of Osler in her diary. They corresponded for some months, as happens after a summer romance, and then drifted apart. Osler explained that he could not get down to see her, 'as year by year I am becoming tied & bound in the chains of my Profession.'[30]

His daybooks show that he had a few patients whom he saw regularly, including the oft-indisposed family of George Washington Stephens, a prominent Montreal merchant. Early in 1878 when Palmer Howard was 'laid up,' as Osler put it, he suddenly became busier. That spring he launched a breakthrough campaign by deciding to stand for appointment as an attending physician at the Montreal General, a position being vacated by Drake of the failing heart.

Osler was still a junior doctor in Montreal and there were members of the hospital's outdoor physician staff who had an arguably better claim to Drake's position. The hospital's board of governors would make the decision. In Montreal as in Britain, these appointments carried so much income-generating prestige in local medical circles that they were always hotly contested. Osler circulated a printed petition listing his qualifications and his major publications, and personally solicited the support of governors and others. He called on scores of prominent Montrealers, a grind he found deeply distasteful. But it paid off when, by a considerable majority, he was elected over three other candidates. A special student petition in his favor was read to the governors, deprecating an idea someone must have spread that he was not acceptable to the students.[31]

The day he got the appointment he sailed for Britain with George Ross for more training and to take his examination for membership in the Royal College of Physicians. He spent most of the summer with leading London clinicians – Murchison ('a model bedside teacher'); Samuel J. Gee ('in whom were combined the spirit of Hippocrates and the method of Sydenham'); Fred Roberts ('showed us how physical diagnosis could be taught'); Bastian; Ringer; Bland Sutton, who held 'Sunday School' on the wards on sabbath mornings; and Sir George Savage, who led rounds among the mentally disordered at 'Bedlam,' the Bethlehem Royal Hospital. Dining regularly at the Savile Club, Osler joined readily in scientific and literary give-and-take, no mean challenge for a colonial still shy of his thirtieth birthday. He made new friends that summer in London and at the annual meeting of the British Medical Association, and he passed his MRCP. The thrust of his summer's work was to prepare to treat patients. So far in Montreal he had spent more time examining the dead than the living.[32]

A kind of blue-ribbon stamp of approval came his way some months later when Peter Redpath, president of the board of governors of Montreal General and a towering figure in Montreal, asked Dr Osler to treat his lumbago. On one of his trips to England Osler had been taught by Ringer that the insertion of needles, the technique known as acupuncture, could relieve lower-back pain. At a meeting of the Med-Chi a few years earlier, acupuncture had been referred to approvingly by one of the city's senior practitioners (who was also the mayor), Dr W.S. Hingston. So Dr Osler inserted ordinary hatpins, as recommended by the mayor of Montreal and Ringer's *Therapeutics*, into Redpath's back. The therapy was not successful, one of Osler's housemates remembered, claiming that Redpath 'ripped out a string of oaths.' (When this story was first published in 1925, Redpath's descendants furiously asserted that he was morally incapable of cursing.) Osler in 1892 testified to the treatment's 'extraordinary and prompt efficacy in many instances.'[33] Neither Ringer nor Osler, and probably not Hingston, had any interest in the history and theory of acupuncture, also known to them as 'needling.'

Montreal General Hospital remained dirty and overcrowded through all of Osler's Montreal years. The patients still slept on straw mattresses, and damp linen from the laundry was often hung up on the wards to dry. The hospital air was a nauseating soup of odors, dominated by the smell of urine because patients' samples were kept by their bedside for the convenience of medical students' testing. Patients were sometimes turned away for want of accommodation, housed in a tent in the summer, or bedded down on the dirty wooden floors. 'The lungs of a suffering tuberculous patient were often filled with smoke from his neighbor's pipe, the neighbor being a strong lusty man with a fractured femur.' The American 'Lady Trainer of Nurses'

who offered this and other scathing criticisms of the hospital had been brought in after a group of imported English trained nurses had given up and gone home. The Yankee girl quit too. Montreal General's attempt to be in the avant-garde of Canadian nursing reform failed. (Osler thought that at least one of the imports had suffered from complete lack of tact; the urine sample issue had pitted good nursing and sanitation against good practice and training.)[34]

Except for Frank Buller, who had taken the specialist position in ophthalmology that Osler had once fancied, the attending staff were still all generalists, often practicing both medicine and surgery, and seeing as wide a range of cases as they wanted. Osler assisted at a few operations, probably administering anesthetic by holding ether-soaked cloths over the patient's mouth. There is no evidence that he ever tried his hand, trained through use of the dissecting knife, at surgery. Each of the twelve attending physicians controlled about a dozen beds. The physicians neither received nor expected payment for treating the charity cases who made up about 95 per cent of the Montreal General's patients, but they had the privilege of offering clinical courses for fees. Osler, for example, began holding summer clinics, in which he gave talks at the bedside and lectures in the hospital amphitheater.

He remained hard up, grossing a total of only $1,369 in 1879–80. On his 1878 European trip, he could not afford to spend £6 ($30) on a work of Virchow's he coveted – until an unexpected £10 gift arrived from his father, 'dear, kind soul! to send it out of his scanty income.' Early in his career Osler met the distinguished and rich British consultant, Sir Andrew Clark, who said that he had worked ten years for bread, ten years for bread and butter, and twenty years for cakes and ale. Osler was still scrambling for bread.[35]

His friends decided to help. Osler was not present at the faculty meeting of 21 April 1880: 'Prof. Howard said that several members of the Faculty had been considering the importance of, by some means, adding to the income at present received by the Professor of Physiology. This matter was discussed, all being unanimous as to the necessity of so doing. It was agreed that the fee for the Institutes of Medicine shall be raised to $16.00

and that the sum of $500 be also paid to the same chair from the funds of this Faculty, annually.'[36]

Osler's university earnings increased just as his reputation was beginning to attract patients, who were usually referred to him by their primary doctor. He grossed $2,778 in 1880–1, $3,884 in 1882–3, bread and butter perhaps, although in the former year he reinvested $1,019 in the department.[37] He might see two or three private patients a day and was now charging five dollars for a half-hour session. He was apparently operating on the model and fee schedule of British consultants, who did not engage in general practice but saw patients when other doctors asked for their opinion. In the winter of 1880–1, for example, Palmer Howard brought him in on the case of Dr Sir Charles Tupper, one of Canada's most distinguished politicians, who had been shocked when a routine life insurance examination disclosed albumin and tube casts in his urine, an apparent sign of serious organic disease. Osler repeatedly examined Tupper's urine but could offer no comfort. Tupper had lived hard, and it looked as though he was washed up at sixty.[38]

Dr Osler lived in rented quarters near the university, usually with congenial landlords. One was a Shakespearian scholar with a fine library, whose chief sin was that he absent-mindedly incorporated young Osler's treasured Shakespeare concordance into his own collection. Osler did not know how to tactfully ask for it back. For several years his landlord at 1351 St Catherine Street was Buller the oculist. Osler had a bedroom and office on Buller's second floor and was soon joined there by a couple of McGill students, Edward Rogers and Henry Vining Ogden. Osler did not think of himself as a men's club man – he did not play billiards, drink very much, or make friends easily outside the profession – but all his life he used clubs as restaurants and hotels. In Montreal he regularly dined at the Metropolitan Club, and once a month a dozen of the young doctors got together for a social dinner. The air would have been heavy with smoke and storytelling, the table groaning with oysters and beer.

Much of the time he had left over from work and meetings was spent with his cousins Jennette and Marian, who loved him like a favorite young brother. Jennette had been as close to him as either of his sisters ever since her first appearance in Canada. She was a highly intelligent slip of a woman, a spinster by choice or default, a case of what was lost by gender inequality in the nineteenth century, and she spent much of her life being 'little auntie' to the children of Marian and other relatives. Plump Marian was a gushing, guileless, and happy soul, despite much to be unhappy about. Her husband, George Francis, seemed to be constantly traveling, spending only enough time in Montreal to sing some duets with Marian and impregnate her. As well, he developed a weakness for drink. The Francis family lived in genteel poverty. The flock of Francis chicks, George (born 1870), May (1871), Gwyn (1874), Brit (1876), William (1878), Gwen (1879), Bea (1881), and Jimmie (1883), suffered mini-epidemics of typhoid fever, scarlet fever, diphtheria, and mumps, usually when Cousin Bill / Uncle Willie / 'Doccie O' was abroad and unable to help.

In good health the Francis children saw more of their one male relative in Montreal than they did of their father. They saw a side of Osler as yet unknown to his colleagues and students – a love of children and childhood and play and fantasy that would stay with him all his life and was reminiscent of no one so much as Lewis Carroll. 'My brothers and I used to watch for him to come home from his lectures,' May Francis remembered. 'He always came down the street at a swinging pace with the spring on the ball of the foot' – though he might be waylaid for a time by a neighboring girl asking him to doctor her hurt doll. 'He entered the house with a cheerful whistle; that was the signal for clapping hands of joy from the children ... "O, the darlings," he would call out gaily and wave to us in greeting. Then he would put his hands lightly on the dining room table and vault across its width. To us it seemed a marvellous feat. He was the Fairy Prince.'[39]

His namesake and godson Willie Francis, effectively a fatherless boy, was particularly attached to him. When Willie was three, Osler stayed for a time with the family at a summer home on Lake Memphramagog and was the best playmate the children ever had. 'As he was leaving,' Jennette recalled, 'little three-year-old Willie F. was sobbing on the verandah, heartbroken at losing him. WO ran indoors, brought down an old waistcoat of his own and threw it into little Willie's lap, saying "There's something of mine for you to keep." The small boy slept with it hugged in his arms every night & whenever he was hurt, or felt sad, we would find him with his face buried in the old waistcoat for comfort.'

Little Bea and Gwen used to run to Osler and climb up on his knees and pillow their heads on his shoulder. 'Every one loved him,' May remembered:

> But none more than I for was he not going to marry me? Yes, we were engaged when I was five years old, and though he was a little older than I, still he had promised to wait for me, and I knew he never broke a promise. We were going to live on a farm on the prairies with horses and cows and chickens and cats and dogs and birds and swings and a merry-go-round, and lots to eat and no bread and butter or rice puddings. And we could go in for a swim when we liked and stay in as long as we liked and in the winter we would live in a log house because they were so cosy and toast marshmallows and pass popcorn and eat it after, too, and skate and toboggan and snowshoe and tell fairy stories in the evening and not go to bed till it was ever so late.[40]

Who *would* Uncle Willie marry? The Francis circle, which quickly expanded to take in Rogers and Ogden (who got a case of mumps for his friendliness and passed it to his classmates), gossiped constantly about the eligible young doctors and their belles. Save for his teenage infatuation with cousin Mary Osler and summer flirtations, Willie appears to have had no love interests. Through his twenties he did not have enough money to think of supporting a wife. With a half-decent income in the early 1880s marriage became a possibility, but where would the right woman be found to look after a man tied and bound in the chains of his profession and loving every moment of it?

A bad marriage could be a disaster. Osler was aware of the great literary example of this, Dr Tertius Lydgate in George Eliot's 1872 instant classic, *Middlemarch*. When Lydgate marries an empty-headed, materialistic beauty, he sets a course that blights his professional career. Osler was set on medicine, science, his microscope, his teaching. 'The lass that marries Willie will have to do the courting,' his father remarked.[41]

Still, Frank Shepherd remembered Osler as having been a favorite with the Montreal ladies. He was a dapper fellow who could be charming and very funny when his mind was not on medicine. His flourishing, drooping, sometimes walruslike mustache was very much in fashion; the fast young woman of the 1880s was said (by Rudyard Kipling) to have compared a mustacheless kiss to an egg without salt. Whether or not she liked her eggs seasoned, a relationship between Osler and Jessie Dow, daughter of a wealthy Montreal brewer, nearly reached the engagement stage, causing much Francis family punning about 'dowering passions' and 'dowry' to come. Some thought old Dow put an end to the affair precisely because Osler, a parson's son with a modest doctor's income, had no dowry.[42] His liberal religious ideas may have been another problem. A poor nonbeliever would be the worst of all gifts from the church!

Osler then moved slightly down the social scale by falling in love with Shepherd's sister, but she married Dr William Molson, scion of an even bigger Montreal brewing fortune. ('Well – another lucky escape,' commented a Montreal socialite forty years later after learning of these Osler dalliances, 'for of all the deadly uninteresting humourless women ever created, Mrs. Molson was the greatest – with a thin high-pitched voice and a silly giggle, *and* stingy! William Osler you were lucky indeed.')[43] Shepherd himself made an entirely successful match with a daughter of the president of the Bank of Montreal. Solely from a dowry point of view, the great coup was that of Jared Howard, Palmer Howard's son, who was following in his father's footsteps in medicine and solved his financial needs forever by marrying Margaret Smith, only child of the fur trader, banker, and railway titan Donald Smith, Canada's equivalent of several Astors and Vanderbilts. Retribution struck, as Howard, who was probably fortune hunting, doomed himself to an unfulfilling narcoticized lifetime in high society.

Osler's bachelor life at 1351 St Catherine was disrupted for good when the landlord himself, Frank Buller, surprised them all by marrying a Miss Langlois, whom nobody knew but who was said, knowingly, to have 'done St. James Street for five seasons.' 'I hope it is all right,' Osler wrote. 'I should not like to see the landlord mated with a shrew.' Buller and Langlois were apparently very happy together. Osler continued to escape entanglements and also to resist Buller's advice to put his money into 'sure-thing' investments. 'I do wish he would marry some wealthy woman, 'twould be a great boon for him,' a flatmate wrote.[44]

What did he do for sex? Many Victorians, certainly many churchmen, would easily have understood Osler's remaining celibate throughout his bachelorhood. On the other hand, as a medical student he would have known a lot about sex and how to get it. One strange piece of evidence, a fragment of a dream he recorded in 1917, might possibly be read to show that as a young man he had visited prostitutes. (He dreams he is attending his own postmortem. Syphilis is found, and in the dream he says he might have got it innocently as a student.)[45] Perhaps Osler lost his virginity in Europe, though I think it unlikely. But if this was the case, he would have been very careful, for fear of disease.

More likely, Osler was thinking of his own experience when he came to write about continence for his textbook in 1892: 'There are other altars than those of Venus upon which a young man may light fires ... hard work of body and hard work of mind. Idleness is the mother of lechery; and a young man will find that absorption in any pursuit will do much to cool passions, which, though natural and proper, cannot in the exigencies of our civilization always obtain natural and proper gratification.'[46] We might presume that Osler masturbated, though his writing suggests that he shared that era's abhorrence of the practice. In matters sexual he probably practiced fierce Victorian restraint. For a discussion of twentieth-century gossip that Osler had a prolonged affair in Montreal with his cousin Marian, you can leap forward to chapter 13, page 494. I do not believe the story contains any truth. Medicine was Osler's mistress. She tied and bound him.

Now that he had added regular hospital work to his continuing pathological investigations, Osler began to know a great deal about many diseases. He saw so much illness in the living and the dead, had so many opportunities to help patients heal and then investigate what went wrong, that by his early thirties he was on his way to becoming an experienced consultant. We can imagine him talking of earlier cases of this condition, drawing attention to the lungs or the liver in cases of that, admitting that this other condition is baffling, trying hard to explain a situation to a concerned family. Perhaps too hard: 'Young man, you talk too much,' an old-timer told him after observing him being earnestly voluble to a patient's relatives. 'For forty years I have practiced medicine with a nod of the head.'[47]

His bibliography swelled with the hospital case reports his students published and his own clinical lectures. Now he could use patients, not just body parts, in his teaching. His bedside rounds with students were remembered as instructive, though perhaps no more so than those of Howard, Ross, Shepherd, or Roddick.[48] We hear him directly in the summer of 1882, giving a clinical lecture in the amphitheater on inherited syphilis:

GENTLEMEN, – In the out-door department and on the surgical side you will have many opportunities of seeing acquired syphilis in its recent forms ... First a word of caution: Do not use the term syphilis before your patients, particularly as in the case just to be brought in of a mother and her child. Many a poor woman has lived in blissful ignorance of the precise nature of her child's affliction until an incautious word has suggested to her the cause, and then, for her, 'farewell the tranquil mind.' We shall use the old term *lues* ...

Now, gentlemen, I would ask you to make a careful study of the child. Do not suppose that it is only in hospital practice that you will find these cases; lues is no respecter of persons, and there is no station in life in which you may not expect to meet it ...

Infantile lues may lead to characteristic appearances in the child; the eruption causing fissures about the mouth, which, when healed, leave scars which radiate from the angle of the mouth to the cheek. In the infant before you the present rash is healing, but during the first year there may be occasional skin eruptions, or mucous patches in the mouth. If the child survives during the first year the disease usually remains latent, but as puberty is approached again declares itself, as you will see in the next cases to be brought in.

Now that the patient has left the room, we may ask the question, Who is responsible for this – the father or the mother? The latter, so far as we can gather, seems healthy; has had no skin eruptions, or throat trouble. The husband is away, and though she says he is healthy, and never had any particular disease which she knows of, I am inclined to think that he is at fault. What about the woman herself? Is she syphilized? Most writers think that a woman who has borne a syphilized child is contaminated in some degree, though showing no positive signs. A strong proof is the fact that you cannot inoculate her with syphilis. If the child you have just seen were given to a healthy nurse, with its conditions of lips, it would give the woman a chancre of the nipple. This is sometimes known as Colles's law.

The next cases illustrate some interesting later manifestations.

Case II. – Girl, aet. 13, showing severe ulceration of throat ...

Case III – Girl, aet. 23 ...

You noticed that I examined the teeth of these two cases with special care. I did so because these organs sometimes give valuable or even positive evidence of inherited syphilis. Mr. Jonathan Hutchinson first called attention to this fact, and I have here for your inspection his Plates illustrating the subject ... At the Congress last year he complained very justly, that men had not sufficiently studied his writings on the subject, and were too apt to regard any malformed teeth as syphilitic.[49]

Osler prescribed the standard treatment for the condition, the regular use of a mercury ointment. Most of his treatments appear to have been standard; he certainly did not hesitate to rely on the five drugs that even Oliver Wendell Holmes had suggested saving from the fishes – opiates, digitalis, quinine, mercury, and ether – all of which had powerful sedative, stimulating, or fever-reducing effects.[50] Where appropriate, he prescribed purgatives and diuretics, to try to help the bowels and kidneys. Never entirely free from old conceptions, he still believed it possible to relieve congestion in organs by applying surface derivatives, such as heated cups and fomentations – which at best were distracting irritants – and he must have reasoned that needles in the lower back somehow drew off pain.

Some of his patients would have been well dosed. For nephritis in pregnancy, he told his students to 'give opiates hypodermically, or by the mouth,' adding: 'Chloral hydrate is highly praised, and Dr McCallum has used it with great success. Bleeding is frequently resorted to, and with good effect. Make use also of the special treatment of the renal symptoms, by cupping, hot poultices, diuretics, and the steam or vapour bath.' His 1877 prescription for the common cold: 'Bismuth, 4 drachms; Acadia powder 1½ drachms. Morphia 1 grain. Use as a snuff. About half of the above should be used in the first 24 hours of a cold, by which time it should be almost gone.' [51]

But from the beginning of his career Osler wrestled with the conundrums of therapeutics. Which treatments worked? Which were unnecessary? What did positive harm? What is the test of effectiveness? What constitutes proof? There was nothing new in these questions, which had occupied physicians for centuries and in their modern form for at least forty years before Osler practiced. He could well have been introduced to skepticism about traditional remedies by his clergyman father. If his materia medica courses at Toronto and McGill had been fairly old-fashioned, his reading of the works of Sydney Ringer and John Brown, as well the training he received in Britain and on the continent, would certainly have familiarized him with the tendency to give fewer medicines and let nature take its course. His work in pathology would have reinforced that predilection, because in many cases postmortems showed that treatment accomplished nothing. Consider a colleague's recollection of Osler at Med-Chi meetings in the 1880s discussing a therapeutic issue that is not without significance to women a century later. The subject was gynecology:

> There was a good deal of talk at the meetings about ... operations; much showing of recently removed ovaries and tubes, and some damping down of undue enthusiasm by Osler, who was constantly asking if ovaries so nearly normal required such heroic treatment. His doubts were due to the frequency with which he found, at post-mortems, ovaries and tubes with advanced pathological changes, in the bodies of women who had never complained much of pelvic pain. [52]

In 1882 Osler published an important clinical lecture on pneumonia in which he gave his students a fully developed set of *principia* in therapeutics:

The *first* is that there is an inherent tendency in many diseases to recovery quite irrespective of any treatment ... [He quotes Jacob Bigelow from 1835 on self-limiting disease.]

The *second* lesson is that nature, in the majority of cases, is quite competent to restore the patient to health. The natural therapeutics, as Professor Harvey of Aberdeen calls the *vis medacatrix naturae*, in contradistinction to applied therapeutics, are capable in 80 per cent of cases of dealing with the disease. As Professor Guebler puts it, 'L'organisme se guèrit lui même' ... Let me advise you, before worshiping at any special therapeutic shrine, to pay your vows to Nature, taking the motto of Edmund in Lear, 'Thou, Nature, art my goddess, to thy law my services are bound.'

The *third* lesson is that the functions of the physician are to co-operate with Nature, to aid her where she fails, and, above all to combat certain tendencies to a fatal issue ... Here arises the importance of an accurate knowledge of the natural history of any disease in order that we may recognize early fatal tendencies and be on our guard against impending danger.

Applying these principles to pneumonia (and ignoring the evils of Edmund's infatuation with nature), Osler reminded the students that the majority of cases do perfectly well when left to themselves, 'and though for the sake of the patient, and still more for the sake of friends, you may have to give a "placebo," the treatment is outside of your own hands; it is in the hands of Nature.'[53] Exhaustion from high or prolonged fever, however, could be fatal, so it should be combated. Osler was beginning to be interested in the use of baths as a therapy, a treatment widely practiced in Germany: 'Some of you may remember two sessions ago the case of a little girl in the children's ward with acute renal dropsy, and how admirably the air baths acted with her without any medication.'[54] But there was resistance in Canada to cold bathing. Palmer Howard had alarmed them with a story about a former student in western Canada who had used baths to treat a member of a prominent family; when the patient died, the doctor was driven out of town.[55] Quinine was Osler's antipyretic of choice: 'We have had numerous proofs of it, and where you have a remedy, the adoption of which has been *tried*, grapple it to your therapeutic soul with hooks of steel.' Osler was wrong; the quinine would have been useless against pneumonia.

Heart failure was another danger. Counter it with stimulants, Osler advised, and the best of these is alcohol. 'When you find your patient's pulse fail, when it begins to flicker; if it runs up and gets weak, begin your stimulants at once. Do not wait; you cannot do any harm by giving a few ounces of whiskey in a day ... Pin your faith, if to nothing else, to alcohol, in pneumonia.'[56] (Notice from these quotations that Osler had learned to offer memorable short summary statements, or epigrams, what he later called 'burrs that stick in the memory' – perfect for note taking. The sound bite predates television.) He freely prescribed alcohol as a stimulant for the aged, including his mother. According to George Washington Stephens' family, his preference was straight gin.[57]

Did the old practice of venesection in pneumonia have any merit? Osler thought the habitual bleeder would lose patients he might otherwise have saved. But his autopsy work had suggested that in some cases the load on the heart in pneumonia could be eased by bleeding, and he had tried it:

> You may remember, two years ago, the case of a man ... whose life, I believe, was saved by [my] timely venesection ... The relief was something remarkable. The only other condition, I believe, in which you can bleed with satisfaction is in the early stage where you have a full, vigorous man, without any vice of constitution. Twenty ounces of blood is neither here nor there in such a man, and it will reduce his pain and fever ... Shall we give arterial sedatives – digitalis, aconite, veratrum viride, and the like? Except at the onset, and in vigorous persons, they are not indicated. Antimony I never use. Local treatment to the chest is often advantageous. We use poultices very much in this hospital, and they are soothing to the pain and grateful to the patient. I never use cold, though I have seen it applied with apparent advantage in German hospitals.

Osler closed his lecture by reassuring the students that he had seen several cases of delayed resolution in pneumonia, so they need not fear a longer than normal course of the disease. But he also showed the diseased lung of a feeble old drunkard who had died in the hospital, and he reminded them of the lesson they had learned at the bedside of another patient the day before: The proper diagnosis of the young man on Osler's ward who had been thrashing around, restrained by two attendants, and talking to an imaginary person was pneumonia, not delirium tremens.[58]

Osler's energies, curiosity, and expanding clinical experience took him riding off in all directions. In the six years after his hospital appointment, he published case studies, analyses, or lectures on pernicious anemia, Bright's disease, Hodgkin's disease, ulcerative endocarditis, tabes, nephritis in pregnancy, aneurysm of the hepatic artery, tubercular meningitis, the histology of tumors, croup, muscular atrophy, fibroid phthisis (lung disease), the impaction of gallstones, empyema, and more. He published his student observations on fresh-water polyzoa, fleshed out with new material from his rambles by lakes and streams in Quebec. Then he contributed further 'Biology Notes' to the *Canadian Naturalist* on the algae in Lake Memphramagog ('fortunately I had my microscope with me and the question was soon settled') and more discoveries of polyzoa in Quebec. In 1879 he was disappointed at there being so few papers of medical interest at the Philadelphia meeting of the American Association for the Advancement of Science, so he took in sessions on chemistry, paleontology, and astronomy, and wrote it all up for the *Canada Medical and Surgical Journal*. He met Thomas A. Edison ('the bogie of gas companies'), who presented to him the very odd notion that one day it would be possible to illuminate the interior of the body by inserting a small electric burner into the stomach.[59]

Working with a brilliant veterinary student, A.W. Clement, Osler organized a major study of parasites in the pork supply of Montreal – they concluded that thorough cooking was the best protection – and carried out the first successful North American experiment inducing 'measly' veal, a calf infected with tapeworm larvae. In the spring of 1882 he toured ten medical museums in Canada and the United States, mainly, it seems, to collect cases of the rare infection of humans with a dog parasite, echinococcus disease. That September he was commissioned to investigate a mysterious

cattle disease in Pictou County, Nova Scotia. He was able to show that the
deaths were not caused by ragwort, a.k.a. 'stinking Willie,' but had no idea
what did cause them. Two years earlier, he and two colleagues had similarly
failed to find the precise origin of a typhoid fever epidemic at Bishop's
College in rural Quebec but had confidently predicted that improved ventilation, perfect drainage, and a pure water supply would end the problem.[60]

'In my Practical Histology class, during the winter of 1881–82, while
the students were working at the blood of the frog, I noticed in one of
the slides a remarkable body like a flagellate infusorian,' Osler wrote. He
was not satisfied until he had searched the literature and written a paper,
which he read to the Montreal Microscopical Society and then published, correcting others' misobservations. Then he was disconcerted to find
himself upstaged when Bizzozero of Turin published further descriptions
of the blood corpuscles Osler had written on in 1874, and named them
Blutplättchen (blood-plates, or platelets), a term that stuck. Osler published a slightly aggrieved review of the matter, urging that the bodies be
known after the original discoverer, as 'Schultze's granule masses.' He may
have mastered sound-bites in the classroom, but he never had a knack for
nomenclature.[61]

Instead of sticking with a research subject, such as the platelets, Osler
restlessly extended his studies to the one great organ he had ignored, the
brain. He and Howard had studied Sir William Broadbent's early neurological work in England, and on his 1878 visit he had come to know and
observe other pioneering British neurologists, Sir William Gowers and Victor Horsley. His reading of the great French clinician J.M. Charcot's *Lectures on Localization of Diseases of the Brain* had stimulated his interest in
the brain's pathology.[62] Soon he was showing his Montreal colleagues how
Giaomini's process made it possible to preserve whole brains as though
they were beautiful wax models, while Dalton's slicing apparatus produced
fascinating transverse and vertical sections. At the 1879 meeting of the
Canada Medical Association in London, Ontario, Osler gave a special lecture on 'The Medical Anatomy of the Brain,' illustrated by diagrams and
specimens. The next year when the CMA met in Ottawa at Canada's Parliament Buildings, Osler had on hand an exhibit of twenty-five specimens

of brain disease. Some doctors must have made the obvious jokes. Having mastered his techniques, Osler was soon reporting on rare brain tumors, cases of hemiplegia and cerebral hemorrhage, and, a first in Canada, multiple sclerosis.[63]

If human brain functions were localized – that is, if they were functions of the physical organ itself – did the structure of the brain therefore determine behavior? Could the hypothesis be tested by looking for physical defects or derangements in the brains of criminals? In 1879 Benedikt of Vienna was one of the first to propound the view that criminal brains were particularly deformed. Osler tested Benedikt's criteria (which had to do mainly with the course of brain fissures) on all the thirty-four pickled brains they had in Montreal. He concluded that the Montreal General either catered to a highly criminal population or Benedikt had failed to test normal brains. Osler had also procured the brains of two Canadian murderers and found them not especially abnormal.

The brain matter troubled Osler philosophically. The extreme determinism of Benedikt's view seemed to negate free will and make criminals, as Huxley had put it, the product of 'theft and murder cells.' Osler was appalled at the thought of 'every rascal pleading faulty grey matter in extenuation of some crime.' In a scientific paper 'On the Brains of Criminals,' we find him quoting Shakespeare's arch-criminal Iago on the mind-body relationship: 'Our bodies are our gardens to the which our wills are gardeners; so that if we will plant nettles or sow lettuce, set hyssop and weed up thyme, supply it with one gender of herbs or distract it with many, either to have it sterile with idleness or manured with industry, why, the power and corrigible authority of this lies in our will.' In this first paper Osler wrote on an issue involving the divide between science and liberal thought, he was trying to bridge the gap.[64]

How would a curious doctor get his hands on murderers' brains? In one case, Osler said, by personally attending the autopsy and persuading the jail surgeon to give him the organ. In the other, Osler sent Henry Ogden to

Rimouski, Quebec, on a similar mission. He armed Ogden with a letter of support from the Canadian minister of justice. So far as Ogden could understand – he spoke not a word of French – the French Canadians in Rimouski saw no reason to pay any attention to Ottawa's dictate and were not inclined to surrender the murderer's brain. Ogden observed the hanging, helped at the postmortem inquest, and with the connivance of the attending doctor got the brain out during the straightening-up before burial. ('No one who has not tried it has any idea of the difficulty of removing the brain in a cold room, your hands so numb you could scarcely hold a knife, and from a head that is virtually severed from the body.') Ogden made it to the train with the brain in his tool bag, then realized it had to be kept cool. Needing a container that locked, he transferred the brain to his Gladstone bag. He told the porter that the bag contained ptarmigan and had to be kept in a cool place. 'I got the brain to Montreal in reasonably good condition. W.O. expressed the greatest delight – but he did not give me a new Gladstone bag.'[65]

Stories like these were the meat and potatoes of medical yarning in Osler's time and afterwards. The Montreal men were unusually rich in anecdotes because the Province of Quebec's Anatomy Act, requiring unclaimed bodies to be given to the universities, was still unenforced. During Osler's years at McGill almost all subjects for dissection were obtained illegally. Frank Shepherd, who became professor of anatomy, told wild and wonderful tales of disinterred bodies being tobogganed down the mountain from Côte-des-Neiges cemetery or arriving from the train station in slightly odiferous Saratoga trunks – and, one winter when the heat was on about thefts from a nunnery, of their being stashed in snowdrifts near the medical school.

'What for you got mine oncle here?' a French-Canadian student said to the professor one day in the dissecting room. Another man found his grandmother on the table. Osler's comment on these 'A1' reminiscences by Shepherd, which he read in the last year of his life, was to add elusively: 'I thought the dénouement came with the stealing of the body of the Mayor of Three Rivers & also of the Bishop.' Like certain of Sherlock Holmes's cases (and also Osler's allusion to 'the case in No. 11 which interested us so much a few weeks ago, too much, in fact, as he got frightened and left the Hospital'), the stories of the mayor and bishop are probably lost forever.[66]

Even in the best of circumstances, inquisitive physicians had a further problem when they wanted to do an autopsy or remove organs against the objections of the deceased's family. If there was any kind of life after death, was it a good thing to cut up the body? Perhaps it was a horrible thing to do. Sometimes no amount of persuasion, verbal or monetary, would move concerned or superstitious relatives. Alexis St Martin, a French-Canadian voyageur who survived for almost sixty years with a hole in his stomach, making possible William Beaumont's classic studies of digestion, died in rural Quebec in 1880. Rumors that Professor Osler was sending a student to take away the historic *estomac* prompted warnings from the local doctor of possible mob action. St Martin's family kept the body at home during a heat wave until it decomposed so badly that the doctors would not dare do an autopsy. Nor, it turned out, would the priests allow it in the church during the funeral service. The grave was dug eight feet deep and armed guards were posted to thwart last-ditch efforts by Osler's resurrectionists.[67]

Osler had been interested in a case of Hodgkin's disease in eastern Ontario, and he was invited to do the autopsy when the boy died. Six local physicians met the distinguished professor to help. But the boy's father, having been forewarned, buried him, not in a vulnerable graveyard but in the orchard right by the farmhouse kitchen. The family physician, one Sherman, felt betrayed and embarrassed. The grieving family gave all the visiting doctors a good breakfast, Osler remembered:

After which the Doctor took the old farmer and his boys aside, and in a few minutes we saw that matters were settled. The body was to be exhumed. It was a most unpleasant situation from which I should have been glad to escape as one could not help sympathizing with the poor people. The body was taken to the barn, and I held the post mortem before a motley gathering of the neighbours, none of whom looked very friendly. I improved the occasion by speaking of the rarity of the disease and got them interested by demonstrating the various organs. We ... parted from the family on friendly terms. On leaving I said to Dr Sherman 'How did you manage to persuade the old man?'

'Manage it,' he said. 'I told the —— that if he did not produce the body, I would foreclose the mortgage on his —— farm. That's how I settled it.'[68]

On another occasion, as Henry Ogden recalled, it was darned hard work dissecting out the brain and spinal cord of a horse at Osler's request, though nobody objected to doing so. But what to do with it next? *Faute de mieux*, the students put the specimen in the bathtub at 1351 St Catherine: 'We had the happy thought of displaying it in such a way that W.O. would see at a glance all its beauty of completeness and entirety. So we carefully laid it out, the brain on the sloping end, the cord running down the mid-line, reaching to the full length of the bathtub, and the spinal nerves spread out on each side – all together we were vastly pleased with the result.' Unfortunately, Buller the landlord arrived home before Osler. Ogden had to hide in his cupboard from the storm of profanity. 'Oh, look at it Buller!' Osler said when he came in. 'Did you ever see anything so nice, see the spinal nerves and all. Oh, isn't that beautiful.' Osler and Ogden made a point of taking the first two baths the next morning.[69]

May Francis told a story about Osler ordering an organ in advance, as it were, by giving an alcoholic street beggar money and then his overcoat ('you may drink yourself to death ... but I cannot let you freeze yourself to death') in return for a promise to will him the cirrhotic liver. Within weeks, both the beggar's liver and the coat came back to the doctor. A further student reminiscence of Osler's passion for a good specimen was deemed too indelicate or apocryphal for his first biographer to use:

It seems that Dr Osler had a patient in the Montreal General Hospital, with Addison's Disease. He was extremely anxious to obtain the specimens of the Supra renals, after the man died; but could not persuade the family to allow an autopsy. He enlisted the aid of the family priest, who was a liberal-minded, scientific sort of a man. But he too was unable to get permission for an autopsy. Then the night before the funeral was to be held, Dr Osler is said to have gone to the Morgue of the General Hospital, greased his arm thoroughly, dilated the Sphincter Ani, broken through the bowel & obtained the coveted Specimens, without anyone being any the wiser.

The joke of it was, that early next morning the priest sought out Dr Osler, quite jubilantly, with permission for an autopsy, if he (the priest) were allowed to be present. Dr Osler had the time of his life performing the autopsy, with the interested priest looking on, & covering up the work of the previous night ... The Specimens were for years in the Medical Museum of McGill.'[70]

Everyone who knew Osler well remembered him as light-hearted, jaunty, breezy. 'He found it difficult to walk in the accepted sense of the term,' May Francis recalled, 'his nature seemed too buoyant to allow him to place one foot in front of the other as is done by more humdrum individuals. He would dance along humming or whistling.' As he became settled and sure of himself in Montreal, the boyhood sense of fun began to re-emerge, first with the Francis children, then with some of his colleagues, especially young Dr William Molson. The friendly feuding may have started when May Francis, in about her eleventh year, was pelting Molson with snowballs as he passed their house. Molson cruelly told her that Osler would never marry her. Osler happened along and formally introduced them: 'This is Miss May Francis, who is going to be my wife. This is Dr. Molson who was never known to tell the truth in his life.' A few days later, Osler dropped in and told the Francis children to invite everyone over for a party. He made them all join hands in a ring and dance round while he sang:

> We'll have lots of cakes and everything
> And we'll steal them all from the goblin king
> And we will dance and we will sing.
> And he will be cross as anything.

Osler knew that Molson was about to hold a party. Taking the Francis kids with him in a cab, he stole all the cakes, cookies, and ice cream from Molson's residence and treated the children to one of the greatest celebrations ever. On another occasion, May remembered, an Osler snowball cleanly removed Molson's fine top hat, leading to a formal charge of assault, appearance before a magistrate, a fine, and much laughter. On the occasion of the first doctors' dinner party after Molson blighted his life by marrying Shepherd's sister, Osler asked Mrs Molson if she might give him a latchkey for their convenience if once again, as commonly happened, they had to carry her husband home. [71]

Osler had become a compulsive writer whose energies were not fully absorbed by his correspondence and scientific papers. Possibly he was inspired by the visits of Mark Twain and Oscar Wilde to Montreal in 1881 and 1882; he helped organize a dinner for the former and took Marian to a performance by the latter. Veteran physicians liked to publish their most remarkable cases, adventures and tales. Shortly after Molson became assistant editor of the *Canada Medical and Surgical Journal,* he cursorily read and approved for publication some 'Professional Notes among the Indian Tribes about Gt. Slave Slave, N.W.T.' by Egerton Y. Davis, MD, Late US Army Surgeon.' They were a set of preposterous stories, 'the outcome of many years intercourse among the natives,' about Indian males' penises being cauterized before marriage to inhibit excessive intercourse, the 'genu-pectoral position' in copulation, dinners of 'baked placenta' to gain strength and courage, and (a practice Osler had seen among medical students in Vienna) of group digital inspection of pregnant women. The mythical Davis's mythical article was set in type and ready for publication when Osler suggested that editor Ross might want to take a look at it. That issue had to be hurriedly reset. [72]

'Joke on Molson,' Osler scrawled over the handwritten manuscript. Molson plotted revenge. William Osler found yet another outlet for his medical writing as Montreal correspondent to the *Medical News,* published in Philadelphia, and E.Y. Davis subsided to think about other strange cases he had seen. Unfortunately, we do not know exactly what happened when Osler went 'skylarking about the morgue' after finishing writing up autopsies. We only know that George Ross would exclaim in exasperation, 'What does Howard think of all this?' Palmer Howard's only weakness, in Osler's view, was that he was excessively serious. [73]

The full dignity of the practice of medicine was on display in London, England, in August 1881 as three thousand physicians and scientists, by one estimate most of the active medical researchers in the world, gathered for the Seventh International Medical Congress. Osler and Howard made a quick trip (relatively quick – about a week's passage each way) to take it in. By luck or design, Sir Charles Tupper was on the same steamer on the way over, and they arranged a special examination of him by Sir Andrew Clark, who was very pessimistic. Tupper was frightened into a period of semi-retirement.[74]

From his first days as a student, Osler had cherished the profession of medicine. The high-flown language he used to describe the congress in his report to the *Canada Medical and Surgical Journal* was heartfelt. The sight of the thousands of medical men 'drawn together for one common purpose, and animated by one spirit ... quickened the pulse and roused enthusiasm to a high pitch.' Sir James Paget's presidential address consisted of 'beautiful thoughts, clothed in the choicest words, and expressed with an ease and grace particularly his own ... such a gifted man.'

Osler heard Virchow again, may have taken in addresses by Huxley and Pasteur, and probably attended as many of the conversaziones, luncheons, dinner parties, garden parties, and open houses as he could. The socializing was always as important at these affairs as the formal sessions, and usually more fun. Osler went to meetings of the pathological, physiological, and medical sections, and gave a paper on endocarditis. He was most impressed by the special museum created for the occasion, some seven hundred specimens on loan from the world's great collections: 'Perhaps as much direct benefit to the working members of congress was obtained during the time spent in the museum as in any of the other departments.'[75] Earlier, as a delegate from the Montreal Veterinary Medical Association, he had attended the British National Veterinary Congress, a less grand affair. Nor could the veterinarians confer upon him any honor as important as fellowship in the Royal College of Physicians of London, to which he was elected in 1883, the first year he was eligible. Only two other resident Canadians had that distinction. Of course, Osler was an original fellow of the Royal Society of Canada, which had been founded the previous year.

McGill continued to stand in the front rank of North American medical schools. By 1883 it was phasing out didactic lectures in the medical sciences for laboratory work, demonstrations, and more time in the dissecting room. Men of Osler's generation had taken over most of the key positions in the faculty. Specialists in gynecology, midwifery, and children's diseases were hired. Donating money as well as his daughter to Montreal medicine, Donald Smith gave the faculty a princely $50,000, and it raised $50,000 more. Plans were afoot to more than double the size of the medical building.

Osler thought the professors still had to cope with the 'excessive drudgery' of too much teaching. In an ideal university, he wrote in an unsigned editorial, well-paid professors and their assistants would be 'placed above the worries and vexations of practice,' and their time would 'be devoted solely to teaching and investigating the subjects they profess.' That perfect Canadian medical school could not be developed 'unless the liberality of individuals is manifested in the manner of the late Mr. Johns Hopkins of Baltimore' or with the liberality of government. But Osler seemed generally optimistic. Proposing a toast to McGill at its fiftieth anniversary dinner in 1882, Osler talked about the need to hire the ablest men possible, 'not only the ablest men that the country possessed, but the best that money could get, the best talent they could get irrespective of nationality.'[76]

The old order at McGill did not pass without incident. In the middle of the 1882–3 term, the first- and second-year students rebelled against the disorganized and irrelevant materia medica classes of the Reverend William Wright, MD. 'The older the remedy and the less used,' Shepherd remembered, 'with the greater elaboration was it dwelt on.' As registrar, Osler was at the center of delicate negotiations aimed at getting the students back in class, Wright pacified, and supplementary up-to-date instruction given. At the end of the term, Wright resigned, aware that his colleagues had not supported him. He gradually lost touch with medicine and as an old recluse twenty-five years later asked Shepherd, 'What are those ten rays [x-rays] one reads about in the papers?'[77]

About the time of the Wright affair, the students also got into a row with Montreal's police. Professor Osler saved the day for McGill by addressing a throng of angry students – who had clubs and thigh bones in hand, ready to riot – and managing to lower their fever: 'He sympathized with us in our grievance, but simply laughed us into good humour.'[78]

Osler had had a splendidly productive career apprenticeship at McGill. Hired because he knew how to use microscopes and was in love with research, and because he had followed Palmer Howard's advice and taken advanced scientific training, he had never varied in his belief that the medical sciences, notably pathology, existed to serve medical practice. Driven partly by the need to make a living, he had seen himself as a practicing physician from the first. He had gone into the medical wilderness to treat smallpox. Then, after getting his hospital appointment, he had begun to come into his own as a clinician and teacher and an amazingly prolific author.

A young man of complete self-discipline, application, and good health and good humor, he had impressed practically everyone with the range of his achievement and his idealism. He had cultivated an enormous circle of medical friends and acquaintances in three countries and seemed equally at home in all of them. Not only was he ubiquitous in the journals and at meetings, but in most of his work he was good – observant, logical, steeped in the literature, and apt at any time to toss off *bons mots* from Shakespeare.

From a raw outsider in Montreal, he had become a member of the city's medical elite and probably its social elite. He had a wide circle of establishment friends, including Donald Smith and the merchant princes who were embarking on Canada's most daring entrepreneurial adventure, the building of the Canadian Pacific Railway to span the continent. Brother Edmund was a member of the railway's board of directors and came to Montreal for meetings. 'At 7, as your brother is down,' Smith's note would read, inviting Dr Osler to dinner. Afterwards, E.B., Smith, George Stephen, R.B. Angus, Duncan McIntyre, and the other businessmen would ignore William as they wrestled with their railroad's latest financial crisis, usually deciding to try and raise more money in New York. Osler was for many years instrumental in raising money for medicine from Smith.[79]

He was a rising star in a rising profession. How bright would he shine? By the time of the international congress of 1881, and certainly with the award of his FRCP in 1883, well-placed Canadian, British, and even American medical men spoke of Osler as a fellow to keep an eye on. Some of his Montreal colleagues thought McGill would lose him sooner or later.[80]

As a scientist he was spreading himself far too thinly. He had no sooner published a pioneering study of platelets or miner's lung or endocarditis or multiple sclerosis than he moved on to something else, never doing the intense follow-ups or staying put long enough to leave a lasting name in the field. He had just missed being the father of blood platelets; if he had thought about and followed up observations on how cells in the lung tried to carry off carbon particles, he might have been a great pioneer in studies of phagocytosis; he came close to being the first to delineate appendicitis. In 1884 he admitted that he was trying to do too much.[81]

In some fields of medical science he was already falling behind. Although the term 'physiology' was replacing 'institutes of medicine' in the description of his professorship, he was much more interested in doing pathology than immersing himself in the new science that investigated life processes through extensive animal research: 'In truth I lacked the proper technique for proper physiology.' He never mastered some of the fancy physiological apparatus installed at his urging in McGill's first lab, he admitted, and 'over which the freshmen firmly believed that I spent sleepless nights in elaborate researches ... I never could get my drums and needles and tambours to work in harmony.'[82]

Even as an apostle of the microscope, the pathological examination, research, and learning, Osler had never in fact thought of himself as primarily a scientist. He was not bound to a discipline, even pathology. His three broad interests were learning about the natural history of disease, teaching about disease, and doing what he could to treat it. Speaking at McGill twenty-five years later, he said of this early period, 'I had become a pluralist of the most abandoned sort, and at the end of ten years it was difficult to say what I did profess: I felt like the man in Alcibiades II to whom are applied the words of the poet: – "Full many a thing he knew; / But knew them all badly."'[83] Osler solved his physiology lab problem by persuading McGill to appoint T. Wesley Mills, a former Toronto classmate who had liked to debate with Bovell, as demonstrator in physiology. Mills, whom they had nicknamed John Stuart, understood physiological techniques, had few teaching and human skills, and was unpopular with the students.

The history of McGill's Faculty of Medicine calls these 'The Osler years.' Perhaps. But even Osler could not prevail against the allurements of Montreal's 1884 Winter Carnival. The students insisted that their classes, like those in the public schools, should be suspended for carnival week. The faculty offered only one day off. Professor Osler announced that he would give his lectures if there was only one person there to hear them. Some days there was one; others, there were three. When the full group returned the next week, Osler began by saying, 'Gentlemen, I am delighted to see you, but I never for a moment imagined that you cared to be classed with school children.' He never mentioned the incident again, nor did he examine the medical men on the work they had missed.[84]

What could a little squabble with the students matter to a professor who planned to leave after his last class for four months in Europe? By 1884 the world of scientific medicine was exploding. 'New discoveries were being announced like corn popping in a pan,' Harvey Cushing would write of these years.[85] Osler was looking forward to leaving Montreal to drink again at the European wellsprings and munch at medical congresses. On March 26 he sailed for Germany. Arduous as it was becoming, the McGill term was still wonderfully short by later standards.

FOUR

The Best Men: Philadelphia

Until the Great War of 1914–18 Osler was a doctor without borders. A man of railroads and steamers and an early automobile enthusiast, he was unusually peripatetic, a medical wanderer geographically as well as clinically and in print. His sense of membership in a catholic profession was more important to him than his national, ethnic, or regional roots. 'By his commission the physician is sent to the sick, and knowing in his calling neither Jew nor Gentile, bond or free, perhaps he alone rises superior to those differences which separate and make us dwell apart, too often oblivious to the common frailties which should bind us together as a race,' he said at a celebration to honor Virchow in 1891.[1] Towards the end of the century he began to show mild traces of an Anglo-Saxon 'race' consciousness and British imperialist fervor, but he was never even casually anti-Semitic. In an age when prejudice against Jews was common among late-Victorian Anglo-Saxons and Americans, Osler had none at all.

He saw and reported on anti-Semitism in Berlin during his 1884 visit: 'The modern "*hep, hep, hep*" shrieked in Berlin for some years past has by no means died out, and, to judge from the tone of several of the papers devoted to the Jewish question, there are not wanting some who would gladly revert to the plan adopted on the Nile some thousands of years ago for solving the Malthusian problem of Semitic increase.' A visitor could not help but notice the prominence of 'Hebrews' in medical gatherings, at the universities, and in any collection of students, he observed. 'Of those I know, their positions have been won by hard and honorable work ... all honor to them!' Osler heard that anti-Semitic agitation was already making it difficult for Jews to advance further in universities, and he meditated on one possible future:

> Should another Moses arise and preach a Semitic exodus from Germany, and should [he] prevail, they would leave the land impoverished far more than was ancient Egypt by the loss of the 'jewels of gold and jewels of silver' of which the people were 'spoiled.' To say nothing of the material wealth – enough to buy Palestine over and over again from the Turk – there is not a profession which would not suffer the serious loss of many of its most brilliant ornaments, and in none more so than in our own.[2]

The material progress of imperial Germany's showpiece city since his 1874 visit astounded him. There had been huge investments in public buildings, including laboratories, hospitals, and university facilities, and the streets had become modern. 'From a dirty, ill-drained, mal-odorous, second-class capital it has changed to a bright, well-drained, bustling metropolis.' At the new obstetrical and gynecological hospital he observed surgeons working inside the abdomen, the advanced frontier of the craft, under stringently controlled antiseptic conditions and with magnificent equipment. 'Nothing appears lacking. The entire building is lighted by Edison lamps.'[3] There were not yet any Edison burners illuminating the stomach.

His trip was partly a revisiting of student days and haunts, with a view to paying homage to Virchow. Osler sat once more in his classes ('what a privilege it was again to listen to ... the great master') and called on Virchow in his private rooms, bringing tribute in the form of four aboriginal skulls. 'Not the warm thanks, not the cheerful, friendly greeting which he always had for an old student, pleased me half so much as the prompt and decisive identification of the skulls which I had brought, and his rapid sketch of the cranial characters of the North American Indian.'[4]

The aging F.T. von Frerichs had just astounded his medical friends by producing a monograph on diabetes, a disorder on which Osler had not as yet had anything to say. The Canadian was impressed by Frerichs's recommendation to treat diabetes with 'mental quietude,' exercise, and a low carbohydrate but varied diet. Osler also attended clinics at the Charité Hospital in general medicine, psychiatric and nervous diseases, and children's diseases, then toured the Royal Veterinary College and visited an abattoir to study meat inspection and add to his collection of parasite specimens. He noted with evident envy that the veterinary professors lived in the college and had no private practice. 'As a consequence, there is much better teaching, and altogether a more scientific tone, than is the case in English or American institutions of the kind. The students, however, do not seem to be up to the average of our own.'

The revolutionary change since Osler's 1874 visit was the explosion of interest in micro-organisms as the causative agents of disease. The age of bacteriology had arrived in a riot of discovery and controversy. Every pathologist was making cultures of this or that bacterium and conducting experiments to study its relationship with various diseases. Two years earlier Robert Koch, discoverer of the anthrax bacillus, had made a stunning breakthrough in isolating a bacillus that causes tuberculosis. Now in 1884 Koch was back in triumph from Egypt and India, where he had discovered the 'comma' bacillus that causes cholera. In this *annus mirabilis* of bacteriology, a congress of German physicians that Osler attended in Berlin was abuzz with Carl Friedlander's claim to have discovered a pneumococcus, the cause of pneumonia. Were there bacterial causes of diphtheria? of puerperal fever? of all fevers and inflammations? Where would it all lead?

The discovery and classification of bacteria in the 1880s caught the popular imagination much as the mapping of the human genome would in the 1990s. 'One is startled by the rapid diffusion of knowledge of these matters among the laity,' Osler wrote from Berlin. 'The properties of various bacilli form subjects for table talk and, naturally, the amount of nonsense and pseudo-science which prevails is what might be expected.'[5]

As a student of parasites, Osler kept far distant from the conservatives who scoffed at the idea of invisible organisms causing disease. He never repeated his student error of identifying blood platelets with bacteria, nor is there evidence that he sided with the 'spontaneous generation' school and others who posited a chemical rather than biological basis of germ action. Within a month of the first full Canadian report of Koch's discovery of the tubercle bacillus, Osler had demonstrated to his students its presence in a tubercular lung.[6]

But neither was this medical Anglican a hot gospeler of bacteriology. Like many of his fellow pathologists and microscopists, he could see too many bacteria, of too many kinds, swarming in tissues living and dead, to be instantly sure of their nature and function. In his letters from Berlin he trod a middle course, weighing evidence and authorities carefully. He recognized that the new German superstar, Koch, with brilliant technical methods and high standards of proof, commanded authority that for many overrode even the great Virchow's conservatism on the cholera question. Still, it was not always clear that bacteria created disease. The micrococci found in pneumonia might still be 'only the normal buccal and respiratory micrococci'; the alleged diphtheria-causing microbe could not be cultivated – one of Koch's own requirements – and so on.

Osler retained aspects of the older, more general approach associated with 'microbiology' in the style of the Louis Pasteur school, rather than 'bacteriology' in the Kochian/Teutonic mold.[7] What an exciting field, anyway! When Osler moved on to Leipzig, he spent his mornings 'going for the bacteria' and working with Karl Weigert on brain slicing in Julius Cohnheim's lab, his afternoons attending clinics or other laboratories. He urged Palmer Howard to have a room at McGill 'rigged up' to do bacterial culturing and promised to bring back cultures if they would stand the heat of travel. If Osler could help it, McGill would not lag in its studies of disease-causing microbes.[8]

The more he worked and lived in Germany, the more he envied the German scientists with their good salaries and accommodation at their labs. He wondered if he and Wesley Mills might get living quarters somewhere in McGill's enlarged medical building. In moods like this, Osler seemed to have lost interest in medical practice. But then he would have doubts. He heard the great German research physiologist Carl Ludwig argue that British physiology had fallen behind because many of its practitioners had drifted off into practical medicine and surgery. Certainly the German institutes catered well to exceptional researchers, he reflected, 'but the rank and file [of students] are not, I believe, so well instructed in their physiological work as with us in England.'

In his puzzlement about the German approach, Osler posed a conundrum about research and teaching that would haunt him for most of the rest of his professional life: 'It is very hard to adjust the two great functions of a University ... The work which shall advance the science, which brings renown to the professor and to the University, is the most attractive, and in German laboratories occupies the chief time of the director. This function is specially exercised, and the consequence is that medical literature teems with articles issued from the various laboratories. On the other hand, the teaching function of an Institute is apt to be neglected in the more seductive pursuit of the "bauble reputation."'[9]

Similarly, Osler could see both sides of the German habit of having hospitals dominated by powerful heads, supported by a staff of assistants. The poorly paid assistants did too much of the work. On the other hand, the wards had become 'clinical laboratories utilized for the scientific study and treatment of disease, and the assistants, under the direction of the Professor, carry on investigations and aid in the instruction. The advanced position of German medicine and the reputation of the schools as teaching centres are largely fruits of this system.'

For Osler, these were still mostly academic issues, of less moment than what McGill might do for him in the way of accommodation. As in 1874, his time in Germany had been professionally valuable; yet he would never be as Germanophilic as many of his later associates. After Berlin and Leipzig, he crossed the Channel to London. 'It is the world. How I should like to live here!'[10]

While Osler was continuing to develop as a man of the world, the medical Brahmins of Philadelphia, Pennsylvania, were debating the limits of professional inbreeding.

For generations, their great city and its premier medical school had been at or near the center of health care in the United States. The Medical Department of the University of Pennsylvania, founded in 1765, was the oldest medical school in the country. The Pennsylvania Hospital, founded in 1751, was the oldest hospital in the country. In the aftermath of the American Revolution, when Benjamin Franklin's Philadelphia had for a time been the political as well as cultural capital of the nation, Philadelphia's Benjamin Rush, professor, philosopher, signator of the Declaration of Independence, had been the most famous physician in the United States. Decade after decade, the Pennsylvania school remained one of America's largest, servicing between three and five hundred students in competition with rivals in other centers and in booming, bustling Philadelphia itself.

Once the Quaker City, once the Athens of America, Philadelphia in the 1880s had become an industrial giant – coaltown, steeltown, railtown, milltown, seaport, all rolled into one. Its population was approaching one million, more and more of the newcomers being recent immigrants willing to do the worst jobs at the lowest pay. In retrospect, its most distinguished resident was probably Walt Whitman, the poet who embraced the coming of age of a lusty, egalitarian American democracy.

Professionally and socially, Philadelphia remained deeply conservative. Sons followed their fathers into law, banking, wholesaling, and medicine, inherited their mansions on Rittenhouse Square, sometimes virtually inherited their teaching chairs at the university. To get ahead in genteel Philadelphia you had to be either a born Philadelphian or a certified one, the stamp of approval being a degree from the University of Pennsylvania.

Many American, Canadian, and British cities were similarly stratified in the late nineteenth century. Everywhere in an uncertain world it made sense to work with kin and kind, not people from far away of whom one knew little. 'No man from Kansas is going to examine my bladder,' a Proper Philadelphian once exclaimed, rejecting the services of a hospital intern. The chauvinism had a sort of medical basis: for the first two-thirds of the century, many physicians would have agreed that the functions of Philadelphians' bladders could be influenced by local conditions, especially the climate. Maybe a Kansan would not have enough intimate knowledge of the locale, the region. Out in Kansas there would have been equal doubts about the qualifications of Pennsylvania-trained doctors. And Osler noted that the diagnosis of tuberculosis was more difficult in Philadelphia than in Montreal because of the possibility of confusing it with malaria in the American city.[11]

In its first hundred and twenty years, the University of Pennsylvania's medical school, one of the best in the United States, had appointed only one faculty member who was not a Pennsylvanian or an alumnus. Most professors were both. The sole exception had done some of his training at the school. 'Inbreeding of a faculty could hardly go farther,' the official history notes.[12]

Quality had not necessarily suffered. Philadelphia and Pennsylvania generated a group of remarkably talented physicians and surgeons through much of the nineteenth century, many of whom won national fame for their work at Penn or its archrival, Jefferson Medical College. Generations of Philadelphia doctors bore famous names – Gross, Agnew, Pepper, Stillé, Wood, Hays, Leidy, Tyson, Keen, Mitchell – blue ribbons of accomplishment and promise. One distinguished graduate wrote seriously of nepotism as 'a form of paternal pride seen in all successful institutions.'[13] Philadelphia arguably remained America's leading medical center.

After the Civil War, the city's medical elite recognized the importance of keeping the university in the vanguard. In 1870 they were instrumental in its decision to move across the Schuylkill River to a spacious new campus in West Philadelphia. In 1874 Dr William Pepper *secundus* (there would be four generations of medical Peppers, plus a sprinkling of Pepper brewers, lawyers, and politicians) took the lead in fundraising to build the first university-owned hospital in America. Pepper and Horatio C. Wood, the ninth-generation Pennsylvanian who was Professor of Therapeutics and Nervous Diseases, then led a movement, against fierce conservative resistance, to reform Penn's teaching. They followed Harvard's move towards a longer term, sequenced courses, and, most controversially, the addition of a third year. Philadelphia would not be outpaced by Boston. Nor, if it could help it, by nearby Baltimore, whose elite were drawing up plans to create a great university, hospital, and medical school, thanks to an amazing $7 million benefaction from merchant prince Johns Hopkins. Pepper became provost of the University of Pennsylvania in 1881 and immediately launched a new round of fundraising, lab building, and general university expansion.

In 1884 one of the medical luminaries of Philadelphia, Alfred Stillé, retired as professor of theory and practice of medicine. Provost Pepper succeeded him in that chair, leaving his lesser chair of clinical medicine vacant. For it, the trustees considered three local prospects, all graduates of the university. Faculty opinion was divided, with no great enthusiasm for any candidate.

One day, at Philadelphia's well-regarded national weekly, the *Medical News*, a group got talking about this situation after their editorial meeting. Why hadn't the medical committee of the board of trustees gone farther afield, looking at talent in other places? Montreal's Osler was mentioned as a possible candidate, probably by the *News*'s editor, Minis Hays, who, as part of his paper's expanding range, had been using the Canadian as his Montreal correspondent. Samuel W. Gross, a Jefferson Medical College surgeon, had attended the London medical congress in 1881 and had either met Osler or heard that his presentation had been a great success. He too was enthusiastic. James ('Urinary Jimmy') Tyson, the professor of pathology and dean of the faculty, also knew Osler but thought it was probably too late to stop the trustees, and in any case Osler was in Europe. The group pressed Tyson, arguing that Penn should find the very best man for its appointment. If a man from Canada would be examining Philadelphian bladders, so be it. Tyson finally agreed to look into the matter.[14]

His only colleague left in town was Horatio C. Wood, temperamentally an enthusiast for reform. Wood volunteered to go to Montreal to sound out opinion about Osler. He visited one of the French hospitals first and found that Osler was highly regarded there – a fine comment on the standing in the city of a doctor who did not speak French – and he then had the opinion reinforced by house staff at the Montreal General. When Frank Shepherd found Wood lunching with the General men he taxed him with having come to spy out the land: 'He admitted the fact, and then asked me about Osler, and he heard the truth. He went home convinced that Osler was the man.'[15]

Osler was working in Leipzig when a letter came from Tyson asking if he would let his name stand as a candidate for the Philadelphia chair. The approach was a complete surprise to him, and at first he thought some of his friends were playing a joke. Then he thought long and hard, weighing friendships and opportunities in Montreal against even greater opportunities at the historic school in the American metropolis. The teaching income would be about the same as in Montreal. 'Of course the temptations are the larger centre and the prospects of consulting work,' he told Ogden. And to Shepherd he wrote: 'After 10 years growth in a place the roots get pretty deep, but I hope I am not too old for transplanting.' Years later, he said that he finally made up his mind by tossing a coin. It fell 'heads' for Philadelphia. When he went to telegraph his decision, he found he had no money, having left his only piece of silver 'as it had fallen' on the table: 'It seemed like an act of Providence directing me to remain in Montreal. I half decided to follow the cue. Finally I concluded that inasmuch as I had placed the decision to chance I ought to abide by the turn of the coin, and returned to my hotel for it and sent the telegram.' Osler may have reasoned that whatever the Americans decided he would not lose, for the possibility of his leaving would spur McGill into a counteroffer.[16]

The Philadelphia situation turned on the judgment of Silas Weir Mitchell, one of the city's and the country's most renowned physicians. Philadelphia born and bred, now in his early sixties, Mitchell was internationally recognized both for his advanced neurological research, arising from a study of gunshot wounds in the Civil War, and as a society doctor who had invented a famous 'rest-cure' for the nervously troubled. He was also an accomplished novelist and poet, a Renaissance or Enlightenment man in the Franklin tradition. One of Mitchell's later novels, *Hugh Wynne*, set in revolutionary Philadelphia, sold more than half a million copies. Mitchell was rich, socially very conservative, a connoisseur of fine food, madeira, cigars, and sophisticated conversation, and a trustee of the University of Pennsylvania. He was traveling in Europe in the summer of 1884. When Osler agreed to stand as a candidate, Tyson and Wood asked Mitchell to interview him. If Osler was acceptable to the grandest Philadelphian, all the obvious questions about his being a stranger, literally a foreigner, would be settled.

Mitchell and Osler spent the evening of July 6 together in London.

'Saw Dr. Osler – pleased,' Mitchell jotted in his travel diary and, according to Osler, cabled home: 'All right! Elect Osler.' In the fullness of later success, Osler playfully amplified the occasion:

> Dr Mitchell ... and his good wife were commissioned to 'look me over,' particularly with reference to personal conditions. Dr Mitchell said there was only one way in which the breeding of a man suitable for such a position, in such a city as Philadelphia, could be tested: – give him cherry pie and see how he disposed of the stones. I had read of the trick before and disposed of them genteelly in my spoon – and got the Chair![17]

It was not exactly that simple, though Osler had, as it were, gone to the core of the matter, and in later years did maintain that this had been the most fortunate day of his life. He and Mitchell had instantly realized that they were kindred spirits. Nonetheless, the Philadelphians gathered other expert opinion on the outsider's qualifications. R.H. Fitz of Harvard, which had also thought of approaching Osler, was cautious:

> With the highest opinion of his qualifications and the knowledge that he is regarded as one of the strongest men in the school, and the information that he occupies a conspicuous position among the younger men as a practitioner, I am in the dark as to his personal relation to students ... The element of uncertainty must exist, and your School should have a man prominent in your own city, if possible ... Montreal expects to lose him sooner or later. He makes an admirable presentation of a subject to the association for the advancement of science. He was admirable in his speeches at the dinner lately given at the McGill celebration.

Then Osler's highly placed acquaintances weighed in with impressive testimonials. He had support from Sanderson, Bastian, and William Gowers in England and from New York's Austin J. Flint, who ranked with Mitchell as a distinguished senior in the American profession. 'Judging by his manner of speaking at a meeting of the New York Pathological Society, I think there cannot be any doubt as to his being a successful oral teacher,' Flint wrote. 'I know of no one who could offer better promise of filling the chair of clinical medicine at your institution.' Gowers, an outstanding neurologist, wrote that no English physician of the same standing had achieved a wider or higher reputation. Minis Hays made sure that his fellow Americans knew of the importance of Osler's fellowship in the Royal College of Physicians; and Osler's invitation to give the Royal College's prestigious Goulstonian Lectures in 1885, an unprecedented honor for a Canadian, was immediately made known.[18]

The icing on the cake came from Mitchell, who had made more inquiries about Osler in England, corresponded with him further, read his testimonials, and on August 17 sent from Switzerland a powerful, revealing statement to his fellow trustees:

> His testimonials ... are of no ordinary character and show that he occupies a quite exceptional position in the eyes of some of the best thinkers among the English physicians. The estimate of him in Canada is singularly high ... Personally he is a gentleman of good breeding, – the son of an English Clergyman resident in Canada, a good linguist, an agreeable and most interesting companion, full of ambitious enterprise, and said to possess a remarkable power to attract and influence students ... His contributions to Medicine are quite numerous and have been much esteemed. As to these and the estimate in which he is held in Montreal and in England, I may leave the documents he presents to speak. As I have seen him, it is more important that I should assure you that everything which can be learned from seeing him socially goes to satisfy me that he is not overrated in the letters of his friends ... I am most anxious about this matter and have carefully weighed every word of this letter, in the hope that it will seriously influence your vote.

Mitchell added that all but one of the medical faculty favored Osler. Their second choice was Juan Guiteras, Cuban born, but trained and teaching in Philadelphia. 'Both are foreigners,' Mitchell concluded. 'But I ought to add that Dr. Osler impressed me as being altogether American in his views and ways.'[19]

McGill tried to keep him. The faculty offered to raise the fees he could collect, raise his fixed salary from $500 to $1,600, and create for him a chair of pathology and comparative pathology. His teacher and mentor, Palmer Howard, wrote eloquently of the sense of loss they would feel if he went:

> The thought of losing you stuns us, and we feel anxious to do all that we can as sensible men to keep you amongst us, not only on account of your abilities as a teacher, your industry and enthusiasm as a worker, your personal qualities as a gentleman, a colleague and a friend; not only on account of the work you have already done in and for the school, but also because of the capabilities we recognize in you for future useful work, both in original investigation which shall add reputation to McGill and in systematic teaching of any of the branches of Medical Science you may care to cultivate; and finally because we have for years felt that vitalizing influence upon us individually exercised by personal contact with you – analagous to that produced by a potent ferment.[20]

Knowing he would probably go, hoping he might not, his colleagues in the Canada Medical Association, elected him their president for 1885.

There was some suspense and more lobbying pending the Penn trustees' decision in October. For a time, Osler and McGill thought he would go south on a one-year trial basis. On October 7, 1884, by ballot of the trustees of the University of Pennsylvania, he was unanimously elected to the chair of clinical medicine. A McGill student remembered Osler pacing back and forth as he tried to explain his regret at leaving, and finally saying, 'Gentlemen – there is no use talking. I must admit that I am leaving McGill for a larger field through *ambition*.' Fifty Montreal physicians attended a dinner to honor the man Palmer Howard toasted as 'the one single disciple of pure science in their midst,' an individual who possessed the instinct of 'social goodness,' and, to boot, the discoverer of 'Osler's granules' in the blood. The students gave him a gold watch and, *en masse*, escorted him to the station.[21]

News that a dark horse, a foreign one at that, had won the race for Pepper's chair astonished many of the Penn medical students and some of the staff.

How could an outsider be better than any Philadelphia candidate? How could a foreigner be better than any American? Osler had a strange, halting, and sometimes clipped way of speaking, probably made worse by jitters in the new setting. His early lectures contrasted poorly with the silver-tongued fluency of his predecessor. 'Every sentence began with a very English "Ah!"' a colleague remembered of an early clinical talk, which did not impress the students. The gossip was that Osler had deliberately picked up speech affectations in England. In fact he had become very conscious of the distinctive high-pitched and nasal American accent, realized that as a Canadian he talked that way too, and may have been trying to change his voice. Perhaps it was literally affected as he attempted to make it borderless, what we would now call mid-Atlantic. Others noted distinctively Canadian usages. With patients, 'instead of asking them a direct question he would generally make a statement followed by an interrogatory grunt, for instance, instead of asking "How are you today?" he would say, "You are better today, eh-,"' one listener remembered. 'I have often noticed that a good many Canadians have this way of putting a leading question.'[22]

His very first lecture at Pennsylvania, the introductory address to the students on October 1, 1884, was a gradgrind effort by any standards, probably a real clunker. It was never published – a rarity in Osler's career – and did not deserve publication. But student grumbling, less serious than the problems of his first year in Montreal, soon subsided. The Americans concluded that while Osler was not the university's most brilliant speaker, he seemed to know his stuff. 'To use a student phrase,' one of them remembered, 'he was "up" – that is, he knew his subject and knew how to teach what he knew, and no one knew a subject better than he did when a show-down of knowledge was to be made.'[23] 'When he drawled out an "Ah-h-h-h,"' another wrote, 'he was stalling for the right word and always found it.' As senior students followed him around on the wards and into the autopsy room, they began to realize they had in Osler a teacher as powerful as the faculty's great American naturalist, Joseph Leidy:

His first ward class was an eye-opener. In it he fairly frolicked in enthusiastic delight, and in a few moments had every man intensely interested and avid for more. Every new specimen that he came to at autopsy, and every interesting manifestation of disease in the living, was to him a treasure, and just as Leidy saw in every flower and stone and bone and worm and rhizopod an inner beauty, so Osler, to change my metaphor, was as the light-hearted child who finding a field of daisies shouts his delight so exultingly that all the other children become interested and gleefully shout with him.

Osler did more than any other man of his day in this city to teach all men that disease is not a horrid thing that some people, called medical men, have to study to earn a living, but a pursuit which a properly trained mind can follow with as keen enjoyment and uplift as an artist can study great pictures or a musician can hear great masters. Before Osler came the student was prone to regard cancer as a cancer; when Osler left the student studied it as an aggregation of cells possessing untold mysteries to be unravelled.[24]

His new senior colleagues welcomed Osler with a round of dinner parties. Dr Hayes Agnew went further and offered what was said to be the greatest courtesy a Philadelphian could extend to a stranger, a seat in his pew at church. Agnew thought a Mrs Osler would also be attending and was famously puzzled to garner from the Canadian that his missing spouse was either pregnant or a Buddhist (the two versions of this story obviously stem from a hand gesture). Strange foreign ways. The Philadelphians did not know how to pronounce his name either. O-sler or Ossler? he was asked. And his reply was straight from Wonderland: 'I will answer to Hi! or to any loud cry.' He attended other Philadelphia churches only to listen to the voices of preachers, apparently in the hope of continuing to improve his own.[25]

He found the Philadelphians 'very kind, but they don't come up to the Northern (Canadian) standard.'[26] His relations with all of them were cordial, and with some, old and young, he formed lifelong friendships. Weir Mitchell became virtually another medical father-figure. As well, Osler spent long hours in conversation with old Alfred Stillé, who had been a student of Pierre Louis in Paris and a pioneer in distinguishing typhoid from typhus fever. He became 'Uncle Osler' to Dr James C. Wilson's children, and a beloved mentor to a young resident, George Dock. Dr and Mrs Samuel W. Gross carried on sumptuous Sunday entertaining in the tradition of Gross's late father, a nationally famous surgeon, and made Osler one of their most welcome guests. In the Gross home he could get a good cup of afternoon tea, perhaps because of the Boston upbringing of Mrs Gross, a great-granddaughter of Paul Revere. Mrs Gross must have been struck on occasion by the strong physical resemblance between Osler and her husband – the same thin face and deep-set eyes, the same receding hairline, the same drooping mustache – the main difference being Osler's comparative youth.

William Pepper, Philadelphia's medical and academic dynamo, was always kind. Stories of emnity or rivalry between the two, of Philadelphia not being big enough for both of them, seem to have been rooted in little more than the normal buzz of academic and medical malice. Harvey Cushing later sloppily repeated some of the innuendoes in his *Life* of Osler, and eventually apologized to offended Philadelphians.[27] 'Osler himself was incapable of appreciating rivalry if rivalry there was and Pepper's position was too secure to have permitted any thought of jealously for the growing popularity of his junior,' Cushing in fact had concluded in his private notes. He also noted, completely without elucidation, 'WO protected Pepper in his scandal.' Nothing has been located about any Pepper scandal – only one tale from a second-hand source of Penn students complaining about Pepper's casual, provostial approach to lecturing and comparing it unfavorably with Osler's thoroughness and scholarship. Osler summed up Pepper's shortcomings in one elusive sentence: 'He was human, and to those of a man he added the failings of a college president.'[28]

In a medical school dominated by a man of Pepper's energies, and by several other vigorous Philadelphians, Osler would not play the leading role he had as registrar and young turk in Montreal. As professor of clinical medicine, he was junior to the teachers of the preclinical subjects and gave no large courses of didactic lectures. His teaching role was confined to clinical work – clinical lectures, ward rounds, whatever he might make of autopsies; and even in the university's hospital, Pepper, the senior professor, had precedence. Osler's basic salary from the university was $1,000, one-third that of the senior chairs. He always managed to double it with fees from extra courses.

Osler was a dutiful faculty man in Philadelphia, but other than serving on a committee that abolished graduation theses, he made no attempt to force the pace of change. Pepper, whose apprenticeship in the dead house and views on medical education were very much like Osler's, was carrying that ball as best he could. His problem was that reform still had a long way to go at the medical school. For fear that students would not come, the formal admission standard implemented in 1881, a one-page essay in English plus a written exam in basic physics, was less rigorous than the Latin-based requirement of 1767. High school graduation was still not a condition of admission, and although a fourth year had been added to the medical curriculum, it was an option hardly anyone took.

The University of Pennsylvania's new campus was a raw and ugly place. The faculty's labs already seemed inadequate, and the university hospital was small, unfinished, and relatively poorly organized and equipped. The Department of Medicine remained divided between young and old, reformers and conservatives, in what one member called a state of 'seething inertia.' H.C. Wood thought the university's veterinary students were getting a better education than its medical students. In his maiden speech at Pennsylvania, Osler indicated his preference for a system of clinical clerks and dressers in medical education. But no significant changes occurred in the Philadelphians' way of organizing their hospitals.

A strong feeler about the chair of clinical medicine at Harvard, only eighteen months into his Philadelphia stay, strongly tempted Osler. 'I should like to live in Boston, and I should feel more comfortable in a university with standards higher than those of the Univ. of Penn.,' he wrote to Harvard's Bowditch, 'but I am, I fear, tied and bound here. I dread another move so soon. Consultation work is beginning in earnest & I can rely upon a rapid increase in income. But what influences me most strongly is the possession here of really first class clinical opportunities. With the completion of the organization of the Univ. Hospital, with wards at the City Hospital and at the Nervous Dispensary, I shall be in command of a material unequalled in richness & variety in any Medical School in the country. I must be content to work on here and hope for a gradual elevation in the standard.'[29]

The clinical material consisted of patients on the wards of the Hospital of the University of Pennsylvania, patients at the Orthopaedic Hospital and Infirmary for Nervous Diseases (an institution dominated by Weir Mitchell), and, above all, patients at the Philadelphia Hospital, the vast complex of almshouse, city hospital, and insane asylum on the old Blockley estate hard by the new university campus in West Philadelphia. With some two thousand inhabitants, all of them charity cases, 'Blockley' was almost as rich in specimens as Berlin's Charité, Vienna's Krankenhaus, or Cootes Paradise in Dundas, Ontario.

As in Montreal, Osler preached the gospel of clinicopathology, showing equal interest in the dead and living. He was happy to do autopsies on the busy Pepper's patients at the university hospital and, in passing, to set up the hospital's first laboratory at his own expense.[30] In the Blockley dead house Osler seems to have ignored procedural protocol, bypassing the two designated pathologists and simply doing whatever autopsies interested him. The Blockley residents, younger colleagues, and students almost literally came running when Osler was about to do autopsies. One of them left an excellent description:

> Osler with his own and any other resident that could get away from his wards repaired to the autopsy room about two p.m. There were three or four tables in the small room – The attendant would place a body on each table. Osler would take one, his resident another & one or two other residents the remaining one or two. After the thorax & abdomen were opened Osler would view the organs in situ the residents following him from body to body. Then we would all return to the task of removing the organs & placing them on platters. Then Osler would examine the groups of organs in turn going over every one of them in the minutest detail. His joy at finding something new or unusual was quickly shared with and enjoyed by us – I

can see him now with his head bent over the table suddenly exclaim '"hoity-toity" boys look at this.'

Sometimes the exclamation may have been sharper or chagrined. Students recalled that Osler was never afraid to admit mistakes. At the end of one busy day on the wards at Blockley, he did a 'rather hasty' examination of a woman admitted with pneumonia, noticed a little dullness on the left side, and passed on. The patient died suddenly the next day. 'To our mortification,' he wrote, they found the patient's chest full of fluid. Osler was sure she could have been saved by timely aspiration. He was probably again embarrassed ten days after giving a clinical lecture on an Irishman with all the signs of pneumonia to learn that the sputum contained tuberculosis bacilli – but it was a kind of progress to be able to correct the diagnosis before death.[31]

In wonderful pictures taken in the Blockley dead house in 1887 we see the young men and one woman, dressed in hospital uniform (said to have been left over from the Civil War) or street clothes, a few wearing aprons, cuffs rolled back, bare hands exposed to all manner of infection, clustering around Osler. In a close-up we see him, sleeves rolled up, inspecting human flesh to find something new or unusual. We cannot see the *Verruca necrogenica* (postmortem or cadaver warts) that he has on his hands, small tubercular nodules caused by the tuberculosis bacilli to which he is otherwise immune. When he grows a new wart, unless he decides to study it for publication, he treats it with oleate of mercury and it soon disappears.[32]

The Blockley 'post-house,' also known as the 'green-room' or 'greenhouse,' was a new two-storey building, opened in 1886. We cannot tell from the photos whether an overflow crowd is looking down from a floor above through the skylight, as sometimes happened. Nor do we know if 'Cadaver Charlie,' the attendant, has installed the severed lunatic's head, with crossed femurs behind it, that had presided over operations in the old autopsy room.[33]

Postmortems could be done immediately on those who died without family or friends. Otherwise consent was required. When Dr Osler wanted

to do an autopsy, undoubtedly to advance the cause of science and humanity, his helpers worked hard to get permission:

> It was considered a distinct disgrace if a resident failed to get an autopsy. We
> travelled to the most remote districts of Philadelphia at great trouble &
> inconvenience to appeal to the families of patients ... If the resident whose
> patient had died failed in his effort the case was invariably referred to my
> room-mate Dr Caspar Sharpless who had an uncanny ability in securing the
> necessary consent when all others failed. All this effort was for Osler. It
> mattered not whether the patient was his – Osler was going to make the
> autopsy & if Osler wanted to make the autopsy that was all sufficient.

When all else failed, Osler would go to a patient's home and plead to be
allowed to make an autopsy there. Pushing his luck, he might then ask to
take an interesting organ back to the university for teaching or display
purposes. If refused, he would ask to at least borrow it.[34]

His passion to dissect interesting cases was of course not unique. It was
said of the great Philadelphia natural scientist Joseph Leidy, who had discovered *Trichinella spiralis* in 1846, that when presented with a dinner of
terrapin at the Biological Club, instead of eating the creatures, he dissected them and discovered three new intestinal parasites. 'Never give Leidy
anything that is edible and worth dissecting,' Weir Mitchell observed. 'We
all know where it will go.'[35]

Complaints about postmortem abuses reached the Blockley trustees, both
from the public and from the pathologists whom Osler and his acolytes
tended to ignore. Before Osler, Philadelphia's most prominent pathologist
and the official pathologist at Blockley was Henry B. Formad, an excitable,
eccentric immigrant from Central Europe, who conspicuously lacked
social graces and standing (and scientific judgment, it turned out, when he
decided to challenge Robert Koch's bacteriology). Whether or not he was
neglecting his terrain, Formad found himself sharing it with Osler and was
not entirely happy. Apparently at Formad's urging, Blockley gradually tight-
ened its procedures to rein in Osler and the residents. The control was
never perfect. After the crowds had departed from Osler's sessions, Charlie

would return organs to the corpses, often hurriedly. When one autopsied body was exhumed on suspicion of death by foul play, it was found to contain three livers.[36] Residents observed that many specimens kept for the museum were ruined when patient-assistants, or possibly Cadaver Charlie, drank the supply of preservative, replacing it with water.[37]

Osler still had to make money from treating the living, in fact had been attracted to Philadelphia partly by that prospect. He had a small office and waiting room in his quarters at 131 South Fifteenth Street, a fashionable address just south of Chestnut. He surprised the Americans by having a consulting practice only. As in Montreal, it developed slowly. Many of Osler's acquaintances doubted that his heart was in it; he seemed much more in his element at the Blockley dead house. Still, as he had told his Boston friends, by 1886 his practice was developing in earnest. His day-books show that normally he saw at least four to six patients several times a week, usually in the mornings, and that he was now charging ten dollars for a basic visit.

Weir Mitchell referred a number of patients to him. Osler was also beginning to be consulted by other physicians and by doctors' relatives, on his way to becoming a 'doctor's doctor.' In July 1886 Philadelphia's dean of American surgeons, William Williams Keen, frantically telegraphed for help with his suddenly ill wife at their cottage on Cape Cod. Osler came, but neither the physician nor the surgeon could do anything. Keen was grief-stricken. 'You sat with me long into the night listening while I bared my very soul to you,' Keen wrote Osler thirty years later. 'What a comfort you were to me you cannot guess.'[38]

Osler did not bill Keen or most other doctors he knew. The loss of income would have been compensated for by other referrals. In Philadelphia Osler's total income, including his practice and his editorial writing for the *Medical News*, rose to about $5,000 annually, reaching $7,330 by his fifth year, 1888–9. His account books show several $1,000 dispersals to brother E.B., probably repaying the cost of his graduate education. In 1886–7 he gave Marian Francis $1,000, perhaps to help her raise the brood, perhaps to repay a loan.

One morning in 1885 Osler received a telegram from a Canadian friend, Richard Maurice Bucke, a McGill graduate who was superintendent of the London, Ontario, Insane Asylum. 'Please see Walt and let me know how he is,' the telegram read. 'Who is Walt, and where does he live?' Osler wired back. Then he remembered how Bucke, at a McGill dinner, had once startled the group into doubts about his sanity by praising an American poet, Walt Whitman, as being in a class with Darwin, Buddha, and Mahomet. Bucke's next telegram supplied Whitman's address, in Camden, New Jersey, a ferry ride across the Delaware River.

Whitman was in his sixty-sixth year and had moved to Camden to be near family after an 1873 stroke had left him slightly paralyzed. Osler found his way to Whitman's unpretentious frame house and was ushered in to see an old man practically buried in a fantastic literary clutter. Many years later he described 'the good grey poet':

> Walt Whitman was a fine figure of a man who had aged beautifully, or more properly speaking, majestically, with a large frame and well-shaped, well-poised head, covered with a profusion of snow-white hair which mingled in the cheeks with a heavy, long beard and moustache. The eyebrows were thick & shaggy & the man seemed lost in a hirsute canopy. The grey eyes had a kindly sympathetic look; the skin was fresh & clear, wrinkled only in the forehead. The nose was large & straight; the mouth was hidden by the moustache. Though high-pitched, his voice was clear and musical, and the words uttered slowly in short sentences ... I could not get much from him about his health. My visit was a surprise as he had not heard from Dr Bucke ... I felt a bit embarrassed, as professional advice seemed superfluous, and our points of contact were few and easily exhausted. I left with the pleasant impression of having seen a splendid old man, and a room the grand disorder of which filled me with envy.

Osler knew nothing about Whitman. That evening after dinner at the club, he opened a copy of Whitman's *Leaves of Grass*. The free verse and the unconventional ideas repelled him: 'Whether the meat was too strong, or whether it was the style of cooking – 'twas not for my pampered palate, accustomed to Plato and Shakespeare and Shelley and Keats.'[39]

Writing in 1919, Osler remembered that he saw Whitman a second time and concluded there was nothing he could do for him professionally: 'His habits were most abstemious, and the man's ailments were those incident to this age.' In fact, Whitman was worried about his eyesight that year, and in October Osler had him examined by a noted ophthalmologist. According to Whitman, the visit was satisfactory – he was not going blind. According to Osler, writing to Ogden, there were signs of deep-seated trouble: 'Walt's eyes are better ... He has ext[ernal] Strab[ismus] & absence of patellar reflex. I expect he has had pretty intimate relations with those prostitutes about whom he sings so joyously.'[40]

Osler found Bucke himself to be a more interesting study when a few months later the Canadian doctor came to visit Whitman. Bucke fashioned his hair, beard, and dress to imitate Whitman. Over dinner at the Rittenhouse Club, his eyes dilated fanatically, almost embarrassingly, as he explained to Osler and other medical friends how *Leaves of Grass* had enlightened him to a new plane of spiritual being. While Osler was also a hero-worshiper, he found it 'a new experience ... to witness such absolute idolatry.'[41]

Osler occasionally went over to Camden with medical friends or admirers of Whitman (Weir Mitchell had been one of Whitman's patrons), and he saw him repeatedly after the poet suffered one or two small strokes in June 1888. Osler once prescribed wine and cocoa for Whitman and urged that constipation be countered, but otherwise treated him mostly with cheerful encouragement. Whitman did not have venereal disease; he was suffering from old age and perhaps the tuberculosis that eventually killed him.

In crotchety moods Whitman would question the doctor's easy optimism, yet he seemed generally pleased with his physician. 'He's a fine fellow and a wise one, I guess: wise, I am sure – he has the air of assurance,' Whitman told his amanuensis. 'I do not fancy the jaunty way in which he seems inclined to dismiss the troubles. Still, that may all be a part of his settled policy – I do not object to cheer. I don't know whether it's from getting down to hard pan or is a theory, but whatever, Osler pursues it.'

Whitman came to like Osler, humanly as well as professionally, and studied his appearance as well as his personality: 'Osler is fine looking: examined, he gains on you: you realize him: his forehead is beautiful: have you noticed the mobility of his eye? Osler, though a Canadian, is yet, as I put it, Southern and French.'[42] It would be many years before Whitman's poetry gained on Osler. And never did he imagine that some day he too would be the object of 'absolute idolatry' similar to Bucke's adoration of the Camden bard.

Another doctor followed Osler to Philadelphia, at least in spirit. In November 1884 the *Medical News* ran a meandering, mildly salacious editorial by an American acquaintance of Osler's on an uncommon form of 'vaginismus,' or spasm of the vaginal muscles. There was a long medical tradition, originating in cautionary tales about the perils of clandestine intercourse in churches, of reporting instances of vaginismus making inter-course impossible or, occasionally, causing the penis to be held captive. Some years earlier in Montreal a case had been reported at the Medico-Chirurgical Society and several members had talked about cases they had seen.

It is hard to imagine that these discussions by the medical men did not have obvious sexual over- or undertones. In any event, the *Medical News* piece bestirred Osler's other self, Egerton Y. Davis, the former U.S. Army surgeon from Caughnawaga, Quebec, to take pen in hand to describe a case he had seen in England. A big, burly coachman had been caught in bed with a wee maid, Davis wrote, and they could not be separated:

When I arrived I found the man standing up and supporting the woman in his arms, and it was quite evident that his penis was locked in her vagina, and any attempt to dislodge it was accompanied by much pain on the part of both. It was, indeed, a case of 'De cohesione in coitu.' I applied water, and then ice, but ineffectually, and at last sent for chloroform, a few whiffs of which sent the woman to sleep, relaxed the spasm, and released the captive penis, which was swollen, livid, and in a state of semi-erection, which did not go down for several hours, and for days the organ was extremely sore. The woman recovered rapidly, and seemed none the worse.

Davis displayed his Shakespearian learning by noting that this was a splendid picture of Iago's 'beast with two backs,' and aired his biblical knowledge by speculating that such cases might explain how Phinheas, the son of Eleazar, was able to thrust a javelin through both the Israelite and the Midianite woman in the inner room, thus saving Israel from the plague.

Davis's letter found its way to the *Medical News*, possibly through Ross and Molson in Montreal, and was not intercepted in proof. It was published in the December 13, 1884 issue. At the time it elicited no special comment. In March, 1886, 'E.Y.D.' struck again, less fancifully, in a letter to the *Medical News* pointing to the absurdities in a recent claim that electrotherapy had somehow transformed an interstitial tubal pregnancy back into a normal intrauterine one. Davis did not think that electricity, though it might move locomotives, could move embryos along the 'Chemin de Fallopius.'[43]

The Philadelphians duly enrolled Osler, not Davis, in their local professional societies and dinner clubs, and he seemed to find more time than any two men to attend meetings and give presentations. As with the Med-Chi in Montreal, he became a bulwark of the Philadelphia Pathological Society, saying or showing something useful at virtually every meeting. As a fellow of the College of Physicians of Philadelphia he formed a special attachment, based on love and duty, to its extremely good library and became a lifelong enthusiast for building the collection. (He had not taken much interest in McGill's library, remembered Shepherd, who had been the librarian; but he did give it his very good collection of recent medical journals when he left.) He gave papers at the Philadelphia Neurological Society, enjoyed the less formal functions of the Biological Club, the Medical Club, and the Mahogany Tree (for high achievers with literary interests), and hung his hat at the Rittenhouse and University clubs. The conservative sense of tradition in Philadelphia, particularly the city's veneration of its medical Brahmins, had a strong appeal to the outsider from Canada. Philadelphia was indeed a 'Civitas Hippocratica.'[44]

From the Pennsylvania parish he moved back and forth to his homeland and out to the wider world, addressing current issues in medical knowledge and politics. He had been in Philadelphia for less than six months when he took leave to go to London to give the important Goulstonian Lectures at the Royal College of Physicians in early 1885. These were traditionally given by 'one of the four youngest doctors in physic' of the college. Osler chose malignant endocarditis as his subject, presenting a state-of-our-knowledge portrait of a little-known and hard-to-diagnose disease, based on the records of two hundred cases at the Montreal General. The lectures were a *tour de force* of pathological and clinical detail about a still-baffling condition. Osler showed his 1884 immersion in bacteriological studies by drawing attention to a micrococcal role in acute endocarditis, with the suitable caveat that only culturing and inoculating experiments, following Koch's methods, could ultimately settle the issue. 'We are only at the threshold of our inquiries,' he concluded.[45]

From practicing pathologist he transformed himself into a medical statesman for his presidential address, 'The Growth of a Profession,' to the Canadian Medical Association in September 1885. In a sweeping overview of medicine and medical education, he roundly denounced unrestricted competition among medical schools as leading to 'free trade in diplomas,' adding that 'free trade in this sense is synonymous with manslaughter.' Canada's tradition of state licensing of physicians through provincial medical boards had saved the profession from the abuses brought on by the wide-open American system, where virtually any quack or charlatan could produce a medical degree. Osler thought of the 'profession' as an organized corporate body, as professions were regarded in England. Professional bodies, such as medical boards, should be charged with maintaining standards, because medical schools had too great a conflict of interest. They simply could not be trusted. The future, Osler thought, lay in continued restraints on competition in medical education, including the closing of many of the weaker schools. Professors in all schools, he argued, had a continuing responsibility to be present at and active in professional organizations, 'to meet their brethren and give to them an account of their stewardship – for do they not hold their positions in trust? – and show by their work and ways that they merit the confidence reposed in them.'

To move into a new age, medical educators would have to find much money for buildings and equipment. 'We should learn a lesson from our brethren of the clergy,' Osler suggested, and obtain endowments from wealthy benefactors 'who feel, with Descartes, that the hope of the amelioration of many of the ills of humanity lies within our profession.' The obvious models were Donald Smith's benefactions to McGill, Pepper's fundraising at Pennsylvania, and Johns Hopkins's princely gift to Baltimore. As early as 1881, Osler had outlined a vision of a 'Model Hospital' and medical school at 'Otnorot' (read it backwards) so good 'that finally one could study better at Otnorot than in cultured and civilized Europe.'[46]

Osler went on from the CMA in 1885 to speak, along with Pepper, at the opening ceremonies for McGill's new medical building. These took place in October while Montreal was being ravaged by one of the worst smallpox epidemics in the history of urban North America. Osler knew that whatever their merits, Canadian medical licensing laws were not saving the children of French-Canadian Montreal from the antivaccination quackery, charlatanism, and ignorance that led to thousands of them dying unnecessarily.

In the 1880s the medical profession was being faced with an unsettling new challenge, as yet unfamiliar to the clergy. The demands of women for medical education were forcing each school to decide whether or not it would admit them. Most faculties and most student bodies, including McGill's and Pennsylvania's, remained closed to women. Apart from issues relating to competition and standards, most of the men would not feel comfortable with women present for their discussions of disorders of the genitalia, including conditions such as vaginismus.

In both Canada and Philadelphia one response to women's insistence had been to create separate women's medical colleges. Osler condemned this experiment for Canada, claiming that such schools would have few graduates because there was so little prospect of women being able to make a living in medicine: 'It is useless manufacturing articles for which there is no market, and in Canada the people have not yet reached the condition in which the lady doctor finds a suitable environment ... Even the larger cities can support only one or two; in fact, Quebec and Montreal have none, and in the smaller towns and villages of this country she would starve.'

But Osler in 1885 did not want to be understood to be 'in any way hostile' to the admission of women: 'On the contrary, my sympathies are entirely with them in the attempt to work out the problem as to how far they can succeed in such an arduous profession as that of medicine.' Compared with most of his colleagues, Osler was fairly progressive on the medical woman question. He almost certainly was teaching students from the Woman's Medical College of Pennsylvania in his hospital clinics, and we even see one woman, identified as Amelia Gilman, in the Blockley dead house picture.[47]

In other addresses Osler applauded the way dedicated women had been working to revolutionize nursing since the days of Florence Nightingale. He had nothing but admiration for the women at the forefront of the movement to replace ill-paid and often uncouth servants from the lower classes with well-mannered, professionally trained – and ill-paid – young women from the middle classes. It came to Blockley in the mid-1880s, when an English nurse, Alice Fisher, fought off local chauvinism and assaults of rotten eggs to bring Nightingale principles to the hospital, only to die suddenly of a heart attack. Nursing seemed to Osler to be women's natural role in health care; he would have much to say about nurses' qualifications and calling.

He cracked many jokes about nurses' attractiveness to doctors and vice versa. As for himself, there was a brief attraction to an unnamed woman (or women) in the early Philadelphia months, but the American women may have been too aggressive. 'I shall have a missus too before long,' Osler wrote to a Montreal friend just after arriving. 'These Yankee girls give a chap no option – it's come on whether you want to or not.' He evidently did not. 'He is only susceptible when idle,' cousin Marian told Jennette. He soon became endlessly busy in Philadelphia and carried on his bachelor routine, still chained by mistress medicine.[48]

How could the medical life be further improved? Osler wanted to spend his time consorting with the very best men in the field, not just the Philadelphians or the Canadians. The development of specialty organizations in American medicine was already well under way. In 1880 the American Surgical Association was formed as a closed-end society of top performers. Within a year Osler had suggested to James Tyson that specialists in medicine (what we now call internal medicine) should form a similar body. Others, including a professor at the University of Toronto, were thinking along the same lines, but nothing happened until a nasty political struggle developed over plans for the Ninth International Medical Congress, scheduled for Washington in 1887.

For almost forty years the American Medical Association (AMA) had been struggling to represent regular practitioners in the United States. Its energies had largely gone into waging war on quacks, sectarians such as homeopaths, and anyone else who refused to follow its formal codes of medical ethics. By the mid-1880s the AMA was pushing to become the profession's quasi-governing body, and in that capacity its president had invited the International Congress to meet in Washington. A special committee created by the AMA to organize the big event began to draw upon the talents of the best-known men in the profession, many of whom happened to be from the great eastern cities: New York, Philadelphia, Boston, Baltimore. But then it emerged that some of the co-opted New Yorkers were anathema to the AMA leadership because of a byzantine ethics dispute. Regionalism also reared its head. The AMA was Chicago-based and at its 1885 convention in New Orleans the delegates voted to disband the eastern-dominated congress committee and created a new one with representation from each state. The medico-political maneuvering involved strong personality conflicts, especially an AMA feeling that the former committee chair, John Shaw Billings, who worked in Washington as assistant surgeon to the army and as director of the army's medical museum and library, had been trying to run the congress show on behalf of eastern interests.

The Philadelphia medical establishment, including most of Osler's new friends and associates, balked at the AMA's high-handedness and, in their view, its parochialism in disbanding Billings' committee. Minis Hays and Pepper led the protest. Osler helped. The Philadelphians saw no reason why the still medically insignificant 'ranches of Texas, the prairies of Kansas, the mines of Colorado, and the forests and wheat fields of the great Northwest' should be officially represented in the planning of an international medical gathering. Their decision to boycott the new committee was endorsed by other leading eastern and Canadian medical men. The upshot of a year of intense controversy was a meeting in New York City in October 1885 at which seven prominent physicians, including Osler, Pepper, and Tyson from Philadelphia, decided to create a new organization.[49]

The Association of American Physicians (AAP) was to have only one hundred members, chosen by internal election. Its aim was the advancement of knowledge in medicine. 'We want an association in which there will be no medical politics and no medical ethics,' the acting chairman, Francis A. Delafield, proclaimed to the first meeting, 'an association in which no one will care who are the officers and who are not; in which we will not ask from what part of the country a man comes, but whether he has done good work and will do more; whether he has something to say worth hearing, and can say it.' By 'no medical ethics' Delafield meant that honorable men had no need to subscribe to anyone else's formal codes. He could also have mentioned that there would be no border: for medical purposes, Canada was (and is) deemed by the Association of American Physicians to be part of America.

AMA loyalists thought the revolt of the 'Eminences' (which doomed the Washington congress to mediocrity) was just another form of eastern sectional snobbery. On the other hand, Philadelphia's Alfred Stillé declared that 'the men of genius, of learning, of skill, in a word of exceptional merit, decline to see themselves placed upon the same base level with men of no talent, attainments, or reputation.' William Welch, pathologist at the new Johns Hopkins University in Baltimore, who was the one-man arrangements committee for the inaugural meeting of the AAP, wrote that it was 'very pleasant, as there were brought together just the men whom I liked to become acquainted with.' Osler, a charter member of course, later referred to the meeting as the 'coming of age party of clinical medicine in America.' An elite had formed a new club, but as the AAP's historian concludes, 'a club of high purpose.' Weir Mitchell was its first president. Osler, whose purpose was sometimes to have fun, told a reporter that the retiring eminence, Delafield, was a fanatical baseball player who, not having time to play on teams, organized street urchins to play the game with him on vacant lots.[50]

Osler made one of the worst nonclinical mistakes of his career during the discussion of William T. Councilman's paper at the first meeting of the Association of American Physicians in June 1886. Councilman, a pathologist at Johns Hopkins University, gave a presentation on the blood of malaria victims. Like Alphonse Laveran in 1880 and several investigators since, Councilman had observed what appeared to be parasites in malarial blood. Councilman was not totally sure of his findings. Osler was even less sure, telling the group he had seen nothing in some cases, only inorganic specks in others.

Osler was fresh from having delivered the prestigious Cartwright Lectures to the alumni of the New York College of Physicians and Surgeons. These had been 'On Certain Problems in the Physiology of the Blood Corpuscles,' a review and elaboration of the blood platelet work Osler had been interested in for more than a decade (he stubbornly refused to speak of 'platelets,' using the French 'plaque' instead). As usual, he was up-to-date and perceptive in drawing attention to the platelets' role in clotting and to the likelihood of the bone marrow as the site of red-cell creation. Osler knew blood. So when he told the elite at the Association of American Physicians that he could not find organisms in malarial blood, they were probably not there.

But Councilman and another speaker suggested he should have tried staining his specimens. Osler had not used many samples; nor was it yet evident how to diagnose malarial blood; nor would Osler have seen much malaria in Montreal. He went back to the microscope that summer, spending long hours examining the blood of Blockley patients suspected of malaria. By September, he was eating crow in print: 'We have been able, without any difficulty, to find these bodies in cases of acute malaria, and the fact of their presence in the blood in this state can be readily demonstrated.' He put together a major presentation on the hematozoa of malaria, fully confirming others' observations of the parasite in its several forms, and arguing strongly that it did have a causal role. 'Two or three years ago, when I first read Laveran's papers,' he admitted, 'nothing excited my incredulity more than his description of the ciliated bodies. It seemed so improbable, and so contrary to all past experience, that flagellate organisms should occur in the blood. The work of the past six months has taught me a lesson on the folly of a skepticism based on theoretical conceptions and of preconceived notions drawn from a limited experience.'[51]

Malaria studies were still in their infancy – the mosquito's role in transmission of the parasite was not yet known – but had taken a huge leap forward. In difficult cases, blood testing could now verify the diagnosis of malaria, in most stages of which quinine was a specific treatment. On two occasions Osler was able greatly to relieve Philadelphians by showing that patients just arrived from the South had malaria rather than the dreaded yellow fever. His interest in malaria continued and by the end of the decade had blended with his other studies of blood cells as the foundation of a major paper on phagocytic action (the war of body cells and invaders), with special reference to malaria. He was still chastened, commenting on the appropriateness of skepticism 'in these days of hasty observation and of still hastier conclusions.'[52]

He had taken his time accumulating other research data, and through his first year in Philadelphia was still publishing studies in Canadian journals based mainly on his pathological work in Montreal. He offered 'Notes on the Morbid Anatomy of Pneumonia,' 'Notes on the Morbid Anatomy of Typhoid Fever,' a consideration of the duodenal ulcer, a study of aneurysm of the cerebral arteries, and more reports, spun off in spare moments, of unusual cases. While he continued to draw on his Montreal experience for the rest of his life – he seemed never to forget a case – he appeared to be losing interest in some of the traditional subjects. His paper on pneumonia tailed off feebly and was, he admitted, 'but a trifling value as a pathological contribution.' In his Philadelphia years, despite the vivid memories of his associates, he did far fewer autopsies: 162 at Blockley, compared with about 1,000 at Montreal General. Often the students seem to have done most of the dead-house work.

He was beginning to rechannel his energies in directions more clinical than pathological, more oriented to neurology and problems of therapeutics. The neurological work was done at the splendidly equipped new 110-bed home of the Orthopaedic Hospital and Infirmary for Nervous Diseases, where Osler saw far more patients with nervous problems than in Montreal. Most neurological disorders posed special problems for pathologically oriented investigators because underlying organic lesions could not be located. In 1887 Osler began a study of chorea, for example, which was broadly defined as uncontrollable muscle spasms, convulsions, twitching, and the traditional 'St Vitus dance' (*choreia*: Greek, dance). Chorea was without a discernible organic base, and it was not clear that it could be considered a clinical entity. Perhaps it was an outgrowth of children's 'growing pains'; perhaps it was a neurosis. Perhaps it was habit forming, or perhaps it did not exist.

Osler ingeniously crept up on the subject from pathology by drawing attention to the frequency of heart murmurs and endocarditis in choreic children, an important contribution to the clinical picture that tended to buttress the view of chorea as a distinct disease. He put together his data from a special follow-up study of the infirmary's patients (postcards were sent out asking them to return for tests), an early example of directed clinical research.[53] He then turned to the study of cerebral palsy in children, a paralysis which by definition did involve brain lesions. Part of the puzzle was to trace the origins of the damage to the motor system of the brain. Osler's analysis of 150 cases tended to stress traumatic causes, including injury caused by the clumsy use of forceps at birth. One of his footnotes directed readers to the ravages of Dr Slop's forceps in Laurence Sterne's

Tristram Shandy. During his cerebral palsy work Osler corresponded on the subject with the Viennese neurologist Sigmund Freud. No Freud-Osler letters have been located, but in Freud's 1897 monograph on infantile cerebral paralysis there are many references to Osler and considerable criticism of his understanding of the disease's etiology.

Osler tried to temper the bleak prognosis in most cases of cerebral palsy with optimism generated by reports from some of the early workers with the feeble-minded 'that with patient training and kind care many of these poor victims may be rescued from a condition of hopeless imbecility and reach a fair measure of intelligence and self-reliance.'[54] The more time he spent on the wards rather than in postmortem rooms, the more thought he gave to therapeutic problems. His reputation as a 'therapeutic nihilist' began to emerge in his Philadelphia years, but neither the term nor the changes Osler rang on it have been particularly well understood. He never subscribed to the extreme view that nothing could be done in the face of disease except wait for it to cure itself, or to the variant that eschewed all extreme, powerful, or heroic treatments. If a treatment could be shown to be effective by significant clinical experience or, better still, by demonstration of its physiological effectiveness (as Horatio C. Wood had argued in his major work on therapeutics), Osler would prescribe it. He supported almost any drug or therapy that obviously relieved suffering or helped to sustain the poor victims of incurable conditions.

It was wonderful that quinine had a specific action on the malaria parasite. Osler convinced himself from experience, aided by new blood-cell-counting devices, that iron supplements worked to relieve certain forms of anemia, especially chlorosis or 'green sickness,' a condition for which others often prescribed only better habits. He experimented repeatedly with one of the oldest workhorses in the pharmacopoeia, arsenic compounds, and published two articles endorsing the use of Fowler's solution (an arsenical) in certain forms of pernicious anemia where iron proved useless.[55]

In Philadelphia he abandoned the Montreal tradition of heavy internal medication for erysipelas and found his results just as good. Nothing worked for leukemia, he had found, whose periods of remission were entirely natu-

ral. If epileptic seizures were due to arterial spasms, as some thought, perhaps nitroglycerine would be useful. Weir Mitchell and other colleagues
were using it. 'Altogether, my experience has not been very encouraging,'
Osler reported in the *Journal of Nervous and Mental Disease* after a series of
nineteen cases. On the other hand the new synthetic coal-tar derivatives,
predecessors of aspirin, at first met with his enthusiastic approval as antifever
drugs. On the basis of twenty-nine cases, he reported in the *Therapeutic
Gazette* in 1887, 'I think we have in antifebrin a prompt and powerful
antifebrile agent, easy to take, and free from unpleasant effects. It has the
advantage also of cheapness.'[56]

There was no curative treatment for the major infectious diseases that
packed his wards. Pneumonia, typhoid fever, and tuberculosis carried off
patients with depressing, predictable regularity. 'A study of the history
of the treatment of pneumonia makes one almost despair of the future of
therapeutics,' Osler wrote in 1886. Therapeutic measures might have an
impact in at best 10 to 15 per cent of cases of typhoid fever. As for tuberculosis, 'the general hopelessness of the treatment of phthisis is shown by the
avidity with which new methods are sought after.' The 1887 antitubercu-
losis fad in Philadelphia hospitals was rectal injections of gas according to
Bergeon's methods. Osler veered between laughing at the absurdity of it
('as the enemy has not yielded to the attack *a fronte,* the tactics have
changed, and we are asked to assault him *a tergo*') and deploring the 'delirium of false' hopes caused by ignorant newspaper publicity.[57]

The therapeutic problem in infectious disease, Osler realized, was not
merely to sweep away useless or harmful measures. It was to find treatments that attacked the specific cause of the disease. If bacteria were the
specific causes, what worked to kill or even arrest the growth of bacteria?
The depressing answer, so far, was that nothing had been found. 'Not a
suggestion is made as to specific treatment, the goal toward which, in this
class of diseases, we are all working ... The outlook is not very encouraging
... So far, the determination of specific organisms in connection with particular diseases has done less than might have been anticipated in modify-
ing our therapeutics.'[58] Osler was optimistic about the long term, but the
antibiotic revolution did not come during his lifetime. What specifics ex-

isted for pneumonia, typhoid fever, tuberculosis? None. Nothing. Nihil. In this sense, every scientifically literate physician had to be a nihilist.

Osler and many of his colleagues were beginning to go further, were starting to question the efficacy of some of the symptomatic treatments in infectious disease, even those that seemed to work: 'New remedies, like new servants, seem always to do well at first, but, with the one as with the other, it takes time before the good and bad qualities can be discovered.' He had no sooner endorsed the new antipyretics than he was beginning to question those results. On careful statistical study – statistics had been a particular interest of Palmer Howard's back in Montreal – they seemed to alter the pattern of fever without achieving real reduction.[59] And what about the function of fever generally? As early as 1888 some German work was suggesting that fever might not be an unmixed evil, but rather a sign of the body's struggle against its invaders. In his Cartwright Lectures that year, the Johns Hopkins pathologist William Welch offered a number of challenges to conventional views about the debilitating effects of fever on the heart muscle and other organs. 'There is no more important question offered for solution,' Osler commented, 'than the definite determination of the respective action on the one hand of the high temperature, and on the other of the infective agent.' His suggestions that sponging and bathing, including the use of cold baths, might be the best antipyretic became more pointed.[60]

He continued to cling to his habit of bleeding certain pneumonia patients in the hope of relieving the strain on the heart. A false hope, he began to suspect, as case after case expired. By the end of 1888 he was admitting that the heroic measure had worked only once in more than a dozen cases, and he was wondering if the problem of heart strain in pneumonia was more than mechanical. But he still thought it a situation that justified resorting to this old heroic practice. A blind spot. Osler clearly understood the phenomenon of the *ignis fatuus*, or therapeutic will-o'-the-wisp, but could not bring himself to apply it to his own views on bleeding.[61] The Osler family had a strain of deep conservatism. In *Medical News* surveys of Philadelphia clinicians' treatments of pneumonia and typhoid fever, Dr Osler was generally in line with his colleagues in stressing diet, rest, and caution in most cases and strong interventions when necessary. But no one else still recommended the use of leeches to treat headache in the early stages of typhoid fever.[62]

On the other hand, bleeding and leeching were forms of quasi-surgical intervention. Knowing when to cut was part of medical expertise. With the wonderful advances in surgery since the 1870s, particularly the ability to work inside the abdomen, certain conditions involving fever, pain, perhaps jaundice, now pointed towards laparotomy. Osler the pathologist had seen the ravages caused by infection of the vermiform appendix. In an instantly classic paper at the first meeting of the Association of American Physicians, Reginald Fitz had put appendicitis on the clinical map, setting out the indications that would lead to appendectomy. With a few minor reservations, Osler was an early supporter of this life-saving surgical intervention. (Life-saving but not life-changing. The story was told of a medical meeting in Canada at which an elderly surgeon, learning of the operation, said that if everyone's appendix could be removed soon after birth, eventually people would be born without them. Osler noted that a like practice had been in universal use among a prominent people, but young Hebrews continued to be born with a prepuce as surely as young Gentiles.)[63]

Relatedly, over the years he had seen several cases of jaundice combined with intermittent fever that seemed to point towards obstruction of the common bile duct by gallstones. By the end of the decade, surgeons had a fair chance of being able to remove the blockage. In 1887 Osler recommended such a procedure for a forty-year-old woman at Blockley and was chagrined when nothing was found and the patient died from peritonitis on the third day. His statement about what followed – that 'friends removed the body at once to Jenkintown, but I fortunately was able to secure an autopsy' – probably hides one of the legendary stories. He found a stone lodged in the common duct, effectively out of surgical reach, and he kept the subject's organs for future reference.[64]

What about sick patients who appeared to have nothing organically wrong with them? Osler and most of his colleagues recognized a category of 'functional' disorders, in which neither lesions nor other physical anomalies could be found. Some of these seemed to flow from excessive strain on or weakening of the nervous system – a concept rooted in old depletion models of disease. No one in America had more experience treating nervous exhaustion or 'neur-asthenia' than S. Weir Mitchell. His 'rest cure' for neurasthenics involved complete bed rest and regulation of diet, and a deliberate effort by the physician to impose on the patient a belief that the treatment would work. Mitchell's powerful personality had an intense impact on many of his patients, particularly females. We do not know whether Osler asked for Mitchell's advice in a case of anorexia nervosa he saw in his private practice in the Kensington area of Philadelphia. The brilliant and promising local doctor who had consulted him, Howard Kelly, had never heard of the condition. Osler stayed to dinner with Kelly, admired his collection of rare medical books, and diagnosed a verminous aneurysm in his horse.[65]

Osler's main Philadelphia excursion into the foggy world of neurosis was to put together thoughts on heart palpitations and related irregularities, a phenomenon Jefferson College's Jacob DaCosta had observed in Civil War soldiers and labeled 'irritable heart.' Osler suggested that in civilian life, irritable heart could have multiple causes. It might develop from toxic stimulants, such as tobacco and coffee, or from overexertion, sexual excess (including masturbation), or neurasthenia. He advised perfect rest, careful diet, and 'removal of the cause.' Osler was the twenty-eighth doctor in three years consulted by a patient at the university hospital for pain around the heart, no other symptoms. 'Treatment should be mental,' he advised. 'Exercise & gradually go back to work. Keep away from Doctors.'[66]

He had a slight problem with boils, but otherwise his own health was almost perfect – if he smoked too much, he found his heart would slow down rather than speed up – so he seldom needed a doctor's services. A colleague told this Osler tale: 'I went into his office one morning and found him struggling in the effort to pass a stomach-tube upon himself, resulting in the ordinary gagging and retching which such a procedure produces in one unaccustomed to it. I said, "what in the world are you doing?" He replied, "well, we often pass these on people, and I thought we ought to find out what it feels like ourselves." Then he offered to let me try it myself, but I declined.'[67]

Osler was too smart and too sensitive not to grow out of his earlier equation of patients with pathological specimens. When he came to Philadelphia he told his students that they would learn to study patients, not cases – individuals, not diseases. His close association with Weir Mitchell and the Infirmary for Nervous Diseases in the next five years reinforced these tendencies. He read Mitchell's books, talked intimately with him about the rest cure, and pondered the secrets of his success. These included, Osler thought, a profound knowledge of human nature and 'the careful consideration which is given to every circumstance in the life and condition of the indvidual.'[68] Such comments were straws in the breeze of Osler's developing bedside skill. So was a note he made one day in January 1888 after visiting Walt Whitman, who had seen a great deal of suffering as a nurse during the Civil War: 'Walt Whitman speaking to-day of peculiarities said that the older we grow the more stress do we lay on idiosyncracies. A doctor does not treat typhoid fever, but he treats the *man* with typhoid, and it is the man with his peculiarities – his bodily idiosyncracies we have to consider.'[69]

We have sampled the cream of Osler's Philadelphia publications. His literary skim milk – his major chapters in Pepper's *A System of Practical Medicine by American Authors*, his several score of editorials in the widely read *Medical News*, his 'Notes and Comments' columns in the *Canada Medical and Surgical Journal*, his book reviews, and his case reports (including chaisson disease or 'bends,' cholesteatoma of floor of third ventricle and of the infundibulum, lesions of the conus medullaris and cauda equina, enlargement and congestion of the right arm, typhitis and appendicitis) – would have been more than adequate for most writers and scholars. The productivity of this period of his life, his late thirties, astonished even legendary workaholics like his friend and biographer Harvey Cushing. Even those who understood the rigid regularity of his habits were not sure how Osler got so much done in mere twenty-four-hour days – especially since he abhorred that new-fangled invention the telephone and did not own a carriage. 'The atmosphere in Philadelphia was literary,' he recalled phleg-matically. 'In College circles everyone wrote, and my pen and brain got a good deal of practice.'[70]

One of his secrets was that he read and wrote constantly – at meals, while dressing, on trains and in carriages, during every free moment on holiday. Hard work was a passion for him, but much of the medical-literary life was not work. Work was seeing patients, doing autopsies, using the microscope, dictating findings to students or secretaries. Most writing was done after work was over, and with the practice of years and the habit of meeting deadlines it came to flow easily – and so quickly that he often literally forgot to dot i's and cross t's.[71] One of his Philadel-phia residents, George Dock, recalled being with Osler on a hot Sunday afternoon in Baltimore when they heard of the death of a former Montreal colleague. In two hours Osler dashed off a five-hundred-word obituary, tag line from Shelley, and sent it for publication.[72] Professional writers develop such habits. Osler had become as professional as a writer as he was a physician.

He was under pressure to write more. The Philadelphia publishers Lea Brothers, whose journals included the *Medical News*, urged him to write a book on diagnosis. He half-promised he would and drafted a couple of chap-ters, but set it aside – 'on the plea,' he remembered, 'that up to the 40th year a man is fit for better things than text books.'[73]

The greatest wear and tear probably came from his traveling routine. He was in and out of Philadelphia constantly, attending conferences, giv-ing papers, visiting libraries, seeing patients, doing autopsies, running up to Canada to see friends and family, dashing off to Europe. In 1886 he took a prolonged holiday that consisted of a several-thousand-mile trip across Canada with brother Edmund on the newly completed Canadian Pacific Railway.

An incident of that trip became legendary in Osler circles. In 1888 he reported in the *Canada Medical and Surgical Journal* that a woman on their moving train in Manitoba had gone into the water closet with diarrhea and given birth to a baby, which fell through the hole onto the track. The train was stopped and the somewhat bruised but living female baby found.

Osler's story was mostly ridiculed as another E.Y. Davis conception. He eventually obtained affidavits testifying to the essential truth of the story – the birth had occurred a few days before the Osler party came through; Osler did see the mother and child. The affidavits were lost for many years. In the 1950s, a Calgary physician discovered a woman nicknamed Railroad Winnie who proved to be Osler's famous 'baby on the track.' She died in the 1960s in her seventy-fifth year.[74]

His mother kept tabs on his comings and goings. Featherstone Osler had retired from the ministry in 1882 and moved with Ellen to a small house in Toronto, where they walked, gardened, and enjoyed the companionship of the ever-growing Osler clan. Sons Featherston, Britton, and Edmund were among the most prominent of Canadians. All had large families and fine homes in Toronto. Worn out by his years of toil, Featherstone gradually became enfeebled. But Ellen, thriving on and continuing her lifetime of hard work, remained a busy contented matriarch, interested in everything, writing sharp-witted, delightful letters to the out-of-towners in the family. Willie's visits to Toronto, she told correspondents, were 'flying,' 'flitting,' 'meteor-like' ... 'We can only be certain of where he is when he is before our eyes.' She worried about his thinness, urged him to rest more often, and prescribed classic stimulants. 'Would not Preparation of Wyeth's Beef, Iron & Wine, be good for you to take & no trouble if you kept it at hand. You know that or good Beef tea would be good for others and if you indulge in Boils you ought also to take the remedies required to heal them.'[75]

Willie's real need, Ellen told his sister Chattie, was a woman: 'I do wish he had a nice wife to attend to little home comforts for him.' But she was thankful for everything about their lives, even fatigue: 'If never tired we should not enjoy our rest.' With the exception of poor Frank, a wanderer and drinker, and underachieving Edward, the boys were doing wonderfully well. When Edmund went to New York on business, he would make a side trip to Philadelphia to see Willie. 'They rush round at a great rate in all directions,' their mother wrote, 'a Kind Providence caring for them and keeping them in safety.' Willie's letters home, often just a few lines as he mastered the use of the postcard (or 'postal'), were destroyed in a fire in

1914. He seldom corresponded with his older brothers, though the Osler men enjoyed each other's company on visits. To the Osler women they seemed mostly strong silent types, who conversed with one another in grunts. Willie never saw Frank, his closest brother in age, though he and Edmund sometimes sent him money.[76]

His ache of loneliness in Philadelphia was for the Francis children, his surrogate offspring and playmates in Montreal. They had now moved to Toronto, spending their summers on its harbor islands. At night in his rooms or his clubs, he dashed off postcards and letters, especially to Bea, Gwen, and Willie Francis, trying to erase distance.

To Bea Francis, age about five, one Sunday from the University Club:

> Dear little Bea
> Chick-a-dee-dee-dee! Chick-a-dee-dee-dee. I hear you singing now. It is Sunday evening 8 p.m. and I see you in your little bed and when I listen very hard I think I can hear you singing. Perhaps it is the little birdies outside. I wish I could see you and be near you. If I had wings I would fly every Sunday to 126 Milton Ave and stay all day with my chessubs. Good bye little darling. Write soon to your loving old Doctor.

To Bea another day:

> ... I send you 50 kisses & Gwendolyn 50 kisses. May 2 punches, Grant a small slap, Gwyn a little poke with your left thumb, Jack a kick with your little toe, Willie a butterfly kiss with your left eye, Joshua a kiss on the right ear, Mammy one on the forehead, Auntie a prick with one of Lizzie's needles, and Mr. Bath – what shall we give him – tickle his toes for me in the morning.

From other letters to Bea:

> ... I love you a thousand pounds ... I would give half my mustache to hear you laugh this minute ... My heart bleeds for you in three places ... You are the apple of my other eye. The left one. Gwen is the apple of the right ... I

love you 1000000000000 pounds and don't you forget it ... Why did I go away and leave you? I have been homesick all the week and wished very often to fly away to the Island. I sing to myself. Who will take her on their knee? & who is smoking my meerschaum pipe? ... I am so glad you are better. Is your nose very sharp? Can you use it as a Knife to cut bread & butter. Glad you liked the ice cream – was it cooked enough?

To the 'Misses Kittiwitty,' c/o the Misses Francis:

My dear little Kitty-witties
You are very welcome and I thank you very much for coming to stay with those sweet little chessubs, as they are darling girllies and you could not have found kinder mistresses in all Canada. My kind regards to your mother & tell her to rub your shut eyes with her rough tongue every day & they will soon open. When you are two weeks old you shall have each, a Mouse on Toast. Just think of that! and when you go to the Island, Rat stew every other day, and Fly biscuits. Please do not mew too loudly, but, as soon as you can, purr little songs to Miss Gwen & Miss Bea, as they both understand our languages. I remain yours very truly. Katamont – King of Kats.

To Willie Francis, age ten, who had had a headache:

> I will to you speed
> If you truly me need
> But meanwhile apply
> three or four crumbs of bread
> To the edge of your head
> If relief does not come
> while you spell the word thumb
> Take a hair of your mother
> Or sister or brother
> Cut it up very fine
> And take it in wine
> No head can withstand

A medicine so bland
The ache will just fly
Like the glance of an eye
For advice thus by post
My charges at most
Are a dollar a word
Mailliw Relso, D.M.

To Willie Francis, age twelve:

Dear Willum. I hope Mammmy arranged for your birthday Kake – do not
let her forget ... You shall have buns, I shriek – do you not hear me – if you'll
be bad yea tons & tons of buns. This day two weeks I shall be in the 'briny'
Ugh! Ugh! throwing up the whole thing perhaps – bkfast. dinner & tea!
right here in the cabin. Keep cheerful old man ... Write often.

'Buns' is a reference to Lewis Carroll. One day in church in Montreal a
preacher had threatened to 'throw up the whole thing' theologically, and
it became a favorite family phrase. On another occasion young Willie,
being teased to tears, got up and left the table, saying the light was too
strong for his eyes. Osler often used that phrase as he told the children of
his thoughts for them. Bea, Gwen, and May were all to move to the United
States to be his wives; Willie was to come down and be his student. A
century later Osler would have lived on airplanes, exceeding all carry-on
limits with armfuls of bounty from Wanamaker's Department Store for his
young Francis friends.[77]

Would the Canadian transplant, blooming in the fullness of his powers,
take root in Philadelphia? He had not been there two years when he paid a
visit to the campus of the new Johns Hopkins University in Baltimore.
'More than delighted,' he told an Ontario friend. 'It is the university of the
future & when the Medical School is organized all others will be distanced

in the country.' The Philadelphians knew that too and were seriously worried. They were being sandwiched by competitors north and south, as Wood and Tyson spelled out in a memorandum to the university's trustees:

> To the North of us the College of Physicians and Surgeons of New York has recently had donated to it over one million of dollars; whilst to the South the Johns Hopkins University is about opening its medical department with a Hospital whose endowment amounts to between one and two million, and whose buildings cost as much more and with laboratories of the most approved character, lavishly furnished not only with apparatus, but also with trained assistants ... We ought to be able to offer sufficient inducement to draw to us the most brilliant men in the United States, but it would appear as though in the future, we could not have better than a second chance.[78]

Wood and Tyson had nothing significant to recommend. In 1887 the thought that Osler might go to Hopkins was being bruited about in the Francis family. The next spring Osler was seen to be spending considerable time with John Shaw Billings, architect of the Johns Hopkins Hospital and adviser to its board of trustees. Sam Gross's wife remembered William Pepper coming to their home one day and saying to her husband, 'We're likely to lose Osler and what in the devil shall we do?' 'Well, Pepper,' Gross replied, 'if the position at the Hopkins is offered him what have we got in Philadelphia that could keep him?'[79]

The philanthropic leaders of Baltimore, as we see in more detail in the next chapter, had decided to try to assemble the best medical talent in the world at Johns Hopkins. Local loyalties and sensitivities were of little interest to them. Once they had decided they wanted Osler, Billings came to him and made the offer. 'Without a moment's hesitation I answered, "Yes."'[80]

The Canadian seemed to have skills no local man could command. On his trip to Baltimore in September 1888 formally to accept the Hopkins offer, Osler was asked by Francis T. King, president of the hospital's board of trustees, to examine his daughter Bessie, who had a long history of medical problems. 'His diagnosis was the same that the celebrated Dr. Kidd of London gave us six years ago,' King told Billings. 'In the meantime we had seen Loomis, Geddings, & DaCosta, & some of our Balto. physicians, but no two of them were alike ... We all liked Osler's candid straightforward manner.' King promptly paid Osler's twenty-dollar fee.[81]

Back in Philadelphia a few months later, Dr Samuel W. Gross lay seriously ill. His doctor, J.M. DaCosta, told Mrs Gross that he wanted a consultation and proposed Roberts Bartholow, a celebrated local therapeutics expert. Gross had told her that he wanted to see Osler, who was just back from rushing to Montreal to be at Palmer Howard's bedside as he died of pneumonia. Mrs Gross told DaCosta she wanted Osler. 'I remember so well – his thoroughly Philadelphian, Jeffersonian Med School reply,' she said many years later: '"Remember Bartholow is a Jefferson Man."'

'My reply was not very polite.'[82]

Osler and other doctors were called in but could do nothing to save Gross. He died in raging fever and delirium, the victim of a bacterial infection, at age fifty-two and the peak of his power, in April 1889.

Two weeks later Osler severed his connection with Philadelphia and the University of Pennsylvania. His final duty was to deliver the farewell address to the graduates. His theme was the physician's need to cultivate imperturbability, inscrutability, or what the dying Roman, Antoninus Pius, summed up as 'Aequanimitas.' For the Philadelphians the occasion was mainly 'Agnew Day,' with students and faculty paying emotional tribute to their retiring surgeon and churchgoer. If Osler was at all chagrined about being overshadowed, he would not have shown it. 'Aequanimitas' soon became a classic in the literature of advice to young physicians. Osler had managed to put into words a description of what every young medical student in the dead house, every intern and resident, every practitioner dealing with the sick and dying, and everyone struggling for self-control under pressure, knew was the right demeanor – the essence of medical cool. He did not say so, but Weir Mitchell was probably close to the model of equanimity Osler had in mind.

William Pepper hosted a farewell dinner for Osler at Philadelphia's Bellevue Hotel on May 4. Harvard's H.P. Bowditch wrote home that the affair was 'quite a festival. It is extraordinary what a hold he has on the profession in Philadelphia. He is one of the most popular men I ever knew.'[83] Three days later, on May 7, 1889, Osler was in Baltimore for the official opening of the Johns Hopkins Hospital.

FIVE

Starting at Johns Hopkins

At last!
This was the most anticipated hospital opening in American history. It had been such a long time in the making. Baltimore's millionaire merchant and financier, Johns Hopkins, had created a hospital trust twenty-two years earlier, in 1867. He died in 1873, leaving $3.5 million, a then fabulous sum, to finance the institution. The university that Hopkins had created at the same time and with equal funding had opened its doors in 1876, but the hospital had seemed to take forever to build, not least because the trustees built it using only the income from their endowment. No borrowing, no entrenchment on principal. Like Hopkins himself, many of them were Quakers, men with an intense sense of stewardship.

They also had an extraordinary commitment to excellence. Johns Hopkins had been persuaded to donate his fortune to create the best possible university and hospital. Giving his trustees a site in 1873, he directed them to erect 'a hospital which shall in construction and arrangement compare favorably with any other institution of like character in this country or in Europe.' It was also to play a major role in American medical education, because, Hopkins directed, 'the institution should ultimately form a part of the medical school of that university for which I have made ample provision.' The hospital and university boards of trustees were to overlap and work closely together, running mates in the competition for American institutional leadership.[1]

Like-minded men were hired to implement the vision. Daniel Coit Gilman, a Yale-trained professional educator, was plucked from the University of California to become the far-sighted founding president of Johns Hopkins University. Pathetically tiny in numbers in the early years, the Hopkins faculty were outstanding in their international connections and their commitment to enlarging knowledge through research, publication, and training scholars at the graduate level. Under Gilman, Johns Hopkins was immediately on the forefront of defining the American university.

When the trustees cast about for ideas on how to make a hospital, an army bureaucrat in Washington, John Shaw Billings, emerged as a medical version of Gilman. Billings had designed hospitals for the government during the Civil War. A scholarly, well-connected physician, the founder of what eventually became the National Library of Medicine and the *Index medicus*, he shared in the 1870s the commitment of reformers to redesigning medical education. Billings convinced the trustees that research and teaching should be at the heart of the hospital's activities: an elite of first-class teachers should introduce an elite of first-class students to the highest quality of medical practice on the hospital's wards. There should be no compromise with excellence in designing a hospital in which patients would get better, not sicken and die from each other's infections. Billings radiated American idealism: 'This Hospital should advance our knowledge of the causes, symptoms and pathology of disease, and methods of treatment, so that its good work shall not be confined to the city of Baltimore, or the State of Maryland, but shall in part consist in furnishing more knowledge of disease and more power to control it, for the benefit of the sick and afflicted of all countries and of all future time.'[2] As adviser to the board, Billings became the key man in the building of Johns Hopkins Hospital and the hiring of its staff.

No one wanted a position at Johns Hopkins more than William H. Welch, BA, MD. Offspring of a line of Connecticut physicians, born in 1850, Welch had graduated from Yale College in 1870 without enthusiasm for any line of work other than being a scholar of the classics. He drifted into the family profession *faute de mieux*, overcoming his revulsion to blood, illness, and cadavers to take a medical degree from the College of Physicians and Surgeons in New York in 1875. Attracted by the microscope and financed by his family, Welch went to Germany in 1876 where, working primarily with Julius Cohnheim, he became a skilled laboratory pathologist and a lifelong Germanophile. Whereas London was 'the world' for Osler after traveling on the continent, for Welch it was 'dull, dreary, doleful, dirty, dismal ... The smallest and most insignificant German nest which I have ever been in is more tolerable.'[3] Welch wanted to spend his life like the great German researchers, working in a pathology lab with a few brilliant students. The Johns Hopkins institutions were the first in America that might give a man such an opportunity. The alternative, Welch found, was to scramble for a living by teaching and doing autopsies and examining specimens for his well-placed physician friends in New York.

In 1884 Johns Hopkins University began to organize its School of Medicine in anticipation of the completion of the hospital. The key appointments would be in basic medical sciences, pathology and physiology. For the latter chair, the trustees chose H. Newell Martin, an Irish-born protégé of T.H. Huxley. (Huxley, the agnostic apostle of evolution, had spoken in connection with the university's opening, a fact which, combined with a perceived absence of prayer, was thought to signal the institutions' commitment to science and secularism, and aroused much critical comment.) Billings, with support from Cohnheim, urged Gilman to hire Welch as pathologist: 'He is 33 years old, unmarried, of good personal address – modest, quiet, and a gentleman in every sense ... activated by the true scientific spirit ... I think he will develop well.'

Welch's New York companions launched an all-out campaign to keep him from burying himself, as they saw it, in a dreary provincial city, far from friends, without prospect of worldly emolument, and in pursuit of 'an ideal which can not ever be realized.' On the other hand, another Hopkins faculty member told him that he would have 'literally perfect' independence: 'Everything for your work that you ask for ... an opportunity ... which can come to a man only once in a lifetime.' Paying a heavy, bitter price in lost friendship and financial opportunity, Welch decided to go to Baltimore.[4]

By 1886 Welch and Martin were welcoming advanced students into their laboratories. Welch's lab was soon moved from the university grounds to the hospital site in east Baltimore, where the medical school would eventually be located and the autopsy room was already built. It was re-named the pathological laboratory. Welch and his students began to inves-tigate the dead while construction of wards for the living went on around them. Welch's assistant, William T. Councilman, supplied specimens that he brought over from a local hospital in pails suspended from the handle-bars of his advanced locomotion machine, a tricycle.

There were still no human patients in the hospital, but here it was – a place where scientists could work on the frontiers of pathology, well-funded, appreciated, left alone, just as in Germany. Martin's and Welch's labs be-came instant magnets for talented young Americans. Johns Hopkins's re-search achievements, most notably Martin's development of a method for perfusing the isolated mammalian heart, were immediate and impressive. Morale among the early Hopkinsites was very high. Young men living the scientific dream in America.

Their spirits were high enough to weather serious setbacks, such as a sharp falloff in the university's income from its endowment when the Bal-timore and Ohio Railroad ran into hard times and cut its dividend in the late eighties. The hospital was at last nearing completion, but the univer-sity would not have money to pay for a full staff for the medical school. It was a perplexing situation, which the trustees navigated according to their founding vision. 'I wish to see no compromises in the standard of the Med School,' Francis T. King, president of the hospital board, wrote Billings. 'The best in the country, or none at all until we can see our way to proceed on our original plans – we have spent too much money on the Hospital buildings & talked too much in America & Europe to do otherwise – at least I have done so. I think my friends would "turn me out of meeting" if I advocated a school of low standard.'[5]

In 1888 President Gilman was asked to serve double duty by becoming Director of the hospital. Its income, mostly from bank stock, was unim-paired. Gilman and King decided to proceed with the hospital organizing and opening, and to worry about the medical school later. The key appointment would be a physician-in-chief. Billings and Welch had known Osler for years and were thoroughly familiar with the man and his work. Another candidate who had been on Billings's mind for some years was Lauder Brunton, older than Osler and perhaps London's most distinguished consultant and teacher. On one of his trips to England, Billings tried to entice Brunton to Hopkins but was rejected for family reasons.[6]

Osler paid a critical visit to Baltimore early in July 1888, lunching with a group that included Welch, Billings, and King. He apparently agreed to throw his hat in the Hopkins ring – it was the opportunity of a lifetime – and King determined to force the matter of getting on with the appointment. On July 25 King wrote Billings of the board's actions at what appears to have been an informal meeting: 'I presented Osler's name & gave the reasons for acting promptly. F. White thought we should first prepare & adopt a plan of organisation – that we were beginning at the wrong end. A long discussion followed before the vote was taken – no one voted in the negative. Could you arrange to meet Osler here – questions may come up.'[7]

In September the hospital board formally approved Osler's appointment as Physician-in-Chief at an annual salary of $5,000. The university board followed suit by appointing him Professor of the Theory and Practice of Medicine (without salary until the medical school opened). Welch wrote his sister that Osler 'is the best man to be found in the country and it is a great acquisition for us to secure him. I know him well and have the highest opinion of him as a scientist and as a man.'[8]

It is said that some eyebrows were raised at this appointment of a man with relatively little clinical experience, who could just as easily have passed as a pathologist. The documents are silent on whose eyebrows – perhaps because, as King and some of the Philadelphians could testify, Osler was more than passing as a first-rate clinician. The only cautionary note we know of as Osler captured the most desirable medical position in the United States came from his mother: 'We congratulate you on the prospect of takeing another upward step up the Ladder. Only dear Willie take heed that as you climb and step firmly on this ladder you get nearer and nearer to the Golden Gate of the Heavenly City and so pass through earthly things, that you lose not the things which are eternal.'[9]

Johns Hopkins Hospital sits on a hill in east Baltimore overlooking the head of Chesapeake Bay. In the early years the hospital was a major landmark, a beacon of hope for the sick and suffering. Its buildings were a pleasing blend of red brick trimmed with West Virginia sandstone. Most of the Queen Anne architectural flourishes – tower, dome, cupola – were lavished on the central administration building fronting on Broadway. It survives today, at first sight a quaint Victorian relic overwhelmed in a medical-educational conurbation. Look again, and you realize that its ornateness, inside and out, is an enduring, handsome testimony to nineteenth-century American idealism and ambition. Francis King hoped the building would stand for a thousand years.

The governing principle of hospital design in the 1870s was to minimize contagion, which was still thought to be primarily airborne. Natural ventilation was fundamental. The Baltimore hilltop was a healthy, breezy site. Wards were housed in detached one- or two-storey 'pavilions.' Other units – kitchen, laundry, pathology, dispensary, etc. – had their own buildings to minimize flows of contaminated air. The Johns Hopkins Hospital complex was originally sixteen buildings plus a gatehouse on the fourteen-acre site. It had 272 patient beds, 212 of them in large public wards. Screened windows and verandahs gave patients access to fresh air; a forest of chimneys dispersed waste gases. The grounds were carefully tended. Here was a pleasing, healthy place from which 'hospitalism,' the tendency of hospitals to harm their patients, would vanish forever.[10]

Built and opened as a unit, the Johns Hopkins Hospital was aesthetically satisfying and reasonably functional; but by 1889, time and the advent of bacteriology had made parts of Billings's design seriously anachronistic. There were no elevators, and no running water was supplied to the wards. The windows were so big that few nurses had the strength to open them; the ventilating system was so complex it was seldom used. Hopkins had to create its own sewerage system, for the City of Baltimore did not provide one until until the twentieth century. The hospital's laboratory and surgical facilities were inadequate virtually from the day it opened. Pressure for improvements to the plant began immediately.

Osler was one of the ground-floor appointments to an organization which, as some trustees had pointed out, was not yet organized. In 1888–9 he worked with the Hopkins leadership in filling other key positions. Osler and Billings tried to hire Lord Lister's successor in Glasgow, Sir William Macewen, as their chief surgeon. He turned them down. Welch had an interesting surgical candidate at hand in the person of William Stewart Halsted, who had been working with him and living in Baltimore. But there was a huge question-mark hanging over Halsted. As a bold surgical experimenter in New York in the early 1880s, Halsted had pioneered in the use of cocaine as a local anesthetic, had taken to snorting it, and, along with all his assistants, had become a full-fledged addict. He twice had to be hospitalized for several months and was then helped back into medicine by Welch. Understandably, the Hopkins trustees made Halsted at first only acting head surgeon, at a salary of $2,000.

Osler hoped to budge a Philadelphian who was working with him, Fred Packard, to come to Baltimore to be his chief resident. 'The father will not consent to his son leaving Philadelphia,' King reported. Osler's next choice, Henri A. Lafleur, a Montrealer of French Protestant lineage whom he had taught at McGill, became the first of many Canadian physicians who worked under Osler at Johns Hopkins. The Superintendent of Nurses and head of the Nurses' Training School, Isabel Hampton, also came to Hopkins from Canada – via New York and Chicago – although her main qualification initially was her physical resemblance to a Greek goddess. Miss Hampton had such an impressive appearance, Osler remembered, that the jaded male hiring committee was persuaded on sight. Osler recommended a Quaker lady from the Pennsylvania Hospital, Rachel Bonner, to serve as the Hopkins housekeeper, or matron. There is no record of Miss Bonner's father objecting to the move.[11]

President Gilman worked out an organizational structure for the hospital. After inspecting hospitals in New York and judging that they were not well governed, Gilman decided to model Johns Hopkins Hospital on a more up-to-date institution, a hotel. He took Osler and Welch to the Fifth Avenue Hotel. 'We saw everything arranged in departments,' Osler remembered, 'with responsible heads, and over all a director. "This" Gilman said, "is really the hospital, and we shall model ours upon it. The clinical unit of a hospital is the exact counterpart of one of the sub-divisions of any great hotel or department-store."' Gilman's instinct proved sound. The idea of strong executive leadership in a departmentalized organization was in accord with the best American corporate practice of the era and very different from the leaderless diffusion of authority commonly found in American and British hospitals. As chief physician at Hopkins, Osler would not share authority with other doctors. He had power over his medical unit comparable only to the chief's sway in some German hospitals. 'I have everything I could desire and more than I could deserve,' he wrote to a friend in the spring of 1890.[12]

He apparently drew on his German observations in creating a strong cadre of senior resident physicians, without fixed terms, to assist the department heads. 'Perhaps the one special advantage which the large German hospitals have over corresponding American Institutions, is the presence of these highly trained men who remain in some cases three, five, or even eight years, and who, under the Professor, have control of the clinical material,' he reported early in 1890. The junior residents, or interns, would not rotate through the departments as in most other hospitals. They would be chosen personally by the chief and would serve their term under him. 'This is not an ordinary hospital for the education of internes.' Osler emphasized personal selection rather than appointment of interns on the basis of competitive examination, as had happened for a time at Blockley, because 'these young men come in contact with us at all hours and it is absolutely essential that they should be persons with whom we can work pleasantly and congenially. I have suffered so on several occasions, from inefficient or ungentlemanly residents foisted on me by the competitive examination plan that I would here enter my warmest protest against it.'[13]

When it formally opened in the spring of 1889 Johns Hopkins Hospital still lacked a chief administrator. The board hired Henry M. Hurd, a gentlemanly, scholarly physician from Michigan who had been managing an asylum for the insane. It had been decided to organize a gynecological service along with the medical and surgical units. Osler chose Howard A. Kelly, the brilliant young physician and surgeon from the Kensington neighborhood of Philadelphia, whom he had come to know there and had tried to advance as his 'Kensington colt' (also nicknamed the 'Boy Laparotomist') for a major appointment at Penn. With Kelly's move to Baltimore at age thirty-one, Philadelphia lost another medical frontrunner.

The most intense frustration at Johns Hopkins Hospital in 1889 was the university's inability to launch the medical school. These brilliant and uniquely well-paid men were in place, and a few score patients were starting to come (it would be several years before all the beds were regularly filled), but they had no students to teach. The future of the medical school was riding on the value of shares of the Baltimore and Ohio Railroad, which seemed to be going nowhere, now paying no dividend at all. Some trustees began to suggest that Johns Hopkins needed another benefactor. 'We must try to endow the Med School, finding some rich man, & call it the — Med School of the JHU,' Francis King wrote Billings. 'I hope that G[ilman] can find one among his many rich friends.'[14]

The hospital had few friends, rich or otherwise, in Baltimore. Baltimore was a sprawling, row-house-and-cobblestone-street semi-southern city of about 425,000, almost uninhabitable in the heat and humidity of summer, with a heavily Germanic working class and a largely black servant class. Unlike Philadelphia, it did not have a proud medical and educational tradition, nor had it been particularly proud of its merchant entrepreneurs such as the late Johns Hopkins. It was Johns Hopkins, not Baltimore, that had created a university and a hospital whose trustees proceeded to hire one non-Baltimorean after another for plum jobs. And what did those big medical brains carry in their carpetbags? Scalpels. The first thing they did up there was pathology. Each Hopkins doctor had the privilege of 'cutting up a nigger,' it was whispered down below. Stay away from there, children. In the early 1880s a colored woman (to use the terminology of the day) had been murdered and sold to the University of Maryland Medical School for fifteen dollars. They'll snatch you too, boy, they'll dig up your body, and they'll cut you up into little pieces and leave cigarette butts and whisky bottles in your empty coffin. Young H.L. Mencken heard these and other grisly stories of the cadavers 'piled up like stovewood' in local university dead houses.[15]

Up on Hospital Hill the young men were too busy in their rarefied atmosphere to worry overmuch about big issues. The residents, all unmarried as a condition of their residency, lived in well-furnished rooms in the administration building and enjoyed the view over the city and harbor. Osler also lived in at times, and it was said that you could set your clock by the sound of his boots being deposited outside his door every night at ten (for shining by servants). He also tried keeping house in Baltimore, bringing one of his nieces down from Canada to be housekeeper. There was fine entertaining at Dr Osler's house until Georgina Osler fell in love with a Hopkins resident and got married; they moved on.

There were hundreds of details still to work out in creating a great hospital. Fortunately, its own endowment income, unlike the university's, remained high. From the beginning, the patients were intensely interesting – though perhaps not the very first patient, a construction worker who broke his leg in 1879 and spent two months convalescing in makeshift quarters ten years before the hospital opened. But the first indoor patient in 1889 had an advanced case of thoracic aneurysm, and Welch went out of his way to compliment the clinicians on their accurate and complete diagnosis, confirmed by the postmortem. Perhaps from a patient's or a Baltimorean's point of view the occasion was not so auspicious – no recovery here – and they would have feared more had they known of Halsted's original Hopkins nickname, 'Jack the Ripper.'[16]

The founding fathers all met every day over lunch – Welch, Osler, Halsted, Lafleur, Kelly, Councilman, and any distinguished visitors who had come to see how the Hopkins experiment was working. The food was superb. Emory the caterer teased the 'nurse girls' unmercifully, and, Councilman remembered, 'Everyone sought to bring something to the feast. There was talk about work, jokes and laughter'[17] – much laughter the day after Osler, having been to a play that included death by apoplexy, announced that there had been a fatality and would be an autopsy, and had 'Counce' stay up late into the night awaiting the fictitious corpse. Then there was the time when Osler told the young surgeon Howard Kelly that he had reassured his patients that the senile tremor would disappear as soon as Kelly began to operate. Osler teased Emory the caterer about crabs causing cancer, terrapin producing impotence, oysters and arteriosclerosis. And there was the day when 'Counce,' possibly on his tricycle, obliviously trailed human intestine twenty feet behind him down the streets of Baltimore.[18] With luck, onlookers might have mistaken it for sausage casing.

The Hopkins men, led by Osler, institutionalized their fraternity by founding a journal club, a medical society, and a historical club. They prepared to tell the world about their work in the *Johns Hopkins Hospital Bulletin,* and the *Johns Hopkins Hospital Reports.* The leaders of the nursing school joined the medico-literary culture, producing a pioneering series of texts and articles. Osler organized the dispensary to service outpatients (and provide some appointments for local doctors), started up his clinical laboratory, and began organizing postgraduate courses so that some teaching would go on in the hospital.

Everyone cherished the wonderful spirit of the early days – the fellowship, the sense of being present at the creation, the very American thrill at a new begining unhindered by the past. 'To blaze a perfectly new road, untrammeled by tradition, vested interests, or medical "deadwood" – best of all, backed by a board of management imbued with a fundamental and abiding respect for scientific opinion and commanding an ample budget – what more could the heart of man desire?' Lafleur remembered. 'The hampering externals of life, the cares, the thought of the morrow,' Councilman wrote, 'were all absent.' After spending a few days at Hopkins, Harvard's R.H. Fitz said it was like a monastery with the unusual feature that the monks cared nothing about the future. And they did often go off to 'the Church' after a day's work. It was Hanselmann's restaurant at the corner of Wolfe and Monument, noted for the host's beer and pretzels.[19]

Osler had not had a long holiday for several years. The first summer, 1889, he stayed close to Hopkins except for a jaunt to Canada, mainly to visit a leper colony in Tracadie, New Brunswick. He took eleven-year-old Billy Francis with him, met up with two Philadelphians, Grace Revere Gross and a friend, and on the train back had to share an upper berth with Francis while a fat Catholic bishop snored below.[20] In the late spring of 1890, with everything working smoothly at the hospital (Osler thought it would be 'quite safe' to give Halsted a permanent appointment, for example), he was able to leave for several months of medical sightseeing in Europe.

He and a University of Toronto friend, Ramsay Wright, racketed around the Bavarian medical schools and hospitals, saw women attending medical lectures in Switzerland, took in lectures and clinics in Strasbourg, visited Laveran (of malaria fame) in Nancy, saw Charcot and Pasteur and many other French medical teachers at work in Paris (also with women attending their classes), and then crossed over to England to spend lazy weekends in country houses with friends, 'doing nothing particular,' Edward Schäfer remembered in a Gilbert and Sullivan vein, 'and doing that remarkably well.' Osler wrote long descriptions from Germany back to his residents, commenting on everything from lecture room decor to methods of doing microsurgery on pigeons, the cause of Christ's death on the cross (after seeing the Oberammergau passion play), dilated stomach in Munich beer workers, and the good results being obtained from the use of cold baths in typhoid fever in Freiburg. He wrote almost nothing about his experiences in France. Instead, his published letters end with a ringing tribute to Teutonic achievement:

The characteristic which stands out in bold relief in German scientific life is the paramount importance of knowledge for its own sake. To know certain things thoroughly and to contribute to an increase in our knowledge of them seems to satisfy the ambition of many of the best minds. The presence in every medical center of a class of men devoted to scientific work gives a totally different aspect to professional aspirations. While with us – and in England – the young man may start with an ardent desire to devote his life to science, he is soon dragged into the mill of practice, and at forty years of age the 'guinea stamp' is on all his work. His aspirations and his early years of sacrifice have done him much good, but we are the losers and we miss sadly the leaven which such a class would bring into our professional life ... The universities of Germany are her chief glory.[21]

More German glory shone at the Tenth International Medical Congress in Berlin in early August, a colossal assemblage of nine thousand delegates from fifty countries listening to some six hundred papers. On August 4, 1890, the whole world was startled to hear that the great Robert Koch, discoverer of the tubercle bacillus, had found a cure for tuberculosis in guinea pigs in his laboratory. 'It is possible,' Koch said, 'to render pathogenic bacteria within the body harmless without ill effect on the body itself.' Osler was in Berlin for the congress and may or may not have heard Koch's speech. Welch certainly did and wrote to his father that if the treatment worked in humans, it would be 'the greatest discovery ever made in medicine.' Johns Hopkins would aim at being in the forefront of applying Koch's amazing news – the equivalent of a Nobel laureate announcing a cure for cancer today – just as soon as details became available.[22]

Osler's main medical interest during early months at Hopkins was in parasites. He continued to study the fascinating life cycle of the malaria parasites. Then, in the summer of 1889, an old man died in the hospital, apparently of pneumonia following sunstroke, 'and to my surprise and chagrin the post-mortem examination of the blood and spleen showed the case to have been one of malarial fever. Had a thorough blood examination been made and full doses of quinine administered, the man's life might have been saved.' Thorough blood examinations were then made routine at Hopkins, to the considerable disgruntlement of the interns who had to do them.[23]

The Baltimore investigators' microscopes also revealed the first American sighting of certain parasites in a case of dysentery. 'They are most extraordinary & striking creatures & take one's breath away at first to see these big amoebae – 10–20 times the size of a leucocyte – crawling about in the pus,' Osler wrote.[24] The residents did most of the clinical, laboratory, and postmortem work at Hopkins, and took the lead in investigation and publication. The hospital became a center for work on malaria and for studies in amebic dysentery, with Councilman, Lafleur, and others gaining prominence and credit while Osler moved on to other subjects.

His subordinates had full authority and independence to act in their chief's absence. For years Osler had been pondering Europeans' use of cold baths to reduce the fever in typhoid. After a new series of favorable results came in from Germany in the late 1880s, he made up his mind to adopt the practice at Hopkins, where therapeutic tradition did not govern. But it would be a labor-intensive routine, objectionable to nurses and, because of the cold and discomfort, to patients as well. In the first year nothing was done. But with Osler in Europe in the summer of 1890 and again writing enthusiastically about the practice, Lafleur took the bit. After a visit to the German Hospital in Philadelphia to study the cold bath routine there, he initiated the hydrotherapeutic regimen at Hopkins. Osler returned to find cold baths at last being used as the preferred approach to high fever in typhoid.

He of course took great interest in the Koch tuberculosis breakthrough. Hopkins sent a senior resident to Berlin to investigate the discovery. About the same time Koch sent small quantities of his extract, soon to be named tuberculin, to John Shaw Billings for American distribution. Billings naturally made it available to Hopkins. Was a new era in medicine about to begin? On Friday, December 12, 1890, the senior staff of the hospital, the house staff, and an invited group of local doctors assembled in the amphitheater to see the history made. Osler and Welch gave preliminary historical remarks, after which Lafleur injected a dose of the still mysterious dark-brown fluid into an advanced consumptive. 'The gathering dispersed with mutual congratulations,' Lafleur remembered.

They began treating ten other patients. At the Medical Society on Monday night, Osler steered a characteristically careful course:

> In the presence of an alleged discovery of such importance, we should neither display a blind credulity nor an unreasonable skepticism. The extraordinary enthusiasm which has been aroused by the announcement, is a just tribute to the character of Robert Koch, who is a model worker of unequalled thoroughness, whose ways and methods have always been those of the patient investigator, well worthy of the confidence which other experts in pathology place in his statements. The cold test of time can alone determine how far the claims, which he has now advanced, will be justified, and

meanwhile the question has been transferred, so far as human medicine is concerned, from the laboratory to the clinical ward, in which the careful observations of the next few months will furnish the necessary data, upon which to found a final judgment.

But he could not resist telling Billings on Wednesday that one of their cases had already 'reacted remarkably' to the injections. This was a hugely premature evaluation; the patient had been misdiagnosed and soon died of cancer of the lymph glands.[25]

Osler paid a daily visit to the wards that winter of 1890–1, but Lafleur and the assistant resident, William S. Thayer, handled all the routine work. Most of Osler's time was given to the most important episode in his 'ink-pot career,' the writing of a textbook. It became one of the great accomplishments of his life and one of the great books in the history of medical education and publishing.

The thought of writing a textbook had earlier crossed his and publishers' minds. With his literary skills and breadth of knowledge, Osler was a natural to do a big book, but he had begged off with jibes about doing better things before forty. Now he had passed forty, and with the opening of the medical school nowhere in sight and his consulting practice languishing in what he called a 'God-forsaken town,'[26] he had time on his hands. He first thought he lacked the energy or persistence for such a hugely grueling job, not unlike running an ultramarathon today. Refreshed by his 1890 European trip, he 'shook myself' and began writing a book on medical practice, starting with a chapter on typhoid fever.

That fall the big New York firm of D. Appleton and Company approached him and suggested that the work become a textbook of medicine. Appleton claimed that its distribution network, through subscribers to its extensive list of medical works, would mean large sales. After some dickering, the firm offered a 10 per cent royalty, rising to 12.5 per cent after 5,000 copies, with a guaranteed sale of 10,000 and a $1,500 cash advance on publication. 'Selling my brains to the devil,' he wrote later, Osler signed the contract in February 1891.[27]

He had made slow progress till then. In 1891 he 'got well into harness':

Three mornings of each week I stayed at home and dictated from 8 a.m. to 1 p.m. On the alternate days I dictated after the morning Hospital visit, beginning about 11.30 a.m. The spare hours of the afternoon were devoted to correction and reference work. Early in May I ... went to my rooms at the Hospital. The routine there was: – 8 a.m. to 1 p.m. dictation; 2 p.m. visit to the private patients and special cases in the wards, after which revision, etc. After 5 p.m. I saw my outside cases; dinner at the club about 6.30, loafed until 9.30, bed at 10 p.m., up at 7 a.m ... The first two weeks of August I spent in Toronto, and then with the same routine I practically finished the MS. by about October the 15th ... The last three months of 1891 were devoted to proof reading. In January I made out the index, and in the entire work nothing so wearied me as the verifying of every reference ... During the writing of the work I lost only one afternoon through transient indisposition, and never a night's rest. Between September, 1890, and January, 1892, I gained nearly eight pounds in weight.

He worked in his shirtsleeves, surrounded by books in time-honored and Whitmanesque authorial style, dictating to his stenographer, B.O. Humpton ('Miss Hump'). At the hospital he took over the sitting room of one of the residents, Hunter Robb. 'I was never able to use the room for fully six months,' Robb recalled. 'Oftentimes right in the middle of his dictating, he would stop and rush into my other room, and ask me to match quarters with him, or we would engage in an exchange of yarns. It was a great treat for me, and except when he would court inspiration by kicking my waste-paper basket about the room, I thoroughly enjoyed his visits.' Robb protected his wastebasket by putting bricks in it. Osler eventually buttered him up with an inscribed copy of the book, in which 'E.Y.D.' apologized on the author's behalf for having, cuckoolike, turned 'the Robin' out of a nest so well stalked, and partaken of his oranges, chocolates, ginger ale, and 'Old Tom.'[28]

The Principles and Practice of Medicine, 'Designed for the Use of Practitioners and Students of Medicine,' by William Osler, MD, was published by Appleton in March 1892. Osler dedicated the book to the memory of his three teachers, Johnson, Bovell, and Howard. He thanked his residents, Miss Humpton, and L.P. Powell, a history graduate student at Hopkins who had gone over the whole manuscript to improve its style. (Powell later said he did very little.)[29] He prefaced the book with quotations from Hippocrates ('Experience is fallacious and judgment difficult') and Plato ('And I said of medicine, that this is an art which considers the constitution of the patient, and has principles of action and reasons in each case'), but otherwise offered no explanation of its provenance or design, and gave no introduction to the principles and practice of medicine. Perhaps he or Appleton deliberately aimed at concision. Perhaps he was completely fed up with what he had described as 'hack labour' on an 'infernal "quiz compend."'[30] Or perhaps he was in a hurry because the woman he had asked to marry him had said he should finish the book first.

It was really a book of diseases and how to treat them. Osler began his 1050 pages with a 270-page section discussing thirty specific infectious diseases, typhoid fever through to leprosy. He followed with sections on constitutional diseases, diseases of the digestive system, diseases of the respiratory system, diseases of the circulatory system, diseases of the blood and ductless glands, diseases of the kidneys, diseases of the nervous system, and diseases of the muscles. A catch-all section included poisoning, sunstroke, and obesity. The final section discussed diseases caused by animal parasites. For most diseases Osler offered material on definition, etiology, morbid anatomy, symptoms, diagnosis, prognosis, and treatment. Sometimes he included a historical note. The book had a full subject index but no bibliography. The publisher cut out the author index that Osler had prepared.

Giving only a few exact citations to the medical literature, Osler drew by name on a large number of European, British, and American authors. He constantly relied on the thousand autopsies he had done at the Montreal General and on his Philadelphia experiences in both the dead house and on wards. He cited cases he had seen as a student in Europe in 1874, cases he had seen with Howard in Montreal and with Mitchell in Philadelphia, cases he had talked over the day before with Welch and Halsted, cases involving Munich beer workers, and cases surviving as specimens in medical museums. He mentioned historical figures ranging from Hippocrates, Mephibosheth, and Sir Thomas Browne, through Montaigne, Oliver Wendell Holmes, Coleridge, and Swift. The book did not cover diseases of the reproductive organs or the eyes. There was no joking discussion of vaginismus, no citation to Egerton Y. Davis, though Osler did offer a line of not inaccurate levity on traumatic hysteria: 'In railway cases, so long as litigation is pending and the patient is in the hands of lawyers the symptoms usually persist. Settlement is often the starting point of a speedy and perfect recovery.' Would Osler on his own have discovered that the material Welch gave him about ergotism, with special emphasis on Romania, was a complete fabrication, a joke on the joker? – who did not like it. Welch confessed before anything damaging was published.[31]

The timing of the textbook was almost perfect. *Principles and Practice* was at once a monument to the achievements of nineteenth-century scientific medicine and a gateway to the twentieth century. Osler had mastered the mainstream clinicopathological tradition of the past seventy years. He was thoroughly up on the bacteriological work of the 1880s that had solved such a central conundrum in the etiology of infectious disease. With a few exceptions, his accounts of the natural history of disease still make sense, in some instances are considered classic. In 1892 the endocrine system had not been understood, the body's immune system was still a mystery, viruses could not be identified, principles of nutrition and genetics were largely unknown, and x-rays, electrocardiographs, and scores of other diagnostic devices had not yet been developed. But exploration produced intelligible maps long before aerial surveying; the Jaguar owner cherishes model-T Fords; and a practitioner who reads Osler from 1892 learns a lot about the etiology and extremes of diseases which the coming of antibiotics and other remedies have effectively conquered, if only, perhaps, for the time being.[32]

Many of the competing medical texts had just been made obsolete, some by bacteriology, others by the death of their authors. Over in England, Sir

Thomas Watson, whose *Principles and Practice of Physic* dated from 1843, had died at age ninety. Many North Americans, including Osler, had thought it time the New World generated its own medical literature. Austin Flint of New York was one of the first and best of the few Americans who had ventured into the field. Flint was gone too; the final edition of his *Treatise on the Principles and Practice of Medicine* had been published posthumously in 1886, largely thanks to his assistant, William Welch. As Osler and everyone else at Hopkins soon realized, Welch could barely answer letters, let alone marshal the energy for sustained academic writing.

William Osler was so well situated and connected that a text might well succeed on his name alone in the 1890s. As the chief physician at America's premier hospital, but English-trained and a British Canadian, he was already something of a one-man North Atlantic medical triangle. Americans, Canadians, and Britons could all buy Osler and feel they were supporting the home publishing industry (though he was particularly conscious of having many references to American authors and must have known the symbolism of beginning with typhoid fever, a disease whose nature had been unlocked by Americans after study in Europe). More important, anyone who bought and read *The Principles and Practice* found he had invested in medical textbook writing at its best. Hack work, perhaps, but Osler had also given birth to a good book.

Its merits, apart from the up-to-date content, were its extreme clarity, Osler's straightforward style, and the sense he conveyed that medicine was anything but cut-and-dried. The clarity and style were influenced by Osler having dictated the book, just as he regularly dictated case notes and autopsy findings. The short uncluttered sentences of *Principles and Practice* were like fresh air to anyone brought up on Flint's rolling, complex phrasings. They contrast favorably with some of Osler's own self-conscious attempts to work in a more literary tradition. He was usually most succinct when he was dictating or talking. At the same time, no one could accuse him of condensing, abridging, or otherwise short-changing his readers. The authors of two other new textbooks that year deliberately omitted history and controversy.[33] Osler delighted in tracing the evolution of medical ideas, outlining conflicts, stating his opinions based on his experience (he used the word 'I' hundreds of times), and admitting uncertainty. He was not the standard textbook author/ity, who knew everything and could answer every question. Instead, he knew the limits of medical knowledge, knew the subtleties and imprecisions of diagnosis, knew how easy it was to be wrong, how hard it is to cure. *Principles and Practice* was a kind of progress report on the current state of an imprecise, evolving, and exciting discipline whose founder had said, 'Experience is fallacious and judgment difficult.'

As he dictated the book, Osler sometimes looked backward, other times forward. He may have been influenced by mood swings during the infernal grind. He may have succumbed to the temptation to relax standards in hack writing. How else to explain his pronouncements on, say, hair color – that blondes are less prone to neurotic gastralgia than brunettes, but are more frequently affected with chlorosis. If Osler realized that the influence of masturbation as a cause of epilepsy was 'probably overrated,' why did he not reconsider the view that it was 'an important factor' in the etiology of hysteria? (Answer: he must have thought masturbation could further functional but not organic impairment.) How could he be a model of common sense in pointing out the number of conditions that were harmless and/or self-limiting, while terrifying the parents of children with enlarged tonsils by claiming that mouth breathing could leave Johnny stupid and stuttering?[34]

Some of his suggestions about pneumonia and Bright's disease have been taken as indications of lingering neohumoralism or perhaps excessive deference to traditional authority.[35] Most of his apparent confusions were in his advice on therapeutics. As a physician thought to be suspicious of drugging, he seemed to prescribe a lot of opium, as in the early stages of the common cold: 'For the distressing, irritative cough, which keeps the patient awake, no remedy can take its place.' There was certainly no harm in trying that 'old-fashioned and sometimes successful remedy' for nosebleed, the insertion of a cobweb into the nostrils, but what about the use of a 4 per cent cocaine solution to relieve nasal catarrh? Sherlock Holmes, indeed. There was good advice for any clubman bothered by constipation – to abjure that 'most injurious of all habits, drug-taking' and learn that 'a pipe or a cigar after breakfast is with many men an infallible remedy.'[36] But there was still the *ignis fatuus*: The medical profession had begun to question bleeding by lancet and leeches in the 1830s; in 1892 William Osler wrote, 'During the first five decades of this century the profession bled too much, but during the last decades we have certainly bled too little.' He recommended bleeding or leeching as a procedure in certain cases of pneumonia, emphysema, stroke, pleurisy ('but a hypodermic of morphia is more effective'), pericarditis, peritonitis, bronchitis, delerium, and mumps. He also suggested acupuncture for lumbago, sciatica, and neuralgia. In the latter two cases the physician could also try injections of distilled water – aquapuncture.[37]

For the most part, there was an underlying consistency to his prescriptions. As he had taught his McGill students, physicians should try to relieve painful symptoms and life-threatening conditions. Patients wanted their pain treated, and doctors had to do it. Occasional lapses notwithstanding, Osler did warn constantly of overreliance on drugs. The ones he prescribed – quinine, arsenic, iron, digitalis, the opiates – were given in simple mixtures, not the polypharmacological or 'shotgun' compounds that were beginning to become fashionable.[38] In his insistence that there were no specifics for bacterial infections and many other diseases, he was blunt and uncompromising:

> Many specifics have been vaunted in scarlet fever, but they are all useless ... Medicines have little or no control over the duration or course of [rheumatic fever] ... We are still without a trustworthy medicine which can always be relied upon to control purpura ... Pneumonia is a self-limited disease, and runs its course uninfluenced in any way by medicine. It can neither be aborted nor cut short by any known means at our command ... To apply a blister to a patient suffering with agonizing headache in meningitis is needlessly to add to the suffering ... There is no method which can be recommended as satisfactory in any respect [for Parkinson's disease]. Arsenic, opium, and hyoscyamia may be tried, but the friends of the patient should be told frankly that the disease is incurable, and that nothing can be done except to attend to the physical comforts of the patient.[39]

In a talk given to a general audience while he was working on his text,

Osler indicated the direction of his thoughts on drugging. To have understood the self-limiting nature of disease was a great step forward by the
medical profession. If only the laity would follow suit!

> A desire to take medicine is, perhaps, the great feature which distinguishes
> man from other animals. Why this appetite should have developed, how it
> could have grown to its present dimensions, what it will ultimately reach,
> are interesting problems in psychology. Of one thing I must complain, –
> that when we of the profession have gradually emancipated ourselves from
> a routine administration of nauseous mixtures on every possible occasion,
> and when we are able to say, without fear of dismissal, that a little more
> exercise, a little less food, and a little less tobacco and alcohol, may possibly
> meet the indications of the case – I say it is a just cause of complaint that
> when we, the priests, have left off the worship of Baal, and have deserted
> the groves and high places, and have sworn allegiance to the true god of
> science, that you, the people, should wander off after all manner of idols,
> and delight more and more in patent medicines and be more than ever at
> the hands of advertising quacks. But for a time it must be so. This is yet the
> childhood of the world, and a supine credulity is still the most charming
> characteristic of man.[40]

Surgery was different. From the beginning of his career, surgical intervention had continually become safer and more successful. As a hospital
practitioner, Osler had always worked closely with surgeons. In addresses
in 1891–2 he proclaimed surgery 'a new art' and condemned 'the conservatism that branded ovariotomists as butchers and belly-rippers.' If he had
any predilection as a medical practitioner it was to call on surgical help
sooner rather than later. The days of simple clinical-pathological dualism
were over: 'The cocksureness of the clinical physician, who formerly had
to dread only the mortifying disclosures of the post-mortem room, is now
wisely tempered when the surgeon can so promptly and safely decide upon
the nature of an obscure case.'[41] Osler thought there was empirical justification for the minor surgeries involved in venesection. In the early 1890s
his recommendation to have surgeons on call in all cases of peritonitis, not

to delay tracheotomy in edematus laryngitis, and to seriously consider the surgical treatment of gallstones were forward-looking. He even recommended exploratory brain surgery where abscess seemed likely.[42]

One of his clearest therapeutical directions by the early 1890s was towards hydrotherapy – bathing, sponging, and wrapping in cold packs – for the treatment of fever. He now disliked the antipyretic drugs on the market, and he had become convinced that cold baths for high fever had better effects, including a reduction in the mortality rate for typhoid fever. In *Principles and Practice* he recommended the use of cold baths, tepid baths, sponging, and icepacks for fever, headache, nervous distress, and insomnia. Therapeutically, Osler was not so much a nihilist as a progressive conservative. His most obvious guiding star was a therapy's effectiveness in easing suffering. In his textbook of medicine Osler carried on arguments he must have had with himself and with Lafleur and the other young turks on the Hopkins wards about those cold baths in typhoid fever:

> This rigid method is not, however, without serious drawbacks, and personally I sympathize with those who designate it as entirely barbarous. To transfer a patient from a warm bed to a tub at 70 degrees Fahrenheit, and to keep him there twenty minutes or longer in spite of his piteous entreaties, does seem harsh treatment; and the subsequent shivering and blueness look distressing. A majority of our patients complain of it bitterly, and in private practice it is scarcely feasible.

Serious disappointment about another new therapy at Hopkins also found its way into Osler's book. Koch's tuberculin, a glycerin extract of culture of tubercle bacilli, had not lived up to expectations:

> Of twenty-three cases in which we have used it at the Johns Hopkins Hospital, only three were benefited; in the others the action was either negative or actually detrimental ... In many cases it seems to aggravate the general and local symptoms.

> We are presently in the reaction wave, after being buoyed up by hopes that at last a remedy had been obtained which was positively curative in all

forms of tuberculosis lesions. It will probably be several years before we can speak with decision upon the true position of this remedy. Meanwhile our knowledge warrants us in urging extreme caution in its use.[43]

More data would soon pour in to evaluate the bathing, tuberculin, and all other treatments. More interesting cases would appear at the hospital and in the literature. More discoveries would be made. The delight of being a textbook author is that you can always make corrections, change your mind, and add new material in the next edition. The requirement to do these things is also the curse of textbook writing, made palatable, however, by the success that creates the demand for more editions. With Osler's book the success was immediate. *Principles and Practice* was enthusiastically received by friends, colleagues, reviewers, and medical students. Its first printing of 3,000 copies was exhausted in two months. In its first two years it sold 14,000 copies, earning Osler a handsome royalty of $10,000. There would certainly be revised editions of what quickly became the dominant medical textbook in the English-speaking world. For the rest of his life the book was a major source of Osler's income. He referred to his balance with Appleton as his 'boodle account.'[44]

Osler did not keep his first copy of *Principles and Practice*. He took it to Philadelphia and gave it to the woman who had refused to marry him while he was writing it. He threw it in her lap, the story goes, saying either 'Take the damned thing' or 'Here's the dirty thing.' Then he may have added, 'Now what are you going to do with the man?'[45]

The woman was Grace Linzee Revere Gross, widow of Dr Samuel W. Gross. She was thirty-seven years old in 1892, childless, reasonably good looking, with fair hair, a fine complexion, sparkling blue eyes, and an erect carriage, albeit a bit square-faced and beginning to add flesh. She had been a Boston beauty, properly brought up and schooled, and never in want, thanks to the family silverware business. In 1876 she and the strikingly handsome Dr Gross had swept one another off their feet. For the next

twelve years she had been hostess and helpmate to Philadelphia's first medical family, not only to the younger Gross but also to his widowered father,
Samuel D., the emperor of American surgery. Osler, we saw, had come to
know her as a frequent visitor to the Gross home. Grace had every social
skill, including warmth, charm, outward self-assurance, and precisely the
appropriate amount of assertiveness. Shopping once on her own in Paris,
she found herself followed by a little Frenchman. She slowed down until
he caught up with her, then suddenly turned round and lunged at him with
her umbrella, saying 'Shoo.' He took to his heels. By birth, breeding, residence, and marriage, Grace Revere Gross was an American blue-blood.
Appropriately for a New Englander, she claimed descent from both sides of
the revolution: Paul Revere told the patriots that the British were coming;
British Captain John Linzee of the Royal Navy bombarded Boston during
the battle of Bunker Hill.[46]

Properly, Grace never spoke of her first husband in later years. One
close friend of the family thought the Gross marriage had been very happy,
but one of her brothers called Gross, who was twenty years older than
Grace, 'a profane old sot.' To colleagues, S.W. Gross had been a high-
achieving, opinionated, authoritarian, profane, and somewhat eccentric
man, but he was suspected of great familial affection. He had published
books on breast cancer and male impotence. His and Grace's only child
had died at birth.

Osler had found Gross a friendly colleague and kindred medical
inkslinger. He had clearly enjoyed being a guest in the Gross household. A
doctor friend from Hamilton, Archie Malloch, remembered Osler taking
him to dinner at the Grosses and saying afterwards that Mrs Gross was the
only woman he would ever marry. Memory plays tricks; perhaps Osler said
she was the only kind of woman he would want to marry. Someone else
remembered him saying in these years that he never wanted to marry anyone other than his childhood sweetheart Mary Osler.[47]

Grace's first impression of Osler must have been of his striking physical
resemblance to her husband, with a considerable advantage in age and
perhaps disposition. We know nothing of their relationship in the four
years after Gross's death, other than the excursion to a leper colony. When

Willie gave Grace the finished textbook and asked what she would do with the man, she agreed to marry him. What did she see in him? At best, a man of delightful personality and unlimited potential; at worst, another hard-working, handsome doctor, a much younger version of her husband, obviously doing well in life. William Osler would be Grace Revere's trophy husband.

They kept their plans semi-secret. When the university's term ended that spring, with the usual speeches and celebrations, Osler told the boys in the hospital he thought he'd go and get married – no one believed him – and went over to Philadelphia. J.C. Wilson, Grace's doctor, knew of the relationship. He lunched with Willie and Grace on Saturday, May 7. They chatted about holidays in New Brunswick and Canadian doctors, and then Wilson went off to work, apparently asking to be invited to the wedding. He got a note dated the next day from New York:

Dear Wilson

That was the wedding breakfast at which you sat yesterday! We went round the corner at 2.30 to a parson and settled matters in a quiet sensible fashion.

Mrs. Osler sends her kindest regards.

It was said that when Grace's servant learned why there was a hansom cab waiting at the door to take them to the church, she exclaimed, 'My God, Mam, only a hansom! Lemme go and fetch a hack.' The newlyweds walked from St James Church to the train station.[48]

They visited his relatives in Toronto, old friends in Montreal, her relatives in Boston. He gave a paper to the Association of American Physicians in Washington, and they took ship for England, where they toured Cornwall and took in the British Medical Association's meeting. Willie had told his mother of their plans, and a few days before the marriage she had written to his sister Chattie giving her views:

I'm sure you heard from Willie of the new life opening before him with a Lady Help at his side. He let me and Father into his secret when he was up, but we were not at liberty to make known the fact – these young things

always think their love affairs are secrets to the outside world, whereas
lookers-on often see things plainly enough. So it may have been in this case
– however I think we all feel glad at heart that there is good hope of Willie
having a loving wife to care for him. When you see Grace I think you will
bid her welcome as a sister-in-law, I feel quite pleased to have her as a daughter in law. And Father is right glad that Willie is likely to have such a good
life partner: the event will make quite a stir in the family.

After the marriage Osler told Lafleur that he would like Grace. 'She is an
old friend of mine and I feel very safe.' He probably meant safe from the
wiles of designing, ambitious, domineering, or unreliable women. He would
avoid Lydgate's fate in *Middlemarch*. 'She is a brilliant and handsome
woman,' William Welch wrote to his sister, 'and it is considered a good
match for both of them.'[49]

John J. Abel, a young American professor with a passion for doing pharmacology in German labs, was en route to Europe in June 1892 and noticed
the Oslers on the passenger list. He had known of Osler by reputation for
years. After some hesitation he struck up an acquaintance, and wrote his
wife about it:

> Mrs. O is from Boston originally, strong fine looking woman, but not enough
> soul or fine edge to suit my taste. Osler is worth meeting, the *only* medical
> man that I have ever met in America who *burns* to know. He began at 18. It
> makes me wild with envy, has been across 8 times to study. Says whenever
> he got 1000 or 1200 dollars he skipped off to Europe. Grand training he has,
> broad & strong. Is not a canny Scot, his people came from back of the
> Lizard light house Welsh & Cornish stock. Very fine fellow but thinks after
> 40 a man's no good. What is to become of me poor soul if that is true [Abel
> was thirty-five]. My talks with him have moved me afresh.[50]

Hold on! Here was William Osler, possessor of the best medical job in

America, author of a just-published textbook, newlywed, fit and healthy, sexually active, age forty-three, telling a young friend that after forty a man is no good. It was not a random or first-time comment. In Europe in 1890, Osler had noted that 'the intellectual digestion usually gets feeble after the crise de quarante ans and new methods are assimilated with difficulty.' In one of his letters home he mentioned 'the theory upon which I am always harping, that a man's productive years are in the third and fourth decades.' In an 1892 speech he referred to 'la crise de quarante ans' as characterized by both declining physical powers ('that lessening of elasticity which impels a man to open rather than vault a five-barred gate') and a 'loss of mental elasticity which makes men over forty so slow to receive new truths.'[51]

Later in life Osler became notorious for his obsessive and pessimistic views of the impact of aging. We see in chapter 8 the furor he caused with thoughts on turning sixty. He was a child of his medical times in holding views about the aging process that seem to have been drawn primarily from pathological work. The nineteenth-century pathologists could not help but note the deterioration of old bodies. They tended to equate aging with physical deterioration, senescence with 'senility,' and increasingly to use 'senility' as synonymous with loss of mental powers. Their views were reinforced by their work in almshouses and charity hospitals with a particularly helpless and diseased group of elders.[52]

Osler wrote little about the aging process per se, but he subscribed to the conventional medical wisdom. He would certainly have read Charcot's *Clinical Lectures on the Diseases of Old Age.* In *Principles and Practice* he helped popularize the notion of arteriosclerosis or hardening of the arteries, as one of the pathological stigmata of age. It seemed to have implications involving a reduction of mental power and quickness. If body and brain (old brains are lighter brains) were actually decaying in the senescent, perhaps ideas about the utility of the wisdom and experience accumulated over the years were wrong-headed. There seemed little doubt that young people had a greater capacity for learning and hard work. Perhaps a person peaked and then began a long downhill slide. About the time he turned forty, Osler had picked up from his reading the notion of men experiencing a turning point in their physical and mental capacities at that age. Whether the idea explained what was happening to his life, whether it helped cause him to make changes, or whether he even had a definable 'crise de quarante ans' is not clear. He certainly did have a sharp turning point.

At age forty Osler had left Pennsylvania for Hopkins and had started afresh as chief of a staff of younger men. In his early forties he stopped frequenting his old workshop, the dead house – Welch and his assistants did the autopsies at Hopkins. At forty-two Osler summed up his medical knowledge in *The Principles and Practice of Medicine*. And he gave up the life of a dedicated bachelor for the responsibilities of marriage. He once observed that as one ages, 'often the mind grows clearer and the memory more retentive, but the change is seen in a weakened receptivity and in an inability to adapt oneself to an altered intellectual environment.' Whether or not Osler became anxious about waning powers, his habits and writings altered significantly. 'Don't count the years,' he said to a young helper on his forty-second birthday. 'I'll get old fast enough.'[53]

In his early forties, the early Hopkins years, Osler broadens his reading, thinking, and oratorical reach. He begins ranging through time more deliberately and self-consciously. Having stopped doing postmortems on people, he turns to the postmortem literary discipline, history, as a way of understanding. His command of good literature increases. His style becomes more self-consciously literary, not always to good effect. He indulges his lifelong penchant for quotation, simile, and metaphor, burdening some of his reflections to the point where meaning becomes obscure and readers and listeners turn away perplexed. He begins to see himself as an elder statesman, or a high priest or bishop of a profession he constantly compares to the clergy. He preaches on the state of his profession, the advancement of science, the march of history. He becomes more interested in preventive medicine and public health. References to aging and reflections on death and the meaning of life become more common, even as his mother continues to urge that he worry about the state of his eternal soul.

He takes time from textbook writing in 1891 to ponder 'Recent Advances in Medicine' at Johns Hopkins University's fifteenth anniversary.

He is in an optimistic mood, arguing that the sanitarian, bacteriological, and therapeutic revolutions have laid the foundation for wonderful progress to come: 'Some of the brightest hopes of humanity are with the medical profession. To it, not to law or theology, belong the promises. Disease will always be with us, but we may look forward confidently to the time when epidemics shall be no more, when typhoid shall be as rare as typhus, and tuberculosis as leprosy ... What has been done is but an earnest of the things that shall be done.'

But he is singularly melancholy a few months later as he addresses the first graduating class of nurses from the hospital's training school. The mission of both doctors and nurses, he says, is to help mankind shelter itself from 'chains of atavism ... legacies of feeble will and strong desires, taints of blood and brain,' the 'frightful tax of human blood' exacted by 'Nature, the great Moloch.' For the most part, he tells the young ladies and their parents, humans are dull, stupid pupils, insensitive to their condition: 'Like schoolboys we play among the shadows cast by the turrets of the temple of oblivion ... Suffering and disease are ever before us, but life is very pleasant; and the motto of the world, when well, is "forward with the dance" ... Perhaps we are wise. Who knows? Mercifully, the tragedy of life, though seen, is not realized. It is so close that we lose all sense of its proportions.' On one of the brightest days of their lives, the nurses are told that in life they, like all of us, will be no more than 'useful supernumeraries ... simply stage accessories.' At best, when they reach the dark river of death, their reward will be blessing for having ministered so well. Osler did delight them by giving each graduate a bouquet of roses. And who ever listens carefully to commencement speeches?[54]

The next year, after finishing *Principles and Practice*, Osler delivered himself of a sweeping lay sermon, 'Student and Teacher,' to the graduating class of the University of Minnesota. He enlisted John Henry Newman, Matthew Arnold, Sir Thomas Browne, William Harvey, Sir James Paget, Dante, Napoleon, Darwin, Plato, the son of Sirach, Sainte Beuve, Rabbi Ben Ezra, Socrates, and St Bernard, among others, in the cause of advising the students to cultivate the Art of Detachment, the Virtue of Method, the Quality of Thoroughness, and the Grace of Humility. A few weeks later he spoke against specialization to an audience of protospecialists at the fourth annual meeting of the American Paediatric Association. Noting that Aristophanes satirized a 'rectum specialist,' Osler suggested that American medicine was producing dangerously narrow-minded practitioners. He quoted Socrates on the need to treat the whole of the patient, not just a body part; this notion, he said, 'embodies the law and the gospel for specialists.' From somewhere in his reading or yarning, he cobbled a superb comparison: 'The man that, year in and year out, examines eyes, palpates ovaries, or tunnels urethrae, without regard to the wide influence upon which his art rests, is likely, insensibly perhaps, but none the less surely, to acquire the attitude of mind of the old Scotch shoemaker, who, in response to the Dominie's suggestions about the weightier matters of life, asked "D'ye ken leather?"'[55]

During his honeymoon touring in England, Osler had a mildly epiphanous experience while listening to a choir in Lincoln Cathedral. The glorious singing led him to reflect on human striving, the quest for 'the ideal State, the ideal Life, the ideal Church ... Such dreams continue to haunt the minds of men, and who can doubt that their contemplation immensely fosters the upward progress of the race?' On his forty-third birthday, Grace gave him a copy of Jowett's five-volume translation of the works of Plato. That winter at Hopkins the medical history group did a special study of Greek medicine. Osler, working on a long paper on 'Physic and Physicians as Depicted in Plato,' steeping himself in European scholarly philhellenism, was drawn to the classic philosophic attempt to contemplate all of time and all existence.[56]

What about his new bride? Where did Grace fit into the changes in his life? Would she change him still more?

Not likely. From long experience, Grace Osler knew her place as a doctor's wife, which was to be a helpmate – and Osler knew she knew it, for he often told medical friends that widows, being broken in, made the best wives. If Grace had forgotten the tenor of medical marriage, she was reminded on their British honeymoon when they took in the British Medical Association's meeting at Nottingham. Grace was abandoned to her own devices in a dismal provincial city while Osler went off with his friends.

Sensibly, she made a point of avoiding getting caught in traps like that again.

But theirs was not a midlife marriage of convenience. Grace became pregnant and gave birth to a boy almost nine months to the day from their wedding. The thought of being a parent, of having a child of his own to play with and cherish, could only have thrilled Willie. Dr and Mrs Osler had begun housekeeping at a big handsome home at 1 West Franklin Street in a leafy, fashionable Baltimore residential area. The birth was unusually easy – Howard Kelly attended – but the baby was 'a little asphyxiated,' Osler observed, 'and I suppose there was slight meningeal haemorrhage, and a subsequent clotting in the veins or sinuses.' On the fifth or sixth day, it went into sudden coma and died. 'One must take the rough with the smooth,' Osler wrote.[57]

Before their marriage, William and Grace had each contributed money to one of the more remarkable feminist crusades in the history of American medicine. At the end of 1888 Daniel Coit Gilman had issued an open appeal for financial help to open the Johns Hopkins School of Medicine. 'Only a man of large means and of large views will be likely to appreciate the situation,' Gilman had written. 'But if such a man can be found willing to consider a plan in detail, it will be easy to shew him that a like opportunity to be of service to mankind has never been presented.' No such man came forward. Instead, a group of women of large views organized a campaign to raise the necessary funds. The condition was that women would have to be admitted equally with men in the new school.[58]

The leaders of the movement were Mary Garrett, Carey Thomas, Mary Gwinn, and Elizabeth King. Their fathers were all Hopkins trustees. They had been lifelong friends, were all unmarried, and shared an intense interest in the advancement of women. Bessie King was in delicate health and often consulted Osler. Garrett was very rich, having inherited part of the fortune her father had made as head of the Baltimore and Ohio Railroad. Thomas, who had been rejected for graduate degree work at Johns Hopkins

University because of her sex, had taken a PhD in Zurich and become dean of the Quaker-founded Bryn Mawr College, just outside Philadelphia. She and her friends also founded the Bryn Mawr School to prepare young women for college.

None of the four women had wanted to go into medicine. (Three of them, Gwinn remembered, had cut up a dead mouse in class, and 'the odour of that mouse forever clung about their fingers.')[59] All believed that women should have the same opportunities as men. By the 1880s quite a few American medical schools, especially those in need of student fees, were open to women, and a number of medical schools had been founded solely for women, including one in Baltimore. Women could get a run-of-the-mill medical training; but they were still excluded from medical education at Harvard, Pennsylvania, McGill, Michigan, and other top North American medical schools. Hopkins intended to position itself at the very top, equal to or better than anything offered in Europe. Women were not admitted to any of the undergraduate or graduate programs at Johns Hopkins University. The Baltimore feminists, who wanted women to have equal access to excellence in all professions, saw a pre-emptive financial strike in medical education as an enormous lever.

Early in 1890 they announced the formation of the Women's Fund Committee to raise an endowment to enable the Johns Hopkins School of Medicine to open. Their goal was $100,000. Supporting committees were set up in Philadelphia, New York, Boston, and Washington; donations came from as far afield as California. Many socially and professionally prominent women contributed, including the First Lady, Mrs Benjamin Harrison, who headed the Washington committee. Grace Revere Gross gave ten dollars to the Philadelphia campaign. The Boston fundraisers received many small sums from unprominent women, including fifty cents from Bridget O'Brien and twenty-five cents from Sarah Birdsall. Mary Garrett contributed $48,000. By the autumn of 1890 the financial goal had been reached. The women would give the money to the university if the trustees agreed to admit women to the medical school.

The men at Johns Hopkins were discombobulated. They were being offered a bribe, and everyone knew it. Women had tried this before in medicine. A decade earlier, Harvard had turned down a $10,000 offer. (Some said it was too small, but when the ante was upped to $50,000 the men still stood firm, though only by a whisker.) Mary Garrett had failed to sway Hopkins in 1887 with an offer of $35,000 towards a coeducational school of science. Now all the stakes were higher. The women's issue at Hopkins was on Osler's mind in Europe in the summer of 1890. He went out of his way to observe female medical students in lectures and clinics, and asked colleagues there how they felt about having women in their classes.

Osler, Kelly, and Superintendent Hurd signed a letter urging the university trustees to accept the $100,000. Welch, who did not believe in coeducation – apparently because he would find it embarrassing to teach women the indelicate parts of pathology – refused to sign. In October 1890 the university board accepted the $100,000 and the condition, but stipulated that the medical school could not be opened until the endowment had reached $500,000. 'Pres. Gilman and some of the Trustees really do not want (sub rosa) the women to succeed,' Welch wrote some months later, 'for they do not like the idea of co-sexual medical education. I do not myself hanker after it.'[60]

It was not clear where the remaining $400,000 would be found. Would the women raise it? Suppose a man produced, say, $500,000? Could the women be bypassed and their money returned? Had the Hopkins educators compromised themselves and important principles by accepting the gift? Many men thought they had. Criticism of the board's action led to a strong rejoinder in the February 1891 issue of the *Century Magazine* from several writers, including Carey Thomas, James Cardinal Gibbons, the Roman Catholic primate in America (who saw no church obstacles to women studying medicine), and one member of the Johns Hopkins Hospital staff, Dr William Osler.

Osler wrote that there were 'diverse' answers to the question of the expediency of women entering medicine, 'the work of which is often disagreeable and always laborious.' But the real matter of principle was clear: 'This is right: if any woman feels that the medical profession is her vocation, no obstacles should be placed in the way of her obtaining the best possible education, and every facility should be offered so that, as a practitioner, she should have a fair start in the race.' Osler's European observations had shown him that medical coeducation was perfectly feasible. 'One of the most distinguished members of the Berne faculty confessed to me that he had not favored coeducation, but that he had not met with any difficulties in his laboratory.' In Paris, where 'the utmost freedom' was given to women, 'it was evident every day that the hearers and seers were considered as students only, quite irrespective of sex.' Osler recommended that Hopkins follow the Paris model of being completely oblivious to the sex of students. 'Many teachers complain that they feel hampered and cannot talk so plainly to a class containing women. This is true, but with practice even the most delicate subjects may be discussed from a scientific standpoint, with the utmost freedom, before a mixed class.' Osler donated his $100 fee from the article to the Women's Fund.

Nothing happened for almost two years. The failure of Johns Hopkins University to launch its medical school was becoming a growing public embarrassment and a matter of deep private concern at the hospital. There was a real possibility that the grand medical vision would crumble and collapse. Superintendent Henry Hurd was particularly alarmed at the failure of the university to find the resources to fulfill the founder's intentions. Over in Philadelphia, Weir Mitchell was starting to boast that it would be only a matter of time before Pennsylvania lured Osler back, and Welch to boot. 'It will be difficult to retain our men much longer,' Hurd wrote as early as August 1890.

The hospital trustees had authorized the launching of postgraduate courses by their staff as a way of both using their resources and putting pressure on the university. The implicit threat, which the university well understood, was that the hospital would create a separate medical school along the lines of those at the great hospitals in London. But these courses did not amount to much. Baltimore doctors may have had little interest in going up the mountain to Hopkins, and some of the Hopkins scientists had little interest in taking on students. In a confidential March 1891 memorandum to the hospital trustees, Superintendent Hurd called for a complete reorganization of the teaching program: 'Although an announcement has been made for two years of the work in Dr Osler's Clinical Laboratory this work has never been conducted in any systematic way and it has amounted to nothing. The defect should be corrected or the announcement should be cancelled. The same is true of the announcement of surgical teaching. It has never been done with any thoroughness or regularity.' Two months later Hurd criticized methods in Welch's pathological laboratory as 'unsystematic and wasteful.' Councilman remembered that in that lab they had deliberately repelled students.

Johns Hopkins Hospital did not have unlimited resources to support a teaching staff without students. Nor, in Hurd's view, were the staff doing 'as systematic work as they would if they had definite teaching to do and felt the stimulus of a class of picked workers. It is also evident that the postgraduate courses now given do not meet the expectations of the country and that the wonderful opportunity which is open to the University to initiate medical teaching of the highest character is being allowed to slip away.'[61]

The Hopkins group had no objection to women doctors taking some of their courses or doing research in their labs. So while casting about for more money, the Women's Fund Committee, led by Bessie King, put pressure on the hospital to appoint women to the resident staff. Osler and Kelly agreed. Mary Sherwood and Alice Hall were to be the first women physicians at Hopkins. But before the scheme could be implemented Alice Hall suddenly got married. The hospital staff would not accept a married woman (or a married man) as an intern and would not break the gender barrier with one woman only. Mary Sherwood was bitterly disappointed. Kelly gave her a job in his private gynecological hospital.[62]

In the meantime, Osler had had the free time to write his text, and even to write several chapters in a new Pepper-edited multivolume text, and the band of brothers at the hospital had happily carried on their research. In the spring of 1891 Osler turned down offers of chairs at Harvard and at Philadelphia's Jefferson Medical College. He had, in effect, a standing offer to come home to McGill – though an 1892 newspaper report that a philanthropist was offering the Montreal school $1 million if Osler returned was probably a huge exaggeration. Referring to such rumors, Osler said he was 'too comfortable here' to think of any change: 'I hope to fill out my twenty years and then crawl back to Montreal to worry the boys for a few years.' His senior resident, Henri Lafleur, did go back to McGill and the Montreal General, eventually becoming professor of medicine. Several other young Hopkins men moved on to good jobs in other institutions. After Welch turned down the chair of pathology at Harvard, it was offered to Councilman, who accepted. Osler himself apparently let well-connected Hopkins folk know that he did not like the 'dry bones' of postgraduate teaching and might have to go somewhere where there were real medical students.[63]

The hospital itself was running smoothly. Its public wards were gradually filling with charity patients, and fees from private patients were helping supplement the endowment income. One major source of what the board called 'mutual discomfort' on the wards was being resolved as the hospital moved to segregate white and colored patients. To the trustee who had done most to build Johns Hopkins Hospital, Francis J. King, this was a major defeat. 'I did my best to avoid the separation of the races,' he wrote to Billings. The sources do not show whether anyone else tried to avoid the separation. King added that he would be a happy man if only the medical school could be opened. 'I hope that some one who wishes to perpetuate his name will turn up soon.' King died in 1892, his hopes unfulfilled.[64]

The funding logjam finally seemed to break at the end of 1892 when Mary Garrett offered to contribute all the money needed to bring the medical school's endowment up to $500,000. But Garrett made her offer contingent on the medical school living up to its original intention of having extremely high admission standards, an undergraduate degree or equivalent. Now, when it came to implementing their lofty visions of years earlier, the medical men faltered. If their admission standards were far higher than any other medical school in America, the vast majority of which still did not require high school graduation, would there be any students? If students did not come – and so far there had not been many postgraduate students – Hopkins would surely have to be free to lower its expectations. If it bound itself forever by the Garrett terms, it would have no flexibility. Even Osler balked at the prospect of Hopkins losing its freedom to adjust its admission requirements. 'The restrictions placed by Miss Garrett as to the preliminary education necessary will limit the number of our students very materially ...' he wrote to Lafleur. 'Welch put it very happily the other day when he said to me that it was lucky we got in as professors; we never would have been able to go in as students.'[65]

After an intense flurry of meetings, statements, clarifications, and re-statements, during which Garrett bent only slightly, the men decided to take the risk, and the donation was accepted. Mary Garrett's total contri-bution to the medical school's $500,000 endowment fund was $354,764.50. She saved everyone from what would surely have been a *crise comique* by not suggesting that the school be named after her. None of the men volun-teered the thought. Johns Hopkins University gave its medical staff ap-proval to begin instruction in October 1893.

The full story of the women's application of what has been called *force monnetaire*[66] to obtain equality while reinforcing elitism may never be un-earthed. Its many layers involved father-daughter relations, deep and protolesbian female friendships and rivalries, excruciatingly delicate aca-demic politics, and, possibly, a desire for first-rate medical care by chroni-cally ill women who felt uncomfortable being examined by men. Mary Garrett and Bessie King were semi-invalids, and Garrett had been treated in New York and abroad by skilled women physicians. The Women's Fund Committee stated that its object was to permit the education of women 'in such manner as to be fully able to care for sick women who may wish or ought to be treated by women.' Carey Thomas described the Hopkins af-fair as 'a tangle of hatred, malice, detraction that beggars description.' That it was more complex than a noble stand for abstract human rights is sug-gested by Thomas's simultaneous efforts to limit Jewish enrollment at Bryn Mawr's prep school.[67]

Osler's constant desire had been to get on with the opening of the medical school. He undoubtedly would have preferred not to have had to deal with the woman question. Once confronted with it, he went to school on the subject in Europe and broke ranks with Welch on the principle at home. Had he been bought by a bribe? 'We are all for sale, dear Remsen,' he wrote to Johns Hopkins University's second president some years later. 'You and

I have been in the market for years, and have loved to buy and sell our ware in brains and books – it has been our life. So with institutions. It is always pleasant to be bought, when the purchase price does not involve the sacrifice of an essential – as was the case in that happy purchase of us by the Women's Educational Association.'[68]

Welch was appointed dean of the Johns Hopkins School of Medicine. The university took over responsibility for one-third of his, Osler's, Halsted's, and Kelly's salaries. To fill the chair of anatomy, Hopkins hired Franklin P. Mall, who had worked for three years as a fellow in Welch's laboratory before moving to Clark University and then to the University of Chicago. Another thoroughgoing Germanophile, Mall was completely committed to laboratory research. The supposition that Hopkins was likely to have very few students was used by Welch as a selling point.

Osler handled the negotiations to lure the pharmacologist John J. Abel, whom he had first met on his honeymoon, away from the University of Michigan. He had earlier encouraged Abel to visit Hopkins to do 'missionary work among our wild pharmaceutical chemists,' telling him: 'Therapeutics is a subject sadly neglected here I am afraid. My function is altogether negative, and largely taken up with the prevention of over-drugging.' Now he added that the atmosphere of Hopkins was 'very pleasant & the idea of organizing a new style of medical school ... very attractive ... You will find a very happy family, no internal troubles ... Tell Mrs. Abel that marketing is easy.'[69]

Abel, who was even more imbued with the love of German research than Mall, wanted leave to work in Germany until January 1, 1894. Mall wanted leave to go to Germany after January 1. Four of the younger residents were abroad for the year. The trustees put their collective feet down. 'The feeling is very strong, perhaps almost morbid,' Welch told Mall, 'that our new professors who will have most of the teaching to do next year, should be here on the ground throughout the year.'

H. Newell Martin, Johns Hopkins's pioneering professor of physiology, could be there for the term but would be of no use. He had become a hopeless alcoholic. In April 1893 he resigned. Osler had been Martin's doctor. Now, Welch wrote,

> Osler had a talk with him and he was led to see that it was the only proper course to pursue. Martin in his day did a great work for this University and for physiology in this country ... He has completely succumbed to alcohol and is no longer capable of making the slightest effort to resist it. Last night he started under the care of Adam, his janitor, for an institution in Canada kept by a physician, a friend of Osler's. He is to remain there six months or a year and probably every effort will be made to put him on his feet again. Fortunately there was no public scandal.

Nor was there an effective cure. Martin drifted back to England, where he died in 1896. One of his Hopkins students, William H. Howell, was hired as his replacement.[70]

They had the splendid hospital, the endowment to fund the medical school, and now the rest of the staff. The Johns Hopkins School of Medicine could at last open. The Johns Hopkins institutions always had a shrewd eye for publicity, but on this occasion they decided not to draw attention to themselves. No formal opening ceremonies were planned for October 1893 for fear that the high admissions standards would keep students away. Suppose you built a medical school and they did not come?

SIX

We All Worship Him

Eighteen students, including three women, registered at the School of Medicine at Johns Hopkins in its first year, 1893–4. One man's mother allowed him to attend only after Dr Osler had assured her that it would be a very, very good school.[1] That was a bold commitment. The school did not have an auspicious beginning. In many ways, it was a disorganized mess. The professors, most of whom were inexperienced as pedagogues, appeared to care little for teaching and little for the students. Male professors and students cared little for the female students, except as prospective brides. And the most experienced teacher, Osler, had little to do with the students until they entered their third year in the autumn of 1895.

At that time, and for the rest of his Hopkins career, Osler became virtually everyone's favorite professor. He could not have helped standing out by comparison with his Hopkins colleagues. But he would have shone in any faculty by the force of what everyone around him saw as a remarkable, charismatic personality. Further, as an organizer of medical education, with *carte blanche* to innovate, he brought to Hopkins what for the United States were strikingly new and important teaching methods, notably the clinical clerkship. More than anyone else, Osler emerged as the man who made Johns Hopkins a very, very good medical school.

The faculty had not published a schedule or calendar of courses, partly because they had thought there might be as few as three students, partly because they were not sure what to teach. Anatomy was the normal starting point, but the professor, Franklin Mall, was having trouble finding bodies for dissection and figuring out how to embalm and store them. Dissection could not begin until Mall had solved his problems with the help of the advent of cold weather, a series of experiments embalming dogs, and possibly some discreet cash payments to obtain human bodies. Makeshift substitute courses in osteology and histology were badly taught. The students thought the instruction inferior and 'dumb,' and complained to Dean Welch. Welch urged patience.

On November 15, the day dissecting was to begin, there was no body to dissect. 'We postponed work until the 16th, and then the 17th,' Mall remembered, 'when, late in the evening, a subject was left in the basement. The next day one came from the State, and a few days later another appeared in the basement ... Toward Christmas ... it was found that cadavers were more abundant and we did not fail to take what came, embalm them well with carbolic acid and place them in a large ice box which had been constructed in the meantime. By spring the box, which was built to hold five cadavers, had in it twenty.'[2]

The greater astonishment for the freshman class was to learn that Mall had no intention of teaching them. He gave no lectures but simply told them to start dissecting. If they had problems, they were to look up the solutions in the literature. He limited his role to wandering around the room from time to time, saying little except to ask irrelevant questions. Students in this and most later classes often floundered, and they complained bitterly. Mall's philosophy, he said, was to force them to learn for themselves. A few did, eagerly. Most survived, many hating the professor. It became Hopkins lore that Mall once said to his wife as she was bathing the baby, 'Why don't you just throw her in and let her work out her own technique.'[3] When a student in the lab complained to Mall that he had nothing to do, Mall gave him a broom. Years later, after the school had become a success and most of the professors much loved, the dour, caustic Mall had the reputation of being a lazy son-of-a-bitch. Even Osler had

complained to him about his failure to teach gross anatomy. Mall stead-
fastly refused to teach 'shoemaker anatomy for the pill doctors.'[4]

The student whom Mall took to most enthusiastically was one of the
three women in the first-year class. As they dissected together, wisps of her
hair would get loose and wave in his face. She dropped out to marry him,
and they lived happily ever after, despite memories of the joke Osler made
in a talk at Harvard. Coeducation at Hopkins was proven a failure, he said,
when thirty-three and a third per cent of the first class of females left to get
married. At that rate, where would they be by the end of the fourth year?

William Welch could be counted on not to take any interest in the
women students, or in most of the male students either. Welch was greatly
loved by those close to him at Hopkins, including Osler. Always affable
and charming, widely read and sophisticated, 'Popsy' Welch was a classic
bon vivant bachelor. His greatest honor, he wrote in 1895, was to have been
selected for the Skull and Bones senior society at Yale. In Baltimore he was
most at home in the Maryland Club, enjoying drinks, the culinary bounty
of Chesapeake Bay, good cigars, and the company of other bachelors. His
duties as dean of medicine and head of pathology were not arduous, and he
usually managed to get them done, but almost never on time. He was notoriously disorganized, a particularly poor correspondent (while others failed
to answer letters, it was said that Welch avoided opening them), and impossible to deal with as an editor. He drove his colleagues near to distrac-
tion as letters went unacknowledged for months, manuscripts unreturned,
decisions untaken. Even Osler got frustrated with that 'lazy devil Welch.'[5]

Most students at Hopkins seldom saw him. He apparently was available
to them only on Mondays. The researchers who worked in his lab seldom
saw him. He was a completely hands-off supervisor. 'Welch paid no attention to me whatever, after having set me to work,' wrote Simon Flexner,
who entered his lab as a student in 1890 and became his senior associate
and ultimately his biographer. 'Welch seemed hardly aware of my existence ... he had nothing to say to me outside of class hour ... He did not
even direct me to reading.' After the early 1890s, Welch did little research
of his own and published less.

Welch was dazzlingly brilliant when he lectured, but he was often late

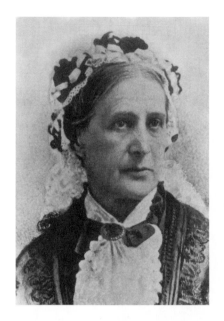

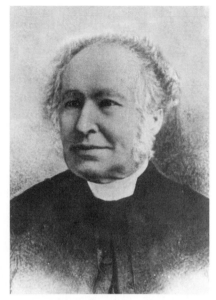

Ellen Pickton Osler (1806–1906).
Mother.

Featherstone Lake Osler (1805–1895).
Father.

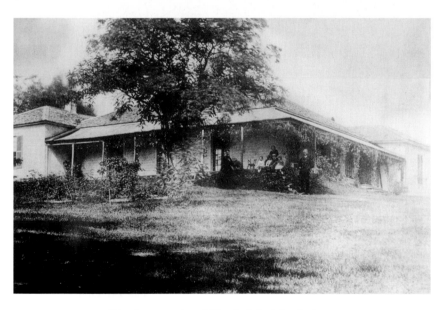

The Rectory, Bond Head. Osler's birthplace.

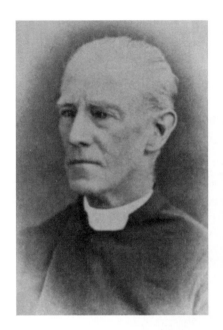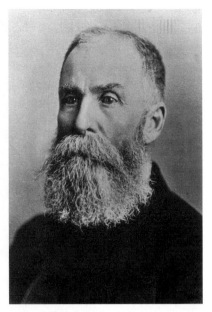

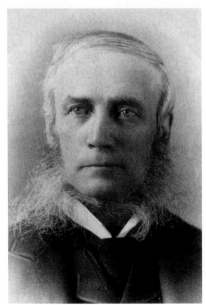

Osler's mentors: W.A. Johnson, James Bovell, and Palmer Howard.

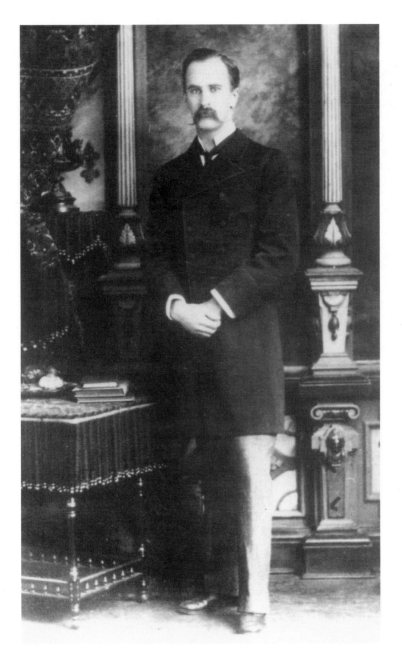

Professor of the Institutes of Medicine, McGill.
A rising star in the North Atlantic medical world.

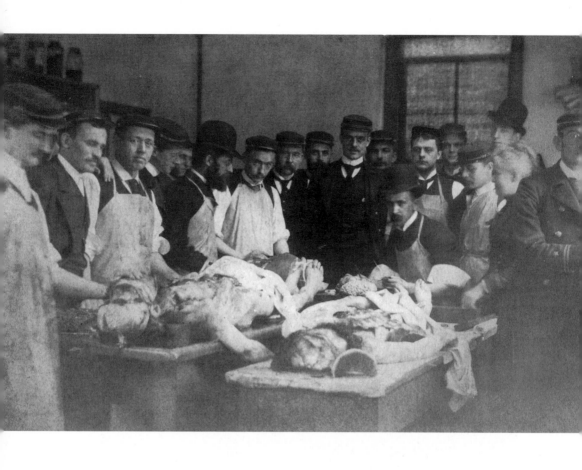

Instructing in the Blockley Dead House, Philadelphia, 1888.
The observers include one woman (second from right).

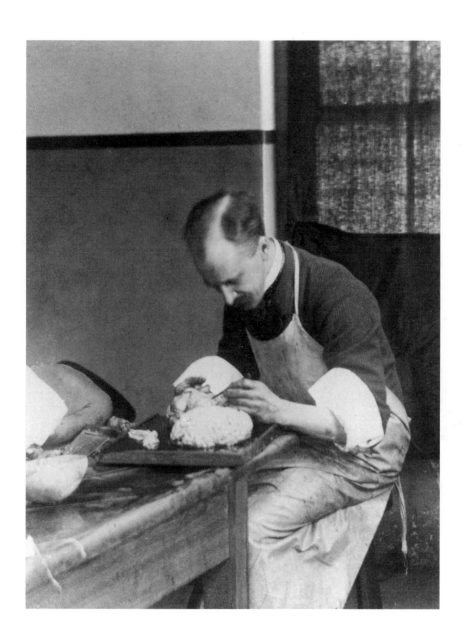

William Osler, pathologist, 1888.

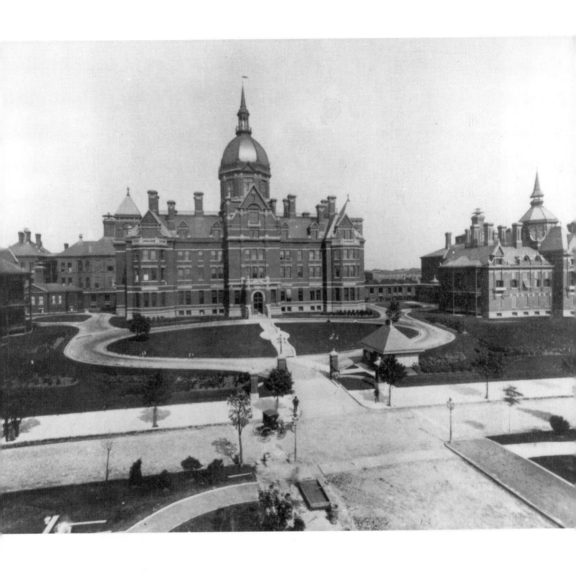

Johns Hopkins Hospital, Baltimore, c. 1892. Built to be the world's best.

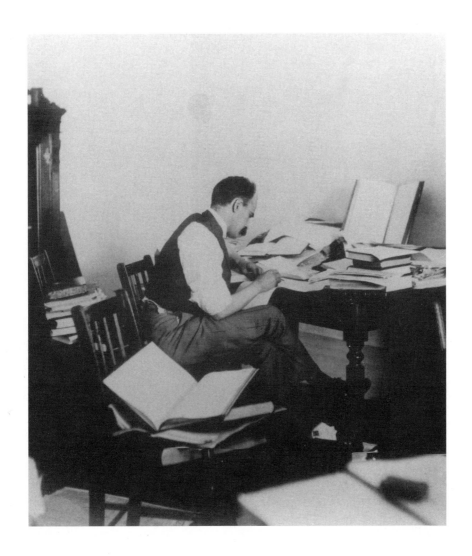

Writing *The Principles and Practice of Medicine*.

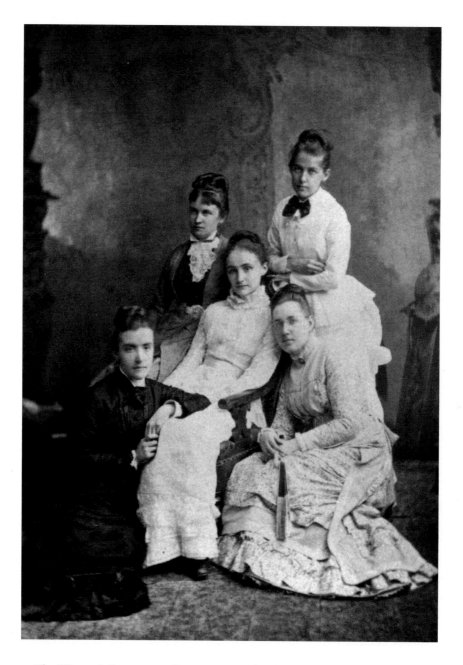

The Women's Committee. Buying into medical education at Johns Hopkins.
No one suggested naming the medical school after Mary Garrett (center).

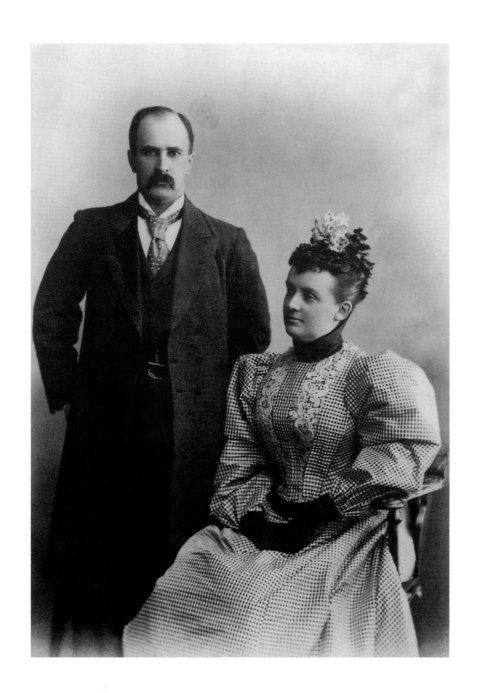

Grace Revere Osler and her trophy husband.

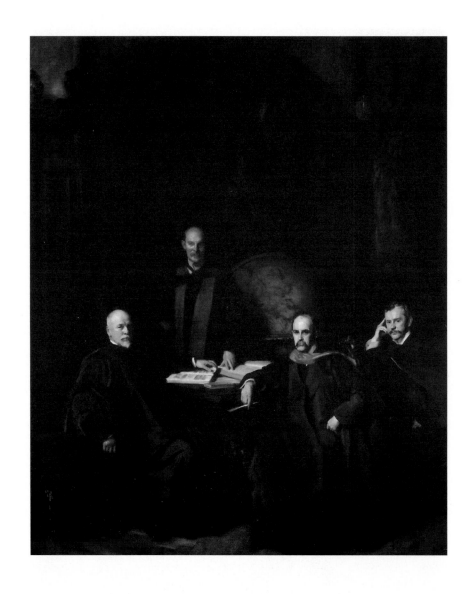

The Four Doctors by John Singer Sargent. Welch, Halsted, Osler, Kelly.

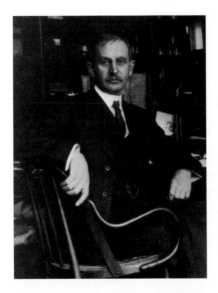

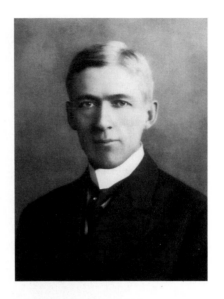

Franklin P. Mall: Osler's enemy.

Lewellys Barker: Osler's successor, and 'devil-may-care Canadian.'

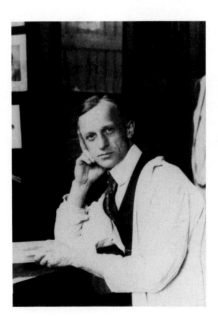

Harvey Cushing: talented, creative, towering, and Osler's biographer.

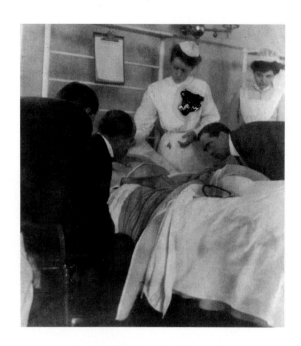

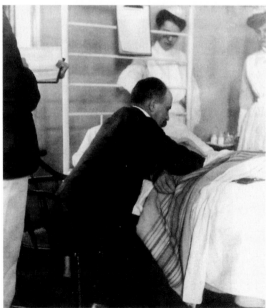

At the bedside: inspection, palpation, auscultation, contemplation.

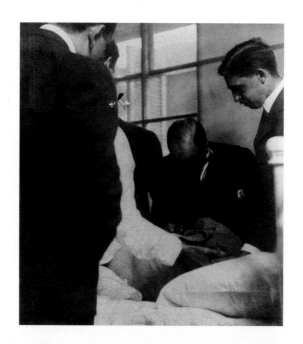

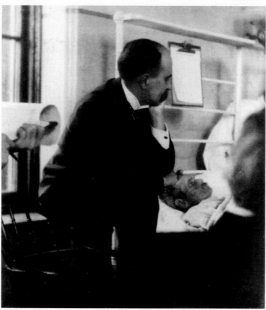

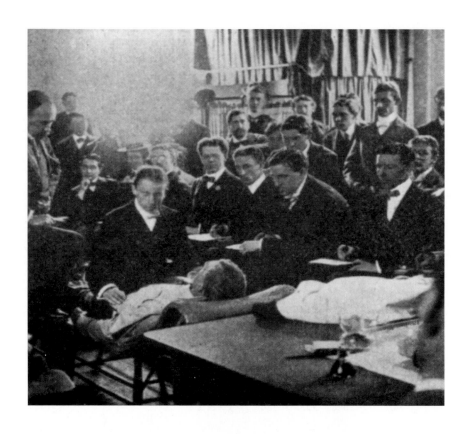

Osler teaching. An 'observation' class, Johns Hopkins.

for scheduled classes and sometimes did not show up at all. Flexner, whom Welch appreciated after he proved himself a talented researcher, covered for him. Their course contained 'too much Flexner, we felt, and too little Welch,' one of the students remembered. Welch was not so much aloof as remote and reticent. He never encouraged the young men to confide in him, and it never occurred to them to invite him to their social events. Osler was always invited and often came, even to meetings of the rowdy Society of Pithotomists (Pithotomists do surgery on kegs of beer). Although Welch was agreeable and ubiquitous in higher professional circles – and was at his genial best hosting gourmet and gourmand feasts for distinguished visitors – he remained a mystery to most of the Hopkins crowd:

> Nobody knows where Popsy eats,
> Nobody knows where Popsy sleeps,
> Nobody knows whom Popsy keeps,
> But Popsy.[6]

A few family members and friends knew that Popsy liked to eat sweets and to sleep at seaside resorts, purging himself of stress by ocean bathing and taking wild rides at the amusement parks. He had a few very close and long-lasting male friendships, including his relationship with W.S. Halsted. In our time, we naturally wonder whether Welch was homosexual; there is no hard evidence.

The reason for William Stewart Halsted's frequent absences from work is no longer a matter of conjecture. Osler realized there was something seriously wrong with Halsted about six months after the latter's permanent appointment; he saw Halsted in a severe chill and began to suspect an ongoing drug problem. Eventually, Osler gained Halsted's confidence and learned that the surgeon had never been able to break the morphine habit he had developed while breaking his cocaine addiction. Through the 1890s the professor of surgery at the Johns Hopkins School of Medicine was addicted to morphia, taking three grains a day, which is nine to twenty times a normal dose.

Nobody knew except Osler and possibly Welch. Osler revealed his knowledge in a manuscript, 'The Inner History of the Johns Hopkins Hospital,' which he ordered to be kept secret for fifty years after his death. It was published only in 1969.[7]

Why did Osler keep silent? Along with his belief in tolerating medical brethren's weaknesses, Osler knew that Halsted was proving himself a surgeon of immense brilliance and influence. Halsted was possibly the most important surgeon in American history, the man who first understood how the sepsis revolution was making it possible to work for long periods inside body cavities with extreme care and respect for living tissue and its healing capacity. Pre-anesthesia, pre-antisepsis, pre-Halsted, surgeons had been quick slashers, doing their bloody work as fast as possible to minimize pain, infection, and shock. Halsted, the exact antithesis of a traditional 'ripper,' taught colleagues to take their time, minimize bleeding and other aspects of trauma, thoroughly remove or excise damaged tissue, suture carefully, and let the body heal. Halsted was so excruciatingly painstaking and so slow that William Mayo once said Halsted's patients were usually healed by the time he completed the operation. If, as has been said, surgeons are either carnivores or herbivores, then Halsted founded the herbivore tradition in American surgery.[8]

He was a philosopher of surgery, an experimentalist who worked closely with Welch's laboratory, perfected his technique on animals, and, despite being thought to have clumsy hands, became a pioneer in vascular surgery, mastectomies, hernia work, and excision of goiters. In Halsted's operating room at Hopkins in the winter of 1889–90, a nurse was given a special pair of rubber gloves, modeled after a pair of autopsy gloves that Welch used, to protect her tender hands from harsh chemicals. The next year an assistant started wearing the gloves. Then Halsted's resident, Joe Bloodgood (of course nicknamed 'Bloody' or 'Bloodclot'), found he could do surgery with them, heavy and stiff as they seemed. Eventually the surgical unit made a huge leap forward in asepsis, pioneering for the rest of the world. The unit was also one of the first to abandon street clothes for clean white cottons.[9]

William Sydney Thayer came to Hopkins from Harvard in 1890, succeeded Lafleur as Osler's chief resident, and became a devoted Osler man. But it was Halsted, not Osler, who made the first and strongest impression on Thayer: 'In Halsted's little operating room, with the old wooden table, the antiseptic technique was so perfect that there was never a moment of anxiety. I could not believe my eyes. It was like stepping into a new world. At this time Halsted's technique was unique, and the sureness and perfection of his results seemed to me then ... the nearest thing to a miracle that it has been given to me to witness.' Halsted's contributions as a research surgeon were more important than Osler's research was to medicine.[10]

Halsted's colleagues had to forgive or overlook behavior that would have had a lesser man fired. 'The Professor' (he hated the appellation, saying it reminded him of dancing masters) was often late or absent from the hospital. Sometimes he offered no explanation. On one famous occasion he asked the scrubbed operating-room staff to excuse a ninety-minute delay because he and Mrs Halsted had been killing rats in their cellar. Sometimes he had to break off operating, claiming he was suffering from a pounding heart (tachycardia) caused by excessive smoking, and turn the job over to Bloodgood. In his dealings with his staff, Halsted was often distracted, uncommunicative, aloof, perhaps shy; or he could be sarcastic and mean-spirited, in either case showing himself painfully inept at human relations. J.M.T. Finney, a distinguished surgeon in his own right and a kindly Christian man, remembered receiving exactly one compliment from Halsted in the thirty-three years they worked together. Nor did he remember Halsted ever complimenting anyone else. In 1891 Henry Hurd reported to the board of trustees that one of the resident surgeons, Hardy Phippen, 'had thrown up his position' and left the hospital without any proper notification: 'His reasons for this hasty and inconsiderate action were the unpleasant attitude of Dr. Halsted towards him. He stated to me in conversation that he could not retain his position with self respect and his only course was to resign. He was earnest, reliable and capable and under more favorable circumstance would undoubtedly have done good work.' Halsted angered another doctor by advising him to take up piles as a specialty because dealing with them did not require much ability. 'I'll make him eat those words,' the offended surgeon remarked.[11]

Halsted's biting, withering sarcasm, said to be unequaled at Johns Hopkins, often caused the performance of those around him to deteriorate. His scorn and bullying was effectively countered only once, Finney remembered. One day some threads from a moistened bandage that was being applied to a patient on the wards became tangled. Halsted held the specimen up and remarked, 'In New York, where I was brought up surgically, a nurse would blush to hand a doctor a bandage such as this.' The little red-headed snub-nosed nurse who had done it shot back, 'Ah, but we are more brazen than they!' Finney, standing behind Halsted, watched the blood mount to the bald spot on top of his head until he became livid. Halsted finished applying the bandage and left the ward without completing his rounds or saying a word. Another time Halsted vetoed the superintendent of nursing's choice of a head nurse for the operating room and she refused to back down. The residents saved the day by hiring a medical student to be head nurse. He was male, which must have caused many jokes, for Halsted had fallen in love with and married his first operating-room nurse, Caroline Hampton, she of the rubber gloves and of a somewhat mannish appearance. The Halsteds had no children and apparently lived in separate apartments in their house.[12]

Halsted made no preparations for teaching medical students. He had announced that students in their second year would receive a course on the surgical aspects of wound healing, but it was never given. For most of the summer of 1895, when he might have been thinking about the major surgical instruction scheduled for the third year, Halsted was literally AWOL from the hospital, causing serious disruptions and a loss of patients. That winter the board of trustees severely censured him: 'His long absence from the Hospital during the past summer contrary to the assurances given by him to the Superintendent, is, in the judgment of this Board of Trustees, subversive of proper discipline and hurtful to the true interests of the Hospital.' Attendance regulations must be 'rigidly observed,' stated the board. In the meantime, the third-year class was without surgical instruction. Welch to Mall, January 11, 1896:

> We must do something for those destitute but deserving orphans, the third year students. They are struggling to learn some surgical pathology, but they have been driven from pillar to post and now have no place to lay their

heads. They have come to me in a body to see if we can not find a room
where they can work with their microscopes, cut sections of tumors, etc.
They are apparently not getting any help from the surgeons or anybody else
in their efforts ... We really must do something ... After I get a room for
them then I am going to come down on Halsted who ought to see that they
have systematic instruction in surgical pathology, as was advertised. Surgery seems to be the only subject which is not satisfactory at present.[13]

Eventually the students had some contact with surgical patients under
what one of them called 'the distant guidance' of Halsted, and under the
closer supervision of his assistants. They did not think the instruction was
very good and were not comfortable. Then again, hardly anyone ever was
comfortable with Halsted – who in pre-addiction years had been a brilliant
undergraduate teacher. When he did teach at Hopkins, he was usually over
the heads of most of the class and everyone was terrified of him. His ward
rounds were known as 'shifting dullness,' a mocking term derived from the
discovery during percussion of fluid in the abdomen. There was no com-
radeship between the professor and most of his residents and interns, some
of whom became his ardent professional disciples. They envied the sense
of fellowship, common purpose, and good spirits everyone enjoyed on Osler's
service.[14]

Howard Atwood Kelly, the professor of gynecology, ranked with Welch,
Osler, and Halsted as one of the 'Big Four' at Hopkins. Kelly was technically the most brilliant of the Hopkins surgeons; everyone envied his skill
with his hands, and he made his mark training his residents in gynecological surgery. He had a heart of pure gold, and a furiously energetic approach
to life that made even Osler look lazy by comparison. Kelly was 'as effulgent
as an Xray tube,' a resident wrote in 1898. 'He is distinctly phosphoresc-
ing.' But Kelly spent little time with undergraduate students. And when he
was not in the operating room at Hopkins or the operating room at the
private hospital he had created in Baltimore, or operating in the homes of
his patients – Osler thought he had the largest income of any surgeon in
America – and when he was not out on the streets trying to save prostitutes or guarding voting booths from corrupt hooligans, or in his library

writing learned books on mushrooms, snake handling, and gynecology, or outdoors canoeing in Canada and founding one of the first boys' camps in America, he was apt to be preaching on street corners, passing out tracts, and asking his associates and students if they had considered the claims of Jesus Christ. 'The only interest he manifested in my classmates,' a student recalled, 'was whether they were saved.' Most of the hospital people found Dr Kelly's evangelism discomforting and many tried to avoid him as a religious crank.[15] His habit of sometimes kneeling in prayer just before his patients were anesthetized disconcerted everyone, from anesthetist to patient, and had to be abandoned (probably to be replaced by a habit of silent praying not unknown even to otherwise unreligious surgeons today). It was one of the few compromises made by a classic fundamentalist, who once asked an assistant to close for him so he could prepare for Bible class. When Harvey Cushing cited Kelly to Sinclair Lewis as an example of scientists' ongoing faith, the writer commented, 'My dear Harvey, what does an obstetrician know about the Virgin Birth?'[16]

Kelly was so interested in specializing in gynecological surgery that J. Whitridge Williams was hired to teach obstetrics. A big gruff man whom the students nicknamed 'the Bull,' Williams laced his carefully prepared lectures with Rabelaisian humor, playing to male prurience and female discomfort. 'He had no use for women students, lived by a double standard for men and women, and could understand no other set of morals,' one of the women students remembered. Some students thought Williams was also anti-Semitic, though Miss Gertrude Stein of the class of 1901 was so generally disliked that it may not have been a matter of race or religion.[17]

The professor of pharmacology, John J. Abel, was a brilliant scientist who was about to become one of the discoverers of adrenaline and was the father in the United States of the discipline that replaced materia medica. Abel was almost a caricature of the eccentrically devout scientist. He shared Mall's distaste for active teaching and when he tried to do it proved himself a thoroughgoing klutz: 'We rather looked on him as a joke,' a former student who admired Abel as a scientist remembered,

> whose lectures were poor, whose class demonstrations almost always failed

& who after lecture or demonstration stood apologetically with a towel over his shoulder, apparently not quite sure why things had gone badly. We had the saying that only one class demonstration was a success, the one that demonstrated gravity when all the corks etc. fell on the floor as he knocked the box off the table, and one almost was a success, the one with apomorphine in which the dog did vomit but missed the basin.

Abel's only advice to his assistants was to put their efforts into research and let other matters take care of themselves.[18]

Altogether, then, it was an odd cast who had been given the mandate to stage a great medical school. They might not have succeeded. In 1897 the arguments used at Harvard to deter students from heading for Hopkins, according to Mall, were 'We have no lectures; we are not organized; we do not make doctors.'[19] But several factors worked in the other direction. First, Johns Hopkins Hospital and University were so well endowed that they were splendid places to work and study, whatever the quality of the teaching. Very small classes, very good equipment, unprecedented access to laboratories – these were conditions that made Hopkins the envy of the world. Second, the elite admission standard, the highest in North America, operated as a self-fulfilling prophecy. Johns Hopkins would be an excellent medical school because it would attract excellent students. Other medical schools still had student bodies that were about as well trained as senior high school students today, and a few were at today's undergraduate level; but Hopkins had the equivalent of a body of outstanding graduate students. Most of them could learn on their own, could learn despite their instructors. A few didn't need to be taught anything.

Third, however inept or uninterested they were as teachers, men such as Mall, Welch, Halsted, and Abel had outstanding reputations as researchers. They stood at the top of their field, were obvious drawing-cards, and, as Mall certainly understood, challenged students to obtain excellence by emulating their professors' love of disinterested study and experimentation. Pedagogically, a lot could be said (and eventually was said by John Dewey and other educational theorists) for the notion of 'learning by doing' as opposed to learning by listening, memorizing, and cramming.

The fourth and most important factor in Hopkins' success was that those who needed to be taught medicine had access to William Osler.

'I was called up yesterday in Dr. Osler's clinic to make a diagnosis of a case and got an old healing appendicitis which wasn't any trouble to recognize. They are the nicest things we go to, for Dr. Osler sits on the table & swings his feet, and asks you all sorts of questions you have never heard of before.'[20]

In second year the students began to creep up on real medicine with a short course on methods of diagnosis taught by Osler's senior resident, Thayer. In the third year Thayer expanded on that subject, another resident supervised systematic work on blood, sputa, urine, and other secretions in the clinical laboratory, and, perhaps to compensate for Mall's shortcomings, there was a special course in medical anatomy. The highlights of the third year were the thrice-weekly noon clinics with Osler in the outpatients' dispensary, what he called his 'observation' classes:

> The student must first be taught to observe [Osler wrote] and can not do better than begin his acquaintance with disease among out-patients. A man with typhoid fever in bed, scoured and cleaned, looks very different from the poor fellow who totters into the dispensary ... Three or four cases are examined in the hour by students taken in rotation. The student asks the questions, repeats the answers and makes the examination. He is taught to use his senses in a simple and orderly manner. The seeing eye and the feeling finger are products of long training. How to see and what to see, how to touch and what to touch constitute the main lesson of the hour ... A diagnosis is not always reached, and the treatment is not necessarily discussed.[21]

Osler had no foreknowledge of the subjects. The patient would be on a wicker couch, Osler at the side, the students in rattan chairs around them. Some gave reports and offered comments as Osler led his 'medical infants,' Holmeslike, through fascinating exercises in medical detection. 'Every case

was a text for Dr. Osler upon which he could talk in the most graphic way,'
W.G. MacCallum recalled. Here are some examples from one student's
notes of the 1896–7 clinics:

> Ask a man of what he complains. Put that down as he describes it in his
> own words. Then take the history ... All patients say they have had 'rheu-
> matism.' Inquire more particularly ... It is most important and most difficult
> to get a history of syphilis ... It is often well to ask: 'How many times a day
> do you drink?' A man who drinks before breakfast as a rule is a heavy drinker.
> This is not true south of Mason and Dixon's line. There a man may take his
> only drink before breakfast.

> E.G., aged 12. He comes in with fever and a swollen tongue. His voice is a
> little muffled and nasal. He looks pale and ill. His external glands are not
> enlarged, except those at the angle of the left jaw which are slightly en-
> larged. There is little mucus from nose. He can not open his mouth widely.
> His tongue is a little swollen, and somewhat coated. It is a plastic tongue.
> The fungiform papillae are enlarged. The tongue can protrude only 2 cm.
> beyond the teeth. The middle of the tongue feels hard and indurated. There
> are not patches in the throat, but a great deal of mucus is present. His gums
> are uniformly white, a little swollen, and covered with a whitish material
> that can be washed off. There is no special fetor. It looks as if he had a
> stomatitis. Give 5 grains of potash and some aconite. Chlorate of potash is
> an interesting drug. It is quite poisonous even in medicinal doses. It pro-
> duces nephritis. It used to be given in too large doses. The patient says a
> good deal of saliva dribbles from his mouth. We see more cases of mercurial
> salivation now with small doses of calomel than we did years ago with large
> doses. This looks like mercurial stomatitis but he says he has not taken any
> medicine.

> Inspection should always precede palpation. He comes complaining of dys-
> pepsia and loss of weight. He is thin. His skin is dry, yet his color is good.
> His abdomen is excavated in the upper umbilical region and in the epigas-
> trium. There is distinct fulness in the lumbar region. First note whether

respiratory movements are present or not. Then note the iliac grooves and lines on the flank. In the normal abdomen one sees only the movement of respiration and the throbbing of the abdominal aorta. In very thin abdomens the outlines of the stomach, liver and even the abdominal aorta with its bifurcations can be seen, as well as the movements of the stomach and large intestine.

Now in this man we can see a distinct swelling corresponding to the outline of the stomach. Waves can be be seen, usually passing from left to right. As the waves pass by, the organ hardens very materially. Changes in outline such as these are called 'patterns of abdominal tumidity,' and often give the diagnosis. The shape of the swelling here gives the diagnosis. The greater and lesser curvature of the stomach are seen. One can make the diagnosis [cancer of the stomach] *de viso*.

A.H., waiter. His whole head throbs and also his neck. He has a remarkable water-hammer pulse in the right radial; the left can scarcely be felt. The whole chest pulsates. This is aortic insufficiency. Nothing else but extreme hemorrhage would give a pistol-shot pulse like this. One could make the diagnosis across the room. The color of his lips could almost give the diagnosis; they are very cyanotic.

Of very few things beneath the skin of the abdomen can we be absolutely certain. This is one of them. It is the characteristic large spleen of chronic malaria.

This is phlebitis ... End results in thrombophlebitis. Possibilities: (1) The thrombus in the vein may suppurate. This is the worst result as death from pyemia usually follows. This outcome is rare. (2) It may persist. If it does the leg remains swollen despite all you can do. It goes on for years. This man will go out better in a month or so and in two or three months will probably come back. Give a guarded prognosis regarding complete cure. You remember when Prof. Edwin Klebs visited the clinic, he pointed to his leg which had been swollen ever since he had typhoid fever many years before (A student remarked that we had not seen him). You are right, it was last year's class that saw Prof. Klebs. Never mind. Tell the story often enough and you will finally believe you saw him ... (3) Cure.[22]

If the patient had a certain disease, Osler wanted the students to know the classic descriptions – Sydenham on chorea, Bell on facial palsy, Addison on the adrenals and pernicious anemia. He had them look up and discuss related diseases. If it seemed in order to prescribe Blaud's pills, Osler asked who Blaud was and assigned someone to report back. Who was Fowler of Fowler's pills? Dover of Dover's powder? What about the follow-up on that case of Hanot's cirrhosis? 'Dr. Osler asked me how the patient was,' recalled Henry Christian, 'and I replied, "I think he is about as usual. I visited him about two weeks ago." With this, Dr. Osler, to my embarrassment, dramatically brought forth a tray containing a large liver and other organs, saying "Christian, he did not continue to do so well. Dr. MacCallum autopsied him this morning."'

On another occasion, a student who was keeping track of an elderly man with aortic insufficiency and angina pectoris, who had been shown at a previous clinic, stated that he had seen the patient at his home and had advised him to take hot baths. With a quizzical expression and in a lugubrious voice, Osler said, 'Is there any danger, Mr. — in ordering hot baths for patients with aortic insufficiency and angina pectoris?' The horrified student, fearing the worst, left the clinic in haste and dashed to the house of his patient, only to find the old man sitting on his doorstep, smoking a forbidden pipe.[23]

In their fourth year the Hopkins students experienced what British and Canadian students had known for generations but Americans had not – the clinical clerkship. Osler at last had the freedom to introduce in Baltimore the system he had worked in at McGill and had not been able to transplant to Philadelphia. Each member of the fourth-year class served for two months as a clerk on the Johns Hopkins wards, rotating through medical, surgical, gynecological, and obstetrical, taking patient histories, doing blood and urine tests, dressing wounds, keeping records – and having to pronounce his position in proper English: 'clark.'[24]

Clerking was a student's introduction to doctoring (he or she would probably be mistaken for a doctor) and to actually having some responsibility for patients. Nowhere else in the United States could medical students have such experience.

Each clerk had six beds. Three mornings a week, Osler made ward rounds. It became a memorable Hopkins ritual. A few minutes before nine – you could set your clock by him – Osler, usually dressed in a gray morning coat and top hat, a flower in his buttonhole, sometimes with walking stick or umbrella in hand, swung down the long corridor, catching up with an assistant or student, taking him by the arm and speeding him up, waving with his free hand at nurses and friends. Residents, interns, visitors, and clerks joined him at the ward doors and swarmed along, sometimes streaming behind like the tail of a kite or comet. They later wagged his rounds in rhyme:

> When William Osler Makes His Rounds
> Haste! Haste! ye clerks, make breakfast brief,
> And follow close your lord and chief:
> With paper blank and pen in fist,
> Let not a single note be missed,
> When William Osler, K.C.B., F.R.S., F.R.C.P.,
> Makes his Rounds
>
> See how the double doors swing back,
> And in he comes with all his pack!
> From North and South, from West and East,
> They flock like vultures to a feast
> When William Osler, K.C.B., F.R.S., F.R.C.P.,
> Is making rounds.
>
> All sorts of folk are in the pack,
> From city swell to country hack,
> Swine-like they crowd each empty space,
> Crowd clerk and interne out of place
> When William Osler, K.C.B., F.R.S., F.R.C.P.,
> Is making rounds.[25]

Everyone agreed that Osler had an uncanny ability to put a patient at ease with a smile or quip or the squeeze of a toe. 'Well! are you feeling nice and fat today?' he liked to say to children (having apparently dropped his Canadian 'eh'). The clerk would read the case history, and Osler would make some remarks or do an examination:

> Osler would often stand at the head of a patient's bed, gracefully using his beautifully shaped, small, brown hands, with their tapering fingers, to accentuate what he had to say. He was fond of enumerating, as first, second and third in order of probability, the situations in which such and such a condition might occur; frequently the last possibility was totally unexpected and entirely irrelevant. In examining a patient, he would sit at the side of the bed, watching the motions of the chest or abdomen and looking for moving shadows in different lights, to which procedure he attached great importance. He told the story of the nurse who, having detected the pulsations of an aneurysm in the chest wall of a patient, changed the position of the patient so that the light brought out the shadow of the localized impulse, which thus became readily visible to the astounded physician. Much time was also devoted to the palpation of the chest and abdomen. Osler was likely to use both hands and to point out the advantages of doing so.
>
> While walking down the long wards, he sometimes stopped to grasp the toes of a patient. As he did so, he would remark that Oppolzer was in the habit of surprising his students by making the diagnosis of aortic insufficiency after feeling the toes of a patient from the foot of the bed. This impressed on us the importance of the 'water-hammer pulse' as a sign of aortic insufficiency.

There are many similar descriptions of Osler on rounds. Henry Christian, who later became dean at Harvard, was particularly good on the fine balances Osler struck:

> Ward visits were an unusual combination of informality and dignity. Students and patients quickly were put at ease by Dr Osler. The discussions seemed very informal, possibly a bit haphazard; yet a surprisingly complete

description of the patient and his disease was left with the students. The combination of informality and dignity in the ward visits probably mirrored the similar combination which was so evident in Dr Osler's own personality. In his frock coat and with his scrupulously neat appearance, he was typically the consulting physician, honored and esteemed by all who came in contact with him, but there was no austerity in this. His twinkling eye, his quick steps his frequent quips, his friendliness of manner, his habit of putting a hand on the shoulder of assistants, students and friends as he talked and talked, all brought into his clinics and ward visits a delightful tone of friendly informality. His criticisms of students and their work were incisive and unforgettable, but never harsh or unkindly; they inspired respect and affection, never fear.

At noon on Saturdays (later on Wednesdays), Osler held a general clinic in the hospital amphitheater, mainly for the benefit of the third- and fourth-year students, but open to everyone. The hospital's experience for the week was discussed, some of their most interesting cases were presented by the clerks, fatalities and mistaken diagnoses were noted, and elaborate blackboard charts of the hospital's experience with its pneumonia and typhoid fever patients were updated. 'I would rather teach medicine from pneumonia and typhoid fever cases than from all other diseases put together,' Osler wrote in 1901. 'They remain the two great acute infections.' He liked to tell the students that in coming to know one disease thoroughly – his other choice was syphilis – they would range through most of the disciplines of medicine.[26]

The clinics were so informal and simple that some visitors couldn't understand Osler's great reputation. To the regulars, week after week, the impact became cumulative. One of the first female interns at Hopkins remembered coming in late, dead tired after a night of attending dying men. Osler hailed her with delight: 'Here's Dr. Reed, she can report on what she's done on the negro wards.'

'Six deaths from pneumonia on the men's ward, sir.'

The clinic rocked with laughter at the thought of what the woman had done.

'I was completely unnerved,' recalled Reed. 'Seeing six young adults die within a few hours was no laughing matter for me. Dr. Osler feeling my distress immediately hushed the outbreak saying that the colored, usually both syphilitic and alcoholics, were the worst risk in pulmonary disease and that it was remarkable that we could save as many as we did. He went out of his way to praise my work.'

Occasionally there would be a special show:

> There was great excitement one day when Osler performed an autopsy. The case was one in which he had made the diagnosis of bilateral congenital cystic kidney. At that time the condition was barely recognized during life, and on this account Dr Osler had asked Dr Welch, as a great favour, to allow him to conduct the postmortem examination. The tiers of seats overlooking the autopsy table were crowded with members of the staff and with students, for the occasion was unique. Dr Osler, protected by a large apron, rolled up his sleeves and went about the job in a professional manner. The climax came when he removed from the abdomen two huge kidneys, filled with cysts.[27]

One imagines that the audience applauded.

On April 14, 1897, and again on February 2, 1898, Osler devoted most of the clinic to the case of Mary S, who had turned up at the dispensary with a disease that had baffled the staff. Dermatological experts had disagreed learnedly on whether the woman's skin lesions were tubercular or syphilitic. Osler had walked in, trailing students, taken a good look, and said it was the first case of leprosy he had seen since visiting New Brunswick. The hospital was agog when a nurse refused to care for the leprous patient – the nurse was eventually dismissed – and no other institution in the city would take the case. Osler related Mary's clinical condition in detail, then gave a mini-lecture on leprosy, mentioning his visit to the colony in Canada, the disease's lack of contagiousness, and the fact that no case had developed among nurses or doctors in Ceylon in one hundred years: 'I may add that it has been to both physicians and nurses of our staff a great pleasure to be able to care for her and make her comfortable.' After ten months in the hospital, Mary S was released, officially as a free agent, though probably as a friendless wanderer.[28]

For comic relief and to illustrate the deceptiveness of appearances, there was the case of the 'pregnant' man:

> A patient was brought in on a stretcher. The patient was completely covered with a sheet. The only clinical feature was a noticeably protuberant abdomen. The spectators looked at one another and smiled, wondering why the 'Chief' was exhibiting a pregnant woman. The patient was brought in and taken out without a word of explanation. After two or three other patients had been brought in and their clinical condition discussed, the first patient was returned, this time without the sheet. The patient was an elderly man and with him was a large bottle containing about 2 quarts of urine.[29]

On Saturday nights Osler entertained the medical clerks at 1 West Franklin Street. Two students were invited for dinner, the rest for 'beer and baccy' and chocolate cake afterwards. The group sat around the dining-room table, smoking, drinking, eating, and talking medicine, and usually Osler showed them some of the fascinating books from his library and talked about great men in the history of their profession. They always broke up around ten o'clock because that was his bedtime. Memorable times. Such faculty-student evenings were not uncommon in the elite atmosphere of Johns Hopkins University, but Osler was the first and for a time the only School of Medicine faculty member to entertain students. Their professional awe of their teacher shaded into deep affection for a professor who cared enough to invite them into his home and got to know them all.[30]

Everyone loved the Chief. He was so warm, so friendly, so happy and charming, so funny, so interesting and interested (in today's jargon, so upbeat and positive) that he enchanted everyone, from patients to his most senior colleagues. To a modern biographer searching for the feet of clay that make subjects credible, the remarkable unanimity of the sources is disconcerting. In later pages a few colleagues will think Osler falls out of date, some that he spreads himself too thinly, and some that he becomes too American; but nowhere is there dislike of Osler. No one thought ill of the man. By the 1890s – and nowhere more than as a teacher of medical students at Johns Hopkins – Osler was on his way to becoming one of the most beloved physicians of the age.

The student 'line' on Johns Hopkins was that if you survived the first two years of hardship in the basic sciences, there were great things ahead in the two clinical years under Osler, and even more if you could get an internship in medicine. Osler was always encouraging his staff to give papers and publish, or advising them on career opportunities and personal problems, and he particularly loved to counsel them on their diseases of the heart. ('Whatever you do,' he would say to young doctors contemplating marriage, 'You'll regret it.') Osler's wards and his staff were said to have a degree of spirit, efficiency, and commitment to teaching not found anywhere else in the hospital. His example infected all his assistants – though, of course, it was even better when he appeared in person. Here is an obscure first-year student at the medical school in 1906, the year after Osler's departure, telling his fiancée about the great man's return: 'Dr. Osler came in the dissecting room the other day. He put his arms round me and the student next to me and made some remark about our dissection. You can imagine how we felt with that great man leaning on us. He created quite a stir among the first year students ... Everyone hates to see him go. He is dearly beloved by all who know him not simply because he is a great physician but because of his personality.'[31]

When Osler came into a room, the room changed. 'I have never known anyone who was surrounded by such a distinctive, attracting, personal "aura,"' Frank Shepherd wrote. 'It was something that was felt as well as seen ... If to anyone, the much abused word "magnetism" was applicable to him in its best and truest sense.'[32] He had a knack most often found in successful politicians (though he despised politicians) of giving you all his attention and interest, perhaps taking you by the arm, listening intently, remarking on an encounter years earlier or on some other bond you had in common, convincing you that for William Osler at this moment you are the most important person in the world ... and then he moves on. If you try to monopolize him, he will slip away. But if you see him again, you will find he has not forgotten your meeting. And few students, patients, or physicians ever forgot having their lives touched by meeting Osler.

To the students he became more than their mentor, more than a great man to be admired. The term 'role model' was not used in those days; perhaps 'ideal' was a near synonym. One or the other exactly describes the way many Hopkins students took to Osler. For them he was everything a physician should be – not only as a diagnostician and teacher and medical writer, but in demeanor, dress, manners, love of good books, Saturday-night sociability, and a near-religious commitment to medicine as a way of life. When one of the pioneering women doctors, Alice Hamilton, took graduate courses at Hopkins, she noticed how all his assistants and the students were imitating Osler's walk, his gestures, his expression, his accent: 'Often I would find myself watching a little crowd of semi- and semi-demi Oslers.' Fetching on occasion, though more than a little annoying when a student tried to imitate Osler's informality with women, throwing an arm around a fiftyish old maid and asking, 'How's the good man and the chicks?'[33]

Osler had to judge all his acolytes at examination time. All the Hopkins professors hated formal examinations. They believed that students should be judged on their work over a long period of time. Where possible, they made examinations informal, quick, and perfunctory – sometimes almost insulting to students who had slaved and fretted in preparation. A common trick in both medicine and surgery, which could be very unnerving to students, was to have them examine a patient who proved to be in good health. Osler once had interns in Philadelphia puzzle over the contents of sputum to which he had added common carpet sweepings (it appears to have been part of his protest against having to choose interns by competitive examination). Oral exams and quizzes could be nerve-racking too, though not if the examiner was helpful: 'Dr. Osler, who could be cutting and severe on occasion, never showed this to his students. His questions were so placed that our knowledge was drawn out of us. He made the poorest student feel at ease and a brilliant student was brought out to outdo himself ... Dr Osler always gave us a break and left us feeling we had not done so badly – even if our knowledge was woefully small. Dr. Halsted – a queer distorted character and difficult to understand – frightened the students to death and made them feel like fools. He never helped to draw us out but scared us into doing our worst.' Examination records in the Johns Hopkins archives suggest that Osler was fairly generous compared with his colleagues but was not greatly out of line. Whereas Mall might write an exasperated 'stupid' in his remarks about a poor student, Osler's pejorative was 'a weak brother.'[34]

Osler almost never gossiped about weak medical brethren, as students or practitioners. His dislike of malicious personal gossip was pronounced. If you began to criticize someone in his presence, he would immediately change the subject – not always to the liking of his less saintly wife. He had strong dislikes, to be sure, and on at least two occasions spoke out openly in medical meetings against second-raters being allowed to stay on in first-rate positions. Privately he knew there were a lot of 'damned fools' in the world and in the medical profession, but publicly the worst the world contained was 'sons of Belial.' To talk behind a person's back seemed to Osler both professionally and personally unethical.

Would he disparage whole groups? Osler once offhandedly remarked, 'I hate Latin Americans,' yet he could not have had much contact with them. We saw him point out to students the propensity of Baltimore's black population to certain diseases, probably an empirical fact. In 1914 he wrote that Canadians had a right to maintain white dominance of their society.[35] These were not unusual views in his time, and Osler could generalize just as wildly about, say, the propensity to syphilis of old soldiers, of men with tattoos, and especially tattooed old soldiers. Osler remained completely unaffected by anti-Semitism. In Augusta Tucker's novel about medical student life at Hopkins, *Miss Susie Slagle's*, it is the brilliant Jewish student who most deeply relates to Osler's image and becomes his 'spiritual grandson.' Nor did he have much to say generally about the great racial divide in America and Baltimore. When Johns Hopkins was considering expanding its colored wards in 1893–4 and perhaps hiring black nurses, Osler was said to have commented that he would have a negro resident – but the context of the remark is murky. Race, although noted, means little in most of his case reports, and there is little sign that he shared his times' infatuation with dialect and race-based humor.[36]

The real 'others,' the strangers, in Osler's medical life were women. Osler had grown up in what was effectively an all-male medical world. In the 1880s the revolution in nursing had begun to change the life of the hospitals Osler attended. Now at Hopkins there were women in his classes. Medical talk and teaching was no longer men's talk. Every day men and women interacted in classroom and clinic, and for many men this was not an easy adjustment. Like athletes suddenly finding female journalists in the locker room, they were uneasy, angry, petulant, and more than a little suspicious of the newcomers' motives. At the very least, as W.T. Councilman said, they could no longer pee in the sink.

Osler had spoken out on the right of women to enter medicine at Hopkins and in 1891 had been willing to take Mary Sherwood as an intern, but he never hid his view that medicine was a hard profession for a woman to follow. Women would be better off staying out of it. Believing in a general sense in the propriety of separate roles for women and men in the world, and that women's greatest fulfillment came in marriage and childbirth while men were breadwinners, he shared a not uncommon view that women had to choose between marriage and medicine.[37] He would not have encouraged a daughter to go into medicine – though he would not have followed one of his British teachers, Sir William Jenner, in declaring that he would rather see a daughter die than become a medical woman.

In 1896 Dorothy Reed, a recent graduate of Smith College, took a trolley out to Hopkins to enroll in the medical school. There was only one other passenger:

> A distinguished gentleman dressed in grey oxford morning coat, striped trousers, and wearing a silk hat ... He literally stared me out of countenance – seeming to go over me from head to foot, as if he were cataloguing every detail for future reference. I decided that he was an oriental – this conclu-

sion brought about by his color and the long, thin rattail moustache that he
kept pulling as he inventoried my charms.

'Are you entering the medical school?' the stranger asked her. She replied
that she was.

'Don't,' he said. 'Go home' – and walked ahead of her into the hospital.
A few days later, appearing before an admissions committee, Reed saw that
one of them was the dark-skinned little man who had discouraged her.
There was no problem with her credentials and she was welcomed to the
school. She was so flustered at being in the presence of the great and mysterious professors, the equivalent of medical royalty, that she backed out of
the room.[38]

Osler welcomed trained nurses as a new breed of practitioners of one
the most time-honored forms of female service. He had a few doubts, sometimes joking about how male patients didn't want women organizing their
sick time ('She will stop at nothing, and between baths and spongings and
feeding and temperature-taking you are ready to cry with Job the cry of
every sick man – "*Cease then, and let me alone.*'"), and he certainly upheld
the notion that nurses were to be absolute medical subordinates of doctors.
They must never be critical, gossipy, or otherwise indiscreet. The trivia of
the austere regulations at Hopkins, such as the requirement that nurses
stand whenever doctors entered, sometimes seemed unnecessary to him,
but he would not have laughed with the brazen redhead who so offended
Halsted.[39]

Most of the Hopkins men, students and staff, were not fond of the 'hen
medics' studying to become 'doctresses.' If women had abandoned the roles
appropriate to their sex, were they desexed? Strangely sexed? Oversexed? 'I
hear that one of our "hen medics" is to be married soon,' a student wrote to
his fiancée in 1906. 'She is following a wise course. I hope that about four
others in our class (and that's all of them) will have some such hard luck as
that. A woman has no business going into Medicine. She can't do it without unsexing herself.' Did Osler sum up all these attitudes in an aphorism
(which has been widely quoted by feminists) that humanity is divided into
three classes: men, women, and women physicians? Did Dr Osler reveal

more misogyny when he moved in 1901 that Miss Gertrude Stein be not recommended for her degree, an unprecedented failing of a fourth-year student? Stein, we know, went on to become a famous writer and *saloniste*, a modernist, and a lesbian cultural icon.[40]

There was a sprinkling of women, as much as 25 per cent one year – it was always well above the national average – in all the classes Osler taught at Hopkins. Some of the women were at times furious about the off-color chauvinism of J. Whitridge Williams's lectures in obstetrics or about the odd raunchy presentation at the medical society. Dorothy Reed remembered one speaker, 'flushed, bestial,' making elaborate comparisons between nasal and penile tissue, and she cried hysterically all the way home. Her companion, Margaret Long, was unmoved: 'She put it down to the natural bestiality of man and ignored it entirely.' (Long, who had no interest whatever in men and in Reed's view should have been a man, kept a six-shooter in her room, presumably as protection against anyone's bestiality running out of control.)[41]

The male students played occasional practical jokes on the women – probably not on Margaret Long – but nothing major, and even they found it all a bit tiresome. Gertrude Stein, an arrogant Radcliffe graduate, was the most actively disliked. She was nicknamed Battle Ax, apparently because of her mannish appearance and mannish habit of smoking. (Other women were known as Buffalo Bill, Strawberry Blonde, and Karyokinesis.) Stein intimidated and irritated men and women alike. In the lab one day, when the students were learning to test samples of their own urine, someone discomfited Stein by lacing hers with glucose. During her clerkship, Dorothy Reed was bothered by what we would now call harassment from an amorous intern, leading to this exchange:

'Dr Fuetscher, please remove your arm.'

'Miss Reed, you forget that you are speaking to an interne.'

'I thought that I was speaking to a gentleman.'[42]

There was serious behind-the-scenes friction in 1900 when Dorothy Reed and Florence Sabin, by virtue of their class standing, became the first female graduates to be offered internships at Hopkins and chose the most popular service, Osler's. Some of the male students thought they themselves should have preferment. Superintendent Hurd was particularly alarmed, telling Reed that everyone would consider that a woman doctor who wanted to take charge of a male ward was doing so to satisfy sexual curiousity. 'When it came to negroes, did I realize that the white nurses were always in danger on the male colored wards and that if anything happened to them by word or deed that I would be held responsible.' Reed remarked that the only serious insult in her four years at Johns Hopkins had just come from the superintendent of the hospital. Osler 'looked very sober when I told him of Dr. Hurd's insinuations but he only said that "Hurd was a crabby soul" ... He commended my work and left me feeling that he was satisfied and that I could depend upon him and Dr. Futcher, the resident, to support me in every way.'

As interns, Reed and Sabin were too shy to use the doctors' lounge in the hospital, going over to the nurses' residence instead. The male interns did not involve them in their midsummer late-night fights with fire hoses and crockery. They felt singled out for professional harassment by one of the residents, Thomas McCrae, but decided he was disagreeable to every-one and was generally disliked. Reed found the colored male patients, who were generally respectful of 'the little white lady doctor,' easier to get along with than the females.

Everyone was alarmed the day a group of colored males awaiting surgery got into a serious fight with convalescing medical cases. (The surgical wards were being particularly badly run that year, McCrae judged.) Dr Reed was summoned by an emergency alarm: 'My entire ward seemed to be a sea of fighting men – with the bed patients yelling and cheering them on. I picked up a crutch I found on the floor and joined the melee. Swinging it to keep anyone from coming close to me, I yelled "Back to your own ward" ... A dozen or more men streamed past me, back to their own quarters. Most of them were bleeding ... and they were limping and tattered.' Reed retrieved the nurses (who had locked themselves in the ward's linen closet), negoti-ated disciplinary action with the resident in charge of the surgical ward, bandaged her wounded, and took much lunchroom kidding about 'the battle of the blacks.'

'On the whole,' Dorothy Reed concluded in her autobiography, 'we women at Johns Hopkins were treated very well.' She singled out the man who had told her to go home for her most extravagant praise: 'Of all the men I have ever known, or even met, William Osler has always seemed to me to have the most vivid personality as well as the finest mind and character. He was the greatest teacher I have ever known; an inspiration to his pupils and colleagues, one of the great gentlemen and influences of his age in the profession of medicine ... No book ... can give a just estimate of his stunning personality and the depth of his influence on all who came in contact with him – patients, nurses, students, doctors. To all of us he was an unfailing guide.'[43]

None of the female physicians in Baltimore had any criticism of Osler. Dr Lilian Welsh, whose memoirs are the sole source for Osler's quip about three classes of humanity, mentions it as a jocular comment that accurately described the social reality she and Mary Sherwood were experiencing in the city. 'We never had any reason to complain of the treatment we received from our male colleagues,' she added in the next sentence, having earlier noted that for Sherwood and herself Osler's friendship was 'one of the rarest privileges life has brought to either of us.' Alice Hamilton used to drop in on Osler's clinic 'just for the pleasure of seeing how admirably he conducted it. He was freer from what the English call swank than almost any other great man I have known,' she observed.

Osler was close to being a role model for the women students too. Another leading Baltimore physician and feminist, and a major art collector, Claribel Cone, took a postgraduate course at Hopkins and found Osler 'the ideal' physician and teacher: 'More than that he was the artist, and with master-stroke he would limn for us case after case. In words rare as they were beautiful, in phrases pregnant with meaning, in manner – at times droll, again almost divine in its subtle suggestion of sympathy – he would assemble the essential facts of each case and create a masterpiece as rich in suggestion, as universal in appeal as a Giotto, a Rembrandt, or a Giorgione.' Like aesthetic taste, students' judgments of Osler could be highly subjective. One of the first three female students at Hopkins, Cornelia Church, withdrew from medicine to practice Christian Science, saying she was influenced by Osler, who was probably a Christian Scientist at heart.[44]

On occasion, the Hopkins medical women mildly asserted themselves. There are several versions of the time Osler had scheduled a discussion of diabetes and the women had the room decorated with (or came wearing) sweet peas. There were howls of laughter when Halsted wandered in and asked 'Why all the flowers?' The women apparently joined in the laughter another day in the amphitheater when a patient was concerned about taking his shirt off in front of ladies, and Osler's resident assured him, 'These aren't ladies; they're medical students!'[45]

Claribel Cone's student friend, Gertrude Stein, had no difficulty at Hopkins until the clinical courses in third and fourth year. Then she found that the practice of medicine held no interest for her and in some ways was deeply repugnant. She was also distracted in her fourth year by a stormy love affair with May Bookstaver. The quality of her work fell off. From Osler, whom she ranked with Halsted as the 'big men' at Hopkins, she received a low passing grade, but she absolutely failed in obstetrics, laryngology and rhinology, ophthalmology and otology, and dermatology. It would have been irresponsible to grant her a degree. The faculty allowed her to stay at Hopkins, studying the brain with Mall and Lewellys Barker, but they too soon found her work unsatisfactory. Gertrude Stein, whose time at Hopkins may have illustrated her own aphorism that 'a difference, to be a difference, must make a difference,' drifted out of their lives.[46]

Nurses did have to be careful when Osler was around, not for fear of sexual advances but because they could never know what he might say or do in a joking or teasing way. He could puncture their dignity with a word or – as on the day he saw the stern Miss Nutting approaching and happened to be standing beside an attendant with a basket of fruit – with a grapefruit bowled down the hall. Only Osler could have got away with it: 'It was Dr. Osler, you know, and his behavior cannot be predicted.'[47]

Sometimes he went too far. The head matron of the new neurological hospital in Philadelphia prided herself on keeping everything in immaculate condition. She also worshiped Osler. One day he confronted her with a skewer containing a cobweb he had found in a far corner of the basement, and with a straight face questioned her housekeeping. Other doctors had to convince the crying woman that it had been a joke. One Hopkins nurse is said to never have forgiven him for pouring all her carefully laid out evening medicines into each other. Another was carrying a bowl of soup with a napkin over it when Osler, on an impulse, put his finger on the napkin and pushed it into the soup. She turned on him: 'I don't know who are you, but I think you're the meanest man I ever saw.' Grace Osler made a special trip to the hospital to apologize for her husband's insensitivity.[48]

No one, male or female, quite knew how to handle Osler when he was being an *enfant terrible*. When he breezed into Halsted's operating room, depositing his hat in one of his sterilizers, cane in another, gloves in the third, and asked how things were going, all the exasperated surgeon could say was, 'Osler, will you never grow up?'[49] Howard Kelly could get better results by smiling and chucking him under the chin. A local girl, Elizabeth Thies, who was hired to organize the Hopkins medical library, dared not use that strategy but did better than most with the abrupt, obnoxious man who never took off his silk hat. One day she just stared at his hat, not at him, until he took it off. When she couldn't understand a request for a technical title, she asked him to write it down. Another time she indignantly refused to climb a ladder in his presence to get a book, so he climbed it himself.

Elizabeth was shocked when he called her Miss Kreis, charmed when he explained, seriously, 'because you are such a saintly woman.' Then she was furious at the medical students who also called her Miss Kreis because they said they followed Osler's lead on everything. Osler gave her good advice about which men at Hopkins to stay away from. And one day, while waiting for a streetcar with her, he made a dive at a passing rooster, saying he was trying to catch a feather for her hat. They became great friends, and when she asked him years later why he had embarrassed her so often in the early days, he said it was to see the color rise in her face. He nicknamed her sister, whom he also delighted, Miss Thesis. Another local Baltimore girl, a debutante who proposed to marry one of Osler's brilliant interns, got into an argument with Osler about whether or not, as he claimed, she would feed on the man's brains: 'I tried to persuade him that men were afraid of brainy girls, which was not far from the truth in the early nineteen hundreds, but after that he always called me Bacilla. I complacently accepted this and thought it rather cute, and it was not for several years that I realized bacilla was a microbe. However, we were always great friends.'[50]

The medical men could be vicious to the women, they could be cold and indifferent, they could be friendly, they could come on to them, or they could be like Osler, paternal, beguiling, and sometimes infuriating. Mabel Southard remembered how he would meet her and Dorothy Reed in the corridor, 'give a hand affectionately to each and say in the most cordial way, "I am *so* sorry, *so* sorry, to see you!" It was his kindly way of registering his protest against our studying medicine,' commented Southard. Rachel Bonner, the first matron of Johns Hopkins, told Harvey Cushing that her whole life there 'was brighter and made possible' by his kind appreciation and support: 'My love and respect for that great and good man is beyond any words that can find in my heart to express.' Elizabeth and Frieda Thies came to love him and hang on every gesture and whistle. Elizabeth endorsed a comment made by one of the Jewish male interns which at first she had thought was silly: 'We all worship him and if it would give Dr Osler any pleasure to walk over me, I would lie on the ground and let him do it.'[51]

Enrollment at the Johns Hopkins School of Medicine rose steadily until by 1900 the entering classes comprised between fifty and sixty graduates from universities across the United States and Canada. The young men and women came to Hopkins thinking it was the best place to study medicine. Their thinking helped make it so. Osler helped make it so. The atmosphere fostered by Welch, Halsted, Mall, Kelly, Abel, and Howell, whatever their personal and teaching limitations, also helped make it so. They all wanted to be the best in America, the best in the world, at medical sciences and the practice of medicine. Their idealism, riding on the stunning achievements of medicine and American economic growth in the nineteenth century, facing the heady possibilities of the twentieth, was very special. So was their intellectual productivity, as measured in volume after volume of articles detailing their scientific investigations, their clini-

cal studies, their therapeutic innovations, and their occasional shortcomings. The senior men at Hopkins became immensely proud of their young
protégés and very happily helped place them in top positions at other
American universities and hospitals.

Osler liked to cite the works of his students as his greatest satisfaction.
What in many of his colleagues was a slapdash, almost casual approach to
teaching was for Osler a carefully thought-out approach to pedagogy. He
had seized the opportunity to bring to the United States what he called
'the natural method' of teaching medicine. At Hopkins he brought his
students out of the lecture halls and amphitheaters and into the hospital
wards, not to be observers but to be workers learning about medicine by
treating patients. It was the clinical version of learning by doing. As Osler
explained it:

> The student begins with the patient, continues with the patient, and ends
> his studies with the patient, using books and lectures as tools, as means to
> an end. The student starts, in fact, as a *practitioner*, as an observer of dis-
> ordered machines, with the stucture and orderly functions of which he is
> perfectly familiar. Teach him how to observe, give him plenty of facts to
> observe, and the lessons will come out of the facts themselves. For the
> junior student in medicine and surgery it is a safe rule to have no teaching
> without a patient for a text, and the best teaching is that taught by the
> patient himself.

In the American context, Osler's methods were radically innovative.
He knew perfectly well that he was bringing to the United States an approach to medicine long practiced in Canada, Britain, and parts of Europe.
In many ways it was a throwback to apprenticeship. For Osler, it was 'the
true method, because it is the natural one, the only one by which a physician grows in clinical wisdom after he begins practice for himself – all
others are bastard substitutes.'[52]

Most of the students were too busy getting on with life to think about
the theory underlying their instruction. They lived at Miss Susie Slagle's
and other boarding houses scattered around old Baltimore. On days off

they took in the sounds and smells of Lexington Market, ate weckers and drank sarsaparilla while cheering for the Baltimore Orioles baseball club – there's Popsy Welch in the grandstand, smoking the cigar, reading proofs of the *Journal of Experimental Medicine* between innings – and they took the streetcar to the end of the line for real fresh air and a country stroll, and slathered hot horseradish on Chesapeake Bay oysters, washing a couple of dozen down with beer. They stayed away from the Back Basin, today's Inner Harbor, which collected much of the city's sewage and smelled like spoiled cadavers. The nurses were under orders to stay away from the medical students, except at special occasions such as commencement, when there were grand dances and, as one of the men put it, 'we all danced until our collars were limp & helpless things.'[53]

Students sometimes broke down – some with 'neurasthenia' from overwork and overworry, others with tuberculosis, malaria, or typhoid fever contracted on the wards or from drinking unboiled Baltimore water. Osler then became their doctor. Most of the young men and women, of course, thrived on long hours, boarding-house fare, real skeletons in their closets, and good German beer at Hanselmann's. 'They all seemed animated by a desire to master all that was known about man and his ailments,' an alumnus remembered. 'The professors made little or no effort to urge them to work. The example ... seemed to be a sufficient stimulus. They had all seen a vision.'

Many of the boarding houses faced on Jackson Place, which has since disappeared. At sundown on a pleasant evening the Hopkins students would gather for a time around the fountain to gossip and banter before drifting back to their rooms. Then, one by one, their lights would come on as they settled down to prepare themselves to be doctors.[54]

The Reverend Canon Featherstone Osler died in Toronto on February 6, 1895, in his ninetieth year, from the effects of arteriosclerosis. He died very peacefully, Ellen wrote. 'There was a gentle sigh, the sigh of a little sleeping child, then one other sigh and without the slightest distress even in look, his soul returned to "God who gave it." My precious one fell asleep in Jesus. No more pain or weariness but "forever with the Lord."' As he had requested, Featherstone was dressed in his surplice and regalia and lay in a plain black coffin as family and friends paid their last respects. '"He yet being dead,"' Ellen wrote, 'preached to all who saw him, true cheerful submission to God's will, and I believe the impression made on the dear grandchildren will be lasting, they all loved him as did his children.' She was in her eighty-ninth year and expected at any time to join her husband in a joyous meeting with the Saviour 'on the other side of Jordan.' In the meantime she carried on, her body invigorated by the draughts of whisky, two teaspoonfuls twice a day, that Willie prescribed.[55]

In Baltimore, Grace Revere Osler gave birth to another grandson for Ellen on December 28, 1895. 'He looks a strong and durable specimen,' the very excited father wrote. This baby survived. The graduate nurses sent a box of superb roses for the young Doctor Osler. The parents considered naming him Palmer Howard Osler but chose the common family names Edward and Revere instead. It was fashionable to have children baptized with water brought from the River Jordan, but Grace directed it be boiled first for hygienic reasons, which reduced the benedictory to a few grains of wet sand. Mother and father doted on Revere, a late and only child (whom Willie nicknamed 'Isaac' or 'Ike,' after the child of Abraham and Sarah's old age), but the baby's routine care was in the hands of a colored 'Mammy.' She was so disgusted by the baptism ceremony that she later performed her own in the nursery with a cup full of water.[56]

Willie had always been a surrogate father to Bill Francis and had told him that when he grew up he could study medicine and live with him. In the autumn of 1895, Bill began studying arts at Hopkins and joined the Osler household at 1 West Franklin. By all accounts it was a happy family circle, constantly open to visiting relatives, doctors, and old friends. 'We would not have felt it strange had we found Montaigne and Laennec there one Sunday afternoon, but should have expected them to greet him as a familiar spirit,' a Canadian Hopkinsite remembered. The Oslers were well-to-do, not rich. Dr Osler did not own a carriage, but always took the streetcar out to Hopkins. Nor would he permit a telephone in his house. When the phone company told him people were complaining about not being able to get through to him and cited their low rates, Osler is said to have replied that he would take a phone when the company paid him that much for the trouble he would have to tolerate.[57]

'I should not like any of Dr. Osler's friends to find him at all changed by marriage,' Grace observed in 1895. Osler once wrote to a medical graduate on the subject of marriage: 'A doctor needs a woman who will look after his house and rear his children, a Martha whose first care will be for the home. Make her feel that she is your partner arranging a side of the business in which she should have her sway and her way. Keep the two separate. Consult her and take her advice about the house and the children, but keep to yourself, as far as possible, the outside affairs relating to the practice.'[58] The Osler household ran on these principles, and within her sphere Grace was sovereign, confident, and competent. She had excellent taste in furnishings and fashion, an independent income of about $5,000 a year, knew how to manage servants (she brought her butler and maid with her from Philadelphia), and liked to do her own 'marketing' – which in those days meant shopping at the market.

There is no evidence of any friction in the family, save for Grace's moments of exasperation at her husband's occasional outspokenness and joking – she could not have appreciated being introduced as 'the widow Grossler.' Some friends thought she had a softening effect on Willie's rough edges, and even he agreed that E.Y. Davis, who would still occasionally sign a hotel register on the Oslers' behalf, had been pretty much drowned in the Lachine Canal in 1884. Bill Francis credited Grace with persuading William to lop a bit off what she called 'the Osler hang-dog mustache.' Grace had largely a wifely interest in medicine and occasionally came across as the grand Boston lady, but she did serve on the Women's Advisory Committee at Hopkins, and she helped with the fundraising for some nursing activities. She would have supported her husband's view that a doctor's responsibilities to the profession and public outweighed his heavy obligations to his nearest and dearest. A triptych of portraits of Linacre, Sydenham, and Harvey hung over the fireplace in Osler's library, which Grace had had copied as a birthday present for him after he had admired it in the rooms of

Sir Henry Acland, the Regius Professor of Medicine at Oxford, on their 1894 visit.[59]

The Oslers seemed always to be entertaining out-of-town medical men, Hopkins colleagues at afternoon tea, or the students on Saturday nights. 'Mrs. Chief' was an excellent hostess, who took a keen interest in the lives of the young men and their women. She seemed 'a little impatient of stupidity or dowdiness,' a close friend recalled, 'a little contemptuous of the advanced woman or the over-intellectual one – but that was merely a traditional mood against their kind, not a conviction against their causes. She thought them awful nuisances and that was all.' Tea at the Oslers was a lovely time of talk and laughter. 'She made his house almost a delightful Club for his friends and in it an inviolable peace and quiet for himself.'[60]

Osler's Baltimore colleagues, like everyone else who knew him, marveled at his ability to chat for a few moments with everyone at afternoon tea – working a room, we now call it – and then slip away. He always had total control of his time. As a traveler – by steamer, train, cab, streetcar – he was constantly reading and writing, and his companions understood. Bill Francis read him the works of Homer and half a dozen other authors in ten-minute intervals while he was bathing in the evenings. If Osler heard someone proposing to do something sometime, he would urge them to action by quoting *Macbeth*: 'The flighty purpose ne'er is overtook / Unless the deed go with it' – referring, of course, to a murder. When he did not want to be disturbed, he would recite the opening lines of Pope's 'Epistle to Dr. Arbuthnot': 'Shut, shut the door, good John! fatigu'd I said, / Tye up the knocker, say I'm sick, I'm dead!'

Marriage and the growth of the medical school did not interfere with Osler's productivity as a scholar of disease. His amazingly high output actually increased as he published more clinical lectures and more cases, and produced revised editions of his textbook in 1895 and 1898. Osler practiced what some were starting to label the 'specialty' of internal medicine. 'At the outset,' he said in an 1897 address on 'Internal Medicine as a Vocation,' 'I would like to emphasize the fact that the student of internal medicine cannot be a specialist.'[61] Not only would the study of any single disease lead through the whole range of medical science, he explained, but sick humans presented a prodigious range of problems, even when whole categories – gynecological and obstetrical ills, eye disease, psychiatric disorders – were passed on to others. Later specialties, such as pediatrics, had barely been conceived. Osler saw a large number of children and by virtue of his interest in many childhood diseases was also considered a pediatrician, at least enough of one to serve as president of the fledgling American Paediatric Society in 1892.

In the middle and late nineties Osler's range included chorea, the diagnosis of abdominal tumors, Henoch's purpura, Raynaud's disease, the classification of tics, angina pectoris (a major interest, discussed below), typhoid spine, paresthetic meralgia, leprosy, a case of enormous heart hypertrophy, and ball-valve gallstones lodged in the common duct. The hypertrophic heart belonged to a little girl who spent most of three and a half years in the hospital; liters of fluid were drained from her peritoneal cavity on 121 occasions. The gallstone quest dated from the Philadelphia patient who in 1887 had died after a futile exploratory operation. The stomach, duodenum, and liver had been preserved. In 1897 Osler displayed them in a clinical lecture arguing that he had since compiled enough similar cases to be able to delineate the symptoms pointing towards a ball-valve-like obstruction of the common duct by a gallstone. Knowing the problem made the chances of successful surgery much better.[62]

The greatest purely medical success story of the 1890s was the introduction of thyroid extract to treat the disease known as cretinism or myxedema. In 1893 Osler was among the first American physicians to use the treatment. He made a special study of the disease, corresponding with physicians across the continent to try to determine its prevalence. In the 1895 revision of his text he hailed the results of thyroid feeding as 'unparalleled by anything in the whole range of curative measures. Within six weeks a poor, feeble-minded, toad-like caricature of humanity may be restored to mental and bodily health.' In 1897 he delivered a major paper, 'Sporadic Cretinism in America,' to a Washington Congress of Physicians and Surgeons in which he used stunning before-and-after lantern slides to show 'marvellous transformations' and 'undreamt-of transfigurations,' and in addition to citing all the medical literature on the subject also referred to descriptions by Milton, Shakespeare, and an instance of 'the brave kiss of the daughter of Hippocrates.'[63]

The conquest of myxedema by thyroid feeding raised the possibility that other diseases might be caused by the absence of vital glandular secretions and be similarly treatable by replacement therapy. The concept of 'internal secretions' of the ductless glands and several other glands was starting to be understood. Many researchers and clinicians were experimenting with pancreas feeding in diabetes, for example. Osler chose to try to treat Addison's disease, a rare disorder of the suprarenal glands which closely paralleled myxedema, with extract from the suprenal medulla. Through most of 1895 a patient in the hospital seemed to be responding very well to the treatment, raising hopes of another breakthrough – hopes reflected in several clinical presentations and the 1895 edition of *Principles and Practice*. But by the 1898 revision the original patient had died and Osler's three other cases had not been improved. A recent recreation of Osler's extract suggests that it would not have been effective.[64]

Cases of malaria and typhoid fever continued to be staples on the wards at Hopkins. Osler made these a specialty in his teaching, writing, and public role as guardian of Americans' health. 'Humanity has but three great enemies,' he proclaimed in a major address to the American Medical Association in Atlanta in 1896: 'Fever, famine and war: of these by far the greatest, by far the most terrible, is fever.' The good news was that the fevers were gradually being defeated. Yellow fever had virtually disappeared from the United States. Smallpox occurred only in isolated outbreaks. Typhus fever and cholera were rarely if ever seen. Even malaria had greatly diminished, especially in the North. 'Typhoid fever is today in the United States *the fever*.'[65]

As a diagnostician Osler continued to be vexed by the failure of the profession to differentiate, especially between malaria and other fevers. Testing for the malarial parasite had become routine at Hopkins, and it showed the disease to be in rapid decline. Many, perhaps most, physicians still clung to old beliefs about chills indicating malaria, the existence of a single typhomalarial fever, or one fever appearing as different fevers in different regions. In article after article, Osler viewed with alarm the consequences of the promiscuous malaria diagnosis: 'During last year I saw in private, or there were brought to my wards, cases with intermittent paroxysms of fever believed to be due to malaria, but which subsequently proved to be the following conditions: abscess of the liver, tuberculosis, influenza, gonorrhea, endocarditis, otitis media, gall-stone fever, post-partum anemia, typhoid fever, and septicemia.'[66]

Except for malaria, treatment certainly lagged far behind advances in etiology. Nothing influenced Osler's views of therapeutics as much as his analysis of the treatment of typhoid fever at Hopkins. If no known medication killed the disease, what could be done? Abandoning the administration of drugs that made patients worse was the first step forward. Careful attention to diet and first-class nursing attention were much more than just counsels of despair or holding actions: 'Good nursing not only means comfort – in all implied in that word – to the patient in innumerable little ways, but it also lessens materially the chances of those complications and accidents which claim so large a percentage of the fatal cases. The mortality has, I believe, been materially influenced by the introduction into hospitals of trained nurses, and would probably be found lowest in those institutions in which the percentage of nurses to patients is found the highest.'

Seventy-five per cent of typhoid fever cases would recover under any form of treatment, Osler estimated. Good nursing, diet, and the abandonment of drugging would save the lives of another 15 per cent, he thought, calculating from the Hopkins experience. And then there was hydrotherapy, the cold-bath treatment about which he felt so much ambivalence. By 1894 the reduction in mortality achieved at Hopkins had convinced him that hydrotherapy had saved an extra 3 or 4 per cent of typhoid patients; the next year he estimated 6 to 8 per cent and dropped from his textbook his *cri de coeur* against the barbarism of the cold bath. Such a convert had Dr Osler become to his residents' enthusiasm for the treatment that he once demonstrated the technique at a clinical lecture. The session, clearly the prototype for Bob Newhart's comic monologues, must have had the students and probably their instructor (though certainly not the patient) suppressing smiles:

> The tub, as you see, is of light *papier-maché* material, and even when filled with water, as at present, is readily portable on wheels. The temperature of the water is 68 degrees ... The patient is given a small quantity of whiskey. Two orderlies will now lift him into the bath ... A cloth wrung out of ice-water is placed upon the patient's head, and with a small sponge the head and face are kept bathed with the same water. You see here an unusually docile patient, who takes the baths without much protest, but, as you have just heard him say, he would prefer them warm. Systematic friction is now applied to the skin either with the hand or by means of a cloth or India-rubber, which for convenience may be attached to a stick. The friction is rightly regarded as a very important element in the treatment, though, as you hear from this patient, he does not at all like it, and prefers to be left alone. Curiously enough Hippocrates laid stress upon this very point ...
>
> I am glad that you have witnessed the little *contretemps* in lifting this patient out of his bath. You see that he is a strongly built, heavy man, and the orderlies were only just able to lift him from the bath to the bed, and you saw that in doing so there was some little difficulty, owing to the catching of one arm on the side of the bath ... Though done, as you see, with the greatest possible care, these little accidents are liable to happen.
>
> The man is now well wrapped up in the [wet] sheet, which is tucked in between the arms and legs, and brought well around the neck ... You see that this man retains a good color in his face; the extremities are cold but not livid; and he is now beginning to shiver. Very often this shivering is distressing while in the bath, and one of the most unpleasant features of the system ... Now, before the patient is wheeled out, he will be given two ounces of hot milk with a little whiskey.[67]

Hopkins' success with hydrotherapy, as well as experiences suggesting that some of the traditional remedies – such as the arsenical compound, Fowler's solution – could be extremely toxic, underlay many of Osler's escalating protests against excessive drugging. He had to take on new therapeutic opponents as well. The apparent success of antiseptic measures in surgery suggested that disinfecting compounds that could kill bacteria outside the body might be reformulated as internal antiseptics. In the 1890s there was a wave of enthusiasm for antiseptic medication, apparently buttressed by reports in the *Journal of the American Medical Association*. In his 1896 address to the American Medical Association on fevers, Osler scathingly dismissed these articles as 'a heterogenous jumble, entirely unworthy of the best tradition of the profession' and as 'midsummer madness' that 'would insult the intelligence of a first year medical student.'[68]

In speaking to the AMA, most of whose members were very poorly trained by Hopkins standards, Osler was reaching out to an organization quite different from the elite groups he normally addressed. In the late 1890s there was another noticeable broadening of his activities as he made more excursions from the cloistered medical hilltop to the everyday world of harried doctors, filthy streets and open sewers, irresponsible newspapers and negligent politicians. He wanted his views on diagnosis and therapeutics to spread throughout the profession. And he wanted his views on public health to spread throughout the country.

From his days investigating *Trichinella spiralis* and pig typhoid, Osler had had a traditional sanitarian's interest in the prevention of disease. Now he was emerging as a powerful neosanitarian and a prophet ('we only demand that the people of this country shall do what Elisha asked of Namaan the Syrian – that they shall wash and be clean') of the second great wave of public-health concern that followed the bacteriological revolution. If typhoid fever and tuberculosis could not be cured, they could certainly be prevented. Comparative statistical studies showed what some communities could achieve and where others, notably Baltimore, fell short:

> Among the cities which still pay an unnecessary Delian tribute of young lives to the Minotaur of infectious diseases, Baltimore holds a high rank. The pity of it is, too, that this annual sacrifice of thousands of lives is not due to ignorance. For more than fifty years this gospel of preventive medicine has been preached ... in the ears of councils and corporations: that *three measures, efficiently designed and effectually carried out, reduce to a mini-*

mum the incidence of infectious diseases; viz., pure water, good drainage, and a proper isolation of the sick. Of sanitary essentials in a modern town, Baltimore has a well-arranged water supply ... It has nothing else – no sewage system, no system of isolation of the sick, no hospital for infectious diseases, no compulsory notification of such a disease as typhoid fever, no disinfecting station, no system of street-watering, no inspections of dairies, no inspection of meat. The streets are cleaned, but so carelessly that for a large part of the year the citizens breathe a mixture of air with horse-dung and filth of all sorts.[69]

His local missionary work included becoming active in the Medical and Chirurgical Faculty of Maryland, the state's Baltimore-based medical society. He addressed it on several occasions, was an enthusiastic member of the library committee, and in 1896–7 served a term as president. His presidential address dwelt on physicians' need for fellowship as a corrective to the effect of daily practice in creating 'an egoism of a most intense kind ... Ten years of successful work tends to make a man touchy, dogmatic, intolerant of correction and abominably self-centred.'

While speaking out often on public-health issues, Osler had as little to do with politics and politicians as possible. (It was left to Howard Kelly of the Baltimore Reform League literally to assault the reactionaries in scuffles at the polls during the 1895 municipal election; E.Y. Davis wrote bad satirical verse about the encounter.) Welch was far more comfortable in the world of medical politics and seemed to glory in wielding influence. Osler did follow his lead on several occasions in the late 1890s to lobby congressmen successfully against proposed antivivisectionist legislation. The 'priceless boon' of thyroid therapy for myxedema, he noted, was 'a direct triumph of vivisection,' easily justifying the sacrifice of hundreds of dogs and rabbits.[70]

Osler the writer was now locked into a lifetime of triennial 'hack work' revising his textbook to keep it up to date. *The Principles and Practice of Medicine* had become a major source of income, some 42,000 copies of the first two editions having been sold. The 1898 revision to produce a third edition was particularly extensive. Osler was up-to-date with important new treatments, such as use of thyroid extract. Sometimes he suddenly touted an old-fashioned remedy, such as the 'Chelsea Pensioner' for arthritis (a compound of sulfur, cream of tartar, rhubarb, and honey in warm wine.) The general therapeutic direction was against drugging. Delightful literary allusions – to corpulence as Byron's 'oily dropsy'; to Eryximachus's recommendations to cure Aristophanes' hiccups, or to Strabo in Plutarch on 'the lisping of the gout' – were accumulating in 'Osler' faster than new remedies.[71]

In his leisure hours Osler wrote papers on medical history. The Johns Hopkins Medical History Club was both stimulus and beneficiary of his interest; in the mid-1890s he gave papers destined for publication on 'Physic and Physicians as Depicted in Plato,' 'John Keats, the Apothecary Poet,' and 'Thomas Dover, Physician and Buccaneer' (the originator of Dover's pills). While researching the literature on malaria he came across the writings and unpublished letters of an obscure Alabama practitioner, John Y. Bassett, whose life of struggle and dedication he immortalized in one of his most famous essays, 'An Alabama Student.' As he told the Medical-Chirurgical Faculty of Maryland in his presidential address, he believed in an obligation to 'knit together the generations of physicians' by honoring the great men of the past in acts of 'filial piety.' Otherwise, as he noted in the Bassett profile, we are all fated to swell, foam for a moment, and then disappear into oblivion. He founded a medical history club at the Med-Chi and became the enthusiatic catalyst in the faculty's development of a first-class medical library.

As the nineteenth century drifted to its end, Dr Osler of Johns Hopkins tempered his criticisms of filthy cities and stupid politicians with overall optimism about medical progress. Who could deny the triumphs of anesthetics, antiseptic surgery, and vaccination, even in a world burdened with human shortcoming and sin? 'The bitter cry of Isaiah that with the multiplication of the nations their joys had not been increased, still echoes in our ears. The sorrows and troubles of men, it is true, may not have been materially diminished, but bodily pain and suffering, though not abolished, have been assuaged as never before ... The pains and woes of the body, to which we doctors minister, are decreasing at an extraordinary rate, and in a way that makes one fairly grasp in hopeful anticipation.'

Osler believed the brotherhood of physicians had done more than any other group to ease human suffering. 'To us as a profession,' he told the American Medical Association, 'belongs the chief glory of the century.' He almost never traded in political ideas, but in a burst of optimism he speculated about the possibilities of larger progress: 'The gradual growth of a deep sense of the brotherhood of man, such an abiding sense as pervades our own profession in its relation to the suffering, which recognizes the one blood of all the nations, may perhaps do it. In some development of socialism, something that will widen patriotism beyond the bounds of na-tionalism, may rest the desire of the race in this matter; but the evil is rooted and grounded in the abyss of human passion, and war with all its horrors is likely long to burden the earth.'[72]

'Fur caps and square hats to Dr Osler's' was the watchword among the porters and cabbies at the Baltimore railroad station. The square hats were the flat-crowned derbies favored by Grace's Boston relatives and Willie's Harvard friends. The fur caps were worn by Canadians, who seemed to be beating a path to Johns Hopkins in Osler's train.[73]

To change the metaphor, he was a magnet for bright countrymen want-ing the best medical training. Both Montreal and Toronto took pride in him as a native son who had excelled spectacularly. What a thrill and privilege to go down to the States, to Hopkins, to work with Osler! His good friends in top positions at McGill and the University of Toronto, some of whom had other Hopkins connections, acted as his talent scouts; his conscientiousness in coming home for all sorts of medical ceremonial occasions kept the network humming. McGill in his absence remained a first-class medical school, though perhaps slipping a bit in competition with the better-endowed American institutions. Since Osler had left Ontario, medical education at Trinity College and the University of Toronto had become very good, with particular strength in the basic sciences. Like-minded Toronto friends, especially the biologist Ramsay Wright, had been sending students to Hopkins for advanced training even before Osler arrived there. The Ontario countryside, rich, socially conservative, and overstocked with human talent, was a fine breeding ground for young men with the same instincts young Willie had had – a desire for professional excellence as opposed to a more obviously American fascination with business success.

If the scientific spirit at Johns Hopkins had many Germanic connections, the accents of the medical scientists were more apt to be Canadian. Osler had brought down Henri Lafleur as his first resident. In the 1890s Tom Cullen, Lewellys Barker, Tom McCrae, Jack McCrae, W.G. MacCallum, John MacCallum, Tom Futcher, Helen MacMurchy, and a large handful of other Canadians, including Bill Francis and another Osler nephew, Norman Gwyn, came to Hopkins as residents, interns, or students. A few eventually went back to Canada. Many stayed. While most of Osler's senior residents had Canadian connections (W.S. Thayer of Boston being the outstanding exception), not everyone from north of the border worked with him. Three of the 'Big Four' – Kelly, Welch, and Osler – were eventually succeeded by Canadian-born-and-educated medical scientists.

Canadian women, a shade less assertive than their American sisters, did not, by and large, come to Hopkins for medical training. Instead, as part of a demographic flow that had little to do with Osler per se, they made up a disproportionate number of the nursing staff – over 20 per cent in the early years. The first two superintendents of the Nurses' Training School were Canadian. Osler once proposed that Canada should levy a $100 export tax on its girls.[74]

Amidst the good-natured bantering about all the 'hyphenated Canadians' at Hopkins, there were occasional murmurs about nepotism or favoritism (and there was an obscure incident in the nursing school in 1893 that caused a trainee from the South to exclaim in a letter, 'Some thing must be done, or the Canadians will overpower us'). Had Osler created what Sandra McRae has called a Canadian Club at Hopkins? Osler once defended himself, with a wink, by saying he came from far northern New York. Years later he commented on how 'well and gently' the Americans had accepted 'the Canadian personality' at Hopkins, attributing the tolerance to Gilman and Welch.[75] None of these men, nor all that many of the Canadian and

American people, took the border particularly seriously in the late nineteenth century. Medically, until the countries began to go separate ways on health insurance in the 1960s, it had even less meaning. For most of the twentieth century, Canada would be a net exporter of talented doctors and nurses to the United States. Why did the U.S. Constitution require the president to be native-born? Canadians quipped. Answer: Because otherwise he would be a Canadian. There was William Osler, the president of American medicine![76]

'There is no border-line with Him who ordereth all things,' Ellen Osler commented apropos of a relative who had gone south.[77] William Osler was one of the many Anglo-Americans about the turn of the century who believed that blood was or should be more important than nationality and that it was too bad the English-speaking people's harmony had been shattered by that unfortunate American rebellion. In 1897, when the British Medical Association met in Montreal, Osler gave a long historical account of 'British Medicine in Greater Britain.' Even listeners who paid close attention would not have been quite sure whether Osler was including the United States as part of Britain's 'American' territory.

In fact he never felt totally at home in the United States. He did not take out American citizenship and always intended to retire back to British soil. In 1895 a minor war scare between the United States and Britain momentarily alarmed him. He was still 'British to the core,' he wrote. 'Damn these politicians: if they raise a war ... I should go back & stand by the boys.' McGill University, of course, wanted him in war or peace. In 1895, much to the alarm of his American friends, a newspaper report said that he was about to take its principalship. He scotched the rumors – apparently there had been some kind of approach if not a formal offer – but talked with Grace about the desirability of some day moving on. Revere's future was an important consideration: 'I do not – nor does Mrs. Osler – wish Revere to be brought up an American.' In 1899 the Oslers brought out an English nurse to take over from Revere's 'Mammy.' Their holidays in England became longer and more frequent. 'I have lost my heart to Oxford,' Osler wrote while attending medical meetings there in 1894.[78]

A northern boy from Cleveland, Ohio – almost Canada – arrived at Hopkins in October 1896. Harvey Williams Cushing was the son, grandson, and great-grandson of physicians, educated in arts at Yale (1891) and medicine at Harvard (1895). He did a year of general surgery at the Massachusetts General Hospital, took a holiday in Canada, and then came to Hopkins to work with Halsted. Nothing had come of an earlier feeler through Thayer to work on Osler's service. Anyway Cushing's bent was now clearly surgical and Halsted was the giant. Halsted's advice to Cushing was to go to Europe and stay there as long as he could, but former Hopkins people told him that a year with Halsted would be worth five abroad.

Cushing was a wiry twenty-seven-year-old, ambitious, intense, and hard-driving. His first impressions of Hopkins in the autumn of 1896 were not favorable: 'Am much dissapointed to find the Hospital a very sloppy place and the work of everyone most unsystematic, i.e. on the surgical side. Dr Halsted has only operated once this month and rarely appears. Hope things will clear up or I can't stand it.'[79] He did stand it, though things did not clear up quickly. 'The surgical operating room during my first year in Baltimore was a circus.'[80] Halsted, who at times did not know who was on his surgical staff, had, sight-unseen, hired a duel-scarred German surgeon as senior resident. The man proved completely incompetent and, before leaving the hospital, challenged the head surgical nurse (still a male) to a duel.

After that first year, during which he took the first Roentgen photographs, or x-rays, at Hopkins, Cushing replaced Bloodgood as Halsted's senior resident. He told everyone, including Halsted, what needed to be done to improve the surgical service. Americans could be almost as belli-cose as Germans: one intern, dressed down once too often in public, challenged Cushing to a fight. Cushing apologized. He also later admitted that he learned pathology and bacteriology for the first time in Baltimore, and grudgingly came to recognize that the 'inartistic rubber-gloved methods of operating' at Hopkins produced far better results than anything he had seen in Boston.[81]

Knowing nothing of Halsted's addiction, Cushing saw him as a dour, mysterious figure who appeared to be lazy, would never make up his mind, and could not be relied on for anything. 'Here I am, a youth, doing surgical work that not one of my school confreres will hope to do for years. It frightens me sometimes. The Chief rarely operates. Today I did all of his private cases.' Halsted had to do an emergency operation on Cushing himself in the autumn of 1897, an appendectomy, which was still risky enough surgery for Cushing to leave postmortem instructions with his friends. He pulled through easily but had a long convalescence as the case that brought to an end the summer's string of 200 operations (mostly by Cushing) without infection. For the rest of his life Cushing carried in his belly several of Halsted's silver-wire sutures.[82]

Sociable, of a literary bent, and eager for fellowship with senior men in his chosen field, Cushing was hardly ever invited to the Halsted home at 1201 Eutaw Place. On the few occasions he got inside it, the residence reminded him of Dickens' Bleak House; it was high-ceilinged, 'cold as a stone,' and furnished with fine old antiques scattered topsy-turvy. Halsted lived on the ground floors; his wife Caroline and their dachshunds above. The Halsteds could have been prototypes for the Addams family. 'She was a strange, unadorned woman dressed in black who affected a masculine garb of the plainest sort,' Cushing wrote. 'Wore flat-heeled, mannish shoes and had her hair brushed straight back and fastened in a bun.' Halsted was personally fastidious to an eccentric degree – though the oft-repeated story that he sent his shirts to Paris or London to be laundered may have come from someone misinterpreting one of his whimsical remarks. When the Halsteds formally entertained – two or three times in Cushing's fifteen years at Hopkins – every detail of the menu and setting, including the wood for the fireplace, was chosen with the most exacting care by the professor, and the conversation was rich and delightful. Otherwise, when the senior resident went round to call on the chief of surgery, there would be a long wait on the doorstep until finally a domestic would open the door a crack to say no one was at home. Once, when Cushing called the servant's bluff, saying he had seen a light in the study, he found Halsted in his dressing gown and slippers, and they had a fine chat about antiques.[83]

Halsted depended on Cushing to carry much of the burden of surgery and surgical teaching at Hopkins in the late 1890s. 'Halsted and all of us have the most unbounded confidence in him,' Osler wrote in February 1899, 'and within five years he ought to have the reputation of one of the best operators and most successful surgeons in the country.' Cushing gloried in his independence and went up and down a scale of feeling for Halsted that ranged from deep admiration to disgust and loathing. He considered leaving Hopkins in 1899; Osler, through Tom McCrae, urged him to stay. In March 1900 Cushing came near his wit's end as Halsted sent in note after note, written in semi-legible scrawl with old goose-quill pens, saying he would not be in to operate: 'I hope that our case of yesterday is not dead' ... 'If my patients for today do not care to wait until Monday please operate upon them & oblige.' Cushing and his assistants did six operations a day, while Halsted did two in about a month before leaving for another six-month summer at his North Carolina retreat. 'If you should break down,' he wrote to Cushing, 'I would be in my grave in a month.'[84]

Cushing finally got away in the summer of 1900 for a 'Wanderjahr' abroad. He had come to know Osler casually in his first years at Hopkins, sometimes being invited over for tea or to drop in and play with Revere, and he saw much more of him that summer in England. Osler was 'kindness itself,' Cushing told his fiancée, and marveled at the way introductions from him opened medical doors in that country.[85] Cushing experimented with growing a mustache just like Osler's. From abroad, Cushing found it unclear whether or not Halsted wanted him back. 'The Chief [Osler] asked me recently what you were going to do,' McCrae wrote to him. 'I said that I thought you were uncertain and that you had no very clear idea of what Dr Halsted thought ("No" said the Chief, "nor has anyone else"). He spoke about your importance to the surgical side as the man who had more "grist" and go than anyone they had.' Cushing found Halsted still vague and unsatisfactory when he came home, had several verbal confrontations with him, and only agreed to stay on at Hopkins after intercession from Welch and Osler.

It happened that Cushing moved into a house at 3 West Franklin, next door to the Oslers, which he shared with Henry Barton Jacobs and Thomas Futcher. As the young doctors moved in, a large case of wine and

boxes of cigars arrived as a gift from 'Professor Hopkins,' in Osler's hand-
writing. Socializing between the medical houses was constant. Would the
doctors come for dinner? lunch? tea? Would they mind if Grace brought
her knitting and her young lady friends over on Saturday night to get away
from Dr Osler's student confab? Did the young doctors have their latch-
keys to 1 West Franklin so they could use the library whenever they wanted?
Why not knock a hole in the fence between the houses to make it easier to
come across? 'It makes life in Baltimore even worthwhile to be next door
to these people,' Harvey Cushing told his father.[86]

The Johns Hopkins Hospital and School of Medicine had been made possible by American economic development in the mid-nineteenth century
– the great merchant fortune Hopkins had accumulated, the railway wealth
inherited by Mary Garrett. While Osler and his colleagues were turning an
earlier generation's generosity into great American institutions in the 1890s,
the country continued its spectacular, sprawling growth. New, almost
unimaginably large fortunes were created in steel, oil, tobacco. Until the
1890s, churches and theological schools had been the favored targets of
well-to-do philanthropists. Now education and health began to come into
their own. Medical schools, universities, and hospitals in Boston, New York,
Chicago, Michigan, California, and dozens of other cities and states benefited from the new philanthropy and the bounty of well-to-do state governments. The Hopkins medical men who chose to be researchers and
teachers, as well as practitioners, slid easily into top positions across the
continent; the women also did well, though with far fewer opportunities.

When American energies were channeled into a short little war with
Spain in 1898–9 and the beginnings of an American empire abroad, there
were still more opportunities for Hopkins medical men. The school had
been in the forefront of the investigations of malaria and yellow fever that
were now focusing on mosquitoes as the vector spreading the organisms
among humans. Two former Hopkins men, Walter Reed and Jesse Lazear,
would be leaders in the U.S. Army campaign that made Havana safe from

yellow fever. Lazear's death from yellow fever during that work gave Hopkins its first medical martyr. Lewellys Barker and Simon Flexner came back in good health from their special Hopkins mission to the Philippines, a kind of safari to exotic microbe country, spreading the word that Americans could now vie with the British, Germans, and Italians in the new field of tropical medicine. Osler would be little more than a cheerleader for such work – he never visited the tropics himself – with nothing but praise for all efforts to make the world safer and healthier for whites and natives alike. One of the most appalling sights of his life had been the arrival in Philadelphia in 1888 of a shipload of workers from the isthmus of Panama whose bodies had been ravaged by malaria and dysentery in the first attempt to build a canal.[87] Scientific medicine, principles of sanitation, and American energies and engineers were about to change all that.

And more. In America in the summer of 1897 a Baptist minister decided to bone up on medicine. On the recommendation of a medical student, the Reverend Frederick Gates selected *Principles and Practice* to take on his summer holiday. He found Osler's style compelling and, medical dictionary at his side, plowed through chapter after chapter until he had finished the book, which he pronounced one of the most intensely interesting he had ever read. What most impressed Gates about the state of medicine, in the Osler version, was how few diseases could be treated effectively. Science had done an amazing job of isolating bacterial causes but had still to produce specific treatments. Suppose medical research were to became more handsomely endowed: 'We might expect,' Gates wrote Osler a few years later, 'in the next generation or two to reduce medicine ... to something resembling an exact science, and we might reasonably expect results as revolutionary, as far-reaching, as beneficent on human well-being as any which have been derived from the practical applications of physical and chemical sciences ... This line of philanthropy, now almost wholly neglected in this country, is the most needed and the most promising of any field of philanthropic endeavor.'[88]

Gates was in a unique position to act on his reflections, for he was no longer active in the ministry but worked as philanthropic adviser to the fabulously rich Baptist oil magnate, John D. Rockefeller. One of Gates's main jobs was to recommend worthy causes for Rockefeller money to support. Most of Rockefeller's givings in earlier years had been to causes sponsored by the Baptist Church. After reflecting on Osler's text, Gates wrote Rockefeller a long memorandum on the glorious achievements of researchers such as Pasteur and Koch, pointing out how little was happening in the United States except at Hopkins and stressing the desirability of creating an American version of European research institutes. Rockefeller and his son saw merit in the argument and authorized planning for what would soon become the Rockefeller Institute of Medical Research. Osler, who was now doing little research as the younger men defined it, knew nothing of Gates's inspiration at the time and had nothing to do with the new organization. Welch, however, became its first chairman and recommended his former student, Simon Flexner, as its first director. Through one connection or another, at home or abroad, Johns Hopkins would lead American medicine and the worship of good health into the twentieth century.

SEVEN

The Great American Doctor

Osler's first private patient in Baltimore was an important elderly gentleman, a Hopkins trustee perhaps. Osler thought he felt a pelvic tumor, diagnosed it as an inoperable sarcoma, 'and in as gentle a way as I could, told his wife, and advised that a surgeon see the case.' The surgeon came the next day, drained the patient's distended bladder with a catheter, and thus disposed of the 'tumor.' Osler used the embarrassment as an object lesson in his teaching.[1]

Otherwise, his private practice flourished. Consultations grew steadily in Baltimore until by the mid-90s he was seeing all the private patients he could handle and had to turn down an increasing number of requests (including, it is said, a man who then came back and read the Hippocratic Oath on his doorstep).[2] He was consulting physician to the huge extended Osler family, to all his old friends back in Canada, to the students, nurses, doctors and their relatives at Hopkins, to the elite of Baltimore, to congressmen and several denizens of the White House, and to cases that interested him up and down the eastern seaboard and as far west as Wisconsin and Iowa.

Like all doctors of his era, Osler often made house or hotel calls, not only in Baltimore but over to Washington, back to Philadelphia, on visits to Montreal and Toronto, and practically anywhere else that a railway or carriage would take him. His fees were high but proportionate with his reputation, and far less variable than those of his surgical colleagues. There was an element of 1890s medical chic in taking your ailment to the great doctor – people joked that it was unfashionable to die or have your appendix out in Baltimore without having been seen by Osler – but he did not become a society doctor on the model of Weir Mitchell, who had become very wealthy treating the neurotic rich. Osler saw all the patients he had to see to satisfy friends, relatives, and professional niceties, and otherwise chose to see mainly cases that interested him. A Maryland doctor once complained that Osler would only occasionally come out forty miles into the country when a large fee was involved but had accepted every single invitation to come out for an autopsy.[3]

By the beginning of the twentieth century and the sixth decade of his life, Osler found that the demands on his time were becoming almost intolerable. Unable or unwilling to cut back on his practice or reduce his obligations at Hopkins, he began to worry about his own health. After his fiftieth birthday he was noticeably more interested in books and bibliography, medical history and biography, and semi-philosophical inquiries into the best way to live and the meaning of death. Some of his colleagues thought he was falling away from the frontier of the profession, a spent force perhaps. Trying to find a calmer berth, drawn back to his cultural roots and congenial society, thinking about his son's future, he spent more of his time in Great Britain. Osler may have become the great American doctor, but he often told his friends that his ideal would be to live within an hour of the British Museum and have the *Times* on his breakfast table.[4]

After morning rounds in the public wards, Osler would visit any patients he happened to have in the much smaller private pay section of the hospital. From 2:00 or 2:30 to 4:30 PM he saw private patients at his home office. He normally saw five patients in those hours, a few more if histories had been taken by a helper or the doctor who had requested the consultation. 'A case cannot be satisfactorily examined in less than half an hour, unless the notes have been taken previously by an assistant,' he wrote in a rare 1895 comment on his private practice. 'A sick man likes to have plenty of time spent over him, and he gets no satisfaction in a hurried, ten or twelve minutes examination.'

A remarkable number of Osler's surviving case notes are in his own hand, but by the nineties he had largely gone over to dictation, for a time using a female 'stenographine,' who was secluded from the patient behind a screen. 'If one never saw a patient the second time, notes might be superfluous, but can anything be more embarrassing in a return visit than to have forgotten name, face, malady, everything?' In 1895 he saw a patient he remembered from twelve years earlier, and his notes proved the fact against the false memories of both patient and attending doctor. He topped that the next year when a man he had never met came in to be treated for extraordinarily noisy breathing; Osler had observed him years before on a train and had made a memorandum about it. Carefully cross-indexed, his patient notes became the basis for still more publications. (Many of Osler's colleagues apparently did not keep written patient records. E.L. Trudeau, the country's most prominent tuberculosis doctor, only began to do it in 1902 after a hint from Osler.)[5]

He saw patients with every disorder, from common colds to mystifyingly strange and exotic diseases, and in every state of health, from normality (Osler witnessed the birth of the routine check-up, what he called the annual over-hauling of the machinery) to imminent death. One of the chief unpleasantries of a consultant's life, he wrote, was

> the passing of judgment on the unhappy incurables – on the cancerous, ataxics, and paralytics, who wander from one city to another ... Still more distressing are the instances of hopeless illness in which, usually for the friend's sake, the entire 'faculty' is summoned. Can anything be more doleful than a procession of four or five doctors into the sick man's room? Who does not appreciate Matthew Arnold's wish? –

> Nor bring to see me cease to live
> Some doctor full of phrase and fame,
> To shake his sapient head, and give
> The ill he cannot cure a name.

He knew he was sometimes used by doctor friends who were going through the motions of leaving nothing left undone, a very old custom. Petronius had written in the *Satyricon*, 'A doctor's really no use except to feel you did the right thing.'

Reviewing a year's practice in 1895, Osler felt he had been useful in four other ways. In certain cases the visit had been crucial to the patient, 'usually in making a diagnosis, upon which succesful treatment directly depended, as in myxoedema or pernicious anaemia.' In a much larger number he felt he had been able to make an important suggestion either in prognosis or management. In a third group of cases he had simply failed, just as baffled as everyone else but having at least learned the wisdom of freely confessing ignorance. Finally, there were the consultations in which his chief value had been to reassure patients that nothing serious was wrong with them and to give them common-sense advice about life and diet: 'Coleridge somewhere remarks that when a man is vaguely ill the talk of a doctor about the nature of his malady tones him down and consoles. It is very true, and to tone down and console are important functions of professional advisers.'[6]

Osler might have added a 'hit-and-miss' category, which most physicians would recognize, in which advice that helps one patient is of no use to another. In 1896 he described two cases he had seen of general bromidrosis, offensive body odor. For a British Columbia man who exuded 'a stale musty smell, not unlike the odour of the parings of the frog of a horse's foot,' he endorsed the use of pilocarpine, an alkaline, and the problem disappeared. He made the same prescription to a Baltimore woman who described herself as being as offensive as the worst Swiss cheese; a few days later, when Osler got into a streetcar, he smelled failure even before he saw his patient down at the far end. She eventually committed suicide. 'I was not surprised as she was in a state of hopeless despair, having tried all remedies in vain.'[7]

Dr Osler's manner with patients was seldom the stone-faced passivity, imperturbability, or inscrutability he is sometimes thought to have recommended in his Philadelphia farewell address, 'Aequanimitas.' Sloppy wording in that talk aside, Osler had actually worried about doctors appearing to be hard or indifferent. Their demeanor should be one of 'good-natured' equanimity, he had advised, and should reflect 'infinite patience' and 'ever-tender charity.' 'To many of a sombre and sour disposition it is hard to maintain good spirits amid the trials and tribulations of the day,' he wrote in a later essay, 'yet it is an unpardonable mistake to go about among patients with a long face.'[8]

The good nature was always dominant. Colleagues who saw Osler with private patients in the hospital remembered a delightful 'round of laughter and gaiety':

> In one room our poor, old, arthritic friend, Mr. D., who suffered through so many months, was always, through some new bit of nonsense, reduced to laughter until he cried from some twinge of pain caused by the physical activity provoked.
>
> And here it was the charming but very loquacious nurse with brittle bones, who suffered, on several occasions, from fractures of rib or arm or leg, who was always greeted by a solicitous inquiry about her jaw.
>
> Or again the sad-faced hypochondriac with a treasured store of questions, who was greeted by some salutation so surprising that his train of thought was exploded as by a mine.
>
> Or the anxious psychasthenic, who was so quickly engaged in a playful discussion of the colour of the ribbons on her nightgown that she quite forgot the number of hours that she had or had not slept – and always he was gone. How? Where? No one wholly knew.[9]

We do not hear much from deceased or disgruntled patients about their doctors. Nor did Osler again see his most articulate Philadelphia case, Walt Whitman, who died in 1892. In general, Osler's patients, like his students, idolized him. He was effectively the family doctor for Harry Reid, a neighbor and Hopkins University colleague; Edith Gittings Reid, a writer, observed Osler closely when Harry was sick with typhoid, when their children were ill, and during her own sicknesses:

> To have been a patient of Sir William Osler's ... was to have obtained an

almost impossible idea of what a physician could be ... It was not necessary for him to be sensitive to a social atmosphere, because he always made his own atmosphere. In a room full of discordant elements he entered and saw only his patient and only his patient's greatest need, and instantly the atmosphere was charged with kindly vitality, everyone felt that the situation was under control, and all were attention. No circumlocution, no meandering. The moment Sir William gave you was yours. It was hardly ever more than a moment but there was curiously no abrupt beginning or end to it. With the easy sweep of a great artist's line, beginning in your necessity and ending in your necessity, the precious moment was yours, becoming wholly and entirely a part of the fabric of your life ...

With his patients he recognized at once the thing or characteristic that concerned him and them; and for the rest, whatever was uncongenial or unattractive he put from his mind and prevented any expression of it. A pose or an attempt at serious chatter about unessentials was intolerable to him. But he was as merciful as he was masterful, and from the very poor and the genuinely afflicted he would even have borne being bored.

Such telling love, such perfect confidence were given him that he could do what he liked without causing offence. Three times in my life I have seen him, when in consultation, smash the attending physician's diagnosis and turn the entire sick-room the other way about; but he left the room with his arm about the corrected physician's neck, and they seemed to be having a delightful time. The reason for this was perfectly evident: every physician felt himself safe in Sir William's hands; he knew that he could by no possibility have a better friend in the profession; that if, with the tip of his finger, Sir William gaily knocked down his house of cards, he would see to it that the foundation was left solid.[10]

Osler's mastery of the uses of optimism, humor, and good cheer, what he sometimes called his 'general cheer-up prescription' or the doctor's 'transfusion of the spirits,' could have an extraordinarily potent effect. Ernest Jones, the psychoanalyst who became Sigmund Freud's first major biographer and had known Osler, remarked in 1928 that Osler had no need for any special knowledge of psychopathology; he could handle mental cases just as effectively on the strength of his own personality. Cushing noted that Osler despised 'the chicanery of psychoanalysis' but was in fact an effective psychotherapist. And Clarence B. Farrer, a former student who became one of Canada's leading psychiatrists, wrote that Osler's 'very presence brought healing. It was immediate unplanned psychotherapy ... There was healing in his voice.'[11]

He usually tried to cushion a grim outlook, a habit some thought he took to a fault in later years. 'The careful physician has but one end in view – not to depress his patient in any way whatever,' he wrote while reflecting on the humor of Rabelais. He cautioned students against saying anything in the hearing of a patient that would increase anxiety.[12] If a man's terror at knowing his chest pains were angina would itself worsen them, Osler told him he had 'a neuralgia of the pneumo-gastric nerve.' On the other hand, he advised telling tuberculous patients the truth about their condition right away. It was 'really not often necessary, since Nature usually does it quietly and in good time,' to tell a patient he was past all hope, Osler maintained, but added, 'and yet, put in the right way to an intelligent man it is not always cruel.'[13]

As a consultant, he would often have left the breaking of news, good or bad, to the attending physician. But many times there was no easy exit. A nurse remembered a tragic case of a mortally ill former Hopkins student clinging to the hope that when Dr Osler came he would have more to offer than the others' despairing palliative, morphine:

> Dr. Osler came, a gentle, tender presence, in a huge fur coat, and sat down by Dr. Swan, who was over six feet in height.
>
> He talked to him like a sorrowing tender Mother for her little boy, and then he put his arm around him and said, 'Now Swan I want you to let this good woman here give you some morphia tonight so that you may relax and sleep, for that is what you need; and, I want you to do this for me, your old Professor and friend.' I will never forget the scene, nor the expression of Dr. Swan's face, tragedy supreme, but so pitiful and no resentment.
>
> The verdict had been given, and from the hand he had counted on to save!

'Now' said Dr. Osler, 'if Miss M. will fix her hypo, you will take it while I am here, and then tomorrow I will find a stronger Swan; and we will talk everything over.' Dr. Swan agreed, he had refused always and everyone to take morphia, the only thing to relax and enable him to lie down.

I gave the morphia, and after a time Dr. Osler left, and Dr. Swan slept all night, feeling much stronger and better the next day, but he did not live very long after that.

Another of his physician patients who lay dying asked for Osler. When an injection of morphia was given him he smiled and said, 'Ah! Osler has come.'[14]

Osler's maxims about treating patients rather than diseases did not cause him to become a sounding-board for people who wanted someone to hear them talk. Psychoanalysis was about to fill that niche. Osler always controlled conversations and usually made them brief, sometimes to patients' (and colleagues') disgruntlement. As a diagnostician, he probably did not attend as carefully to patient narratives as physicians do today, their lab tests and instruments doing much of the rest of the work. While soothing troubled souls with a little wit and sympathy, Osler spent most of his visits examining bodies for signs of organic disease.

The classic ritual was inspection, palpation, percussion, auscultation: look, touch, listen. Osler wrote many thousands of words on the interpretation of sounds heard with the stethoscope and the ways in which the body, including its toes, revealed itself to the physician's touch. Stories of Osler at the bedside most often focused on his visual acuity. As Welch once put it in a slightly different context, 'How much his eyes will see that would escape most of us!' Osler's gaze was first into your eyes, then over every inch of your body. Both children and adults remembered that he seemed to be able to look inside or through them. 'He could see more in five minutes than we in twenty-four hours,' a young doctor recalled. Thayer described him making a first quick glance, then 'calling for a chair, sitting down and looking across chest or abdomen of his patient, with his head at the level of the body, as he pointed out to us that there are many things that one can see in this fashion which cannot be made out by other manoeuvres of eye, ear or hand – the descent of the lungs, retractions or pulsations in chest, peristaltic movements of stomach or intestines, the rounded fundus of an almost or quite impalpable gall bladder moving up and down with respiration.'[15]

With students, he worked on a more basic level. So we have looked at the patient's chest. What next? Palpation, says the student. What about inspecting the back? says Osler:

Many years ago at the Girard Hotel, Philadelphia, I saw a remarkable case which illustrated the value and importance of the point. The patient had a large area of pulsation in the lower front of the chest, extending almost from one nipple to the other, with distinct prominence. There was a double murmur at the base of the heart, and the case had been regarded as one of aortic insufficiency, which condition was present. He had paroxysms of great distress and orthopnea, and there were peculiar features about the case, so that one or two of the leading physicians in Philadelphia had expressed themselves as somewhat puzzled about its nature.

Fortunately, after finishing the inspection in front, I turned the patient's back to a good light, and the diagnosis was made at a glance. There was a pulsating aneurysmal tumor in the left interscapular region, which had given him no pain whatever, and which had not attracted the attention of his physicians.

On another occasion Osler was the first physician to ask a certain patient to remove rather than just tuck up his undershirt – he found the aneurysm at a glance. And there was the case of the priest suffering from pain primarily in his arms and legs:

He was a large framed, well built man. After he had removed his night shirt I stood at the foot of the bed to get a general survey, and my attention was at once attracted to his right breast, which stood out prominently. He had not noticed it himself, nor had any of his physicians. He had had no pain, and nothing to call attention especially to it. On examination he had a firm, hard tumour, evidently a scirrhus ... Finding the breast tumour, there was no question then as to the nature of the spinal cord trouble. I did not hear of the subsequent history of the patient.[16]

Incidents like these created the legend of medical master who could stand at the door and say what was wrong with every patient on the ward. Remember the famous leprosy case. Similar stories were told of the elite clinicians at the great British hospitals. It wasn't such a hard knack, Osler would tell his students. You don't necessarily have to have vast experience with obscure cases. Just be up on the literature:

It is astonishing with how little reading a doctor can practise medicine, but it is not astonishing how badly he may do it. Not three months ago a physician living within an hour's ride of the Surgeon-General's Library brought to me his little girl, aged twelve. The diagnosis of infantile myxoedema required only a half glance. In placid contentment he had been practising twenty years in 'Sleepy Hollow,' and not even when his own flesh and blood was touched did he rouse from an apathy deep as Rip Van Winkle's sleep. In reply to questions: No, he had never seen anything in the journals about the thyroid gland; he had seen no pictures of cretinism or myxoedema; in fact his mind was a blank on the whole subject. He had not been a reader, he said, but he was a practical man with very little time.

In 1901 a doctor's wife came to Hopkins with symptoms that had baffled physicians all over the country. Osler instantly diagnosed a liver abscess. Halsted drained it, and the patient made a good recovery. 'Any one at all familar with recent work on the liver could have made [the diagnosis] easily,' Osler told the hospital medical society. 'In fact my secretary, to whom a young physician dictated the notes of the case in my absence, made the diagnosis from his description.' With her other doctors, the poor woman had been 'seeking a diagnosis but getting only treatment.'

During her internship at Hopkins, Dorothy Reed witnessed one of its best physicians missing a diagnosis, and Osler, drawing on his Montreal experiences, saving the hospital from a potential disaster:

> One day I found a husky black man had developed over night a remarkable rash. Under his very dark skin were shot-like lumps over his entire body. Calling Dr. Futcher, the resident, at once he pronounced the case 'chicken pox' – and said that Dr. Osler would be delighted to show it to the 4th year students. So we got all ready for rounds, and Dr. Osler blew into the ward followed by 30 to 40 students and doctors. When all were grouped about the patient, Dr. Futcher threw back the sheet showing the man's entire body. Dr. Osler's face changed from an expression of gay and whimsical humor to a grim visage. 'My God, Futcher, don't you know smallpox when you see it?'
>
> What a scramble followed. The patient sent to isolation and all the contacts on the ward – nurses, doctors, students, had to be vaccinated. The ward was isolated for 6 weeks, 2 or 3 more cases came down with the infection, and altogether it was a tiresome time. I certainly learned all the symptoms and appearance of the rash in the negro, but as I have never seen smallpox again it was of no practical use ... Poor Dr. Futcher who had been the innocent cause of the exposure of most of the 4th year class and many others, was frightfully embarrassed.[17]

Osler was notoriously gentle with the ignorance and mistakes of attending physicians. He may have consoled poor Futcher by telling him of his own embarrassing confusion of a smallpox case at Blockley with secondary syphilis. Inevitably, the great Zadiglike diagnostician had a hilarious comeuppance in front of his third-year observation clinic. When a student thought he had exhausted the possibilities of observation, Osler exclaimed, 'Look at his eyes, man – I can see it from here.'

'Oh, yes, one pupil is larger than the other.'

'Cheese it, Gov'nor,' the patient whispered loudly. 'That's a glass eye.'

On the other hand, his private and sometimes public judgments could be very harsh. The father of the myxedemous daughter may well have recognized himself in print. So would these doctors:

A patient ... was brought to me only a few weeks ago, supposed to have a protracted fever after typhoid. Her father, a physician, her husband a physician, and it is scarcely credible that neither of them had the faintest idea that the poor soul had advanced consumption, though it had reached a stage in which there was shrinkage of one side of the chest, and the diagnosis could almost be made by inspection alone ... A very distinguished and careful physician brought his daughter to me a few years ago to have her blood examined, as he felt sure she had a chronic malaria. She had little or no cough, but an afternoon rise of temperature, and it turned out to be the usual story – quite pronounced local disease [tuberculosis] at her left apex.

Osler told his students that if they did not do their business properly, when they got to heaven they would be met by large numbers of little children, shaking their fingers and saying, 'You sent us here.'[18]

Osler's medical art was informed and controlled by all the assistance science could give. He did not discuss diagnosis as a matter of intuition. Every scientific aid was welcome. He had always been a champion of urine testing, blood testing, and bacteriological studies, and he made a point of insisting that examination was not complete without at least a glance through the microscope at blood and urine. In 1896 it was Osler who recommended that Johns Hopkins purchase its first x-ray equipment. In 1902 he described a case in which a thoracic aneurysm could not have been found without an x-ray – though, with typical balance, he then emphasized how much the physician could find by looking at a bare chest in a good light and with good eyes.[19]

Osler sometimes seemed to disparage reliance on laboratory findings. 'What I wish to emphasize,' he said in a 1901 paper, 'is the importance of basing a judgment less on the urine than on the general condition of the patient.' He described how one of his most distinguished private patients, later revealed to be Sir Charles Tupper, had continued to lead an exceptionally vigorous life for twenty years after being scared almost into retirement by the discovery of traces of albumin and tube casts in his urine. The story illustrated the old adage, 'The urine is a harlot or a liar,' Osler wrote. Then he concluded with one of his 'let me not be misunderstood' qualifications: Urine tests disclosed potential problems ahead; the problem for the practitioner was to differentiate more clearly the problems' range and susceptibility to treatment. One did not just toss the lab work down the drain. The year after writing this article, Osler supervised pioneering studies of the blood pressure of his typhoid and pneumonia patients, using the apparatus just developed by Howell and his students in physiology. They were refining an early sphygmomanometer that Cushing had brought back from Europe. (Cushing's studies of blood pressure and surgery were particularly important. The Hopkins nurses were having trouble keeping up with the technology – at least, one flustered student nurse was. When told by Cushing to take a blood-pressure reading during an operation, she began to apply the pneumatic cuff to his leg).[20]

Sir Charles Tupper and many of Osler's other private patients were strikingly different from most of his hospital cases. In his years as a hospital physician he saw mostly poor or working-class people who were being ravaged by organic disease. He saw a much broader range of afflictions than specialists in internal medicine do now, including many grotesque and advanced maladies – massive tumors, blocked and distended organs (the obscenely swollen megacolon of the patient they called the Balloon Man is still on display in Philadelphia), and bodies rotting with infection. Today ready access, early diagnosis, and powerful therapies have practically eliminated these in North America. Most of these patients were suffering, in various ways, the stigmata of nineteenth-century poverty. Osler's private patients, by comparison, were usually from affluent backgrounds. While many kinds of illness and breakdown strike indiscriminately, a large number of Osler's clients suffered from ailments not requiring or amenable to hospital treatment.

Cases of neurasthenia or nervous exhaustion, for example, had no organic cause and often few treatable physical symptoms. At the other extreme, severe bouts of chest pain or angina pectoris led to sudden death more often than to hospitalization. Osler did not see a single case of angina pectoris during his hospital-based work in Montreal, had only two cases under his charge at the university hospital in Philadelphia, one at Blockley, and four during the first seven years at Hopkins. But so many came to him in his Baltimore practice that by 1896 he was able to publish an important series of lectures based on sixty cases.[21] He estimated that he was seeing privately more angina pectoris than appeared at all the Baltimore hospitals combined.

He had done a great deal of clinical and pathological work on diseases of the heart valves and endocardium, but angina, still fairly mystifying to the profession, was different. It was 'not a disease,' he wrote, 'but a syndrome or symptom group (without constant aetiological or anatomical foundations) associated with complex conditions, organic or functional, of the heart and aorta ... We employ the term generically, qualifying the varieties by such names as true, false, hysterical, and vasomotor.' Partly because of the lack of hospital and pathological material, Osler and his colleagues were still groping towards an understanding of myocardial infarction and related conditions.[22] 'The opportunities for observing the paroxysm do not come very often,' Osler wrote dryly, 'and when they do the condition of the patient is such that our efforts are directed rather toward his relief than to the study of special points in the case.' Even so, drawing on the results of animal research, he was very close in 1896 to outlining the concept of the heart attack.

Not surprisingly, given the nature of his practice, Osler thought angina pectoris occurred almost entirely in men, usually in high-achieving men, and disproportionately in doctors. He was particularly impressed by the extreme anxiety many sufferers experienced – a 'mental anguish' so overwhelming that it could take on a life of its own, leading to varieties of the syndrome based on and accentuated by worry and stress. Arteriosclerosis was often enough discovered in angina sufferers, but the total picture seemed to involve a more general pattern of chronic misuse of the body – too much eating, drinking, work, and worry – leading to its deterioration.

If public health measures could stave off infectious disease, good personal habits were called for to avoid or minimize bouts of heart pain. In his metaphoric way, Osler had always advised young men against worship at the shrines of Venus, Bacchus, and Vulcan. Now he varied false-gods images with advice not to overstrain the human mechanism. In the early twentieth century his favorite image of the body was as a machine. Like the transatlantic steamers Osler and his well-to-do patients so often took, no doubt using the crossing to rest and reflect on their health, the body would give out if the engines were overstoked, driven too long under high pressure, negligently maintained. During actual malfunction, you worked desperately to get things going again. Otherwise, for signs of overexertion, ranging from chest pains to nervous exhaustion, the prescription was often simply to reduce speed. Osler found himself telling patient after patient (for his angina consultations continued to increase) to eat less, drink less, smoke less, work less, worry less. Look after the machine. Cut back from twenty-five to fifteen knots: 'Go slowly and attend to your work, live a godly life, and avoid mining shares ... I doubt if quinine could have very much influence.'[23]

Such advice shaded into general maxims for healthy living. These fitted with and reinforced Osler's dislike of unnecessary drugging as well as his personal temperance. To the Johns Hopkins graduating class of 1900 and at the Historical Club in 1901 he preached lay sermons about how the progress of the past century had culminated in 'a new school of medicine,' based on a return to natural methods for both the treatment and the prevention of disease. Hydrotherapy and massage were important in treating disease. Diet and exercise, he argued with a touch of hyperbolic fever, were crucial in preventing it:

> Some one said he cared not who made the laws, so that he could write the songs of a nation, which I would paraphrase by saying, I care not who physics the people, provided that I could train their cooks. From the kitchen must come one of the great needed reforms in medicine. The besetting malady of this country is dyspepsia ... From it about one half of the income of doctors is derived, and at least two thirds of that of the patent medicine vendors ... If the women of the country whose energies are at present engaged in the problems of temperance, the suffrage, missions and millinery, would take a year off and spend it in the kitchen something might be done ...

With the introduction of light beer there is not only less intemperance, but we see much less of the serious organic disease of heart, liver and stomach caused by alcohol, and less of the early general degeneration ... How few cases, comparatively, of alcoholic cirrhosis of the liver one sees. I wish that I could say the same of intemperance in eating ... We physicians are beginning to recognize that the early degenerations, particularly of the arteries and of the kidneys, which we formerly attributed in great part to alcohol, is due to too much food. The clinkers kill, and we all, I fear, habitually have clinkers and ashes in our machines which clog the workings, rust the bearings, and lead to premature break-down ...

The remarkable increase in the means of taking wholesome out of door exercise goes far to counteract the universal malignity of the American kitchen. Golf and the bicycle have in the past few years materially lowered the average incomes of the doctors of this country as derived from persons under forty. From the senile contingent – those above this age – the average income has for a time been raised by these exercises, as a large number of persons have been injured by taking up sports which may be vigorously pursued with safety only by those with young arteries.[24]

In other talks Osler sometimes warned against the excessive use of tobacco, but it was not in the foreground of his neopuritanism. In 1896 he remarked on the rarity of tobacco's toxic effects despite its widespread use. He believed there was a form of angina, 'tobacco heart,' brought on or aggravated by tobacco, and a tongue condition, 'tobacco tongue.' Otherwise, he sided with lovers of the precious weed and attacked a writer in the *British Medical Journal* who condemned cigarette smoking: 'As a cigarette smoker of some twenty-four years standing, I would like to make the counterstatement, that to smoke a cigarette (a good one, of course!) is to use tobacco in its *very best form,* and that in moderation it soothes physical irritability and corrects mental and moral strabismus.'

Osler proscribed all forms of tobacco for youth. Tom Cullen told the story of Osler one day persuading a young man to give the vile habit up and throw away his box of cigarettes. 'Dr. Osler walked down the step to the lawn, picked up the box of cigarettes, took one out, lighted it and put the box in his pocket.' When an older convalescent patient asked him if he was allowed to smoke, Dr Osler said, 'You may,' and handed him a good cigar.[25] His own smoking habit had become two or three cigarettes a day. The ability to use a highly addictive substance in moderation for years is a striking marker of Osler's constitutional capacity for self-control. Cushing, by contrast, was a chain smoker, and the cigarette burns may still be seen on his desk at Yale.

Osler was a moderate drinker, a glass of sherry and a few sips of wine of an evening, and he ate lightly. He got most of his exercise from walking, always briskly. A keen swimmer on his seaside holidays, he took up golfing in 1901, but was so time-conscious that he golfed almost literally on the run. Never a sports spectator, he did find time to join many others in viewing with alarm the state of American football. In 1904 he persuaded the Johns Hopkins Hospital board of trustees to support a demand that American colleges change the rules of football to reduce the number of injuries and fatalities.[26]

A moderate health reformer in those years, Osler today would have eschewed the extremes of modern food and exercise faddism, though he surely would have stopped smoking. He would certainly have endorsed devotion to good health as an almost religious pursuit. The very origin of his profession had been in the cult of Aesculapius, the worship of health. 'In the old Greek there was deeply ingrained the idea of the moral and spiritual profit of bodily health.' It was too bad, Osler wrote at the beginning of the twentieth century, that 'the beauty and majesty of this old therapeutic worship' had degenerated into the sordid superstitions of Lourdes and other shrines to modern faith healers.

As a physician he thoroughly understood the uses of faith, faith as confidence in authority. Johns Hopkins Hospital's reputation and atmosphere made it almost shrinelike, he wrote in an essay on 'The Faith That Heals.' 'Faith in *St. Johns Hopkins*, as we used to call him, an atmosphere of optimism, and cheerful nurses, worked just the same sort of cures as did Aesculapius at Epidaurus.' Osler did not normally expect his patients to think medically for themselves. He expected them to believe and to comply. One day, when he found a patient with a box of

forbidden candies, he scattered them all over her bed. In treating tuberculosis, there was to be 'a rigid regimen, a life of rules and regulations, a
dominant will on the part of the doctor, willing obedience on the part of
patient and friends.' Weir Mitchell's success with neurasthenics, Osler
concluded, came mostly from his ability to inspire patients with faith in
his power to cure. If a physician could come across as 'a strong man
armed with good sense, and with faith in himself,' Osler said, he could
seemingly work miracles:

> As Galen says, confidence and hope do more than physick – 'he cures most
> in whom most are confident' ... Faith in the Gods or in the Saints cures one,
> faith in little pills another, suggestion a third, faith in a plain common doc-
> tor a fourth ... The cures in the temples of Aesculapius, the miracles of the
> Saints, the remarkable cures of those noble men, the Jesuit missionaries, in
> this country, the modern miracles at Lourdes and at St. Anne de Beaupré in
> Quebec, and the wonder-workings of our latter day saints are often genu-
> ine, and must be considered in discussing the foundations of therapeutics.
> We physicians use the same power every day. If a poor lass, paralysed appar-
> ently, helpless, bed-ridden for years, comes to me having worn out in mind,
> body and estate a devoted family, if she in a few weeks or less by faith in me,
> and faith alone, takes up her bed and walks, the Saints of old could not have
> done more.

On reflection, he added in the published version of these comments
that faith could not raise the dead, put in a good eye in place of a bad one,
cure cancer or pneumonia, or knit a bone. 'In spite of these ... restrictions
... faith is a most precious commodity, without which we should be very
badly off.' The 'poor lass' had been a real case, a New Jersey girl who had
lain paralysed in bed for ten years, but when brought to St Johns Hopkins
and assured that she would soon get well, had within a fortnight walked
around the hospital square.[27]

By all accounts, Osler's good-natured equanimity blended with his air
of authority and with knowledge of his great reputation to give him enormous influence over his patients. Thomas McCrae, whom Osler treated

for typhoid fever, remembered having 'absolute confidence' in him and thought other patients responded similarly: 'There was the certainty that there would be no failure from lack of skill or interest on his part. His cheerfulness had much to do with this and the ability to give the desire to fight to those who had lost courage and hope.' (Memory sterilizes: McCrae may have trusted Osler, but the word around Hopkins was that his experiences with the typhoid tub turned him against cold baths. Early sponge bathing in typhoid was introduced, and bath temperature raised by fifteen degrees.)[28]

There were bound to be exceptions and specially hard cases. J.M.T. Finney once observed Osler visiting a distinguished old Baltimore doctor who was suffering from angina. The doctor started berating Osler for doing so little to help. He was in pain and wanted effective medicine:

> Dr. Osler, in his characteristic manner, began twitting him about what poor patients doctors make, but the old doctor was insistent. 'What's the use,' said he, 'of having the supposedly best doctor in the country as your physician when he doesn't do anything for you? I'd rather have a fifty-cent doctor from South Baltimore who would do something to relieve my pain than the best in the land who just comes in and jokes and pats you on the back, and then goes out without leaving you any medicine to make you feel better.'

On his way out Osler prescribed the medicine and told the nurse to make sure the patient got enough to be comfortable.[29]

No fee can be found listed in Osler's account books for such a close colleague or, of course, for treating any of his relatives or friends, or for treating poor patients such as Walt Whitman. Most such appointments appear not to have been recorded. Nor did Osler charge medical fees for patients of his who stayed in the paying rooms at the hospital. Being a consultant to physicians and their families has been described by a physician as 'the most arduous, flattering, unremunerative, and time-consuming of all kinds of practice.' Osler once studied the records of two of his busiest weeks in practice and estimated that 15 to 20 per cent of his work had been without remuneration. 'Yet they were people whom it was a pleasure to be able in any way to help.' Quoting Thomas Browne, he labeled a physician's gratis work 'Loans to the Lord.'[30]

In the 1890s his basic fee for a thirty-minute consultation appears to have been constant at $10, the equivalent of about $300 a century later. Sometimes he charged a patient $20 or $25, apparently for taking a bit more time. Osler's accounts show that he occasionally charged very large fees, on the order of $1,000–$3,000, but careful study shows that they invariably involved several days' travel; most of the charge was for traveling time. In 1898 Osler told Thayer that his minimum 'all-day,' twenty-four-hour fee was $500 (and advised Thayer to charge on the order of $250–$300). In 1900 he told Lafleur that his basic fee for a trip to Toronto or Montreal – two days by train – would be $1,000. His frequent trips to Washington, less than an hour from Baltimore by train, were usually billed at $100. He seems generally to have billed his time at $20 an hour, for all who could afford to pay. A British consultant friend noted that 'distant journeys at high fees' generated the best kind of professional income.[31]

Should the rich pay more for their doctors? Thayer claimed that Osler never speculated on the size of a person's income but stuck to his fee schedule. If there were abuses in soaking the rich by the Hopkins group, they tended to come from Osler's surgical colleagues, who appear to have set fees based on patients' means. Both Halsted and Kelly became notorious for their charges. Kelly, Osler wrote in his 'Inner History' of Hopkins,

> had probably the largest professional income among surgeons in the United States. He charged very large fees, $10,000 to $12,000 for some of his more important operations. He seemed conscienceless in the matter, & yet men have told me that after conversation with him they were glad to get away without making an assignment of their estates. He was exceedingly liberal and gave with great freedom both to the Hospital, to his assistants & to general charities.

Halsted caused more problems:

> He was not very popular with the Trustees, partly on this account, as they
> heard so many comments on his high charges. The natives were simply
> aghast at them – in fact I used to think them high but I never 'went back on
> him,' though he often got me into trouble. He charged a patient of mine
> $10,500 for a gall-stone operation – a most serious & protracted case, with
> two operations – but the woman got well. The people were wealthy & I
> stood by him & told the artist story to the old man [we do not know the
> artist story], who at the last felt thankful that the fee was so small. He really
> had not much conscience in matters of charges but he had the feeling of a
> high class artist about the value of his work. He was a liberal fellow, without
> an 'itching palm' and was always ready to 'hand out' for all sorts of pur-
> poses.[32]

Superintendent Hurd thought the one good that accrued from the reputation Kelly and Halsted got for their fees, 'deservedly or otherwise,' was
extra work for the younger surgeons who charged less. Halsted's traveling
fee ranged from $20 to $75 an hour; he submitted one bill for $13,825. Bill
Francis told a fine story of Halsted once taking his whole operating-room
staff to Washington to carve an immobile tycoon, then being implored to
stay on for the night, but refusing. 'He wasn't interested, he politely explained, in an extra $5,000, nor would his first assistant be tempted by
$1,000, nor his 2nd by $200. Besides he needed them both at 9 the next
morning in Baltimore. Then he looked across the room and for the first
time took notice of the raw intern whom he summoned and introduced,
"But here's our Dr. So & So; I'm sure he would be delighted to stay for five
dollars!"'[33]

The highest fee recorded in Osler's accounts is $3,000, charged on sev-
eral occasions. The best-documented one involved Captain Frederick Pabst
of the Milwaukee brewing family, on whose behalf Osler made a four-day,
Sunday to Wednesday, trip in December 1903. He made the trip at a time
when he was feeling the strain of overwork. 'I am just off to Milwaukee to
put a bung in old Pabst,' he had complained to a medical friend, perhaps a

bit sourly. News of his visit got out in the local press, which said he had charged the family $10,000. 'What a pity it is I had not charged it,' Osler wrote to his old friend, H. V. Ogden, a month later after Pabst had suddenly died, apparently of causes different from the condition Osler had treated. His estate paid Osler's fee, though not before he joked about his only compensation being a keg of Pabst's Blue Ribbon beer.[34]

The growth of his private practice, supplemented by textbook royalties, catapulted Osler from comfort into prosperity, from bread and butter to chocolate cakes and ale. In 1893 his practice income more than doubled, rising to $7,560. By 1897, in an era of falling prices, it had grown to $12,796. That year he also had his regular $5,000 salary from Hopkins and $5,644 in textbook royalties, for a total income of $23,440, or about $700,000 by today's standards (and with yesterday's freedom from income tax). Osler had nothing to show in the way of savings from the first twenty years of his professional life. Now he would never again have cobwebs in his pockets or red ink in his bank book.

Osler had no false modesty about money, the value of his services, or the pleasures of living well. The personal attention he gave his accounts and some later comments to Grace ('I fear the time when my income will be very small, & expenses the same') suggest that he paid as close attention to his financial position as his father had in the Upper Canadian bush. So much of his income was contingent on royalties and moonlighting that he may never have felt fully secure. But he seldom talked or wrote about fees, except to deplore physicians' quest for the wretched guinea. Thayer remarked on his horror at the commercialization of medicine. When Dorothy Reed moved on to a residency in New York, her new chief badgered her about what made Hopkins so special. 'Well, sir,' she finally burst out, 'it is hard to point out the essential differences, but you may understand when I say that in six years in Baltimore I never heard money mentioned in regard to the practice of medicine. Here, when any attending or a visiting physician is taken around the hospital, the conversation always reverts to the almighty dollar, how much a man received for an operation or how much less or more was being made this year or last.'[35]

One of Osler's many donations was a gift of several hundred dollars a year to help support Hopkins' special work on tuberculosis. This was the disease that most obviously cut across class and social lines, infecting rich and poor alike. Osler knew phthisis/consumption/tuberculosis from his earliest days in Montreal; he had seen it in every week of hospital work in Philadelphia, and he saw it in Baltimore and in a large number of his private patients. Some of the most depressing cases were medical students and residents at Johns Hopkins – particularly susceptible because of their work – whose careers were blighted and lives destroyed. Over the years several members of Osler's family, including Bill Francis, became tubercular. The 'white plague' could strike anybody, anytime; no one with a deep nagging cough and a mild fever could escape the fear of having contracted a terrible wasting infection that would eventually destroy body and soul. John Bunyan had called the disease 'the captain of the men of death.'

In early years Osler was mainly interested in the pathology and diagnosis of tuberculosis. While Koch's discovery of the bacillus raised hope that a specific treatment would soon emerge, the much-trumpeted tuberculin had been an embarrassment. Like many others, Osler was impressed by the late-1880s research of Edward L. Trudeau, a consumptive New York doctor who had moved to the Adirondacks for the pure air that was thought to be helpful. Working with tubercular rabbits, Trudeau seemed to have proved that animals kept in damp, dark quarters fared much more poorly than those allowed to roam around in fresh air. The rabbit tests were the scientific justification for Trudeau's promotion of his Adirondack Cottage Sanitarium at Saranac Lake, New York, as a haven for consumptives. He became the American leader of the growing sanitarium movement.

Osler sent patients who could afford it, including Hopkins staff and his own relatives, to Trudeau's establishment. The apparent success of a natural therapeutic approach over tuberculin and many other failed drugs fitted nicely with his own evolving views. As early as 1891 he realized there was a social dimension to the TB therapy problem in that many of the urban poor were as confined in their cramped and poorly ventilated housing as some of Trudeau's rabbits. In the first edition of his text, Osler called on cities to build sanitaria, within easy access by railway, for poor consumptives.[36]

It did not happen overnight. The vast majority of victims had to stay at home, and because they were contagious they stood a good chance of infecting people close to them. What could be done on an interim basis to treat and prevent the spread of tuberculosis? As part of his evolving interest in the social dimensions of disease, Osler decided to improve Johns Hopkins' handling of its tubercular patients, most of whom were serviced through the outpatient dispensary. In 1898 he used his own money and contributions from the sisters of a patient to set up a Fund for the Special Study of Tuberculosis and hire a young Canadian doctor to develop a program.

The main initiative came to be a series of visits by female medical students to the homes of all the consumptives treated at the dispensary. Blanche Epler, Adelaide Dutcher, Elizabeth Blauvelt, and Esther Rosenkrantz functioned as the first hospital-based 'social service workers' in America. They gave advice to patients and their families about sanitation, the care of sputum, and the need for fresh air, rest, and as much milk and eggs in the diet as possible, and they reported back to the hospital on the conditions they saw. Osler founded a Laennec Society at the hospital for the study of tuberculosis, had Trudeau come and give talks, and became an early publicist for the 'home treatment' of consumption.[37]

He was in the forefront of a gathering medical-social crusade against tuberculosis throughout the Western world. In Britain in 1899 and 1901 he attended special meetings on the subject. He worked with Welch in Maryland to lobby politicians. The Baltimore workers linked up with other pioneers, notably Lawrence Flick in Philadelphia, who had important financial support from a local philanthropist, Henry Phipps. Phipps soon came to admire Osler (who treated one of his children) and in 1903 supplied a very handsome $20,000 to expand the Hopkins work through the creation of a special tuberculosis dispensary. Osler's student visitors gave way to professional nurses, hired by the dispensary with fundraising help from Grace Osler, who became trailblazers for similar programs across North

America. By 1904 the leaders of the American profession had worked through a thick tangle of medical politics to found the National Association for the Study and Prevention of Tuberculosis. Trudeau was the first president, Osler vice-president.[38]

With rates of morbidity and mortality from the disease falling, there was to be no more fatalism about consumption in the new century. Tuberculosis could be beaten. Osler was 'tuberculously daft,' Grace wrote of his enthusiasm during the great British Congress on Tuberculosis in 1901. He predicted to it that the captain of the men of death could be reduced to a lieutenant, then a private, and finally drummed out of the regiment. He demoted TB symbolically in his textbook that year by giving the captaincy of the men of death to pneumonia. 'Were I a woman,' he once said, 'I had rather be a district tuberculosis nurse than anything in the world.'[39]

Osler never had a political agenda, aside from his lobbying on medical issues and his vague dreams about medical internationalism and brotherhood as a model for humanity. He had no vote in the United States and no fixed party allegiance in Canada (where brother E.B. became a Conservative Member of Parliament) or in England. Nor was he in any serious way a social critic, except on public-health measures. Issues of the affordability of health care seem not to have troubled him: those who could, paid; those who could not pay were looked after anyway. To the poor and downtrodden he was a Good Samaritan with a streak of realism. One night in Baltimore he happened on a broken-down mother with a sick child. He put them in a cab for Johns Hopkins with a note that the child was 'Mrs. Osler's youngest' and was to be well cared for until he could come. Telling the mother her child would be well looked after, he gave her a five-dollar bill and told her to go home and get drunk.[40]

'I cannot go to press without your name.' Clifford Allbutt, the Regius Professor of Physic at Cambridge, one of the most distinguished of all British physicians, pleaded with Osler in 1894 to contribute to the *System of Medicine* volumes he was editing. The peripatetic Canadian had risen to become one of the best-known physicians in the English-speaking world, claimed as virtually a native son in the United States and Great Britain as well as Canada. Universities in all three countries considered him an outstanding candidate for honorary degrees. McGill was first off the mark in 1895. Michigan and Philadelphia's Jefferson Medical College tried in 1897, but he declined, saying he had not yet reached the LLD stage of imbecility. A participant at the British Medical Association's extraterritorial meeting in Montreal in 1897, the year of Queen Victoria's Diamond Jubilee and Britons' height of enthusiasm for all things imperial, remembered Osler as the most prominent physician there.[41]

Whether or not he felt more imbecilic in 1898, Osler accepted LLDs from the two great Scottish universities, Aberdeen and Edinburgh, quipping that the letters warranted adding a 'Mac' to his name. The school he had dropped out of, Trinity College in Toronto, honored him with a DCL.

The year 1898 became his *annus mirabilis*, Osler wrote. That spring he received word of his election to fellowship in the most distinguished scientific body in the world, the Royal Society of London. As a young scientist he had aspired to such standing, but in his clinician years had assumed he would never be considered. The joke was that the letters FRS would stand for Fees Raised Since. 'Two LL.D.'s, a D.C.L. and the F.R.S. make 1898 a pretty full year in the life of your old man,' he told Grace from London that summer. Then echoed Kipling: 'But keep humble – lest we forget!'[42]

'Get some rest lest we break down' might also have been his motto that year. In the spring he complained about the pace of his life, about being 'horribly driven' and the strains of travel.[43] As soon as classes ended in May, he began the annual round of society meetings, dinners, commencement speeches, and visits to Canada, always taking work with him (a major textbook revision was at hand). He had also become dean of the medical school, replacing Welch. In July he was off to Britain to get his honorary degrees and go to endless dinners and meetings and on hunts for information about Thomas Sydenham, leaving Grace and Revere to summer in Maine. He joined them at Bar Harbor in August, just missing the funeral of William Pepper, who had died of a heart attack at age fifty-five. Osler was promptly laid low with a cold. Weir Mitchell and other Philadelphians tried to persuade him to come as Pepper's successor. 'I should only be worried to death by practice in Philadelphia,' Osler told Thayer – and then set off 'on the road,' practicing medicine across half a continent:

> One of my assistants Dr. W. Davis was very ill in Minneapolis & they telegraphed me to come out. I could not refuse of course. It was in the midst of that hot spell in Sept and I was rather knocked out. Poor chap died – Addison's disease. I got back to Mrs. O & found a telegram from my bro. Edmund saying that his son Jack was very ill (acute polyneuritis) so I had to retrace my steps to Toronto. I got back to Balt. Sept. 15th rather used up. Then I had a call to Mass. Returning in the train Sept. 15th I sat up all night [in the baggage car] with a labor case & caught cold, which hung about me for a week, got better & then on the 30th I was knocked out completely with an acute bronchitis & some broncho-pneumonia of left base – defective resonance but no tubular breathing or rusty sputa. Fever for 7 days – for no day continuous, dropping every morning to normal, cough disappeared with the fever, but I was very much used up.[44]

He had to spend more than a month recuperating from his first moderately serious illness since boils in Montreal. Friends and family would have feared tuberculosis. Osler was a grumpy uncooperative patient who did not like being nursed. The setback gave him an excuse to resign his deanship, though it had not really been onerous. As Cushing put it, the medical school had a way of running itself.[45]

Osler passed another milestone by turning fifty in 1899. He normally paid no attention to birthdays but apparently resolved to try to go a little slower, or at least not be so spry. On a golf course one day he came across a little stream, not a yard wide. He started to jump it, then stopped, and went around by the bridge. 'I made up my mind that at fifty I would stop jumping streams,' he told his companions.[46] He was back in England again in the summer of 1899 to give the Cavendish Lecture to the West London Medico-Chirurgical Society (on the etiology and diagnosis of cerebrospinal meningitis; in the votes of thanks he was called a modern Hippocrates), to take in the British Medical Association meeting and have the usual

round of luncheons and dinners with old friends. Being abroad gave him
an excuse to miss his LLD ceremony at the University of Toronto. Grace
and Revere were with him in England, and on the advice of Lord Lister
and Clifford Allbutt the Oslers took a cottage in the beautiful village of
Swanage on the Dorset coast, where they enjoyed a two-month summer
idyll of swimming, golfing, cliff walking, excursions to historic places, and
a comparatively new interest, hunting for rare books.

The good times in Britain, where Osler saw few patients, were a sharp
contrast to his hectic pace in America. In this golden autumn of Victoria's
reign, when the sun never set on the British Empire, when London was the
capital of the world and the British upper classes enjoyed a quality of life
unequaled then and perhaps since – and when it was just a matter of time
before the wretched little South African business with the Boers was cleared
up – Osler's consciousness of being 'British to the core' increased. Where
else would a man want to live if he had a choice? He and Grace talked of
retiring to Britain in another eight or ten years.

Osler's old friend Edward Schäfer held the chair of physiology at the
University of Edinburgh, and in the spring of 1900 Edinburgh's chair of
medicine became vacant. Schäfer and other friends urged Osler to apply
for what was arguably the leading professorship of medicine in the British
Empire. Osler, a product of an Edinburgh education as transplanted through
McGill, considered this the chair he most cherished in the English-
speaking world, but he loathed the thought of applying for a position and
having to solicit testimonials. Osler was not a snob, but neither was he
falsely humble. He no doubt assumed that he had earned a place in the
medical world beyond testimonials. He had certainly earned immense im-
portuning and flattery ('you might do for us in medicine what Lister did in
surgery'),[47] along with assurances that his appointment would be virtually
automatic – after all, he had written the chief text used at Edinburgh. But
the Scots insisted that he go through the ritual. In a season when work and
travel were again getting him down, Osler finally agreed to be a candidate
for the Edinburgh chair.

He immediately faced in Baltimore what Cushing, on the spot, characterized as a 'perfect hullabaloo.' 'I had no idea that they would make it such

a personal matter,' wrote Osler, 'and my special associates and assistants in the Medical Department were so stirred about it that my feelings were terribly harrowed ... I had no idea ... These men have stood by me for ten years in getting the School organized and the Hospital in working order.' On the other hand: 'Mrs. Osler ... very willing to go. All my friends in Canada have been very excited about it.' The deciding factor may have been the influenza, his first bout ever, that attacked him at exactly the same time. Sick and depressed, under pressure from everyone but Grace to change his mind, he worried about how his health would stand up to the cold, gloomy, damp Edinburgh climate (Baltimore's heat had been more agreeable to his slight frame than Montreal winters) and whether he really wanted to start all over as a teacher: 'I am 50+ & the fear of changes perplexes me now as it did not 10 years ago.' Within a week he changed his mind and took his name out of the running. He handed the withdrawal telegram to Bill Francis saying, 'There are 2,000 medical students to teach in Edinburgh, and in winter the street lamps are lit at three in the afternoon.' He later mused, 'I wonder what would have become of me at Edinboro. Whiskey or John Knox? I think I could have got on with the men, as I have always liked the Scotch.'[48]

'We should have been brokenhearted if he had gone,' Welch wrote, 'and never could have filled his place.' Over in Britain, Schäfer and his other supporters, the cream of the profession, were deeply embarrassed and not a little angry. But when the Oslers appeared in London for meetings and another holiday at Swanage the next summer, all was forgiven. Cushing, on the spot again, marveled at Osler's popularity. 'His name would make way for one anywhere over here and to run about with his cards means to have people fall over themselves with attentions.'[49]

Osler was called back from Britain in the summer of 1900 to attend to his brother Britton Bath in a serious illness. B.B. Osler, who had become the most famous trial lawyer in Canada, died of heart disease in February 1901 at the age of sixty-one. 'Dr. Osler has felt his brother's death very much,'

Grace wrote. Two years later his sister Nellie died from cancer at the age of sixty-two. Ellen Osler, who had turned ninety-five in 1900, lived on in Toronto. Although her sight and hearing had deteriorated, she remained 'very chipper & bright,' Willy wrote, 'full of fun & most interested in everything.'[50] Ellen lived, as she always had, in perfect assurance that her physical death would be a passage into life eternal spent in the company of her loved ones.

One patient might die calmly at Johns Hopkins, another in agony, a third in a restless drugged stupor. For each hospital death from March 1900 into 1902 a nurse or intern would fill out a printed card for Osler with information on the following points:

The act of dying:

If sudden

Did respiration stop before pulse – how long?

Coma or unconsciousness before death – how long?

If any fear or apprehension, of what nature –

Bodily, ie Pain

Mental

Spiritual – ie remorse, etc.

N.B. The object of this investigation is to ascertain, the relative proportion of cases in which (1) the death is sudden; (2) accompanied by coma or unconsciousness; (3) by pain, dread or apprehension. Prof. Osler requests the intelligent co-operation of the members of the medical and nursing staff. Please note fully any other special circumstances connected with the act of dying.

Osler's life had been lived in the shadow of death in many obvious medical ways – the hours at the bedside of thousands of patients, the thousands of hours cutting up and examining bodies in the dead house, the reflections on death as a failure of his science, or on death as a relief from pain and suffering, and the many times he had to console the living and grieving. All this after his upbringing as a child of devoutly religious parents who believed there was no such thing as ultimate death. The absolutely central message of the Gospel that had guided Featherstone and Ellen Osler through their lives on earth was the hope and promise of life thereafter: 'For as in Adam all die, even so in Christ shall all be made alive.'

The mask of cheerful equanimity almost always hid Osler's deeper emotions and religious beliefs. People who knew him intimately disagreed on whether or not he had retained a basic Christian faith, including belief in personal immortality. To some, his jauntiness seemed a thin cover over an underlying spiritual melancholy. No one doubted the reality of Dr Osler's grief at the loss of a relative, a friend, a promising Hopkins student, or a patient he thought could be saved. At times he admitted to whistling that he might not weep, like Uncle Toby in *Tristam Shandy*.

Marriage brought him back to occasional church attendance, but he would never discuss issues of religious belief. Instead, he hid behind a response he had read about:

> 'What is your religion, sir?'
> 'Mine is the religion of all sensible men.'
> 'And pray, what is that?'
> 'Why all sensible men keep religion to themselves.'[51]

No one could hear Osler talk for five minutes on most subjects without concluding from his biblical language and allusions and his Christian imagery that he had a religious cast of mind, though it was also obvious enough that he had distanced himself from any particular creed. His clearest statement of his true beliefs, I think, was his quotation in a talk entitled 'The Faith that Heals' from what he considered a 'wonderful poem,' Swinburne's 'The Altar of Righteousness':

God by God flits past in thunder, till his glories turn to shades:
God to God bears wondering witness how his gospel flames and fades.
More was each of these, while yet they were, than man their servant seemed:
Dead are all of these, and man survives who made them while he dreamed.[52]

The main objects of Osler's worshipful habit came to include great literature, Greco-Roman culture, great physicians through the ages, and the practice and profession of medicine.

As a practitioner, and probably in his family and personal life, Osler was intensely conscious of the aging process, the decline of mental and physical powers, the growing uselessness of the old, the inevitable advent of senility (a term he used as a synonym for age), and, of course, the inevitability of death. In the late 1880s, about the time of his own 'crise de quarante ans,' he had read and endorsed William Munk's *Euthanasia: or, Medical Treatment in Aid of an Easy Death*, which argued that death normally comes painlessly and with serenity, and doctors should calmly, albeit passively, facilitate the transition.

In the 1898 third edition of *Principles and Practice*, Osler made a remarkable and obviously considered change in his discussion of the etiology of pneumonia. He had called it 'the special enemy of old age.' Now he wrote, 'Pneumonia may well be called the friend of the aged. Taken off by it in an acute, short, not often painful illness, the old man escapes those "cold gradations of decay" so distressing to himself and to his friends.'[53] As he meditated on achievement in history, Osler was conscious that for most humans death means being forgotten, the slow or sudden descent into 'dull oblivion.' He ended his account of 'An Alabama Student' with lines from Matthew Arnold's 'Rugby Chapel':

> No one asks
> Who or what we have been,
> More than he asks what waves,
> In the moonlit solitudes mild
> Of the midmost ocean, have swelled,
> Foam'd for a moment, and gone.

One of the few measurable aspects of death was the attitude of people as they face it. Do they fear death? Do they die in terror? In pain? Are they conscious at the moment of death? Osler's death survey at Hopkins was meant to test Munk's conclusions about the placidity of most deaths. Osler never wrote up the survey for publication, but his notebooks show that he did consider writing about death, one idea for a title being 'The Inevitable Hour: A Discourse on Death & Dying.' He also came to own many books on death and the possibility of life afterwards.[54]

Harvard had been given a grant to support an annual lecture on immortality. When President Charles Eliot first asked Osler to give one of these Ingersoll Lectures, he declined, as had Welch. (Welch had told Eliot that so far as he could see, science had nothing to do with immortality, to which Eliot replied that he should come and say that; Welch said it would not be possible to fill an hour saying so.) Osler, pressed repeatedly, concluded that it would seem 'ungracious, even cowardly,' not to accept. The paper he delivered at Harvard on 'Science and Immortality' in May 1904 was one of the most carefully prepared of his essays, and it became one of the most widely circulated.[55]

Most of his lecture was a demonstration of the irrelevance of belief in life after death. In the real world, the vast majority of people are indifferent to the issue, he argued: 'Immortality, and all that it may mean, is a dead issue in the great movements of the world ... A living faith in a future existence has not the slightest influence in the settlement of the grave social and national problems which confront the race to-day ... Over our fathers immortality brooded like the day; we have consciously thrust it out of lives so full and busy that we have no time to make an enduring covenant with the dead.' For the most part, science had made up its mind. The battle to put man at the center of the universe had been won; the 'mental cataclysm' of the past forty years had seen a revolution 'from the days when faith was diversified with doubt, to the present days, when doubt is diversified with faith.' Psychology had dispensed with the soul. The scientific search for the spirit had been futile.

As a physician, 'whose work lies on the confines of the shadow-land,' Osler could only contribute the observations they had made at Hopkins. Were people terrified of the transition?

Popular belief is erroneous. As a rule, man dies as he has lived, uninfluenced practically by the thought of a future life ... I have careful records of about five hundred death beds ... Ninety suffered bodily pain or distress of one sort or another, eleven showed mental apprehension, two positive terror, one expressed spiritual exaltation, one bitter remorse. The great majority gave no sign one way or the other; like their birth, their death was a sleep and a forgetting. The Preacher was right: in this matter man hath no preeminence over the beast, – 'as the one dieth so dieth the other.'

Then he appeared to slip the net. Osler allowed for a realm of faith, unmixed by and unmixable with science, the faith of mystics, idealists, the Saint Theresas, 'more often for each one of us the beautiful life of some good woman' (surely his mother). He told his audience that men of science were in a 'sad quandary' and that all men had to tread alone the winepress of doubt. Finally, Osler became autobiographical, even as, in the mode of Sir Thomas Browne, he remained elusive:

On the question before us wide and far your hearts will range from those early days when matins and evensong, evensong and matins, sang the larger hope of humanity into your young souls. In certain of you the changes and chances of the years ahead will reduce this to a vague sense of eternal continuity, with which, as Walter Pater says, none of us wholly part ... Some of you will wander through all phases, to come at last, I trust, to the opinion of Cicero, who had rather be mistaken with Plato than be in the right with those who deny altogether the life after death; and that is my own *confessio fidei*.

Insofar as he retained a personal faith, Osler seems to have been saying that it was of little moment in his life as a scientist or citizen. By his selection of authorities, he suggested that he was more of a Platonist than a Christian. Mostly, he was saying that these big questions, so vitally important in the life of his parents, were practically unanswerable: 'A majority of sensible men will feel oppressed by the greatness of the subject and the feebleness of man, and it is with these feelings I close.'

Osler later joked about the impossibility of talking about immortality when his wife and mother-in-law were in the audience, and he appended to one copy of the lecture a story about a dying bishop who lost patience with his chaplain's soothing words and muttered, 'Don't be a fool! Pass the syphon!' But 'Science and Immortality' was the closest he came to a comment on his parents' and his own deepest beliefs. Intellectually he had abandoned belief in personal immortality. His sense that this is our only life infused his practice, his use of time, his notions of history and duty.[56]

President Eliot was disappointed with Osler's Ingersoll Lecture, seeing it as a literary rather than medical presentation. That was not quite accurate, but Eliot, like many other listeners, would have felt smothered by Osler's literary references. Osler began the essay with five quotations – two from Plato, the others from the *Rubaiyat of Omar Khayyam*, the *Diary of the Reverend John Ward*, and Tennyson. In the first four paragraphs of his text he mentioned Job, Dean Swift, Byron, Browne, Plato, Oliver Wendell Holmes, Tennyson, Aristotle, and Shakespeare. Eight pages of further notes and quotations were appended to the published version. Appropriately, Osler donated his fee for the lecture to a library.[57]

He was becoming markedly more bookish early in his sixth decade. He spent more of his time studying historical records and preparing biographical essays on American and European medical greats: William Beaumont the physiologist, Rhode Island's Elisha Bartlett, physician and philosopher John Locke, Sir Thomas Browne, and, a new discovery, Robert Burton, author of *The Anatomy of Melancholy*. (Although Osler valued Burton's descriptions of melancholy, he was never prone to the condition himself. He often quoted Burton to support cultivation of the *aequus animus*, or even-balanced soul: 'If unhappy – have hope. If happy – be cautious.')[58]

A good and growing friend of libraries and librarians, Osler was in 1898 a founding father of the Association of Medical Librarians, serving as its president in 1901–2. In a lecture on 'Books and Men' at the Boston Medical Library in 1901 he offered what became a famous literary-medical credo: 'Books have been my delight these thirty years, and from them I have received incalculable benefits. To study the phenomena of disease without books is to sail an uncharted sea, while to study books without patients is not to go to sea at all.' In his Ingersoll Lecture he did not presume to dictate religious beliefs to anyone, but he did urge a program of reading: 'To keep his mind sweet the modern scientific man should be saturated with the Bible and Plato, with Homer, Shakespeare, and Milton.' Men did win a form of immortality by living on through literary works in memory, he observed. Through reading they could be communed with, honored, venerated. Osler thought that every medical library ought to have 'a select company of the Immortals set apart for special adoration ... a sort of alcove of Fame, in which the great medical classics were fathered.'[59]

A collector and classifier of specimens and cases, Osler now succumbed to another kind of collecting mania. He had always bought medical journals and books, the former more than the latter because most new work appeared in article form. (Osler's early use of libraries, Jennifer Connor has noted, was parallel to his use of laboratories.)[60] On leaving Montreal and Philadelphia he had given most of his journal collections to McGill and Penn. Over the years he had taken an interest in old medical books and had purchased the odd gem or bargain, but until at least the mid-1890s he could not be classified as a collector, if only because of his limited resources.

Medical bibliography, an interest in medical books as books, and medical bibliomania, the passion for collecting them, were established avocations among elite physicians.[61] John Shaw Billings's achievement building the collections of the U.S. Surgeon-General's Library and publishing its *Index-Catalogue*, had been gargantuan, and Osler had appreciated it from the early 1880s. Weir Mitchell, W.W. Keen, and other Philadelphians were ardent bibliophiles. At Johns Hopkins, Welch appreciated old and beautiful books, and so especially did Howard Kelly, who was in the field building a great private library well before Osler and may have been particularly influential. One of Osler's oldest British friendships, going back to student days in the seventies, was with Joseph Frank Payne, one of the finest medical scholars and book collectors in England.

Osler's serious collecting began in the late 1890s when he at last had the necessary discretionary income:

I began to buy, first the early books and pamphlets relating to the profession in America; secondly, the original editions of the great writers in science and in medicine; and thirdly, the works of such general authors as Sir Thos. Browne, Milton, Shelley, Keats, and others. Catalogues – German, French, and English – appeared at the breakfast table, and were always in my bag for railway reading. Summer trips to England and the Continent ... gave time for reading, and my interest got deeper and deeper in the history of medicine and in the lives of the great men of the profession.

The association with Billings and Welch was a stimulus, and the Historical Club of the Johns Hopkins Hospital awakened no little enthusiasm. In the classroom more and more attention was paid to the historical side of questions, and at my Saturday evening meetings, after the difficulties of the week had been discussed, we usually had before us the editions of some classic ... Buying freely English and foreign books and subscribing to more than forty journals, I soon had the house overrun ... I was really fonder of books than anything else.[62]

One of his first indulgences, dating from 1899, was to collect a complete run of the editions of Browne's *Religio Medici*. (He also paid for a glass casket in which Browne's skull would be displayed in Norwich.) He decided to make a collection of the one hundred greatest medical works and by 1901 was buying up all the medical classics that became available. On a quick trip to the Netherlands in 1901 with Grace and his friend George Dock, Osler snapped up volume after volume at prices Dock thought ridiculously low but could not himself afford. Grace was amused when Willie looked at only one picture in an art gallery and then rushed off to an old bookstore. The fee from a consultation in England, she noted, 'will cover many indiscretions.' Back home in Baltimore, Harvey Cushing and the other latchkeyers were invited to inspect the new treasures. 'I never saw such a man ...' Cushing enthused to his father. 'Dr. O has brought back a great pile of old books: very rare most of them and elaborately bound ... Old Linacres, Harveys works, more Lockes etc.' Cushing, who shared his father's deep literary interests and was also a compulsive writer, decided to become a collector too. Osler got him interested in the works of the great sixteenth-century anatomist, Vesalius.[63]

One precious night at 1 West Franklin, the Johns Hopkins Historical Club was treated to a display of five copies of the Editio Princeps of Vesalius's *De humani corporis fabrica* on display from the collections of Osler, Kelly, and Cushing. 'We cannot have too many copies in America & no Medical Library is complete without one,' Osler wrote Cushing. The rich and successful American physicians were buying the medical treasures of the Old World. They were also reclaiming their own heritage. One morning Osler opened an Edinburgh catalogue that offered a collection of medical theses written by American students at Edinburgh between 1760 and 1813. He cabled an order for the 126 theses ('Do you mean all of them?' the dealer cabled back) and just beat the Surgeon-General's Library, the College of Physicians of Philadelphia, the New York Academy of Medicine, and William Pepper. He gave the thesis collection, all of it, to the Frick Library of the Medical and Chirurgical Faculty of Maryland.[64]

The fees continued to pour in to support the book purchases, the donations to many good causes and needy relatives, the wages of the servants at 1 West Franklin, and the long holidays abroad. By 1901 Osler had developed the habit of annually taking stock of the plenitude of his life. That year he saw 780 new patients, 402 of whom came from Baltimore, the others from thirty-one states, the District of Columbia, three Canadian provinces, Mexico, and the West Indies. He was out of town thirty-three times professionally, most often to Washington: 'Two consultations at the White House and several Cabinet Ministers are responsible for a considerable increase in patients from the Capital.' His total income passed $30,000 in 1900, and $40,000 in 1901, including almost $28,000 from practice. That year's honorary degree came from Yale, which at its bicentenary celebrations honored sixty notables from around the world, including President Roosevelt, a brilliant professor at Princeton named Woodrow Wilson, and three Hopkins men. 'I am bothered to death with practice,' Osler wrote Frank Shepherd in October, 'hard to keep it within decent limits so as to have time for teaching & private work.'[65]

He again earned $40,000 in 1902 and complained more often about the pressures of work. Bronchial and sinus infections laid him up from time to time – Grace and Revere suffered more often – and he also recorded feeling 'when hard pressed several days of sub-sternal tension, a warning of too high pressure.' He had to cancel his English holiday because of a load of writing commitments; these including the production of an emergency fifth edition of his text because Appleton had failed to copyright the fourth edition in Britain and a pirated version was undermining the market. Osler did much of the literary work that summer in pleasant circumstances at Murray Bay, Quebec, renewing many old acquaintances and making new ones, including the William Howard Taft family. He teased Taft about Canada being formed by the best Americans, the United Empire Loyalists, who had moved north after the revolution. Grace made him promise not to see any patients at Murray Bay, and he almost kept to it.[66]

Wherever he went he was in touch with the climate at Hopkins. In 1901–2 he heard stories that young Cushing was given to openly criticizing some of his surgical subordinates and colleagues, and he took the time to write Cushing, warning that such an attitude would be 'absolutely fatal' to his success there: 'The arrangement of the Hospital staff is so peculiar that loyalty to each other, even in the minutest particulars, is essential. I know you will not mind this from me.' Much to everyone's disappointment, he cut his Hopkins rounds from three to two mornings a week in the autumn of 1902 and his observation classes from two to one.[67]

In this busiest period of his life he wrote some of his best essays about the medical calling. 'Chauvinism in Medicine,' delivered to the Canadian Medical Association in September 1902, was Osler's hymn to the profession, a fraternity more appropriately called 'universal' than even the Catholic Church:

> It is not the prevalence of disease or the existence everywhere of special
> groups of men to treat it that betokens this solidarity, but it is the identity
> throughout the civilized world of our ambitions, our methods and our work.

To wrest from nature the secrets which have perplexed philosophers in all ages, to track to their sources the causes of disease, to correlate the vast stores of knowledge, that they may be quickly available for the prevention and cure of disease – these are our ambitions. To carefully observe the phenomena of life in all its phases, normal and perverted, to make perfect that most difficult of all arts, the art of observation, to call to aid the science of experimentation, to cultivate the reasoning faculty, so as to be able to know the true from the false – these are our methods. To prevent disease, to relieve suffering and to heal the sick – this is our work. The profession in truth is a sort of guild or brotherhood, any member of which can take up his calling in any part of the world and find brethren whose language and methods and whose aims and ways are identical with his own.

Osler condemned the chauvinistic spirit that built barriers between parishes, provinces, countries: 'Nationalism has been the great curse of humanity. In no other shape has the Demon of Ignorance assumed more hideous proportions; to no other obsession do we yield ourselves more readily.' Parochialism was running riot in North America, he warned, as state and provincial licensing boards put outrageous barriers in the way of medical mobility. Parochialism led to inbred medical schools and laboratories closed to outsiders.

The antidotes to chauvinism were openness, travel, liberal culture, and a sense of international fellowship. With 'widened sympathies and heightened ideals' medical men might develop 'something perhaps of a *Weltculture* which will remain through life as the best protection against the vice of nationalism.' Whatever the threats posed by the spirit of intolerance, the contributions of medicine were Jovian, Godlike, Promethean:

Search the scriptures of human achievement and you cannot find any to equal in beneficence the introduction of Anaesthesia, Sanitation, with all that it includes, and Asepsis – a short half-century's contribution towards the practical solution of the problems of human suffering, regarded as eternal and insoluble ... There seems to be no limit to the possibilities of scientific medicine, and while philanthropists are turning to it as to the hope of humanity, philosophers see, as in some far-off vision, a science from which may come in the prophetic words of the Son of Sirach, 'Peace all over the earth.'

Never has the outlook for the profession been brighter. Everywhere the physician is better trained and better equipped than he was twenty-five years ago. Disease is understood more thoroughly, studied more carefully and treated more skilfully. The average sum of human suffering has been reduced in a way to make the angels rejoice. Diseases familiar to our fathers and grandfathers have disappeared, the death rate from others is falling to the vanishing point, and public health measures have lessened the sorrows and brightened the lives of millions.

Relatively free of literary clutter, Osler's essay included a line from Browne that exactly described the Canadian: 'I am no plant that will not prosper out of a garden; all places, all airs, make me one country; I am in England, everywhere, and under any meridian.'[68]

A nice blow was struck against medical particularism in Osler's home province, Ontario, when Trinity College and its medical school merged with the University of Toronto in 1903. A state-of-the-art building was erected for the enlarged faculty. Osler, of course, was invited to give the celebratory address. He began it with genial reminiscences of his student days and his teachers, hoped the University of Toronto would be allowed to absorb the rival faculties at Kingston and London as part of becoming 'a school of the first rank in the world,' and then gave the best of his many talks on the medical student life. His description of 'the master-word in medicine' became one of his most quoted passages:

Though a little one, the master-word looms large in meaning. It is the open sesame to every portal, the great equalizer in the world, the true philosopher's stone, which transmutes all the base metal of humanity into gold. The stupid man among you it will make bright, the bright man brilliant, and the brilliant student steady. With the magic word in your heart all things are possible, and without it all study is vanity and vexation. The miracles of life are with it; the blind see by touch, the deaf hear with eyes, the dumb speak with fingers. To the youth it brings hope, to the middle-aged confidence, to the aged repose. True balm of hurt minds, in its presence the heart of the sorrowful is lightened and consoled. It is directly responsible for all advances in medicine during the past twenty-five centuries. Laying hold upon it Hippocrates made observation and science the warp and woof of our art. Galen so read its meaning that fifteen centuries stopped thinking, and slept until awakened by the *De Fabrica* of Vesalius, which is the very incarnation of the master-word. With its inspiration Harvey gave an impulse to a larger circulation than he wot of, an impulse which we feel to-day. Hunter sounded out all the heights and depths, and stands out in our history as one of the great exemplars of its virtue. With it Virchow smote the rock, and the waters of progress gushed out; while in the hands of Pasteur it proved a very talisman to open to us a new heaven in medicine and a new earth in surgery. Not only has it been the touchstone of progress, but it is the measure of success in every-day life. Not a man before you but is beholden to it for his position here, while he who addresses you has that honour directly in consequence of having had it graven on his heart when he was as you are to-day. And the master word is *Work*, a little one, as I have said, but fraught with momentous sequences if you can but write it on the tablets of your hearts, and bind it upon your foreheads.[69]

Osler's own work in 1903 was prodigious by even his standards. He saw more patients than ever, made more money than ever (a total of $47,280), wrote his usual dozen clinical papers, helped his mother through a serious illness in her ninety-seventh year, helped Revere through a bout of whooping cough (though it was said that he could not bear to hear his son's whoops, and we can imagine Grace doing much of the doctoring), sat for a portrait and a plaque, and spent three weeks in Paris studying hospitals, attending lectures, and buying books, two months holidaying with Grace and Revere on the Isle of Guernsey, and a few days visiting Phipps the philanthropist at a castle in Scotland. From his income the Oslers spent about $19,000 in 1903, saved $20,000, and gave away $9,000. 'I have got to my limit so far as work is concerned,' he complained in November, not long before rushing off to Milwaukee to see Pabst the brewer. 'He pretends

to not like it,' Harvey Cushing wrote his fiancée about Osler's busyness
with consultations. In May 1903, Cushing organized a dinner in Osler's
honor at the Maryland Club. The Hopkins house staff presented him with
a set of the just-completed sixty-three-volume *Dictionary of National Biography*. Egerton Yorrick Davis, Jr, was present and spoke.[70] The Davis spirit,
or what has been called the 'sub-umbilical' aspect of Osler's sense of humor, inspired him to write to the *Boston Medical and Surgical Journal* on
Valentine's Day to report a case of Peyronie's disease, or penile strabismus
(or 'squint of the cock'), under the signature of a Philadelphia surgeon
friend, J. William White. White then wrote in as E.Y.D. Jr. suggesting that
the case had come from a 'scotch and soda' clinic in Baltimore.[71] It is now
known that penile curvature is relatively common in men after the fourth
decade. It was said (by Paula Jones) to be a distinguishing feature of President Clinton.

The output of clinical case studies from Hopkins was almost as high as
ever. Some broke new ground, such as Osler's 1903 paper to the Association of American Physicians on 'Chronic Cyanosis, with Polycythaemia
and Enlarged Spleen: A New Clinical Entity.' Ten days after he described
this condition of excessive red-cell production, enlarged spleen, and deep-
red facial coloring, the *Medical News* dubbed it 'Osler's disease,' one of the
fastest uses of an eponym in medical history. Too fast, in fact. H. Vaquez
had anticipated Osler in 1892 – Osler knew of and acknowledged his precedence – and it became known as Vaquez-Osler or Osler-Vaquez disease.[72]

William Stokes and Robert Adams preceded him in the description of a
syndrome characterized by slow pulse, susceptibility to vertigo and syn-
cope (fainting), periods of chest pain, and sometimes sudden death. Osler
had noticed what the French called 'la maladie Stokes-Adams' in his early
work on angina pectoris, and in 1903 he returned to the subject in the
Lancet with a careful study of thirteen cases, 'On the So-Called Stokes-
Adams Disease (Slow Pulse with Syncopal Attacks, &c).' He stressed the
variety and irregularity of manifestations of the symptoms, their tendency

to run in families, and, despite the possibility of living with the disease for many years, the generally bad outlook from 'a condition not much within the scope of our art.'

The paper was an important contribution in its own right to knowledge of a rare, little-studied condition. What no one noticed at the time or afterwards was that the details of the history of 'Case 4' in Osler's paper matched exactly and irrefutably what is known of the fatal illness of his brother, Britton Bath. Other documents disclose a belief that the Osler family had a slow pulse rate, and William himself had commented that excessive tobacco use caused his heart to slow down rather than increase. In his 1903 paper he stated, 'I know a family most of the members of which have a pulse-rate of about 60; one son died from Stokes-Adams disease, another, perfectly healthy, has sometimes a pulse rate of only 48.' This was clearly a reference to his family and himself.

Was Osler still perfectly healthy? He had noted 'sub-sternal tension' in 1902, the year after his brother's death. Whether stimulated or not by B.B.'s fate, his studies of Stokes-Adams syndrome suggested to him that it might have a hereditary component. He must have begun to wonder if he was a candidate for a condition not much within the scope of his art. All he could prescribe in 1903 for Stokes-Adams syndrome was 'a quiet, well-regulated life' in which 'emotional disturbances and over-exertion are to be avoided.'[73]

No one noticed that Osler had any interest in leading a quiet, well-regulated life. Although he had cut back slightly at Hopkins, he was a whirlwind of energy in the hospital, as outgoing and friendly as ever. His textbook remained always up to date. His attendance and presentation record at medical meetings was exemplary. There was no slowing of the entertaining at 1 West Franklin, and he always made time for play and pillow-fighting with Revere.

Still, an undercurrent of critical talk was developing in Baltimore. Was Osler as good as he was made out to be? Was he as good as he used to be? Everyone could see he had been canonized. The incomparable Hopkins medical artist, Max Brödel, had drawn a wonderful cartoon of him as 'The Saint,' from whom all the microbes except the typhoid bacillus are fleeing.

It was natural for the tough-minded young to ask probing questions about the great man up there on the pedestal, the great man doing very well with his textbook and his practice. Was he past his peak? Was he losing his edge in his fifties? More than anyone else, it was Osler who kept telling them that a man went downhill after forty.

Some of the medical scientists at Hopkins knew he had drifted away from the leading edge of their disciplines. Pathology was evolving into a study of the processes that caused lesions, whereas Osler remained mainly a student of gross pathological lesions. Bacteriologists knew that he had not really progressed from his studies of much larger parasites to learn modern staining and culturing techniques; and by the late 1890s he was beginning to lag in accepting some of their new findings, such as the possibility of a second bacillus causing another form of typhoid fever, or the distinction between the pneumococcus and meningococcus. Yes, he had been a groundbreaking advocate of laboratory studies in clinical medicine, but by the twentieth century Osler's idea of laboratory work as mostly urine, blood, and sputum studies seemed passé. He did not seem interested in using his clinical laboratory for the active experimental work that seemed to be the future of medical science at the bedside.

He seemed fundamentally an observer and classifier of disease, a great nineteenth-century natural historian. Rufus Cole, one of his medical residents at the beginning of the new century, remembered much discussion in those years about the desirability of new approaches. 'Questions were constantly arising that could be answered only by more fundamental investigations than could be carried out at the bedside or in the primitive clinical laboratories,' Cole wrote much later. 'It is not enough to study phenomena as they occur in nature; nature must be put in chains, and the phenomena must be studied under controlled conditions. Many men realized that if medicine were to retain its place as a real university discipline it must become experimental, as other sciences had done.'[74]

Franklin P. Mall, the professor of anatomy, was the most disapproving of Osler's colleagues. Mall was a complete disciple of German research science, and by the early twentieth century he was campaigning more or less openly for the transformation of elite American medical schools into

university-based research institutes. He believed that all the teachers, including the clinicians, should be full-time professors, on salary. They should
be devoted to science, not to making money or even to doing very much
teaching. Their main job, perhaps their only one, should be to organize
research and publish scientific papers. Johns Hopkins should lead the way
in America.

Mall did most of his grumbling and proselytizing behind the scenes and
was careful never to provoke an open quarrel with Osler. But he let some of
his students know who he thought stood in the way of progress at Hopkins.
'We want an entirely different breed of men to fill our practical chairs,'
Mall wrote in 1902 to his former student Lewellys Barker, who had become
professor of anatomy at Chicago. 'Kelly, Osler even Halsted were taken
into the JH on account of their extensive private practices. The practices
followed & instead of aiding them in their teaching & in the hospital work
rather retards them.' Mall chafed at the 'very conservative faculty' at
Hopkins and thought Osler's department was particularly out of touch.
'We want a university professor who will conduct his medical work along
laboratory lines & will not continue publishing cases,' he wrote in 1905.
'The man must have his chief interest in the work of the university &
develop a strong staff. So far the members of the Faculty do not think that
this has been the case. Nothing but reports of cases & no real problems.'[75]

Resentment at the physicians' and surgeons' large private fees was also a
simmering issue at the hospital. Were the high-profile men neglecting their
hospital responsibilities to go off seeing private patients? If they stayed
around the institution, were they exploiting the hospital by admitting to
its modestly priced private wards patients from whom they then collected
very high fees? Idealism and the notion of unselfish service ran very high
at Johns Hopkins. Was it being undermined by the lure of the almighty
dollar?

To some at Hopkins, Osler certainly seemed too busy. You could not get
a word alone with him or be sure that he had made or even remembered
making decisions.[76] But this seems to have been the only complaint. I have
not found a whiff of criticism of Osler's income, private practice, or other
comings-and-goings in these busy years, except by Osler himself, who both

then and later wondered if he had not gone too far with some of his long trips to see patients. Welch said that Osler never neglected his duties. And he could not be criticized for taking fees from private patients in the hospital because he did not take any. It is tempting to portray a resentful, malevolent Mall, who had few opportunities for moonlighting, envying Osler's success and spreading calumnies about him. But the evidence cannot be found. Harvey Cushing, who knew practically everything about Hopkins in those years, thought Mall's and Osler's differences were philosophic, understandable, and never led to live sparks between them.[77]

On the other hand, some junior staff at Hopkins did resent their seniors' absence on visits to paying patients.[78] That most did not may have had something to do with their realization that their turn would come. Henry Hurd and the hospital's board of trustees were naturally the most concerned about the institution's well-being. Apart from the special problems Halsted posed, the main issue seems to have been the surgeons' fees and practices. Was the hospital losing out on revenues it might properly claim? Was the publicity that Kelly's and Halsted's charges generated bad for the whole institution? Hurd was deeply and permanently angered by a large fee Kelly charged a patient in 1896.[79] Why shouldn't the hospital set, collect, and keep all medical and surgical fees, paying its staff a fixed annual stipend?

Fees were a perennial topic with the board. It gradually stopped most residents and interns from taking payments and outlawed the use of private nurses in the hospital. It earnestly considered putting limits on fees charged by senior staff, but knew they would respond by directing their private patients to other Baltimore hospitals that would be happy to have them. Howard Kelly already had his own private hospital and could move his patients around virtually at will. Come down on him too hard and you would lose the services of one of the best surgeons in America. Besides, many patients thought they would have a better relationship with their doctors and get better care, even in hospital, if they paid their fees directly and personally.[80]

Osler himself said little about such issues in these years, but he always knew the pulse of the hospital and of the profession. The idea of research

as the leading edge of medicine was very much in the air. Osler's stimulus
to the men around John D. Rockefeller had culminated in the creation of
the Rockefeller Institute for Medical Research. Welch's and Mall's protegé,
Simon Flexner, was its first director. In 1902 Lewellys Barker gave a much-
noticed address to Hopkins alumni in Chicago, 'Medicine and the Universities,' in which he more or less spelled out Mall's ideas about the desirabiltity
of clinicians becoming full-time research scientists. Osler wrote Barker that
his paper put the question well. 'Whether a Professor of Medicine could
ever keep "whole & undefiled" I doubt ... 'Tis hard to serve the public and
the best interests of the school.'[81]

Osler kept on serving them as best he could, mornings and noons in the
hospital, afternoons with private patients, evenings for socializing, reading, and writing, six and seven days a week, often feeling utterly 'used up'
and wondering how long it could go on.[82] He was a superstar in the medical
firmament, certainly the best-known physician in America, soon to be
even better known with the publication of a collection of his essays under
the title *Aequanimitas*. He was also probably the best-known American
physician abroad.

The Johns Hopkins Hospital and School of Medicine were clearly the
best-known American medical institutions abroad. By the turn of the century it was possible to detect the beginnings of a great reversal in the transatlantic search for medical excellence. 'I think at last we have got the
Germans stirred up to the conviction that there is good work being done
on the other side,' Osler would soon write. The medical world wanted to
see what was happening at Hopkins. Everyone had a foreigner to entertain, Harvey Cushing remarked in 1904.[83] Visitors wanted to see what happened when Dr Osler examined patients.

Osler had his usual fun with the crowd that followed him. One day at
the bedside:

'Whose case is this?'

'Mine sir.'

'Well, Mr. Freeman, what is the first thing you would do in examining this patient?'

'Take the history, sir.'

'No, that's already been done. What next?'

'Inspect the patient.'

'Not yet. What before that?'

The student gives up.

'Well, the first thing to do is to ask Dr. Lambert to stand out of the light.'

But the problem was becoming serious. 'Dr. O's rounds are assuming frightful proportions,' a postgraduate student wrote in 1902. 'On Monday I counted 48 people, not including the interns, the staff, and the nurses; of the 48, sixteen were fourth year students for whom the teaching rounds are primarily given. You may imagine how much is seen at the bedside. I slip off & follow Dr. McCrae. I see more.'[84]

EIGHT

Leaving America

February 7, 1904. The business district of Baltimore is ablaze, a terrible fire completely out of control. A strong south wind drives the flames towards the fashionable residential district where the Oslers live. From their dining-room windows, they can see the fires lighting up the early evening sky. Having trouble with his equanimity, Osler smokes more than usual and twiddles nervously with his watch chain. He goes over to 3 West Franklin and brings back Harvey Cushing's baby and young wife Kate. Cushing and the other latchkeyers are out of town, but Halsted joins the group. A policeman comes and tells them to prepare to evacuate, as one of the nearby blocks will soon be blown up to try to stop the fire. Grace has hired a wagon to stand by, and supervises the packing of the most precious books, silver, clothes, linen, and china. The servants prepare a final oyster supper as burning brands begin to fall on nearby roofs. Revere is awakened and dressed.

The wind suddenly shifts, and the danger to 1 West Franklin subsides. The blaze had come within two blocks. Before it finally ended the next day it had gutted commercial Baltimore, destroying some seventy blocks of buildings. Many of these were properties owned by the Johns Hopkins Hospital as part of its endowment. 'Poor Baltimore is ruined and we are all weary,' Grace wrote. The hospital was thrown into the most serious crisis in its young history. The trustees implemented an austerity program while urging the doctors to admit private patients to help increase income. Characteristically, Osler sweetened letters about the fire with comments about Phoenix tricks and the uses of adversity. He offered to donate his $5,000 salary to the hospital for ten years in order to maintain its publications.[1]

More important, Osler and Welch drew on the respect their work had garnered in the circle around the world's richest man, John D. Rockefeller. Osler wrote Frederick Gates, the adviser who had been so impressed with his textbook, asking if Rockefeller could help Hopkins recover from its losses. Welch, who was president of the Board of Scientific Directors of the Rockefeller Institute, approached John D. Rockefeller, Jr. The family responded. In April it was announced that John D. Rockefeller, Sr, would give Johns Hopkins Hospital $500,000 to cover the income and capital lost from the great fire. The Maryland legislature simultaneously contributed $40,000, and the Rockefellers generously did not reduce their grant accordingly. Sweet the uses of adversity: Johns Hopkins rose from the great Baltimore fire of 1904 richer than before.[2]

Across the Atlantic another troubled medical school, if it could be called one, was locked in conflict with its graduates. Degrees in medicine had been obtainable at the ancient University of Oxford for many centuries. In 1546 King Henry VIII had founded a regius professorship of medicine, and for a time in the seventeenth century Oxford had led the world in experimental science. Through much of the next two centuries, Oxford medicine had been, like much of the rest of the university, stagnant to the point of irrelevance; and by the nineteenth century, as we saw with Edward Osler's training, the teaching of medicine had come to center in the great London hospitals. Oxford students could still get a bachelor of medicine degree, but only by doing all practical work in London and then being examined back at Oxford by the regius professor, who otherwise had practically nothing to do. The preliminary work at Oxford was so resolutely classical and unscientific that by the early nineteenth century very few students, about one a year, took this route into medicine.

In the late nineteenth century Oxford gradually came alive to the sciences, including the medical ones. Sir Henry Acland, regius professor from 1857 to 1895, fought a series of good and largely successful fights to develop biological sciences at the university, overcoming the objections of anti-Darwinians, antivivisectionists, and others committed to tranquil inertia. Acland helped found the University Museum. Another notable advance was the 1875 appointment of John Burdon Sanderson, Osler's former supervisor in London, as Oxford's first professor of physiology. In 1895 Sanderson succeeded Acland as Regius Professor of Medicine. Other medical sciences, including anatomy and pathology, were strengthened, the curriculum and organization of Oxford medicine was reformed, and by the 1890s it was possible to get a decent training in the preclinical medical sciences at Oxford, walk the wards for a year or two in London, and, upon examination by a regius professor who still had very few other duties, get an Oxford medical degree. While not professionally as impressive as a stamp of approval from Edinburgh or the University of London, the Oxford initials were respectable enough and usually signified a doctor of some cultural breadth.

The aging Burdon Sanderson decided to give up his chair in 1903. Who would be Oxford's next Regius Professor of Medicine? The only widely favored candidate, Sir William Church, president of the Royal College of Physicians, was not interested. While Oxford's regius might have a great deal of prestige – second only to the regius in divinity – and very little to do, he would earn very little income, a royal stipend of only £400 annually, unless he scrounged around for consulting work. Oxford had recently constructed its first up-to-date pathology laboratory but could only afford to offer James Ritchie, its pathologist, a reader's stipend. Sanderson and his scientific colleagues came up with the idea of elevating Ritchie to professorial rank and a decent total income by having him appointed regius professor. In one deft move Oxford pathology would become well established.

When word of the impending maneuver leaked out, prominent Oxford medical graduates in London blew a loud public whistle. In their view, the scientists were about to run off with the regius chair in medicine. Indeed, it would be captured by one science, pathology. By the time Ritchie, a comparatively young man with no reputation outside his discipline, retired from the chair, it would be lost forever to the world of clinical medicine, even though the regius's one important function was to counterbalance the preclinical sciences with assurance that degree holders had the ability to practice.

Prime Minister Arthur J. Balfour was to make the appointment in the King's name. The Oxford medical scientists and the London clinicians squared off, publicly and privately, in brilliant and occasionally bitter epistolary conflict. The Londoners had enough influence with the prime minister to block Ritchie's appointment but could not find a suitable candidate of their own. They saw the regius professorship as one of the most prestigious chairs in the medical world. They wanted it filled by an Oxford man of great experience in clinical work and teaching, thoroughly familiar with all facets of medical education, 'a man ... who could worthily uphold the dignity of the University in the estimation of the profession and the public.' But they had to admit that only 'old fossils and incompetents' seemed to want the chair. The prime minister let it be known that he would not be rushed into making a second-rate or stopgap appointment. 'Name your man,' the scientists taunted the clinicians. Observers must have wondered whether either the regius chair or Oxford's Faculty of Medicine had much of a future in such a climate of fundamental division between scientific researchers and active practitioners. Certainly Oxford medicine would be unlikely to present its best face when the British Medical Association convened its annual meeting there in the summer of 1904.[3]

Back in America, Harvard was renewing its old courtship of the Johns Hopkins professor of medicine. When Osler gave his Ingersoll Lecture at Harvard in April, President Eliot sounded him out on coming over for a year to inaugurate their new chair of hygiene. Osler joked that his wife would not want to live so near her relatives, and more seriously said that his clinical opportunities were so attractive at Hopkins that he did not want to be away even for a year. W.T. Councilman told Eliot that perhaps

clinical opportunities could be found for Osler in Boston. Harvard continued the wooing, sending flowers, as it were, in the form of an honorary
degree, to be given at the end of June 1904. The citation was to 'William
Osler, Anglo-American, the leading medical consultant, author, teacher,
and orator of this continent.'[4]

By that time someone in England – it is not clear who – had suggested
the name of William Osler for Oxford's regius chair. Osler was an outsider
who met every other qualification, and would satisfy every faction, would
be a brilliant appointment if he were interested. When he heard the suggestion, Sanderson is said to have clapped his hand to his forehead and
exclaimed, 'That's it – the very man!' This story may be apocryphal, inasmuch as Sanderson proceeded to tell Osler in a sounding-out letter of
June 8 that his first choice was Ritchie. Approaching Osler was 'the next
best course.' Would Osler come if invited?[5]

Grace was visiting her Massachusetts relatives. On her birthday,
June 19, Willie suddenly arrived in town. On the drive from the station he
quietly showed her the letter from England. 'As I read the letter I felt a
tremendous weight lifted from my shoulders as I had become very anxious
about the danger of his keeping on at the pace he had been going for several years in Baltimore.' She wanted him to wire his acceptance right away.
He teased her about being so eager to leave America. He cabled Sanderson
that he would like to talk about the situation when he came over for the
BMA. In a June 21 letter he weighed the pros and cons:

> In many ways I should like to be considered a candidate. While very happy
> here and with splendid facilities, probably unequalled in English-speaking
> countries, I am over-worked and find it increasingly hard to serve the public
> and carry on my teaching. I have been in harness actively for thirty years,
> and have been looking forward to the time when I could ease myself of
> some of the burdens I carry at present. With the income from my book we
> have a comfortable competency, so that I am in a measure independent.
>
> My only doubt relates to the somewhat relative duties of the Chair. I am
> interested in clinical teaching, am fond of it and have acquired some degree
> of aptitude for bedside work which gives me a certain value in the profes-

sion. I should miss sadly the daily contact with the students ... On the other hand ...[6]

Grace had chosen to stay in America that summer. Osler collected his Harvard degree, had a quick holiday with the family at Murray Bay, and sailed on the *Campania* on July 16. Cushing and McCrae traveled with him, sharing a cabin. Osler would spend long, quiet mornings in bed reading and writing, then be ready for socializing. The doctors enjoyed splendid fellowship with other traveling medicos, including James Tyson from Philadelphia, Toronto's young Herbert Bruce, and the ship's surgeon. Osler's proposed contribution to the 'Programme' of the 'North Atlantic Medical Society' was a paper on sleep and obesity at sea.

His first impression of the Oxford opportunity, perhaps gleaned from Sanderson, was that it would be a sinecure. At a dinner in London on his second day there he casually asked a leading British physician, 'Do you think I'm sufficiently senile to become Regius Professor of Oxford?' That day he told a surprised Cushing about the prospect, and Cushing promptly told his wife:

> Dont you dare tell but Dr. O has been offered the Regius Prof at Oxford. May take it. Says it will be a great place for Mrs. O to become a fat dowager and himself too. A synecure – no work big salary – nothing to do but give one lecture a year and drink port the rest of the time – perhaps write the history of Medicine.[7]

As the BMA settled in for its Oxford meeting there must have been a fair amount of gossip about Osler's potential candidacy. Insofar as he was still being looked over, the impression he made was very good. Seconding the vote of thanks after the association's presidential address, Osler not only referred favorably to Oxford's traditions and ideals, but pointed out that the president's listing of Oxford medical greats had omitted John Locke. No wonder the Oxonians were impressed, if not embarrassed by their ignorance of their own history. On its part, the BMA had named Osler as one of six medical notables to be honored with an Oxford LLD. The convocation in the Sheldonian Theatre was splendidly colorful and rich with the sense of tradition that had always pleased Osler. The applause the Canadian received was unexpected and prolonged, Cushing noted, to the point where even his dark skin could not hide the blush.[8]

Osler spent a week in Oxford socializing, conferring, and pondering the future. The British decided they wanted him. Highly placed and independent leaders of the profession told the Oxford people that it would be a brilliant, magnificent appointment, though they could not understand why Osler would walk away from the best position in the world at Hopkins. There was no need to collect testimonials. But he himself was uncertain. When Grace learned he was wavering, she wired back, 'DO NOT PROCRASTINATE ACCEPT AT ONCE.' In a later version of the story, Osler said she added, 'BETTER GO IN A STEAMER THAN GO IN A PINE-BOX.'[9] Osler showed Cushing and McCrae only the 'DO NOT PROCRASTINATE,' covering up the rest of the cable. Prime Minister Balfour had made up his mind, obtained the King's assent, and, just as Osler was leaving for America, offered him the Oxford chair. Not procrastinating, Osler at once accepted.

He spent much of the voyage home writing scores of letters to relatives, colleagues, and old friends, explaining his decision to take 'a quiet easy berth for a man whose best work is done.' Perhaps because he was at sea, perhaps because he was a naval officer's son, or perhaps because his whole life was a series of journeys, he used nautical imagery: 'I have been sailing very close to the wind and it does not seem possible to reef in Baltimore & Oxford is really a snug harbour in which to refit for a few years.' In effect, he was retiring after thirty years of hard work as a teacher and practitioner, retiring because he doubted he could maintain the pace of his American life without destroying his health. In one letter: 'I was riding for a fall.' In another: 'I am tired of the hunted life.' In another: 'The racket of my present life is too much for me. I am going down hill physically & mentally.' He had always planned to retire at about sixty, and fifty-six was close enough (he was to stay at Hopkins for the 1904–5 year). It would be heartbreaking to leave the best medical job in the world, and to leave his friends in

America, though of course he had strong attachments in England. To his ninety-eight-year-old mother he added, 'It will be much better for the boy [Revere] in every way.' They would come out every year, he assured her, 'and I daresay see more of you than we have done of late.'[10]

Privately, Grace was torn. She was terrified of leaving her friends, her lovely home, and her aging parents; and she also hated the damp, cold English climate, having had respiratory problems during recent visits. But she had been unwavering in her support of the move as the one way for her man to break out of his routine. 'You can never know what a struggle it has been and such hard work for me to encourage Dr. Osler to do what I knew was really the best for him,' she wrote a medical friend. 'What could I do?' she told her sister. 'Reverse the circumstances & any one must agree that an American would be glad to come back to American traditions etc. having been brought up in them.'[11]

The news, which came without warning, depressed everybody at Johns Hopkins. 'Every one is in mourning over Dr. Osler,' Florence Sabin wrote a friend: 'One of the trustees has said that his leaving is worse than the fire ... Dr. Hurd is terribly used up.' Welch wrote Osler: 'Your letter drove me into a fit of the blues ... I shall miss you, we all shall, more than can be told, and I do not like to think of it.' Hurd told Osler that he, too, was thinking of resigning, and was gracious in his tribute:

I have thought for a long time that you were driving the machine much too hard and that you must inevitably break down if you did not find some way to slow up ... If talents, self-sacrifice and high devotion to the good of the Profession deserve any reward you have certainly earned the promotion ... I feel that the success of the Hospital and Medical School has been largely your achievement and that you have done the most to hold together the different departments and to establish a high standard of professional work. In fact if it had not been for your breadth and liberality of view we could never have attained our present position.

Weir Mitchell had been on the point of writing Osler urging him to cut back. Now to cover up his sorrow, he teased Osler about the future: 'Very soon you will be saying raily for really and H's will be lost all over the house, and you will say Gawd for God ... Do be careful of your English.' 'As to Jn. Hopkins,' Mitchell added, 'perhaps you do not know that the Med. School at J.H. is or was Wm. Osler.' W.S. Thayer was in seclusion in a Washington hotel trying to get some writing done, so he did not receive Osler's personal letter explaining the move. He read about it in the newspaper: 'I was completely overcome. I could think of nothing else, and, despite myself, I lay down on the bed and wept like a child.'[12]

H.L. Mencken thought that it was the sick doctors of America, arriving on every train to be examined by Osler, that drove him out. Cushing thought that if Osler had had to make up his mind about Oxford from Baltimore, where everyone would have pressured him as they had over the Edinburgh offer, he might never have gone. This time the decision was never reconsidered.[13]

Life would go on at Hopkins, of course, and so would the Oslers go on in America for another eight or nine months. There would be ample time to say goodbye, to get a successor in place, to get to work on the new *System of Medicine* Osler had just agreed to edit for a Philadelphia publishing firm, and for many patients to have a final Stateside consultation with their doctor. After returning to America, the Oslers spent the last weeks of summer ostensibly holidaying at Pointe-au-Pic, Quebec, answering thirty to forty congratulatory letters a day and still falling behind. En route to Baltimore they did a round of family visiting. Grace soon found she was 'weary of the triumphal procession through Canada of the Regius Professor and his family.' His mother's advice was to keep his sense of proportion: 'Remember William, the shutters in England will rattle as they do in America.'[14]

Franklin Mall may have been the one Hopkinsite pleased at Osler's departure. As the champion of getting on with research (a certain kind of research, for it was not clear that Mall, who was repelled by disease, ever understood the clinical research Osler's department had done on, say, malaria and typhoid), he felt that the deadwood was cleaning itself out of medicine at Hopkins. The opportunity and challenge would be to make sure the right man was appointed to succeed Osler so that his department could be elevated, Mall put it, 'to a higher level – one on a par with the leading departments of medicine in Europe.' Most others felt that no one could be found anywhere who could do more than shuffle around in Osler's shoes.[15]

Well, William Welch had a standing about as high as Osler's, especially among the researchers, for whom he was a genial godfather. And he had taken a medical degree many years ago. The first thought of some Hopkinsites was to have Welch succeed Osler as Professor of Medicine and Physician-in-Chief. Although in most ways a ridiculous idea, it was taken seriously for a time as a kind of grand Hippocratic gesture. The Professor of Medicine would stand at the pinnacle, under whose auspices all the other departments would function. Welch himself was dubious. Cushing remembered that after Mall teased him one day about being the modern Hippocrates, Welch would have nothing more to do with the proposal.[16]

Why not promote Osler's assistant and closest protégé at Hopkins, W.S. Thayer? Osler's own first thought was that Thayer had an unassailable claim to the job: 'I do not see how I could go back on Thayer.' The fact that Thayer was a pure clinician, a cultured and literate New England brahmin, very much cut from Osler's cloth, had made them compatible over the years. It also made Thayer uninteresting to Mall and most of the other scientists. Primarily a diagnostician, a little disorganized and dreamy, Thayer had not done much in the way of research as they understood it; his appointment would simply offer more of the same. It also might set a disturbing precedent for Hopkins, the apparently automatic promotion of the leading associate when a chair became vacant.[17]

No need to advertise the position or have a formal search, of course. Everyone knew everyone. The two leading outside candidates were George Dock, Professor of Medicine at Michigan, and Lewellys Barker, Professor of Anatomy at Chicago. Dock had worked under Osler in Philadelphia; Barker had worked with him at Hopkins and was a fellow Canadian, an original latchkeyer and friend. Dock had more clinical experience than Barker, who had never practiced, but he was a cold fish of a scientist, of whom it was said that he could never be accused of having a bedside manner. Barker was brilliant, extremely personable (Dorothy Reed, who did not much care for him, described him as 'a devil-may-care Canadian') and ambitious, a feverishly hard worker who might have the makings of a great clinician as well as a first-class scientist. Welch, Halsted, and Mall supported him in the faculty's Sanhedrinlike deliberations. Mall was especially enthusiastic.[18]

Osler took a great but not controlling interest in the matter. He was in the delicate position of probably being able to have his way about a successor if he used his influence, but knew he should not try unless he felt very strongly. He canvassed some of his associates about the situation and finally decided to do little, probably after learning that there would be no exodus from Hopkins if one or the other candidate was chosen. Osler may have indicated that he leaned to Barker over Dock, who had support from Abel, Howell, and Hurd, but that something should also be done for Thayer. After several meetings early in 1905, thirty-seven-year-old Lewellys Barker was chosen to try to fill Osler's shoes. Thayer was promoted to the new but subordinate position of Professor of Clinical Medicine. Osler stayed away from the final meeting.[19]

Barker knew he had been chosen over Thayer because he had more varied scientific interests and more laboratory experience. Nothing was stipulated at the time, but Mall and probably Welch did not expect him to practice much medicine privately. As Barker had suggested a few years earlier, it seemed desirable to put him on a full-time salaried basis as soon as funds were available. In the meantime, Mall advised him to get on with 'the higher work.' Mall to Barker, March 4, 1905: 'You will naturally carry over into the Clinic what you have done in the Laboratory, that is what we all want you to do ... Get real workers ... Do not have a teaching program like a house of cards ... Have problems going. Reporting cases is like reporting anatomical variations. There is nothing in it ... Use the metric system.'[20]

'Every invalid in the land wants to see him before he gets away,' Cushing wrote home about Osler during his lame-duck year. Osler cut back on his practice as best he could, turning down many 'long distance calls' in the winter of 1904–5 to try to save his strength for the farewell ceremonies in the coming spring. Soon enough he was caught up in the elaborate, exhausting business of saying goodbye. 'His portrait is being painted every few days for some university or society,' Cushing observed. 'He has several addresses to write and deliver; every body wants to give him a dinner; and as usual his house is constantly full of visiting friends and patients that will not be turned away.' On November 5, 1904, as in previous years, the Osler house was full of strange noises and dark maneuvers. A gunpowder plot was discovered in its very basement, and Guy Fawkes himself, who looked uncannily like Harvey Cushing, was discovered hiding on top of the furnace.[21]

Gunpowder-sized renal calculi probably caused the attack of lower left lumbar pain Osler experienced one night late in December while reading an article in the Medical and Chirurgical Faculty library. By the time he got home he felt faint and had to go to bed. The pain subsided in an hour or two. When Thomas Futcher examined two urine specimens the next day, he found what first appeared to be five (!) passed kidney stones. He soon realized that Osler had salted the specimens with quartz particles from his front walk.[22]

Osler kept saying he would be back to Baltimore often as a visitor, but he and most of his colleagues treated his leaving as a great break. He was not only departing from America but seemed to be effectively retiring from the profession. He wrote three formal farewell addresses, each a summary and elaboration of his most deeply held views. The least of them got him into the most trouble.

The longest was given to students at McGill and Philadelphia, and eventually published as 'The Student Life.' It was really about the medical life, which Osler urged should be lived as a perpetual student, a seeker after truth, 'a lover courting a fickle mistress who ever eludes his grasp.' It was a sustained plea for broadmindedness: neither students nor practitioners should become bookish, overly specialized, set in their ways, or parochial. They should be always learning, reaching out, alive to the poetry of life. Perhaps the ideal physician, Osler suggested, would be 'the cultivated gen-

eral practitioner.' The example he cited, a Scottish village doctor who
spent all his spare time translating Greek medical texts, must have seemed
unreal to North American students at the dawn of the new century. More
down-to-earth were Osler's triadic recommendations for education – 'a
notebook, a library, and a quinquennial brain-dusting' – and for the three
well-stocked rooms which it should be every doctor's ambition to have in
his house: 'the library, the laboratory, and the nursery – books, balances,
and bairns.'

The quiet life of the country medical parish could be perfectly fulfilling.
Osler went out of his way to urge students to resist the temptation to move
to a larger center: 'In a good agricultural district, or in a small town ... you
may reach a position in the community of which any man may be proud.
There are country practitioners among my friends with whom I would rather
change places than with any in our ranks.' On the other hand – always, the
other hand – his most cherished belief was that doctors must eschew chauvinism. 'Get denationalized early,' he told his audiences. 'The true student
is a citizen of the world, the allegiance of whose soul, at any rate, is too
precious to be restricted to a single country. The great minds, the great
works transcend all limitations of time, of language, and of race, and the
scholar can never feel initiated into the company of the elect until he can
approach all of life's problems from the cosmopolitan standpoint.'[23]

Osler broke down in the middle of 'Unity, Peace and Concord' – another beautiful psalm to medicine that was his farewell to the American
profession, delivered at the Medical and Chirurgical Faculty of Maryland.
The phrase was taken from the Anglican Litany ('that it may please thee
to give to all nations, unity, peace, and concord') and was Osler's parting
hope for the future of the profession. He was never more eloquent on the
greatness of the church of healers:

Medicine is the only world-wide profession, following everywhere the same
methods, actuated by the same ambitions, and pursuing the same ends. This
homogeneity, its most characteristic feature, is not shared by the law and
not by the Church, certainly not in the same degree. While in antiquity the
law rivals medicine, there is not in it that extraordinary solidarity which

makes the physician at home in any country, in any place where two or three sons of men are gathered together. Similar in its high aims and in the devotion of its officer, the Christian Church, widespread as it is, and saturated with the humanitarian instincts of its Founder, yet lacks that catholicity – *urbi et orbi* – which enables the physician to practise the same art amid the same surroundings in every country of the earth ... In a little more than a century a united profession, working in many lands, has done more for the race than has ever before been accomplished by any other body of men.

So great have been these gifts that we have almost lost our appreciation for them. Vaccination, sanitation, anaesthesia, antiseptic surgery, the new science of bacteriology, and the new art in therapeutics have effected a revolution in our civilization ... a revolution which for the first time in the history of poor, suffering humanity brings us appreciably closer to that promised day when the former things should pass away, when there shoud be no more unnecessary death, when sorrow and crying should be no more, and there should not be any more pain.

Never was he more priestly than in his final benediction:

> I would give to each of you, my brothers – you who hear me now, and to you who may elsewhere read my words – to you who do our greatest work labouring incessantly for small rewards in towns and country places – to you the more favoured ones who have special fields of work – to you teachers and professors and scientific workers – to one and all, through the length and breadth of the land – I give a single word as my parting commandment ... CHARITY.'

Osler was ashamed at having lost his poise, but according to Cushing, who was there, there was not a dry eye in the house.[24]

He intended to elicit more laughs than tears in his farewell to Johns Hopkins, given to a capacity crowd at the university's anniversary ceremonies on February 22, 1905. Half his talk was an earnest summing-up of what they had achieved medically:

Personally there is nothing in life in which I take greater pride than in my connexion with the organization of the medical clinic of the Johns Hopkins Hospital and with the introduction of the old-fashioned methods of practical instruction. I desire no other epitaph – no hurry about it, I may say – than the statement that I taught medical students in the wards ...

American scientific medicine is taking its rightful place in the world's work ... But let us understand clearly that only a beginning has been made.

The longest part of the address was a fairly light-hearted defense of his decision to leave. Hopkins would not be the worse for it, he argued. Like polyzoa or beehives, organizations always survived the defection of individuals. Change was the nature of things and professors should change around more often:

It passes my persimmon to tell how some good men – even lovable and righteous men in other respects – have the hardihood to stay in the same position for twenty-five years! To a man of active mind too long attachment to one college is apt to breed self-satisfaction, to narrow his outlook, to foster a local spirit, and to promote senility. Much of the phenomenal success of this institution has been due to the concentration of a group of light-horse intellectuals, without local ties, whose operations were not restricted, whose allegiance indeed was not always national, yet who were willing to serve faithfully in whatever field of action they were placed. And this should be the attitude of a vigilant profession. As St. Paul preferred an evangelist without attachments ... so in the general interests of higher education a University President should cherish a proper nomadic spirit in the members of his faculties.

Osler warned of two academic diseases: intellectual infantilism, caused largely by minds never cutting loose and growing up; and progeria, or premature senility, which seemed specially to infect inbred and narrow faculties. 'It takes great care on the part of any one to live the mental life corresponding to the phases through which his body passes.' American universities normally made professorial appointments for life. Osler thought men should be hired for a fixed period, so that they would have to leave when they had lost their usefulness. 'It is a very serious matter in our young universities to have all the professors growing old at the same time. In some places, only an epidemic, a time limit, or an age limit can save the situation.' Then, in ill-chosen words, he spun out some of his stock notions:

I have two fixed ideas well known to my friends, harmless obsessions with which I sometimes bore them, but which have a direct bearing on this important problem. The first is the comparative uselessness of men above forty years of age. This may seem shocking, and yet read aright the world history bears out the statement. Take the sum of human achievement in action, in science, in art, in literature – subtract the work of the men above forty, and while we should miss great treasures, even priceless treasures, we would practically be where we are today ... The effective, moving, vitalizing work of the world is done between the ages of twenty-five and forty – these fifteen golden years of plenty, the anabolic or constructive period, in which there is always a balance in the mental bank and the credit is still good. In the science and art of medicine young or comparatively young men have made every advance of the first rank ... The young men should be encouraged and afforded every possible chance to show what is in them ...

My second fixed idea is the uselessness of men above sixty years of age, and the incalculable benefit it would be in commercial, political and in professional life if, as a matter of course, men stopped work at this age. In his *Biathanatos* Donne tells us that by the laws of certain wise states sexagenarii were precipitated from a bridge ... In that charming novel, *The Fixed Period*, Anthony Trollope discusses the practical advantages in modern life of a return to this ancient usage, and the plot hinges upon the admirable scheme of a college into which at sixty men retired for a year of contemplation before a peaceful departure by chloroform. That incalculable benefits might follow from such a scheme is apparent to any one who, like myself, is nearing the limit, and who has made a careful study of the calamities which may befall men during the seventh and eighth decades. Still more when he contemplates the many evils which they perpetuate uncon-

sciously and with impunity. As it can be maintained that all the great advances have come from men under forty, so the history of the world shows
that a very large proportion of the evils may be traced to the sexagenarians
– nearly all the great mistakes politically and socially, all of the worst poems,
most of the bad pictures, a majority of the bad novels, not a few of the bad
sermons and speeches. It is not to be denied that occasionally there is a
sexagenarian whose mind, as Cicero remarks, stands out of reach of the
body's decay ... It is only those who live with the young who maintain a
fresh out look on the new problems of the world. The teacher's life should
have three periods, study until twenty-five, investigation until forty, profession until sixty, at which age I would have him retired on a double allowance. Whether Anthony Trollope's suggestion of a college and chloroform
should be carried out or not I have become a little dubious, as my own time
is getting so short.

Osler excepted women from his proposals because he thought their influence on their sex after sixty could be 'most helpful, particularly if aided by
those charming accessories, a cap and a fichu.'[25]

The speech was a great success, and was preceded and followed by heart-
felt tributes to Dr Osler. He was awarded Johns Hopkins University's only
honorary degree of that year. If anyone noticed that he had misremembered
parts of Trollope's obscure novel – the method of euthanasia was venesection, not chloroform, and it was to happen at sixty-eight, not sixty-one – it
hardly seemed to matter.

The great angle on Osler's talk was instantly obvious to reporters with
an eye for a good story. Men over forty useless! Chloroforming sexagenarians! This is not some two-bit quack but William Osler, the great American doctor, saying these things. What do the forty-year-olds, what do the
sixty-year-olds think about it?

The newspapers had grand sport. 'Useless at Forty' ... 'Professor Osler
Recommends All at Sixty to Be Chloroformed' ... 'Lethal Chamber for the
Aged.' 'Sexagenarii in Panic,' claimed the New York *Daily News*, listing
some of the prominent New Yorkers who would be eligible for chloroforming, including John D. Rockefeller and Andrew Carnegie. 'I am very glad

nobody thought to chloroform me thirteen years ago,' the seventy-three-year-old Hopkins classicist Basil Gildersleeve told a journalist, while Senator Chauncey Depew noted how energetically he had been out campaigning at seventy. Large numbers of judges, congressmen, and clergymen seemed eligible for euthanasia. Worse – or more fun -- every man over forty had been dismissed as 'comparatively useless.' What long lists it was possible to generate of comparatively useless high-achievers, including Demosthenes, Aristotle, Plato, Spinoza, Cervantes, Cromwell, Leonardo, John Hunter, Pasteur, Mohammed, George Washington (on whose birthday Osler had spoken), Abraham Lincoln, Dr. Osler himself, and Cy Young, who had pitched a no-hitter at forty. 'Dr. Osler declares that men are old at 40 and worthless at sixty,' the *Washington Times* noted. 'There must be an age at which man is an ass. What is the Doctor's age, anyhow?' Grace teased him as 'the shattered idol.'[26]

The humorists predicted a boom in hair dye, wigs, and false teeth. How about an Osler cocktail, guaranteed to keep a man under forty? And one might have asked whether the great American symbol, Uncle Sam, should be put out to pasture.

> Brother I am sixty-one,
> So my work on earth is done;
> Calm should follow after storm
> Reach me down the chloroform.

How about 'oslerizing' the aged as a euphemism for chloroforming them? Jokers issued invitations to oslerizations – the word would eventually get into a number of dictionaries. ('The ogry Osler will oxmaul us all,' James Joyce later wrote in *Finnegans Wake*.) In a serious vein, the newspapers reported several instances of sexagenarians who were said to have committed suicide after reading about the doctor's comments.[27]

We cannot be sure of the accuracy of such stories, but Osler, inundated by angry reaction, began to realize the matter was serious. He gave interviews and wrote letters to the editor denying that he had recommended chloroforming the elderly, trying to explain that he had been making a joke. On the other hand he was not going to recant what for him was a considered view: he reiterated his opinion that the world's best work was done by men under forty and that men should retire at about sixty. The good work being done by men still active beyond sixty could probably be better done by the young. 'Poor man!' Cushing wrote from next door. 'He little thought what a bomb he was going to spring ... He has been showered with abusive and threatening anonymous letters – the house besieged with reporters – telegrams galore from newspapers everywhere asking for amplification of his views. The local papers have been full of it – many amusing and many serious things. We have been in at No. 1 W. Franklin this evening, reading some of the extraordinary letters ... The misunderstandingness of people passes comprehension.'[28]

Osler's and Cushing's misunderstandingness was considerable too. The 'fixed period' remarks made such good press not just because it was a slow news time and not just because some reporters may have gloried in getting back at a snooty medical bigshot, or just because American reporters had (or had not) a perverse sense of humor, or just because it was risky to be 'politically incorrect' even in 1905. Osler in fact was advancing and determinedly clinging to a set of fixed and clear ideas about the relative value to society of youth, middle age, and old age. To everyone except the young, they were fairly depressing ideas.

Osler's 'fixed period' speech fed right into the anxieties of every middle-aged man in the workforce, right into men's fear of losing their powers and becoming useless and unwanted. It was certainly true that Dr Osler had loved and venerated specific older people all his life – some of his best friends were old – but he was nevertheless passing severe judgment on the normal consequences of aging. In his obituaries of grand old men of his profession, he often remarked on their exceptionalism in old age. *In general*, Osler was saying, old people were not to be deferred to and consulted as fonts of superior wisdom. Old people were not generally venerable. Old age was demonstrably a pathological condition. In general the aged were to be shunted aside as effectively useless.

Historians of age and retirement in America point to the debate Osler caused in 1905, which echoed through the periodical press for several months, as a revealing moment. The speech had really been a call for com-

pulsory retirement for professors in order to make way for the young. It fed
into a growing sense in many industries that older workers, being less productive, should be forced to retire. Was this an example of the desire of a
competitive, hard-driving, efficiency-conscious generation to begin pushing aside a group whose numbers were growing because of the achievements of medicine and public health?[29] This was exactly the attitude in
England that Anthony Trollope in his old age had seen fit to satirize in *The
Fixed Period*. It was also the attitude Osler had acted upon in a notorious
incident at the 1895 meeting of the American Medical Association when
he had been hissed after speaking loudly in favor of replacing its sixty-
three-year-old secretary as being inefficient.[30] To his credit, Osler had at
least suggested 'a double allowance' by way of pension for aged professors.
Possibly he had some influence, along with others, on philanthropist Andrew Carnegie's decision later that year to create the Carnegie Teachers
Pension Fund, endowed at $10 million, to provide basic pensions for retir-
ing college teachers. Few of them would have as satisfactory a retirement
berth as a regius chair at Oxford.

Otherwise, his vision had been sadly constricted. As though to illustrate his very point, Osler at fifty-six had become a prisoner of his own
preconceptions, both pathological and professional – scientific medicine,
like most fields of science, had been largely the domain of the young; Huxley
had once suggested strangling all scientists at sixty. Osler was remarkably
short-sighted, for example, about the possibility that the medical progress
that he invariably celebrated and predicted might have an impact in de-
laying the ravages of the years. He thought and read about the act of death,
but medically he seemed uninterested in developing a special knowledge
of age. He was not in touch, for example, with some of the work that was
laying the foundation for the development of gerontology.

While Osler is not on record as supporting active euthanasia, his desire
to let people die peacefully would put him in the camp of those of today's
physicians who like to see the light of life go out cleanly and neatly. 'All
reasonable people must deplore the increase of suicide in our modern civilization so often a selfish and cowardly act,' he wrote in a note on Donne's
Biathanatos, only to add that among the scores of suicides he had seen,
there were a few that he 'could not condemn' and others that he 'could not

but admire and even, maybe, approve.' Was it surprising, he wondered, to find in an age when for many death was the 'be all and end all,' that there were men like Shakespeare's Brutus 'who, when beaten to the pit deem it more worthy to leap in than tarry to be pushed.'[31]

Another reason for his pessimism, I suspect, was his having lost any belief in aging as a progress towards a heavenly reward after bodily death. For Osler, age was a time of physical and mental decline towards nothingness, death as end-all. Professionally, he preached the virtues of turning away from age and the aged, an attitude that would later be crudely but accurately labeled 'agism.' Personally, while accepting his limits and going into retirement, really a form of early retirement, he could not look forward in his own old age to many developments other than gradual decline, death, and nothingness. No wonder he never celebrated birthdays. The prophet of medical progress, the Ingersoll lecturer on science and immortality, must have realized that his and his generation's life expectancy was infinitely less than that of his parents.

Cushing marveled at Osler's equanimity as he juggled all his obligations – a textbook revision, getting the new *System of Medicine* series underway, keeping his ward rounds punctiliously, and attending to sick doctors and doctors' sick relatives, along with all the farewells. That spring Osler also plagiarized an idea of Cushing's. Young surgeons wanted to watch each other operate rather than listen to papers, and in 1903 Cushing had been a founder of the American Society of Clinical Surgery, which held its first meeting at Hopkins. Osler, being Osler, invited all the members to dinner. In the spring of 1905 Osler invited 'a few of the younger men' in Boston, New York, Philadelphia, and Baltimore to form an Interurban Clinical Club, primarily to study one another at work. Its first meeting was at Hopkins on April 28–9. A highlight, of course, was when the younger men, many of them Osler's former students, observed their departing chief on ward rounds and at an amphitheater clinic. Interurban clinical clubs gradually spread across America and will soon celebrate their first hundred years.

On May 2 the blue-blooded elite of North American medicine – every living notable Osler had ever known it seemed, some of whom had traveled across the continent – gathered six hundred strong at the Waldorf-Astoria in New York to say good-bye. The men dined on Mousse de Jambon à la Vénitienne, Filet de Bass de Mer à la Ferzen, Suprême de Volaille Archiduc, Carré d'Agneau, Pintade du Printemps, Gelée de Groseilles, Glaces de Fantasie, and more, accompanied by wines, three kinds of champagne, and liqueurs. James Tyson of Philadelphia chaired the assemblage, possibly the most glittering in the history of medical America. In the fashion of the time, beautifully dressed wives watched from the balconies – they at least got to hear the speeches – with Grace, her mother, and Revere in a special box. Francis Shepherd spoke about Osler's Montreal years; J.C. Wilson, the wedding-day friend, recalled the Philadelphia period; Welch, of course, stood for the Hopkins era. At the end of Welch's speech, 'The Saint Johns Hopkins Gastric Quartette' led the company in 'Our Regius Professor,' sung to the American tune 'My Country, 'Tis of Thee,' which is the British tune 'God Save the Queen':

> Our chief, we turn to thee,
> Beloved from sea to sea,
> To thee we sing.
> We love thy genial ways,
> Thy wit and merry plays,
> Thy matchless eyes' dark rays,
> And tribute bring.

> CHORUS: God save the mighty chief,
> We part from him in grief,
> God save our chief.
> God save our Regius Prof,
> Our hats to him we doff
> God save our Regius Prof,
> God save our prof.
>
> ...

May he find tophi there,
Bardolphian noses rare,
Undiagnosed.
Long may his eye be keen,
His touch to feel the spleen,
To auscultate the Queen,
This is our toast.

Abraham Jacobi, one of the grand men of the American profession and the father of pediatrics, drew a word-picture of the ideal physician and made it indistinguishable from Osler. The other dean of American medicine, Weir Mitchell, presented Osler with a 1744 edition from Benjamin Franklin's press of Cicero's treatise on old age, *De senectute*. Mitchell offered to Osler 'the hope that you will have no age which will be old, except in years. I, my friend have found old age both happy and productive and so, I trust, may you when that far-away autumn comes upon you.'

In reply, Osler stressed how unusually happy he had been in his friends, his profession, his patients and students, and above all in his home. He told about coming to the United States after Mitchell had approved his method of handling cherry stones and thanked his colleagues, general practitioners throughout America, and 'the inspiration of my life,' his students:

> I have had but two ambitions in the profession: first, to make of myself a good clinical physician ... My second ambition has been to build up a great clinic in this country on [the] Teutonic lines ... which have placed the scientific medicine of that country in the forefront of the world ...
>
> I have had three personal ideals. One to do the day's work well and not to bother about to-morrow ... The second ideal has been to act the Golden Rule, as far as in me lay, towards my professional brethren and towards the patients committed to my care.
>
> And the third has been to cultivate such a measure of equanimity as would enable me to bear success with humility, the affection of my friends without pride, and to be ready when the day of sorrow and grief came to meet it with the courage befitting a man.

Applause and cheers, often prolonged, punctuated all the speeches. The audience also applauded Jacobi's comment: 'I take the man I speak of to be an American, one of us.'[32]

The Oslers gave furniture, books, journals, china, and other mementos to the latchkeyers and other friends. There is a story that after his last rounds at Hopkins, Osler gave his stethoscope to Thomas Boggs saying, 'Now carry on my work.' There is another story, possibly also apocryphal, that as Osler was leaving his last faculty meeting he turned and remarked to Mall, 'Now I go, and you have your way.' Willie got out of Baltimore on May 16, leaving Grace to supervise the final packing. 'Willie's motto may well be aequanimitas,' she told the Cushings, 'because he always flees when things like this are going on.' The house was to be demolished for redevelopment of the lot immediately after the Oslers left, yet Grace insisted that it be left spotless. She gave the doorplate with their name on it to Harvey Cushing.[33]

Osler took part in the annual meeting of the Association of American Physicians in Washington on the sixteenth and seventeenth. He finished the preface to the sixth edition of *The Principles and Practice* on the seventeenth, noting that it was in many respects a new book. On the eighteenth he spoke to the National Association for the Study and Prevention of Tuberculosis on the need for public education. On May 19 he, Grace, and Revere sailed from New York on the *Cedric*, heading for retirement in the Old World. One of Featherstone Osler's sons was going home. 'Almost dead!' Willie exclaimed in his daybook.

NINE

A Delightful Life and Place

Oxford, England. Saturday, May 27, 1905. The pace of transatlantic travel depends on the weather, and because it has been good the Oslers have landed a day early. They telegraph ahead and come on by train and then carriage. Later in the afternoon Dr Osler, Mrs Osler, Revere, and a secretary-governess arrive at 7 Norham Gardens, a big brick pile of a house on a pleasant street in a newer part of town. They are renting it from Mrs Max Müller, widow of the Sanskrit specialist famous for having brought Teutonic philological scholarship to England and for apparently discovering the common origins of all mythologies.

The rental includes the servants. A butler named William meets the American party at the door. The maids stand ready in the hall. The bedrooms have been made up, and the cook has made a delicious meal. A happy beginning.

On Sunday morning the Oslers attend service at Christ Church Cathedral. A few old acquaintances come to call. Then nothing happens. Despite the beautiful gardens and the birdsong of Oxford in May, Willie, Grace, and Revere find the tranquillity oppressive. 'I was blue as indigo for the first two or three days,' Osler will recall. 'Do let us go out and shout,' Revere suggests. 'It will take months to shake down & feel at home,' Osler writes back to America. 'Evidently I shall have to settle down into a quiet academic life but in time I shall like it very much.'[1]

The mood indigo gradually lifts as he runs up to London for a dinner party, has his first private consultation, does some fishing and punting with Revere on the Isis, and is caught up in Oxford social life. The Oslers find an acceptable tutor for nine-year-old Revere, who seems much better adjusted to life in England than to life in Baltimore. 'Goodness – if Revere does *not* grow up a man of tender refined feeling it will not be from lack of surroundings from nine years of age,' Grace exclaims to her mother. Grace takes instantly to the beauties of Oxford – the flowers and gardens, the colleges, the rituals, and most of the people – even as she decides that English women, especially professors' wives, have no idea of how to dress or present themselves. 'Such *awful* looking women I have never seen – Wives of scientists mostly ... perfect frumps.' At a glorious summer garden party at Blenheim Palace, the Duke of Marlborough spends most of his time with Grace and young Marjorie Howard, their first houseguest. He likes them, Grace reasons, because they are not run-of-the-mill university women and 'because we have straight teeth I suspect ... All the people here have crooked teeth.'[2]

Basking in summer sunshine, the peaceful university town at the center of the British Empire welcomes its new 'Reggie' and Mrs Reggie with social calls, receptions, luncheons, dinner parties. Night after night they dine in academic splendor at tables laden with silver that Grace Revere Osler admits would cause great-grandfather Paul to take a back seat. She finds it a bit intimidating to be placed between 'terribly learned men' at these affairs but notes that the Russo-Japanese war is always good for worldly conversation and at Oxford one can always fall back on the weather and gardens. In any case the secret of the Oxford social routine is that dinners are short and everyone is home before ten. In a later season the Oslers will have to take their turn as hosts; this summer it takes all of Grace's energy to begin repaying the ritual social calls. By the end of July she has visited or left her card at 113 addresses and is only two-thirds of the way down her list. The British women continue to strike her as so timid she hardly dares speak to them for fear of causing fright.[3]

Willie settles into the regius professor's quarters at the University Museum and into rooms at Christ Church College, where he is officially a

Student. He fancies that John Locke and Robert Burton had these very rooms. He browses in Oxford libraries and attends his first meeting as a curator of the Bodleian Library. He arranges to do some clinical work at the Radcliffe Infirmary, Oxford's hospital, where he will actually be the informal chief of staff. 'Our dear Reggie is very giddy,' Grace tells the Cushings. 'He has two new gowns – one all scarlet & another scarlet habit which he wears over a black gown on state occasions – also lovely surplices for Sunday etc. at Christ Church.'[4]

Much of his gowned time is spent up in London, sitting with his former Hopkins colleagues, Welch, Halsted, and Kelly, while the renowned Anglo-American portraitist, John Singer Sargent, whose father was a doctor, paints *The Four Doctors* on a commission from Mary Garrett. The work is an artistic immortalization of the school's founding fathers, who of course have fine sport commenting on Sargent's characterizations. Appropriately, Sargent consigns Kelly to one side of the painting and has Halsted towards the back, masked in shadows. Osler is the foremost; at the center of the painting is Osler's right hand holding a quill pen. No medical implements or patients are on display, only books. In the background there is a faint representation of El Greco's *St Martin of Tours Dividing His Cloak with the Beggar*. The doctors are in front of a globe, for they belong not to Johns Hopkins but to the world. Perhaps anticipating biographers to come, Sargent has more trouble painting Osler than any of the others. His skin seems to change color every day. 'He has caught my eyes and the ochrous hue of my dour face,' Osler finally decides.[5]

Even in these first weeks the world begins to beat a path to the Oslers in Oxford. Hopkins colleagues, former students, Canadian relatives, a new breed of students known as Rhodes scholars, former patients, new patients, Hopkins nurses, and others arrive at 7 Norham Gardens for tea, company, advice, good cheer. The servants, who thought the Oslers would know no one, are astonished and a bit disconcerted at the extra work. 'I believe William the Butler thinks we are all quite mad,' Grace writes, 'I have already had to pay all the servants extra.' 'Madam,' the upstairs maid tells her in September, 'I think we better keep all the beds always ready in this house.' The Oslers have not been in England two months, yet they are already complaining of feeling fatigued by the social whirl and needing to get away.[6]

The getaway possibilities are delightful. London, the capital of the world, is an hour by train; the Oslers run up so often for business or shopping or socializing that even Grace has to have her club. His is the Athenaeum, hers the Empress. For super tranquillity, only fourteen miles outside Oxford lies the beautiful village of Ewelme, with its fifteenth-century church and an almshouse founded by a granddaughter of Geoffrey Chaucer. From the early 1600s the Regius Professor of Medicine has also been Master of Ewelme Almshouse. The Oslers delight in excursions to a country site that predates the discovery of America, and they open a safe there chock-full of documents hundreds of years old. They decide to modernize and use the master's rooms at Ewelme. On their first visit they arrive with tobacco and newspapers for the residents of the almshouse. 'I am sure Willie will make them all fond of him & be good to them,' Grace writes. They talk about using a motor car for future excursions.[7]

They are guests of the Regius Professor of Physic at Cambridge, the Clifford Allbutts, on their first visit to the other great university town. Allbutt, inventor of the clinical thermometer and said to be George Eliot's model for the good points of Dr Tertius Lydgate in *Middlemarch*, is a much older man, less outgoing than Osler, but very distinguished as a clinician, scholar, humanist, and mountaineer. Early in August the Oslers are guests of a steamship owner on his yacht at the great regatta at Cowes. King Edward VII looks 'frisky and well' as he runs about the fleet in his gig, Grace reports. Then the Oslers go to the Highlands of Scotland, to spend a week with the American millionaire and philanthropist, Henry Phipps, at his rented castle. Fishing, shooting, and house partying are in full sway. 'It is always so amusing to be doing the things exactly as one reads about them in English Novels,' Grace writes her mother. The scenery is stunning. 'I never imagined anything so wonderful as this.'[8]

They have a week to themselves on the Isle of Skye. Then the Canadian millionaire and philanthropist who is High Commissioner (ambassador) to Great Britain, Lord Strathcona, formerly plain Donald Smith, tops the Phipps's hospitality by entertaining the Oslers at Colonsay, one of the Inner Hebrides. Strathcona owns the whole island.

The long summer ends with a week in Paris for a tuberculosis congress. The city is full of Americans, including innumerable Baltimoreans. The once-fashionable shopping at the Bon Marché has become dull by America's rising standards, Grace finds. But French food is the best she has ever tasted. Willie organizes a party of the American physicians to go on a pilgrimage to the tomb of Pierre Louis, the great clinician and pioneer of medical statistics. They track down Louis' mausoleum in the cemetery of Montparnasse; Osler lays a wreath of autumn leaves on its steps and says a few words of appreciation; pictures are taken. Many of the participants are genuinely moved at this highly symbolic act of medical ancestor worship.[9] Back in Oxford, Osler receives the one hundred thousandth copy of *The Principles and Practice of Medicine*, now in its sixth edition. He gives it to Revere, who will be his heir. He participates in several ceremonies to mark the three hundredth anniversary of the birth of another medical ancestor and hero, Sir Thomas Browne. Browne's example shows, he suggests 'that the perfect life may be led in a very simple, quiet way.'[10]

Acting on the advice he gave to other hard-driving middle-aged men, Osler really did slow down after moving to Oxford, if not from 25 to 15 knots, perhaps from 40 to 25 knots. He was a dutiful regius, but the duties were relatively light, and he did little to expand them. He turned his back on doing clinical work or teaching at any of the great London hospitals and sharply reduced his consulting practice and the income it had generated. He kept his hand in with one or two clinics a week at the Radcliffe, five or six private patients a week ('chiefly stranded Americans & colonials'),[11] and the usual constant reading and shop-talk with other doctors. After a considerable rest from writing in his early Oxford months, he took up his pen to describe some of his more interesting cases and begin preparing a few formal lectures. The regius professor was always good for a short homily at prize-giving ceremonies and for exhortations to county medical societies, and the Oslers' house was always open for visitors. About the time of his sixtieth birthday he took a sabbatical on the continent, which was particularly refreshing, for he followed it with some of his very best writing.

'Willie's delight in the college life is a joy to see,' Grace wrote one day in 1905 after they had enjoyed a romantic walk home in moonlight and mist after dinner at Corpus Christi College. Year after year, in letter after letter, Osler exclaimed at his happiness in England. 'This is a delightful life and place,' he enthused to Grace one night in 1910 after coming home from Christ Church.[12] He continued to be prone to bronchial infections and other minor ailments, but his worries about his heart and slow pulse seem to have dissipated. It was the perfect life and place for growing old graciously, for spending more of his days in his library, and for being father to Revere, to other young children who dropped in, and to some of the Oxford students looking for mentors and models in life.

British friends joked that the Oslers liked to weekend in America. No sooner had their first academic term in Oxford ended in December 1905 than they headed over for Christmas and hectic weeks of visiting and traveling. Grace and Revere came back in January, but Willie stayed an extra month, doing still more traveling, taking ward rounds at Hopkins, seeing old patients, and conferring with Tom McCrae on the *System* volumes they were putting together. He wore himself out and knew it, coming down with a respiratory infection when he got back. 'I was rather knocked out by the racket in America. I am evidently reaching a state of pre-senile enfeeblement.'[13] Grace vowed that she would never again let him loose in America during winter.

The next winter their trip was even more exhausting, Cushing judged. Its magnificent highlight was Ellen Osler's hundredth birthday party in Toronto on December 14, 1906. Most of her six living children, twenty-six grandchildren, and twenty-one great-grandchildren were able to attend. It took two men to carry the hundred-candled, five-layered cake – one layer for each of the British monarchs of her century – up to her room. Special souvenir plates and spoons were given to all her descendants and have become treasured family memorabilia. Ellen's eyesight was dim, but she still read her Bible, said her prayers, and signed her checks. 'She was wonderfully well in mind and body and no one enjoyed the festivities more than she did,' Willie wrote. She attributed her longevity to having lived a simple life and told reporters that Willie's views about old age were just one of his jokes.[14]

Official Toronto wanted Dr Osler to stay on permanently. The University of Toronto was in the midst of a major modernization, which included ongoing improvement of its medical school. The Toronto General Hospital was about to be rebuilt as a world-class teaching hospital for the university. Inspiration for much of the Toronto reform agenda had come from the Johns Hopkins experience and the views of the world-famous native son, William Osler. The businessmen-philanthropists engineering the momentous changes knew the Osler family well. When the cantankerous incumbent president of the University of Toronto decided to exit with the old order, there was one obvious candidate to take his place. In the summer of 1906 Osler was asked by the Premier of Ontario if he would assume the presidency of the University of Toronto.

His immediate reaction was negative. 'I am not fit to be president of a college. I have no executive gifts, and I am 15 years too old. All the same it is most gratifying to be remembered by one's native province.' He was uncertain enough, though, to let the matter hang until his Toronto visit at the end of the year. He was made a formal offer, thoroughly discussed the university and hospital situation, thought carefully about the remarkable opportunity he was being given to lead what could become one of the world's great universities and medical schools – the opportunity to realize the vision he had had for 'Otnorot' a quarter-century earlier – and reasoned back to his starting point. He had neither the training nor the disposition for the job, and he turned it down.[15]

Osler was not able to return to Toronto when his mother slipped away from earthly life a few months later. Ellen had stayed mentally alert to the last, and she died surrounded by relatives, including daughter Chattie and niece Jennette. 'A more delightful old age could not be imagined,' Willie concluded.[16] Ellen died in the belief that she was passing on to be united with Featherstone, B.B., Nellie, and little Emma. One tasteless American newspaper obituary observed that she had survived to a hundred because her son had not chloroformed her at sixty. The 'fixed period' speech haunted Osler on his American visits like the lingering odors of flatulence.

In 1906 the Oslers bought the big Victorian Gothic red-brick house at 13 Norham Gardens, down the street from the place they had been renting. They spent months and many thousands of pounds having the thirty-year-old house thoroughly renovated, installing American-style central heating and three new bathrooms. Grace created a local legend in Oxford when she climbed into a porcelain tub at a shop to try it out for length. The Americans must have seemed obsessed with washing and keeping warm. They were certainly obsessed with haste and were driven nearly mad by the snail's pace of British labor. Despite or perhaps because of their frustrations, the Oslers finally gave a wind-up dinner in their garden for the more than hundred workers who had done the job. Externally, 13 Norham Gardens was (and is) architecturally undistinguished. Its virtues for the Oslers were its large size and its terrace, tennis court, and large garden fronting on the University Parks. Norham Gardens is still a peaceful street of English country houses in easy walking distance of academic and medical Oxford.

Osler's sense of family was almost literally all-embracing. His siblings and their spouses and children and grandchildren were always welcome in Oxford. So were more distant relatives, but especially his particular favorites, the Francis children. They had grown to adulthood and begun to disperse across North American and Europe, but Willie always remained surrogate father, confidant, and generous subsidizer to his special favorites, Gwen, Bea, and Bill. He sometimes enthused, sometimes worried about the girls' matrimonial prospects; and he worked quietly behind scenes to have his Montreal friends give a helping hand to Bill, who had done some pathological work after graduating from Hopkins and then tried to make a go of practice in Montreal.

None of the Francis children had easy lives or unalloyed success. Most teetered on the edge of the genteel poverty they had always known. Bill, for example, was not really cut out to be a doctor. He loved detailed literary work, like editing, checking texts, doing a little versifying, much in the tradition of his Osler and Francis grandfathers. Willie enlisted his help with some of his textbook revisions. Bill led a bit of a harum-scarum bachelor's life, blowing hither and yon, keeping irregular hours, and 'looking more than ever like a third rate variety showman,' according to an unusually critical comment of Uncle Willie's. When Bill came down late for breakfast, Osler would say to him, 'Never mind, ... You'll be in time for the afterbirth.' In 1911 Bill's prospects were further blighted when he went down with tuberculosis.[17]

Osler cheerfully acted as replacement dad to anyone else who seemed to need it, and he was particularly close to the children whom his own mentor, Palmer Howard, had fathered during a second marriage. After the death of their parents, Marjorie and Campbell Howard found loving substitutes in 'Doccie O' and 'Aunt Grace.' 'I should like to stand to you in the same relation your father did to me,' he wrote to Campbell, for whom he was godfather, in 1897. He had guided Campbell through medical school at McGill, brought him to Hopkins as a resident, advised him on presenting and publishing papers, and enthusiastically supported a move back to McGill. Marjorie Howard, who came to England with the Oslers to attend school, was one of their first and most constant houseguests. The ulterior motive for the Oslers' visit to Lord Strathcona's island, Colonsay, in 1905 was to re-establish relations with Jared Howard, the older half-brother of Campbell and Marjorie, who was Strathcona's son-in-law. For years there had been a rift between the Jared Howards on the one hand and the Oslers and younger Howards on the other. It was patched up by the visits.[18]

Grace shared Willie's love of family. Other Reveres, including sister Susan Chapin and her family, were always welcome in Oxford; 'Aunt Grace' or 'Tante Grace' happily looked after Oslers, Howards, Cushings, and all the other favored young men and women. She also liked to claim to be the mother of the Rhodes scholars. As older folk were wont to do in those times – see the novels of P.G. Wodehouse – Willie and Grace kept a close though not oppressive eye on the youngsters' matrimonial prospects. They were always more than happy to introduce eligible young men and women, especially if they could have a hand in selecting the most attractive eligibles. Both Willie and Grace delighted in being physicians, midwives, and even surgeons in the young people's 'cardiac' affairs. Given a free hand, they would have created elaborate marital networks of MDs, nephews and nieces, and other special favorites, and Osler would have recommended all the worthy men for jobs in Montreal or Baltimore.

During the Baltimore years they had given plain gold rings to some of their American protégés to wear as a way of discouraging the attentions of 'designing women' during their studies abroad. When Marjorie Howard was being courted in Germany, 'W. Reggie Davis' warned her to be careful: 'I do not like German husbands for English or American girls.' All the boys who frequented Norham Gardens were longing to see her, he wrote: 'Good old Mange is so sweet. I really wish you could marry him in May ... I would give you away.' Then an even better outcome: Thomas Futcher, the Oslers' former resident and neighbor in Baltimore, decided during an Oxford visit that he was in love with Marjorie and, with prodding from the Oslers, pursued her to Colonsay and proposed. '*Dee*lighted,' Osler exclaimed to Marjorie:

> I knew all would go well. You have a good man, not quite as good as yours devotedly, but with possibilities under your guidance. You are just the girl for him ... We really managed well. A.G. the old darling says she made the match but we know! She is so happy ...
>
> How delighted you father would be! ... There will be all sorts of worries getting things settled but I will give you a few doses of 'aequanimitas' ... I see you a great success at B[altimore]. I will map out a programme – domestic, social, and charitable – for you. Love and blessings.[19]

Willie nicknamed the new house the Open Arms and quipped that Grace had missed her calling in not running a summer hotel. One guestroom was nicknamed Baltimore, another Philadephia. Cecil Rhodes, the great empire builder, had died in 1902, and by 1905 his scheme to fund scholarships for elite students from the Anglo-Saxon nations, including Germany, was well launched. There were nearly one hundred and fifty Rhodes scholars at Oxford. A Canadian acquaintance of Osler's, George Parkin, was the secretary of the Rhodes Trust, and 13 Norham Gardens became virtually a social center for 'Rhodesians,' especially on Sundays. After a quiet lunch one Sunday early in their stay, according to Grace:

> In the afternoon WO trotted off to look up some newly arrived Rhodes Scholars and brought back 2 for supper – one from Prince Edward Island and another from Watertown N. York – The former evidently very clever – the latter a perfect bumpkin. He said, 'I've been about very little' ... and then said to Amy 'Well – Miss Gwyn I guess you're soaking in knowledge here.' Now really it does seem a very great pity to have such men represent an American gentleman – doesn't it?

Amy Gwyn, a niece, was over for a visit. 'She is so pretty I should think all men would fall in love with her,' Grace added. After she left, Grace described another Sunday: 'About 30 undergraduates called Sunday afternoon – Billie [Francis] was here and we had some nice music. I think I must always have *a girl* here it makes it very attractive for the men.'[20] Someone once called the Norham Gardens girls 'Mrs. Osler's decoy ducks.' In 1905 Osler was toastmaster at the American Thanksgiving dinner, a feast of roast turkey with mountain corn, thrown by the Oxford Rhodes scholars.

'Scarcely a day passes without someone of interest turning up,' Osler wrote to Weir Mitchell.[21] As unofficial North American ambassadors in Oxford, the Oslers constantly offered hospitality to visitors, ranging from the American ambassador to Great Britain, to Mark Twain, both of whom were in town for a grand Oxford pageant in 1907. Rudyard Kipling also attended and accepted the Oslers' invitation to stay with them – his wife was a distant relative of Grace's. Seventy-one-year-old Mark Twain behaved very badly at a luncheon thrown by the Oslers, deliberately snubbing one of Grace's American guests who had been invited on his behalf. But Kipling proved a delightful house guest, taking Revere for a walk, allowing Osler to persuade him to cut down on his smoking, taking an interest in medical history. On another occasion, Lord Baden-Powell, founder of the Boy Scouts, came to tea before giving a lecture on Scouting. There was great anxiety about how Kaiser Wilhelm of Germany might behave during his British visit in the autumn of 1907, but it went well in every respect, including the special ceremony at Windsor Castle to confer an Oxford honorary degree. As regius professor, Osler was one of the party attending the ceremony, which was presided over by Oxford's chancellor, also a great imperialist, Lord Curzon. The Kaiser asked Osler about Lord Lister's health.[22]

As regius professor, and because of his great reputation, Osler was invited and expected to sit on many university and professional bodies, and of course was invited to join some of the elite dining clubs of London and Oxford. No single commitment seemed particularly arduous, so Osler accepted most of them. Soon, of course, he was regretting all the obligations he had accumulated. The most important of these at Oxford were membership on the Hebdomadal Council, which was the university's governing body, membership on the Delegacy of the University Press, its governing body, and his work as a curator of Bodley's Library. As well, he served as a member of council of the Royal College of Physicians and was on its library committee; he was a sometimes councilor of the British Medical Association, and was a hearty supporter, amounting to a moving spirit, of the 1907 amalgamation of several London societies into the Royal Society of Medicine, on whose council and library committee he also served. In 1906 he was one of the founders of the Association of Physicians of Great Britain and Ireland, an elite body modeled after the Association of American Physicians.

Every spring, Osler spent several weeks examining medical students at Oxford and reciprocating at Cambridge with Clifford Allbutt, his fellow regius (the two were famously announced at a reception in London as 'The Brothers Regii!'). Instead of giving lectures, he completed his professorial duties with a weekly clinic at the Radcliffe Infirmary, for medical students and local doctors; some terms, he gave medical students his observation clinics. During term, he dined regularly at Christ Church. 'I am settling down to the life of a pre-senile Don,' he wrote Thayer in early 1908, 'only I am quite unable to do justice to Port! Councils & committees. 'Tis often a bore but it is interesting from an educational standpoint. I am afraid nothing short of a French Revolution will modernize Oxford & Cambridge.'[23]

Being both a tradition-loving Englishman and a make-our-own-tradition American, Osler was ambivalent about Oxford's ambivalence towards change. In medical education he was generally content with the status quo, in which students did their preclinical work at Oxford and their practical training in the London hospitals. He supported ongoing efforts to elevate the sciences in the classics-drenched university, the first achievement being full funding of the chair of pathology, although James Ritchie, who professed no disappointment in not getting the regius professorship, moved on. By 1912 Osler had become instrumental in having pharmacology established at Oxford, and the next year was influential in having Charles Sherrington, who would enjoy a brilliant career, appointed to the chair of physiology. He was also responsible for the creation of a small clinical laboratory at the Radcliffe Infirmary, its first. Generally, Osler's years were transitional in the institutional evolution of Oxford medicine, which shone while Osler was there mainly because, as Gertrude Stein might have put it, Osler was there. He must have smiled at the irony of being regius professor at an institution that was widely believed not to have a medical school. He was apparently responsible for a 1906 article in the *British Medical Journal* reminding the profession that Oxford did have one.[24]

As a Delegate to the Oxford University Press, Osler helped supervise one of the largest academic publishing enterprises in the world. 'The meetings form a sort of literary seminar, & we really have great sport, particularly with the expert opinion sent in upon works which are offered.' Osler enjoyed everything about the world of books, new as well as old (for a time he tinkered with the idea of creating a 'College of the Book' at Oxford), and was influential in Oxford's expanding into medical publishing; he was the founding, figurehead editor of its *Quarterly Journal of Medicine*.

The problem for Oxford's great library, the Bodleian, was to keep up with all the books it accumulated. The largest university library in the world was desperately trying to enlarge its storage space and catalogue its collections. Osler supported all schemes for expanding and modernizing the Bodleian – perhaps there was a symbolic import in his gift to it of the clock that still sits under the bust of Bodley in Duke Humfrey's Library – and, as a member of the standing committee of the curators, he was closely involved in library management. In 1906 he dunned Lord Strathcona and several other friends for much of the £3,000 required to purchase the first folio edition of Shakespeare, a volume the library had once owned but had disposed of in the 1660s as superfluous. The twentieth-century librarian E.W.B. Nicholson wept with gratitude for Osler's help in raising what was then an immense sum of money to buy a book. He told Osler he deserved a statue in the Bodleian quadrangle.[25]

Osler joined in other fundraising efforts, notably the new University Endowment Fund, aimed at marshaling resources above and beyond what the colleges might offer to support such university institutions as the Bodleian, the museums, and Osler's own projects in medicine. It had mixed success. Through his American connections, especially Henry Phipps, Osler was able to bring in some money, but he was not sufficiently aggressive, persistent, or fawning to be a great fundraiser; and he spread himself too thinly, for he tended to support every good cause at every institution he had touched. Would the millionaires please help buy book collections for Hopkins? Can the Rockefellers help McGill rebuild after a devastating fire? (They won't, but Strathcona will.) Would Mr Carnegie consider the needs of Oxford? How wonderful that Henry Phipps has agreed to fund a psychiatric clinic at Hopkins! 'It is very hard to get money out of English people.'[26]

Osler wanted to see change at Oxford. He sided early with the reform group locked in perpetual conflict against those resisting virtually all changes. In Osler's years the issues included trying to strengthen university governance to make the institution more than the sum of its colleges, strengthening the sciences and research, phasing out compulsory Greek, providing pensions for professors, and granting degrees to women. Osler first identified with a plan to have radical change imposed on Oxford from the outside, then supported the elaborate proposals for internal reform presented by the chancellor, Lord Curzon. These progressed very slowly. 'I wish you were 50 and here as President,' Osler wrote to Daniel Coit Gilman, his retired leader at Hopkins. 'How we could make this old place hum! There are such possibilities, & it is such a delightful spot, that it seems hard to have essential changes blocked by antiquated machinery.' Osler's taste for the higher levels of university politics quickly faded, and he resigned from the Hebdomadal Council after three years. Most of the reforms he supported came to Oxford after his death.[27]

In 1908 Osler became involved in the higher politics of another British university with the least possible investment of his own time. He went along with the request of a group of students at the University of Edinburgh to put his name forward as a candidate for Lord Rector. They would campaign on his behalf. Most rectorial candidates had been active politicians, supported by their party organizations. Osler was a rare independent, contesting against the Rt. Hon. George Wyndham, a Unionist, and the Rt. Hon. Winston Churchill – at the time, a Liberal cabinet minister. Osler did not have to go to Edinburgh or do anything during the campaign, though he did cough up £50 towards the students' expenses, and brother E.B. sent £100. The campaigns consisted mostly of giving out free beer at smokers and fighting pitched battles against other candidates' partisans in an orgy of Scottish student rowdyism. 'The motto of the Oslerites before a battle was "Get hurt,"' the gentle doctor was told. 'Fortunately none of us were detained long in bed, the severest case being ten days.' The Oslerites claimed to have won all the battles, but the graduates' votes decided the war. Wyndham got 826 votes, Churchill 727, Osler 614. It was judged a remarkably good showing for an independent.[28]

Osler turned down an invitation to be a member of a Royal Commission on Vivisection. Such outside activities 'take the leisure I need for all sorts of work,' he told Cushing.[29] He had arrived in England with case reports from Hopkins that he wanted to write up and with a major new publishing commitment, a textbook to keep current, and ideas for all sorts of investigations into the history of medicine. His idea of leisure was to have time to write.

Two days before the Oslers left for England, German researchers had announced their discovery of the spirochete that generates syphilis. While Osler might slow down, the growth of medical knowledge would not. Its frontiers now included principles of genetic inheritance, understanding of the immune and endocrine systems, biochemical work on metabolism, and the development of neurophysiology. Osler was still determined to keep abreast of it all in his publications.

The *System of Medicine* he had agreed to edit for Lea Brothers in America was to be a multivolume series of specialized articles by the best authorities he could sign up. The models were the *Systems* edited by William Pepper in the 1880s and Clifford Allbutt in the 1890s, to both of which he had contributed. Working physicians bought these series to supplement their textbooks and journals, and the works sold on the editor's name, a guarantee of quality. The publisher urged Osler not to go overboard with English contributors and to make sure that his authors emphasized practicality, 'for the reputation of being erudite is commercially disasterous [sic].'[30]

Osler used Tom McCrae as his assistant, and after Osler had signed up the authors, McCrae did most of the work. Osler supplied an introductory article, 'The Evolution of Internal Medicine,' for volume 1, which appeared in 1907 under the British title A *System of Medicine* and the flashy American moniker (which Osler did not like) *Osler's Modern Medicine*. Six more thousand-page volumes were issued by 1910. Osler enlisted many of his old friends, most of whom were leading experts in their fields, as contributors. He wrote five articles himself – four on heart disease and a collaborative study of syphilis. A few relative newcomers contributed, such as a Japanese-American researcher, Hideyo Noguchi, and the fellow in pathology at McGill, Maude Abbott.

Abbott, a graduate in medicine from Bishop's College in Quebec, had found a niche as the first female faculty member at McGill (which still did not allow women medical students). From her first encounters with Osler – 'I shall never forget him as I saw him walking down the old Museum towards me with his great dark burning eyes fixed full upon me' – Abbott worshiped him. As curator of McGill's medical museum she became almost literally the keeper of his body parts. Osler encouraged Abbott to write for the *System* on the neglected field of congenital heart disease, an area in which the museum's collection was particularly useful. He praised Abbott's work to the skies as the best thing done in English and the making of volume 4. The article did make her a considerable reputation. Maude Abbott was the only woman among Osler's 104 authors.[31]

Osler could not understand how Gordon Holmes, a distinguished London neurologist, could do such a bad job on diseases of the peripheral nerves. It was more puzzling when Holmes denied knowing anything about his alleged contribution. It turned out that Osler's original request had been delivered to an undistinguished London physician also named Gordon Holmes, who had happily signed on and duly produced. Osler resolved the 'Gordon Holmes Jekyll and Hyde Episode' by buying out the accidental contributor. The real Holmes appeared in volume 7 in the company of such experts as Lewellys Barker and Harvey Cushing. Cushing wrote on tumors of the brain. In the years since Osler had left Hopkins, Cushing, working with ferocious energy, had made himself the best-known neurosurgeon in America and the most creative teacher at Johns Hopkins.

The books had a reasonable success in a very competitive marketplace, going into a five-volume second edition and apparently making money for the publisher. Osler did very handsomely with the *System*, collecting $10,000 on publication of the first volume and another $10,000 when the last was issued. McCrae earned about $1,100 a volume; the contributors were paid $4 a page.[32]

What Osler scoffed at as the old 'quiz-compend,' *The Principles and Practice of Medicine*, continued to dominate the textbook market. It was the required text at most of the better and many of the mediocre medical schools in North America and the United Kingdom and had been translated into several languages, including Chinese. Osler had seen *Principles and Practice* into its sixth edition before coming to Oxford, and in 1908 he dutifully made the revisions for a seventh.

Osler always grumbled about the time he had to spend on textbook revision, and in the preface to each new edition stressed how much he had altered. Textbook work is always a grind, though, and authors always try to hype the current edition. Despite the improvements Osler made with each revision – changing the order of chapters in one, switching a disease to a different category in another, adding new findings, especially on vaccines, the use of serums, and other therapies, improving the literary quality of single sentences or paragraphs, and eliminating some literary allusions only to add more – *The Principles and Practices of Medicine* was still fundamentally the same book in the 1909 seventh edition that it had been in the 1892 first edition. It remained an unusually well written guide to the clinicopathology of disease, with a heavy emphasis on infectious disease, and with up-to-date information on treatment by a physician whose skepticism about specific remedies had continued to grow. In the section on treatments for neurasthenia in the seventh edition he added a long paragraph on the utility of faith healing. On the other hand, he was now suggesting that gallbladder patients were 'much safer in the hands of a surgeon than when left to Nature, with the feeble assistance of drugs and mineral waters.'[33]

He incorporated such recent findings as the discovery of *Spirocheta pallida* in syphilis and August von Wassermann's development of a test for its presence. When Ronald Ross nailed down the mosquito as malaria carrier, Osler began recommending the use of mosquito netting (on visiting 1 West Franklin in Baltimore, Ross exclaimed loudly about the mosquito larvae he found infesting Osler's premises). Cushing's expertise could be detected in the updating of the sections on neurological disorders and diseases related to the pituitary. The measurement of blood pressure was becoming common and an important indicator in various conditions. Beginning with the fourth edition, the presentation of Hodgkin's disease had been greatly clarified by the new histological picture that had emerged from Johns Hopkins, thanks to the work of Dorothy Reed, the woman whom Osler had advised to 'go home.' The distinctive malignancy in Hodgkin's disease is the presence of what are still called Reed-Sternberg cells.

Like its author, the text was becoming storied in its own lifetime. Physicians corresponded with Osler about fine points ranging from pathological and therapeutic exotica to Greek exegesis and the differences between cats and dogs. Americans packed it off to Europe as their traveling medical companion. Medical students drew up gag exams about *Principles and Practice* ('Who was convinced that more wise men than fools are victims of gout? ... How did Eryximachus treat the hiccough of Aristophanes? ... Who had a translucent head? ... On what occasion was a surgeon entrapped by a neurotic physician?') and celebrated it in many stanzas of bad verse:

But when of the names we are weary
(Directories muddle the brain),
We're provided by you with philosophy too
In the trite Aphorisms of Cheyne.
Geography also you teach us,
Until I came under your thrall,
I don't mind confessing that Conoquenessing
I never had heard of at all.[34]

The stream of royalties remained an important source of income now that Osler's regius stipend was his only fixed income and he had cut back on his practice.

His real literary love at Oxford was the history of medicine. He had told Cushing that he might use his regius professorship to write it, and he got off to a magnificent start in 1906–7 with his two most important historical excursions, a far cry from the easy, feel-good *historia amabilis* he would later be accused of fostering.[35] The first foray, in October 1906, was what Cushing called the 'blue-ribbon event of British medicine,' the Harveian oration at the Royal College of Physicians. It was steeped in tradition, a lectureship founded by William Harvey himself in 1651. Each year's orator was directed to offer an address in Latin (that part of the tradition had ended in 1865), 'wherein shall be a commemoration of all the Benefactors of the said College by name ... with an exhortation to imitate these Benefactors ... and to the Fellows and Members to search and study out the secrets of Nature by way of experiment.' A general feast was to follow.

Many Harveian orators used the occasion to talk about recent medical achievements. With his reverence for 'the mighty minds of old ... the illustrious dead,' Osler chose to make his an historical talk. But it was more than another set of profiles of the illustrious dead or a paean to medical progress. Osler had become interested in the evolution of scientific knowledge, what he called 'the growth of truth,' and he used Harvey's announcement of his discovery of the circulation of the blood as a case study of the problem of establishing new truths in the teeth of received authority. Osler was not a naive believer in the easy progress of science through the overthrow of one idea after another. He clearly understood what modern generations see as the problem of the paradigms underlying scientific discourse and the relationship of discovery to paradigm shifts:

> All scientific truth is conditioned by the state of knowledge at the time of its announcement ... The growth of Truth corresponds to the states of knowledge described by Plato in the *Thaetetus* – acquisition, latent possession, conscious possession. Scarcely a discovery can be named which does not present these phases in its evolution ... Long years of labour gave us a full knowledge of syphilis; centuries of acquisition added one fact to another, until we had a body of clinical and pathological knowledge of remarkable fullness. For the last quarter of a century we have had latent possession of the cause of the disease ... The conscious possession has just been given to us ... But when these stages are ended, there remains the final struggle for general acceptance. Locke's remark that 'Truth scarce ever yet carried it by vote anywhere at its first appearance' is borne out by the history of all discoveries of the first rank. The times, however, are changing; and it is interesting to compare the cordial welcome of the pallid spirochaete with the chilly reception of the tubercle bacillus ... The seniors among us who lived through that instructive period remember well that only those who were awake when the dawn appeared assented at once to the brilliant demonstration. We are better prepared today.

The bulk of his lecture was a beautifully wrought portrait of Harvey's brilliant demonstration and its chilly reception by his mentor Fabricius, by Sir Kenelm Digby and Sir William Temple in England, and by Guy Patin and practically everyone else in France. Sir Thomas Browne shone almost alone in declaring that he preferred the circulation of the blood to the discovery of America.

Eventually, of course, Harvey's work was the foundation of a new paradigm. 'Once accepted, men had a feeling that so important a discovery must change all the usual conceptions of disease ... More important than any influence upon treatment was the irresistible change in the conceptions of disease caused by destruction of the doctrine of spirits and humours, which had prevailed from the days of Hippocrates.' More important still, Osler argued, was Harvey's methodological breakthrough, his use of experiment:

> While Bacon was thinking, Harvey was acting ... No longer were men to rest content with careful observation and with accurate description ... Here for the first time a great physiological problem was approached from the experimental side by a man with a modern scientific mind ... To the age of the hearer, in which men had heard, and heard only, had succeeded the age of the eye, in which men had seen and had been content only to see. But at last came the age of the hand – the thinking, devising, planning hand; the hand as an instrument of the mind ... from which we may date the beginning of experimental medicine.*[36]

Osler followed this train of thought in a 1907 address to the Congress of American Physicians and Surgeons on 'The Evolution of the Idea of Experiment in Medicine.' As he ranged forward in history, Osler acknowledged his own datedness. The work of the French school and Virchow, so inspiring in Osler's life, had been a last flourishing of the old Hippocratic art of observation, an illustration of what the 'rigid inductive method' could accomplish. Only in the second half of the century had the experimental

---

*Osler concluded his oration with another of his melancholy meditations on the dead who are not remembered. A few years later its references to the poppy and to rolls of names must have seemed haunting: 'While we are praising famous men ... the touching words of the son of Sirach remind us: "Some there be that have no memorial, who are perished as though they had never been, and are become as though they had never been born." Such renown as they had, time has blotted out; and on them the iniquity of oblivion has blindly scattered her poppy ... For the immense majority on the long roll of our Fellows – names! names! names! – nothing more; a catalogue as dry and meaningless as that of the ships in Homer, or as the genealogy of David in the Book of Chronicles ... Much of the nobility of the profession depends upon this great cloud of witnesses, who pass into the silent land – pass, and leave no sign, becoming as though they had never been born. And it was the pathos of this fate, not less pathetic because common to all but a few, that wrung from the poet that sadly true comparison of the race of man to the race of leaves!' Osler donated his fee from the Harveian oration to the college to enable it to put it order its collection of Harvey documents.

method come into its own in medicine and been recognized as the basis of science.

Osler slid from past to present in a plea for clinicians to cultivate the sciences and an admission that his own progress from science to the clinic was no longer a likely career path:

> One thing is certain; we clinicians must go to the physiologists, the pathologists and the chemists – they no longer come to us. To our irreparable loss these sciences have become so complicated and demand such life-long devotion that no longer do physiologists, like Hunter, Bowman and Lister, become surgeons, chemists, like Prout and Bence-Jones, clinicians, and saddest of all, the chair of pathology is no longer a stepping-stone to the chair of medicine. The new conditions must be met if progress is to be maintained.[37]

Osler included in this essay an important statement of the fundamental ethical issue in research. 'The limits of justifiable experimentation upon our fellow creatures are well and clearly defined. The final test of every new procedure, medical or surgical, must be made on man, but never before it has been tried on animals ... For man absolute safety and full consent are the conditions which make such tests allowable. We have no right to use patients entrusted to our care for the purpose of experimentation unless direct benefit to the individual is likely to follow. Once this limit is transgressed, the sacred cord which binds physician and patient snaps instantly. Risk to the individual may be taken with his consent and full knowledge of the circumstances ... Enthusiasm for science has, in a few instances, led to regrettable transgressions of the rule.' Osler's statements on scientific ethics are so few because he was usually in the company of physicians like himself who did not need to discuss them. These issues were on his mind in 1907 because of the Royal Commission on Vivisection, to which he had testified, mainly about the wonderful achievements of experimental research on animals in making possible the defeat of yellow fever and the consequent construction of the Panama Canal.

Osler's thoughts on history kept leading him to the present, which was where most of his audiences wanted him to be. On prize-giving days, he gave advice to graduates; to county medical societies he talked about the role of the country medical society; in hospital talks, he spoke about the future of hospitals. To the students of the London (Royal Free Hospital) School of Medicine for Women on July 4, 1907, he talked about the future of women in medicine. It was a satisfactory profession for women, he now believed, so long as they realized it was about much more than getting money. The greatest problem women faced in medicine, he suggested, was that other women did not trust them, which made their aptitude for work on diseases of women and children difficult to apply. He recommended that women get good advice from experienced female doctors before going into general practice, and that they consider such alternatives as medical missions in India and institutional staff work.

Osler told the medical women that there were excellent openings for their sex in laboratory work and in studies related to scientific medicine. To the male students at St Mary's Hospital a few months later, he also urged adopting the missionary spirit in medicine, but otherwise primed them with his usual advice as they prepared for the 'Derby' of medical education, 'where the field is large, the scratchings numerous, and the pace killing.' The key to their training would be learning the art of managing patients and curing disease. In an unusual reversal of field, Osler went out of his way to warn the St Mary's students against the advice of one of their distinguished professors, Almroth Wright, a bacteriologist and vaccine maker, who predicted that most medical problems would be resolved by lab work and immunization. 'Stop your ears with the wise man's wax against the wiles of that Celtic Siren, Sir Almroth, who would abolish Harley Street and all that it represents. There is still virtue, believe me, in that "long unlovely street" and the old art cannot possibly be replaced by, but must be absorbed in, the new science.'[38]

Osler still had contributions to make to both art and science. He gave fewer original papers in these years but, as befitted an elder statesman, was often an active participant in clinical discussions at medical meetings, especially sessions of the British Medical Association. Certain rare clinical conditions continued to interest him especially. In 1907 he gave the Royal

Society of Medicine an update on 'Splenic Polycythaemia with Cyanosis' (Vaquez-Osler disease) of which forty or fifty cases had been reported since his trail-breaking 1903 paper. On his first visit back to Hopkins he was excited to see on the wards a patient who had a hereditary condition of multiple capillary lesions, or telangiectases, similar to three patients he had described in a minor paper in 1901. He saw the patient again the next year, and in October 1907 pulled together all the case reports in an article 'On Multiple Hereditary Telangiectases with Recurring Haemorrhages' for his new *Quarterly Journal of Medicine*. This condition, which most often led to recurring nosebleeds, became known as 'Osler-Weber-Rendu disease.'[39] In the next issue of the *Quarterly Journal*, Osler collaborated with the brilliant London clinician and scientist Archibald Garrod to discuss a rare case of ochronosis, or blackening of the cartilege, fibrous tissues, and urine. They had both published previously on the disorder; eventually, Garrod's studies of this and other rare urinary disorders would be recognized as pioneering work in metabolic errors and the concept of biochemical individuality.[40]

Continuing a remarkable series of clinical publications for a man allegedly in semi-retirement, Osler completed a quarter-century study of endocarditis with an important article describing the subacute bacterially caused form. He drew particular attention to the appearance of painful nodular spots on the hands and feet of sufferers; these became known as 'Osler's nodes.'[41] Finally, in a new edition of Allbutt's *System of Medicine*, he returned to Stokes-Adams disease, not only updating his 1903 paper with more cases but coordinating his work with the brilliant pathological findings of Arthur Keith and utilizing observations made by the new electrocardiograph machine. The Osler-Keith study for the first time located Stokes-Adams symptoms as products of lesions in the 'Bundle of His.' Osler had little to say in this paper about heredity in Stokes-Adams, nothing that referred to his own family. His good health since coming to England may have convinced him that he did not have to worry about his slow pulse.[42]

His only regret about life at Oxford was the relative lack of students to teach. There was nothing to compare with the scores of bright acolytes he had trained and worked with at Johns Hopkins. But there were always a few, and for some of them Osler made a huge difference. He had not been at Oxford two months, for example, before he was approached by Miss Mabel Purefoy FitzGerald, a young woman who had been allowed to do research in physiology at Oxford, though not to take a degree. She needed access to the Radcliffe Infirmary for experimental work. Osler made it happen, encouraged and befriended her, and helped her obtain a Rockefeller Travelling Fellowship for work in America. Catching up with one of its pioneering female scientists, Oxford finally granted Mabel Purefoy FitzGerald her degree in 1972 at the age of one hundred.[43]

Gertrude Flumerfelt, daughter of well-to-do Canadians, was probably in the audience for Osler's address on women in medicine at the London School in 1907. A student there, she got to know Osler, was a regular guest at the 'Open Arms,' and probably had Osler's help in getting admitted to clinical studies at Manchester. Osler called her Trotula, an appellation that mystified her until she learned of the sixteenth-century female surgeon who had first been accused of quackery but was vindicated and became a great success. 'In every stage of my medical life, from the day of my first meeting, Sir William stood by me, a very present help in all days of need,' Gertrude recalled. The modern Trotula – her husband and many friends adopted the name for her – was not accused of quackery; she became a distinguished consultant in her own right and married a leading British neurosurgeon, Sir Geoffrey Jefferson.[44]

'We are in clover,' Osler wrote from an American relative's apartment on the avenue d'Iéna in Paris in November 1908.[45] He had decided to have a winter's sabbatical, his first since beginning teaching. The sumptuous accommodation included a beautiful library and two servants. With Revere in school, Grace joined him. They took conversational French lessons over breakfast, Oxford got on without its regius, and the delightful break coincided with the publication of another major anthology of his literary work, *An Alabama Student and Other Biographical Essays.*

They avoided the American colony in Paris, 'everybody in fact, as I wished to be in seclusion as much as possible & Mrs. Osler has had such a busy year that she needed rest.' Osler visited hospitals and attended lectures in the mornings and buried himself in libraries after lunch. He went through the expected professional motions – assisting at clinics, earnestly studying and writing about French medical education ('the work done is first class, considering the wretched state of most of the hospitals'),[46] witnessing and writing about student and intern riots against changes in the examination system, and doing a modicum of socializing with his French colleagues. The brain dusting also took him far from wards, clinics, and medical libraries. He attended a course on Rabelais and lectures by Henri Bergson on Bishop Berkeley, bought old Berkeley editions that Bergson had said were unobtainable, and immersed himself in Swinburne, the most francophile, sensuous (and tedious) of English poets. Despite the lessons and his Montreal background, he could never speak more than a few words of French or any other foreign language – perhaps because, as he put it, he had never acquired the best aid for learning a language, 'a sleeping dictionary.'[47]

He took a special and revealing interest in French appreciation of the dead, as reflected in the celebration of *Toussaint*, All Saints Day, on November 1. Osler made it a three-day ritual. On October 31 he went back to Montparnasse Cemetery to lay another wreath on the tomb of Louis. Standing inside the 'Gates of Grief' at the entrance to the cemetery, he watched a procession of flower-laden visitors:

A group of young schoolgirls passed, each one bearing a bunch of chrysanthemums to lay on the tomb of a fellow pupil or of a loved teacher; close at hand were two Sisters of Mercy arranging wreaths on a vault that looked one of the oldest in the cemetery – perhaps the annual devotion of the guild to a loved member. A little laddie of eight hurried by with a bunch of violets in his hand, running with the ease of one who knew his road. A young mother in deep mourning with a baby in her arms, an aged couple arm in arm, each with a little basket of flowers, two young students, a little old lady with her daughter followed by a footman carrying large wreaths, workmen in rough clothes, soldiers, sailors – a motley group, a touching sight, but on the whole not a sad one ... The general impression was of a cheerful festival, and the glorious sunshine, the bright flowers and the merry voices of the children helped to dispel the gloom of the city of the dead.

Osler spent the next two days among the hundreds of thousands of Parisians who were strewing with flowers the famous cemetery of Père La-chaise. He succeeded in a special mission to find the grave of the great pathologist-anatomist M.F.X. Bichat and was pleased to see that it was adorned with flowers; he added his own bunch of pansies 'for thoughts.' Osler later told American readers that the strongest single impression left by his sabbatical was of the reverence of the French. 'There are more stat-ues to medical men in Paris than in Great Britain and the United States put together ... Every Frenchman is a hero worshipper, and has a master, dead or alive, whom he adores.' *Toussaint* seemed to him a magnificent demon-stration of loyalty and reverence, obviously a quasi-religious ceremony: 'To the cold-blooded Anglo-Saxon this festival of the dead is a revelation, which he can not witness without profound emotion and without a regret that England and America miss in great part the moral and intellectual inspiration associated with such celebrations. France sings one song: 'Glory to Man in the highest! for Man is the Master of all things,' with which words Swinburne (who has been of all modern Englishmen the most sym-pathetic interpreter of the French) ends his famous "Hymn of Man."'[48]

He found time in Paris to take in an aerial demonstration by the Wright brothers and to sit for a portrait by Seymour Thomas, another fashionable American expatriate artist. Most portraits and photographs of Osler after the 1880s feature a stiff, wooden figure, larger than he was in life, whose mouth disappears behind his mustache – a codger from the age of Colonel Blimp who bears little resemblance to the free-spirited little man-in-motion everyone remembered. His dress is always fashionable. His pate is mostly bald, his remaining hair and mustache are beginning to gray. The difference in the Thomas portrait is his eyes, which are particularly shad-owed, dark, and intense, as in some pictures from his McGill years. Osler has taken off glasses to see more clearly. 'I feel that you can look clear through me and see the wall on the other side,' Thomas said to him during the sittings.[49] The Thomas portrait became the Oslers' favorite; the artist kept it for his own collection.

In mid-January 1909 the Oslers moved south to Cannes, where Willie was sick for two weeks but 'delighted with everything ... I am thinking of settling at Monte Carlo ... I lost $25 in five minutes & then stopped ... So far as women are concerned this is the Remnant Counter of Europe.' In February it was 'Rome at last!' Their breath was taken away, Grace put it, 'by the wonders of Rome – and by the horrors of modern Rome.' The Italian holiday was filled with visits to shrines, including the ruins of an Aesculapian temple, to churches, bookshops, and, thanks to special connections, to the Vatican Reading Room. Osler delighted in its treasures, of course, but the most powerful impression came from 'the odour of unwashed humanity to a marked degree, that smell of clothes soaked with sweat ... On entering the room it was evident, & it became intensified as the morning wore on.'[50]

Osler's belief in the healing power of faith was reinforced by seeing the crutches, braces, trusses, and other instruments scattered before the Madonna del Porto, the madonna who helps pregnant women. The toes of her left foot were worn away by the kisses of the faithful. He also made a pilgrimage to the mother church of Saints Cosmos and Damian, the patrons saints of surgery, where he 'burnt a candle – a small one' for his surgical colleagues. The instruments with which they cut off a leg which had a cancer & transplanted the sound leg of a just dead man are carefully preserved in the church – with an arm of each saint and a bottle of the milk of the Virgin Mary.'[51]

They went on to Florence, Venice, Bologna, Padua, and Milan before returning to England in April. On his travels Osler had won the lifelong love of several little girls and their dolls, whom he had befriended, played with, and written to. He had also been called on to help several sick Americans. He 'sanctified' one of his fees by spending it on three copies of the 1543 edition of Vesalius's *Fabrica,* one for himself, one to give to McGill, the third for the library of the Maryland faculty. In Rome he saw a remarkable case, a robust Australian doctor who suddenly became severely purpuric from hemorrhaging blood vessels, turning plum-colored everywhere except under one patch of skin where he had put a mustard leaf. The patient died fifteen minutes after Osler saw him. The regius wondered whether it could have been a case of malignant smallpox; perhaps he recalled poor Neville in Montreal thirty-five years earlier.[52]

He wound up his sabbatical with a strenuous two months in America, visiting all his old cities and friends. The most important ceremonial occasion was the opening in May 1909 of the Medical and Chirurgical Faculty of Maryland's new building, one of whose rooms was named Osler Hall. Osler gave the main oration, noting, of course, the rarity of participating in a dedication to oneself. Europe was on his mind as he explored the relationship of past and present, the need for all institutions to blend old with new. He quoted William James's recent remark, 'We live forward, we understand backwards,' and struck his usual balance in preaching reverence for the past and relevance and leadership in the present. He concluded with another statement of his near-mystical sense of the way in which the living were bound by the dead:

> The best of all old things about this Faculty is that subtle force by which the
> men of the past influence us today – not by tradition, by the spoken word
> handed on from father to son, teacher to pupil; not by the written record in
> which one generations reads of the deeds of another, but by that intangible,
> mysterious force hard to define but best expressed in the words *noblesse oblige*
> – that obligation to act in a certain way, to foster certain habits, to conform
> to certain unwritten laws – a sacred obligation, as potent now as in the time
> of Hippocrates, the alchemy of which at once turns to gold whatever may
> be leaden in the new of today.[53]

Looking forward, Osler spent several days in Boston, where medical history was coming close to repeating itself in Peter Bent Brigham's legacy to build a great new hospital that would be associated with the Harvard Medical School, a second Johns Hopkins. Osler rebuffed feelers to come back as medical director. One of his former students, Henry Christian, was dean of the Harvard Medical School, and the Bostonians were probably already scheming to lure Harvey Cushing to be the Brigham's marquis surgeon.

'What an age of growth everywhere!' Osler exclaimed towards the end of his North American stay.[54] By 1909 the spirit of what everyone called 'modern' medical education was sweeping the United States and Canada as universities and medical schools made plans to join forces, lengthen courses, raise admission standards, pour millions into laboratories and hospitals, introduce clinical clerkships, and hire the best scientists and clinicians they could find. Splendid new medical buildings were rising from the ashes at McGill. The University of Toronto was about to get a great teaching hospital in the rebuilt Toronto General. Philanthropists and their foundations were about to pour resources into medicine, betting with their money that it offered more hope for the future than theology. The Carnegie Foundation, working with the American Medical Association, had commissioned a special study of medical education with a view to certifying the most progressive schools and stamping out the laggards.

Osler ended his sabbatical and summed up much of his career with a sweeping address to the Ontario Medical Association in June 1909 on 'The Treatment of Disease.' He talked of the revolution in his lifetime in the conceptualization of disease – how the discovery of microbial causes had led to wonderfully successful campaigns, not for cure but for prevention; how the understanding of etiology had led to the realization that the body could be strengthened to resist and throw off infection, as in the modern treatment of tuberculosis; above all, how the profession had learned to accept its limits, be honest, and turn its back on 'quack-like promises to heal.'

Osler thought he saw the prospect of a new era in the triumphs of metabolic therapy. He speculated to his audience in Toronto (more presciently than he could ever have dreamed) that 'as our knowledge of the pancreatic function and carbo-hydrate metabolism becomes more accurate we shall probably be able to place the treatment of diabetes on a sure foundation.' In the meantime, he warned against false and misleading therapies, whether peddled through the old-fashioned faith in polypharmacy or through the new products and pamphlets of the pharmaceutical houses. 'Far too large a section of the treatment of disease is to-day controlled by the big manufacturing pharmacists, who have enslaved us in a plausible pseudo-science,' Osler warned in 1909.

He gave his audience detailed advice on the knowledge medical students should have of drugs that relieved suffering, and he meditated on the uses of the kind of faith he had seen in shrines and temples in Europe. He had no regrets about his opposition to indiscriminate drugging that had led to his being branded a therapeutic nihilist. 'The blind faith which some men have in medicines illustrates too often the greatest of all human capacities – the capacity for self-deception.' No one should delude himself that medicine could do much for cancer or pneumonia. Were such dashed hopes an indictment of all the wonderful developments in medicine?

> Some one will say, Is this all your science has to tell us? Is this the outcome of decades of good clinical work, of patient study of the disease, of anxious trial in such good faith of so many drugs? Give us back the childlike trust of the fathers in antimony and in the lancet rather than this cold nihilism. Not at all! Let us accept the truth, however unpleasant it may be, and with the death rate staring us in the face, let us not be deceived with vain fancies. Not alone in pneumonia, but in the treatment of certain other diseases, do we need a stern, iconoclastic spirit which leads, not to nihilism, but to an active skepticism – not the passive skepticism, born of despair, but the active skepticism born of a knowledge that recognizes its limitations and knows full well that only in this attitude of mind can true progress be made. There are those among us who will live to see a true treatment of pneumonia.[55]

Having finished his sabbatical, having done his duties and seen his friends and summarized medical progress to audiences in America, Osler sailed for home on the *Empress of Britain*. He read a life of the Brontë sisters during the crossing. On June 26, 1909, less than three weeks from his sixtieth birthday, he returned to Oxford to pick up the rhythms of that delightful life and place.

Back in his study at 13 Norham Gardens, Osler would have opened parcel after parcel of books shipped home from the antiquarian shops of France and Italy. Book collecting and the study of medical bibliography was now edging off his agenda the clinical case studies that had long ago overtaken the pathological work. Bibliomania was the hobbyhorse Osler rode for the rest of his days. In a talk about it, he suggested that one of the best features of British life was the tendency of physicians to have hobbies. 'No man is really happy or safe without one ... Anything will do so long as he straddles a hobby and rides it hard.' The continental wandering prepared Osler for much hard riding to come with book dealers and at the auction houses (though at a Paris auction in 1908 he was still too shy to bid among all the dealers), for it stimulated his interest in medical incunabula, the scarce and often obscure products of the infancy of printing in the latter half of the fifteenth century. He also continued to build a good collection of English literary works.

Just as he had done in America, he promoted medical reading and libraries. At the Belfast meeting of the British Medical Association in midsummer 1909, Osler became the first president of a new Medical Library Association for the United Kingdom (it proved short-lived) and gave a major talk on books and libraries for physicians. At Oxford he gloried in his access to the Bodleian. 'Very soon there was a feeling that a day had not been well spent if altogether away from Bodley. I envied the men who could be there all day and every day.'[56] At his college, Christ Church, he found that the books from Robert Burton's library were scattered indiscriminately through the collections, and arranged to have them reassembled and shelved together under Burton's portrait. On January 23, 1910, he was a guest in Cambridge for Magdalene College's annual dinner in honor of Samuel Pepys, whose library was splendidly preserved there. Osler became a last-minute substitute for a missing speaker. 'Such a delightful occasion.' Such experiences caused him to begin to reflect, as all hard-riding hobbyists must, on the fate of his own horse. What would happen to his library when he died?[57]

The thought that it would pass to his son and heir was tempered in these years by Osler's concern that young Revere was no scholar. In letter after letter, he referred to the boy's trouble learning Greek and Latin and his apparent disinterest in books and other studies, despite his happiness with English life. What Revere really liked, in fact loved with a passion, was fishing. So now, to his dad, Revere's nickname Isaac (or Ike) had angling as well as biblical connotations (his other nickname, Tommy, may have come from Sir Thomas Browne, or Browne's son Thomas, or from the British Tommy craze of the 1890s). Revere would have owned and read at an early age a copy of Izaak Walton's *The Compleat Angler*. His father would certainly have longed to buy the pristine 1653 first edition of Walton he saw auctioned, 'amid suppressed excitement,' at Sotheby's in 1907. Osler jotted down the bidding as the book finally went for £1,290, three times the previous record price. Medical books were much cheaper: Over the years, Osler picked up several copies of Harvey's *De mortu cordis* (1628) at prices ranging from £8 to £48. At the end of the twentieth century, Harvey sold at Christie's for over $550,000.[58]

Osler often took Revere fishing, in and around Oxford and especially on the family's regular vacations to the ends of the British Isles. Hard as he worked and traveled, an annual vacation in a secluded resort town was part of Osler's ritual. He swam and took 'headers' (dove), walked, golfed, fished, and, of course, read and wrote. In 1908, very much against Grace's inclinations, the Oslers bought a Renault motor car and hired a chauffeur to drive it. Their first long excursion was up the Great North Road to Scotland for fishing in Highland streams, with a week in the Lake District and an excursion into North Wales on the way back. The weather was glorious and 'the river was so low & clear that the trout winked at Revere & passed the time of day with his flies.' Wordsworth's granddaughter kindly showed them all the treasures of the house at Grasmere. 'We have had such a happy time,' Osler wrote.

Next summer they went about as far south as one can go in the United Kingdom, spending a week at Sennen Cove, a mile from Land's End. Osler and Revere went ocean fishing and both got seasick. The waters were probably more accommodating off Swanage, the Dorset port they had enjoyed so much a decade earlier, where they now spent another week. In 1910 the summer holiday was at Pointe-au-Pic, Quebec, immediately after arriving in America. Revere fished the month away while his parents rested and then went on their visiting rounds to Montreal, Toronto, Hamilton, Boston, Baltimore, Washington, Bar Harbor, Newport, and New York, 'trying to see the new generation of babies everywhere.'[59]

Osler's health was fairly good as he entered his sixties. 'I have kept very well, only when pressed or worried the sub-sternal tension returns,' he wrote after the sabbatical.[60] Colds and bronchial infections periodically immobilized him, but he used those days busily in bed, catching up on reading and writing. In January 1910 he had a recurrence of the kidney colic of eight years earlier. There were no practical jokes this time as the physician observed himself and his pain to the limits of his tolerance:

> Periods of complete freedom, extending from two to three, to eight or ten hours, attenuated with three types of disturbance of sensation – a dull, steady, localised pain, the situation of which could be covered with a penny. It could be imitated exactly by firm pressure with the handle of a knife, or, indeed, with a finger upon a bone, particularly upon that tender spot on the sternum just a little above the ensiform cartilage. Lasting for hours and unmoved it was fairly bearable. Now and then, when free from pain, there were remarkable flashes, an explosive sort of sensation, not actually unpleasant, and accompanied by a glow-like wave along the course of the ureter and out through the flank, as it were through the muscles. And then abruptly, or working out of the steady pain, came the paroxysm, like a twisting, tearing hurricane, with its well-known radiation, followed by the vasovagal features, the pallor, cold extremities, feeble pulse, sweating, nausea, vomiting, and in two attacks, a final, not altogether unpleasant period, when unconsciousness and the pain seemed wrestling for a victory reached only with the help of God's own medicine – morphia.[61]

His 'rocky experience' took 'a week of squirming,' he wrote a medical friend. 'It only bowled me over twice into the faint & puking stage but it bored for hours at a time.' He thought gout was at the bottom of his troubles and said he would have to live on distilled water and grits. Surgery was a possibility, but the pain subsided, apparently as a stone passed. Through 1910 Osler continued to feel loose rocks rattling at the end of busy days, or Gibraltar about to chip, he wrote, and apparently cut the 1910 American trip short because of them. Examination by x-ray did not show any large stones, but in later years Osler felt occasional twinges of gout: 'I cannot take a glass of champagne without feeling it in my great toe.'[62]

Not a pebble stirred on long donkey rides the next winter as Osler joined brother E.B.'s Canadian group on a lavish Egyptian tour. For a month they cruised the Nile on a deluxe launch arranged by Thomas Cook & Sons, stopping every so often for donkey-back excursions to pyramids, temples, and tombs. One night the donkeys took them in full evening dress to a dinner party with the local pasha, who had two sons at Oxford. 'I looked they said like the picture of the white Knight in Alice.'

Grace, who hated heat and dust and did not think they should both be that far from Revere, stayed home. Willie sent her and everyone else a blizzard of letters and cards describing the sights, the weather, the boatmen (he thought they all looked like descendants of Ramses II), and his observations on medical and bibliographical Egypt. The Egyptian Hospital in Cairo reminded him of Blockley in Philadelphia, 'only smellier & dirtier.' The khedival librarian tried to interest him in trading ornate Korans with the Bodleian in exchange for certain manuscripts 'taken' from Egypt in the seventeenth century. He read Herodotus on the voyage up the Nile to Assuan (Aswán) and found the journey into history breathtaking: 'Heavens what feeble pigmies we are! Even with steam, electricity and the Panama Canal.' The modern Egyptians were less impressive: 'If the ordinary Egyptian could be made sanitary the country would be a paradise but it is dirty beyond description & the amount of ophthalmia & hookworm disease is appalling.' Osler thought that Egypt, a British dependency, would do better under German authority.[63]

Early on the trip he had to take time to examine the Canadian millionaire Sir James Ross, who was making the same tour and had an attack of pericarditis. Ross's boat shadowed the Oslers' for the rest of the trip as the old tycoon vowed to stay close to his doctor. Osler saw him almost every day – 'He says I have saved his life' – and the fees more than paid for his share of the trip's cost. After the Egypt trip Ross insisted that they cross the Mediterranean on his private yacht.[64]

'What sights we have seen!' Willie wrote Grace towards the end of it. 'I am choc-a-bloc full. I shall read nothing but Egypt for the rest of my days.' He added: 'I will not have lost much by being away. There are always a good many expenses about me – town & taxies mount up in the course of a month. Only we must save the money for the boy. On the whole we have not done badly but I fear the time when my income will be very small, & expenses the same, or with the boy starting, even larger. Still if anything happened to me you would have £18,000 and the house – which would enable you to live & keep up my contributions to the family ... We have done pretty well. And you have been an angel! How you have borne with me all these years!'[65]

These Egyptian letters are William's only surviving correspondence with Grace. In them, husband chats to wife familiarly. He teases her about all the world coming to visit this summer and having only invited every other person he has met.[66] He tries to reassure her about Revere, who seems to have been in danger of having to leave Winchester school: 'Please do not worry, that boy will come out all right – good health, sweet disposition – hang the brains – they might only get him into trouble ... Dear lad – No one could help liking him when one got under that Oslerian shell of re-serve ... He may pull up now & do well. We must not be discouraged.'[67] He reassures her that the souvenir presents he is bringing back are not trash and that the thousand Egyptian cigarettes are good value. He makes jokes about missing her – 'I am just furious that you are not here. I have no one to squeeze – I cannot squeeze my blood relatives and Elsie B. is too thin' – and imagines her as 'poor patient Grizal – sitting quietly at home, spinning while I am loafing.' He often signs off 'Your loving Egerton.' The fees from further consultations lead to more presents, including dress fabric, 'that nice camel hair & silk stuff, all embroidered.'[68] He brings back a mummi-fied crocodile for Revere.

Revere was now a struggling student at Winchester College, one of Britain's great boarding schools. None of the father's letters to the son have survived from these or earlier years. There must have been many, and they would not have been anxious; they would have been full of love and play, and fish stories. Osler delighted in children's company even more as

he aged. Here are two letters he wrote to the little girls and their dolls he
had befriended in Paris and Rome:

Dear Susan:

It was so sweet and kind of you to send that nice photograph, I have got it in
my room next the great big one which shows you feeding the pigeons; only
I do feel a bit sad that you have not on your lap my darling Rosalie, instead
of that stuck-up, overdressed, disagreeable, plain Marguerite! I do hope you
have washed Rosalie's face for the year, & given her a clean petticoat &
some new gloves! I am sending you a photo. Revere is at home, but is just
going back to school ... I hope to see you in the summer, & then I shall bring
back Rosalie to live with me. Please tell her & give her a kiss. Yours
affectionately, Wm. Osler. O O O O for you O O O for Rosalie.   for
Marguerite.

Dear Muriel-Marjorie-Maude!

... I cannot come to Rome this spring; on the even-alternate years my wife
is very cross in the spring, and only allows me out every day, and I could not
possibly get away as far as Rome ... I have not had a decent cup of tea since
last winter with you and those angelic friends of yours. Give them my love.

My boy is so horrid – has turned into a Winchester man! He has just
come home. I had to go on in ink with this, as my fluffy-headed stenographer struck her fist on the table, and said she did not come here to take
down nonsense – not she, not from any man! What do you think I said?
Nothing – but I gave her a basilisk look, & she fainted dead away & is
groaning with her fluffy head in the waste-paper basket & there she can
stay until I finish this.[69]

While Willie was in Egypt, Grace looked after the mail. She was glad
she had avoided the Egyptian heat. 'And another reason I am glad,' she
wrote home to America, 'is that I have read in his absence letters from
young doctors, old doctors, men of all ages, which made me feel more than
ever how wonderful an influence Dr. Osler has been in the profession.
How proud I am of him *no one* can believe.'[70]

TEN

Sir William

Some of his American friends had cynically predicted that Osler would end up in England with a title. Regius professors were ideal candidates for honors, and soon after Osler arrived in Oxford the King's physician, Sir William Broadbent, had told him that the wheels had been set in motion. Osler asked him to stop the wheels. 'I was a stranger, regarded as an American, and it was hardly fair to give me any titular distinction in so early a period of my residence.' He knew it would be said he was a title hunter. Broadbent died and Osler thought nothing more about titles. He was apparently taken by surprise in June 1911 to hear from Prime Minister H.H. Asquith that it was intended to confer a baronetcy on him in the honors list accompanying the coronation of George V.

'What excuse are you going to give for declining it?' Grace asked him. 'You always have said you would.'

'I think I'll have to accept – Canada will be so pleased – there's only one Canadian baronet.' In his autobiographical notes for that year, Osler also stressed the Canadian and family connection: 'I am awfully glad for the sake of the family in Canada. It has been a long pull from the parsonage at Tecumseth to a Baronetcy of the United Kingdom. I only wish father and mother could have lived to see it, and my brother BB and my sister Nellie.' To his sister Chattie he said it was really a matter of swimming with the tide. 'These court honours mean so much here ...

I am glad for the family ... It is wonderful how a bad boy may fool his fellows if he once gets to work.'[1] In 1912 E.B. Osler was also knighted.

He would become Sir William Osler, Bart., and the title would pass to Revere and later male heirs. There was an instant flood of congratulatory messages from three countries, more than a thousand in all. Eventually, the Oslers thanked every correspondent. Osler said to many friends that he had had much more than his share in life and didn't need this. Grace Revere was bemused, telling the Cushings, 'It seems all very nice but *never* can he be anything but "Dr. Osler." It seems unnatural otherwise ... Lady Osler!!!!! Gosh!!!!!!' A little girl whom Osler had treated for diabetes and charmed with his magical nonsense exclaimed on hearing the news, 'Oh dear. They should have made him King.'[2]

Osler skipped the coronation ceremonies, partly because of the illness of a friend and patient, E.A. Abbey, a prominent Anglo-American artist. J. William White, the distinguished Philadelphia surgeon, who had known Abbey and Osler for years and probably introduced them, crossed the Atlantic to be present at exploratory surgery on Abbey. Nothing could be done, and Abbey soon died.

In an almost literal way, everyone Osler knew became his patient. White himself, a man of fanatical energy and enthusiasms, especially for strenuous exercise, consulted Osler several times about his chest pains. Osler advised him to slow down. 'I wish I hadn't asked him to examine me,' White grumbled good-naturedly. He would reduce throttle, become deeply unhappy, and then go right back to full speed. Osler apparently decided his troubles were purely neurotic but kept touting the merits of a quieter life on general principles. White continued mostly to ignore him, though Osler did manage to persuade him to retire gracefully from his chair of surgery at the University of Pennsylvania. [3]

Another American, the distinguished philosopher William James, had turned down an Osler offer of hospitality during an Oxford visit (to give the Hibbert Lectures) because he was suffering from nervous fatigue. In fact he had serious angina, and at some point during his 1908 stay in England, Osler was called on to treat him. Soon afterwards Osler received a letter from James's younger brother, Henry, who felt he too had symptoms of heart disease. Osler referred Henry James to Sir James Mackenzie, a London consultant, who told the novelist that he was mainly suffering from the dread of the unknown that he had so beautifully immortalized in his story 'The Turn of the Screw.' William James's daughter also came to see Osler – about a stomach pain she thought might be appendicitis. Osler diagnosed nervous fatigue and prophesied that the pains would disappear with rest. They did.[4]

In 1910 Henry James fell into deep depression, simultaneously expecting, fearing, and wanting death. A relative's suggestion that he see Dr Osler, in James's words 'a very high authority – the highest, doubtless' – had an immediately cheering effect. In London in March 1910 Osler gave Henry James (who had been following the fad of overchewing, or 'Fletcherizing,' his food) the most complete physical examination he had ever had. A nephew described the occasion and the outcome:

> Uncle Henry was in a bad way with his digestion and his nerves. He'd been Fletcherizing for several years, was getting old and beginning to go to pieces. Osler frisked round him, jollyed him, poked fun at him, cheered him up; told him (in Greek) that his only trouble was that he was revolving round his belly-button etc. He prescribed a reasonable regimen & imposed a nurse who was to massage. But that involved the sort of mistake that I don't believe Osler made often. It would have required constant and authoritative supervision to make my Uncle stick to any regimen (he was too old, too domineering and too far gone nervously) and the nurse – as a matter of fact – lasted less than 24 hours after I'd turned my back. Still it was a reassuring and refreshing episode.[5]

Osler did not bother to charge for seeing William James's daughter, but he did send Henry James a bill for his normal London consultation fee, £44, which he regretted on hearing a rumor that the novelist was short of money. The story was an exaggeration, the bill was paid, and Henry James eventu-

ally pulled out of his depression and lived until 1916. William James died
of heart failure in North America in the summer of 1910.[6]

Osler examined Henry James the day before he delivered the second of
his three Lumleian Lectures to the Royal College of Physicians of London.
He was revisiting angina pectoris, having seen another two hundred cases
since his 1896 lectures. While saying little that he had not anticipated on
the basis of his first sixty cases (his angina population continued to be
heavily weighted by worried middle-aged male physicians), Osler was witty,
expansive, and medically humble: 'Fullness of knowledge does not always
bring confidence; the more one knows the more timidity may grow.' He
had seen too many men live for years with severe angina, too many apparently mild cases die suddenly, and, now that postmortem data was coming
in, too many confusing and contradictory pathological findings to be confident in a prognosis. Angina kept reminding him of the Hippocratic dic-
tum: Experience is fallacious and judgment difficult.

With angina, as in so many areas of his medical thinking, Osler was bridging a gulf – in this case, between those who saw it as a reflection of measurable cardiovascular lesions and a newer school of physiologically oriented
heart men who were interested solely in the system's ability to keep pumping. He spanned both models by zeroing in on angina as a pain that could
have multiple causes. Later heart specialists who reduced their notion of
angina to a simple symptom of blocked arteries or infarction would miss some
of the complexities of the condition, and of the heart's disorders, that Osler
had catalogued through long and patient observation.[7]

While he now had considerable experience in emergency treatment of
heart problems – and, in severe cases, used such powerful drugs as nitro-
glycerin and chloroform – for most of his patients Osler could only continue to fall back on lifestyle advice: Slow down the machine, care for it
better, and hope for the best. But he did vary his imagery, more often comparing the body to an automobile than a steamship. As both a doctor and
an automobile owner, he understood the pecularities of machines sold as
though they were identical. As he explained in a later lecture,

Take a dozen of 1911 Napiers turned out of the same shops, on the same pattern, with the same parts, and of the same horse power, and driven with the same make of petrol. Not all will last the same time, not all will wear as well; one will run 20 miles to the gallon, another only 16. One is in the shops every few months, the other is as good as new at the end of the year. And it is not a matter of the chauffeur alone, in the way the machine is driven, or the care which is taken, there are curious differences in spite of the similarity, indeed of the identity of the machines. And the same is true of men.

After the Egyptian trip, where he had seen huge irrigation systems in action, Osler favored metaphors of pumps and piping systems, sluices, drains, and canals to describe the workings of the heart and arteries. With these he could accommodate blood-pressure data and the beginnings of work on the physiological response to stress, as well as having an even better model for encompassing both structural and functional problems.[8]

At the end of three long state-of-the-art Lumleian Lectures on a disease central to his private practice, Osler was uncertain. He had 'unmixed satisfaction' at his professional experience with typhoid fever, totally opposite feelings about pneumonia, and only guarded satisfaction about angina. 'No known disease kills so peacefully, so painlessly and there has been real and solid progress in the advance of our knowledge of how to treat it.' On the basis of a case he had seen in Italy, Osler made the prescient forecast that heart disease in women would increase as they took up smoking. Otherwise the formula stayed the same: 'I usually give two prescriptions – "Go slowly," "Eat less" – on which I find a great many patients put about the same value as did Naaman on the prescription of Elisha ... Like longevity, angina pectoris is largely a question of the arteries. It is an old story, this association of a long life with a small intake.'

Osler felt by 1910 that he was 'no longer in active work, rather in the rear guard than in the van.' In that very year a younger American, James Herrick, gave the first of his great papers delineating the concepts of coronary thrombosis and myocardial infarction.[9] British colleagues who saw Osler practice in those years judged that some of their countrymen, such as

Clifford Allbutt, had better clinical skills, but Osler was still near the top
of the heap. When even his vast experience played him false, there was
the extraordinary personality to fall back on, a reserve Allbutt did not
have. Some Britishers thought Osler was simply too good to be true; others
joined the congregation. Here, in the recollections of a son of one of his
colleagues, Osler misses a prognosis and recoups wonderfully:

> One remembers a young brother with very severe whooping-cough and
> bronchitis, unable to eat and wholly irresponsive to the blandishments of
> parents and devoted nurses alike. Clinically it was not an abstruse case,
> but weapons were few and recovery seemed unlikely. The Regius, about to
> present for degrees and hard pressed for time, arrived already wearing his
> doctor's robes [gowns]. To a small child this was the advent of a doctor, if
> doctor it in fact was, from quite a different planet. It was more probably
> Father Christmas.
>
> After a very brief examination this unusual visitor sat down, peeled a
> peach, sugared it and cut it in pieces. He then presented it bit by bit with a
> fork to the entranced patient, telling him to eat it up, and that he would not
> be sick but would find it did him good as it was a most special fruit. Such
> proved to be the case. As he hurried off Osler, *most uncharacteristically*, pat-
> ted my father on the back and said with deep concern 'I'm sorry Ernest but
> I don't think I shall see the boy again, there's very little chance when they're
> as bad as that.' Happily events turned out otherwise, and for the next forty
> days this constantly busy man came to see the child, and for each of these
> forty days he put on his doctor's robes in the hall before going in to the sick
> room.
>
> After some two or three days, recovery began to be obvious and the
> small boy always ate or drank and retained some nourishment which Osler
> gave him with his own hands. If the value of personal approach, the quick
> turning to effect of an accidental psychological advantage (in this case
> decor), the consideration and extra trouble required to meet the needs of
> an individual patient, were ever well illustrated, here it was in its finest
> flower. It would, I submit, be impossible to find a fairer example of healing
> as an art.[10]

Oxford students were as dazzled as Americans had been by Osler's evident love of and enthusiasm for his profession and by his conduct of ward rounds. He would talk to them about how he recognized no difference between a duchess and a cook in his attitude to patients.[11] One student did not realize how unusual Osler was until he went up to London, to St Thomas's Hospital, for his clinical work. The doctor who could wield the magic of robes of authority when necessary was a friendly democrat compared with London colleagues:

> The nearly complete absence of humanity in the handling of patients in this and other major London hospitals was a cruel contrast to the medicine I had seen taught and practised in Oxford.
>
> Physicians, in particular, conducted their teaching rounds in frock coats, pin stripe trousers and wearing top hats, their diamond tie pins and gold watch chains glinting in the sunlight ... Here were our teachers exhibiting all the crude paraphernalia of social distinction and wealth to humble, poverty-stricken and ailing members of their own community.
>
> Humanity and friendliness were rare towards their students, and even rarer in the handling of their patients ... That these sick folk were beset with natural human anxieties, never seemed to enter into the clinical appreciation of the patient's problems as a whole, of the which the factual disease was merely a part. At the bedside, all too often, the full implications of a disease were discussed without inhibition or limitation, almost regardless of the fact that in the bed there was a sentient human being in reasonably full possession of all the faculties, even if poorly educated and elementary.
>
> Much too much was talked about the affluence and pecuniary rewards which came to the 'successful' members of the Staff – it all sounded very mercenary. I can only remember one occasion on which Sir William ever referred to money, when, characteristically, he said that 'no doctor should ever worry about the fees which were not paid because they would be credited to his account in heaven'!
>
> Thankfully, gratefully, one looked back with longing thoughts to the gay and completely delightful medical 'family parties' in the Radcliffe Infir-

mary, with Sir William as host and the patient as the most honoured and important guest.[12]

Along with his regular Radcliffe work, Osler was a founder and enthusiastic supporter of the Oxfordshire County Association for the Prevention of Tuberculosis. He set up a special tuberculosis dispensary at the Radcliffe which became a model throughout the Kingdom. With tuberculosis Osler continued the public health missionary work he had begun in America, propagandizing for outreach to the poor in their own communities, dunning rich friends for financial support, urging governments to be more active, and seeing patients himself.

Inevitably, he became doctor to many distinguished Oxonians. 'See that fine old man over there,' Osler said to Bill Francis on one of his visits. 'He's Sir James Murray. The University pays me my stipend as Regius Professor to keep him alive till the Dictionary is finished.' Osler failed, despite prescribing for 'Dictionary' Murray, the founding editor of the *Oxford English Dictionary*, a heroic regimen of x-ray therapy for his prostate troubles. Murray died in 1915 at the age of seventy-eight while still on the t's.[13] Nor was there a happier outcome with the Bodleian librarian E.W.B. Nicholson, an Oxford fixture whose health began to collapse in 1910. After sporadic and unsatisfactory attempts to return to work, Nicholson was eased into retirement by the curators in an atmosphere of vicious librarian rivalries and intrigue. Then he broke down completely and became, as Osler put it, 'mad as a hatter.' Nicholson believed spiritualists had summoned spirits to conspire against him, and one night he went rushing out into the street in his nightshirt with a knife to fight them off. Osler engaged in kindly discussions with Nicholson about the reality of the spirits. 'I promised to send him a secret answer if he wrote for any special aid, but to deceive the spirits if I meant what I wrote a cross would be on the envelope and if it was the opposite a circle.' After a few more bouts with the spirits, Nicholson died in 1912, aged sixty-three. Osler contributed £50 to the fund that Oxford friends raised for Nicholson's widow.

Osler chronicled these events for posterity in his copy of W.D. Macray's 1868 *Annals of the Bodleian Library*. He also recorded the decision to elevate Nicholson's hated rival, Falconer Madan, to the librarianship. Osler abstained from the discussion of the various candidates, 'nor did I feel it right to speak of the risk of putting a man of 61 in charge of so big a job.' Five years later, Osler added a note: 'I was mistaken. He was not old and has made an A1 librarian.'[14] In the Oxford milieu, after the mess he had made with the 'fixed period' statement and now a sexagenarian himself, Osler had little more to say in public about old age.

(He did not get along with another aging Oxford fixture, Robert Bridges, a physician and contemporary who in 1913, at the age of sixty-nine, was appointed Poet Laureate. In a written comment that his friends later suppressed, Osler called Bridges 'a hopeless man to meet, either from constitutional shyness or from rudeness, I never could make out which.' Grace thought it was rudeness, that Bridges was the rudest man she had ever met, and apparently let him know it. For his part, Bridges was extremely annoyed in the Bodleian Library one day to overhear Osler point him out to visiting Americans in the same breath as he introduced the Shelley relics. Bridges became one of Britain's least memorable poet laureates – everyone thought Rudyard Kipling held the title – whose reticence on an American visit led to the splendid headline: 'King's canary refuses to chirp.')[15]

The heir to the British throne, Edward, Prince of Wales, began attending Magdalen College, Oxford, in October 1912. The King, who was anxious about his son's health and about what seemed to be a daring experiment in allowing him to live on his own (in special rooms and with special servants, to be sure) requested that Sir William act as his physician. Edward got through his first winter satisfactorily but came down with influenza in the spring when Osler was away in America. Osler saw him for the first time on May 28, 1913, as he had had some 'circulatory symptoms.' Osler wrote this memorandum about the future king (who abdicated in 1936 and became the Duke of Windsor):

He is a small, delicately-built lad of 19, with good colour, but very thin, weighing only 7st. 8 lbs [106 lbs]. The muscles firm, superficial glands a little large, pulse only 48 but regular. It has been only 36 and heart's action regular, sounds clear, nothing in abdomen, lungs clear. Blood pressure 89.

V[aso] m[otor] reflex anaemic. Knee jerks difficult to get. He is a bit nervous and apprehensive and worried that his father and mother should think
that he does not eat enough and does not try to get fat. The probability is
that he will always be undersized, but he is developing mentally and takes
an interest in his work. He does not impress me as a very strong organism.

Edward had a good summer in Germany but gained only a few pounds, and
the next fall the King asked that Osler examine him again. Neither the
prince nor the physician probably thought it was necessary:

They fuss and worry about his being so thin and this distresses him. He is
not so nervous and has been less depressed. He has promised to take milk
and malt. [Edward told Osler that he hated milk and when prescribed it had
thrown it down the toilet.] The truth is he is undersized and ill developed
and can never be expected to be much of a man physically. He is happy at
Magdalen, and should do well if he is not fussed into a state of depression.
The poor lad feels that he is not up to much and this re-acts upon him
injuriously.[16]

As befitted an Anglo-Canadian who had become a regius professor and
a baronet, Osler respected the British monarchy and social system, but he
had no special interest in rank. He took little interest in his baronial coat
of arms, asking that it include fish because of Revere's interest, a beaver for
the Canadian background, and the motto 'Aequanimitas.' He declined a
Court appointment, telling Grace that he did not care to be 'at the mercy
of every little royal belly-ache.' One day when the Archbishop of Canterbury excused himself from an Oxford meeting saying he had to be at Court,
Osler is reputed to have queried, 'Co-respondent?'[17]

Well-to-do patients of Dr Osler stayed at the Randoph or the King's
Arms in Oxford. Osler employed A.G. Gibson, a local clinician who became his medical factotum and disciple, to take blood and urine samples
and blood pressure readings, and to stand in for him during his continental
sabbatical. He certainly took no fee in the case of a medical student from
Keble College who died of tuberculosis. We do not know whether he ex-

pected payment from Williams the Welsh masturbator – 'an unusually bad variety' – with whom he had plain talk and for whom he prescribed rest and exercise. Nor do we know how he responded to the concerns of a big burly undergraduate who was in despair, Osler reported, about his erotic infatuation for another student. It appears that Osler was called in by the much-annoyed subject of the boy's affections.[18]

Osler charged the same consulting fees he had in America, raising them by 5 per cent in 1913 to keep up with inflation. He saw far fewer paying patients, usually no more than one or two a day, and his annual income from practice averaged only about £2,000 (or $10,000 at the fixed conversion rate), about one-third his take during the busy years in America. He continued to earn substantial royalties and received significant dividends from American investments (it is possible he had made a handsome capital gain when his Baltimore house was sold for redevelopment). His Oxford salary and incidentals added about £600 a year. His annual gross when he was not on sabbatical was about £6,000–£7,500, about 20 per cent down from the good years in Baltimore. It was a very good 'cakes and ale' income, though perhaps not in the medical champagne category. Osler's largest single billing was $4,000 to a Manhattan lady he saw sixteen times in London in 1910 at £50 a visit. There was no bill to the Canadian Leader of the Opposition, Sir Robert Borden, whom Osler saw at the Hotel Cecil when Borden was in town for the coronation in 1911. There were no bills for treating paupers or princes. The Prince of Wales sent an inkstand and a framed photograph.[19]

Back in America, Johns Hopkins Hospital and School of Medicine seemed to have gone from strength to strength after Osler's departure. To Franklin P. Mall, William Welch, J.J. Abel, and other researchers at Hopkins the appointment of Lewellys Barker as Osler's successor heralded a new era in clinical research at the institution. The age of collecting cases, à la Osler, gave way to purposeful experimentation to study and treat disease. Barker, primarily an anatomist and pathologist, more than fulfilled expectations as he immediately founded not one but three new clinical research laboratories, one each for biological, physiological, and chemical studies. All were headed by full-time clinical scientists. Over in surgery, Harvey Cushing had built a similar experimental capacity, founding the Hunterian Laboratory as a center for experimental studies and surgical teaching using animals. From this point of view, William Osler was hardly missed.

The public reputation of Johns Hopkins never stood higher than in 1910, five years after Osler's departure, when the Carnegie Foundation's landmark report, *Medical Education in the United States and Canada*, treated it as the model towards which all other medical schools should evolve. The fact that the report's author, Abraham Flexner, was a graduate of Johns Hopkins University and was the younger brother of Simon Flexner, William Welch's student and protégé, was by no means the only reason why the institution was so commended. Almost everyone believed that the university and hospital founded by the Baltimore philanthropist had been a brilliant success. By 1910 the medical school faced a crisis of popularity as incoming classes of one hundred students strained its resources.

Over in England, Osler heard private rumors from time to time that things were not so rosy at Hopkins. Barker, trained in pathology and anatomy, had stepped into the most prestigious clinical position in America, perhaps in the world, without paying much in the way of clinical dues. The scuttlebutt among the Hopkins students, and among such professional giants as Weir Mitchell, was that Barker had had to be taught how to percuss a chest by his resident and that the medical side of Hopkins was not keeping up with the surgical and scientific side. But Barker had also, by virtue of his position, inherited much of Osler's private practice. In great demand from private patients, he appears to have learned fast and well, had a good bedside manner, was treated decently by Thayer and other members of the Osler old guard, and soon was significantly augmenting his hospital income through practice (though sick Hopkins students preferred to be seen by Thayer).[20] Barker was the man who in 1902 had popularized Mall's vision of putting clinical teachers on a 'full-time' basis – on salary only, no private fees. Now he was going down exactly the same road Osler and the other clinicians had taken. Would anything be done about it?

Publication of the Flexner report was a disaster for the weak American medical schools condemned in its pages, many of which soon closed. Ironically, the strongest school, Hopkins, was thrown into a severe time of troubles by the impact of its success. Andrew Carnegie, who sponsored the Flexner Report, concluded from it *not* to give more money to the business of medical education. This was not in fact a problem, because the officers of the Rockefeller philanthropies also read Flexner carefully and saw in medical education another field, close to the research area they had recently entered, that would surely repay sowing. Frederick W. Gates, the major-domo of Rockefeller giving, who had been so influenced by Osler's text, asked Abraham Flexner what he would do if he had a million dollars to spend reorganizing medical education. Flexner said he would give it to William Welch: 'With an endowment of four hundred thousand dollars, Dr. Welch has created, in so far as it goes, the one ideal medical school in America. Think what he might do if he had a million more.' Flexner soon was in Baltimore studying the Hopkins situation with a view to reporting to the Rockefellers how Welch and company could make the best use of a major new grant. This was the beginning of their troubles.

Flexner's confidential report about Hopkins to Gates, the head of Rockefeller's General Education Board, was frank to the point of indiscretion. Welch somehow got a copy, which he treated indiscreetly, and the document was soon read and copied and circulated throughout the hospital, where it caused a sensation.

Flexner had nothing but praise for the productivity of the laboratory and scientific departments, both in terms of research and in training staff for other institutions. Turning to the hospital, he argued that the private wards had become 'in large measure high-priced sanitaria for the well-to-do private patients of the prominent clinicians connected with the hospital and medical school.' These clinicians, Flexner charged, had effectively sold out:

> As contrasted with the instructors on the laboratory side, the clinical staff has been on the whole less productive and less devoted ... The clinicians have with very few exceptions proved too easy victims to the encroach-

ments of private practice. Not only has productive work been sacrificed to private professional engagements – routine teaching and hospital work go by the board when a large fee is in prospect. Classes are turned over to subordinates in order that the chief may leave town to see patients, not because they are scientifically interesting, but because they are pecuniarily worth while ...

While the laboratory staff was fluid, Flexner charged, the hospital's clinical roster was very rigid. Many clinicians had been around for many years, largely, he thought,

because they have long ceased to be scientifically significant and hence outside institutions do not desire them; at the same time, these men have developed in Baltimore lucrative private practices which they would not abandon to accept an academic call elsewhere ...

Whether the extremely prosperous physician or surgeon should have a place in such an institution as the Johns Hopkins Hospital seems to me most doubtful. Once there, he will invariably exploit his prestige for his own pecuniary benefit. He thereby brings the institution into disfavor with the local profession, who very rightly believe that he is using his position to collect more and larger fees than those lacking such a connection. Moreover, the spectacle is not a wholesome one for students to witness.

The answer, then, was to put the main clinical chairs on a salaried full-time basis, as Mall had been urging for years, as Barker had seemed to endorse back in 1902, as Welch and Halsted now supported, and as most private businesses employed their executives. No private practice or private fee income would be allowed. Of course the change would necessarily involve higher salaries to compensate for lost outside income. Flexner suggested that the chiefs of medicine, surgery, and the new departments of psychiatry and pediatrics should be paid $7,500 a year rather than $5,000. Obstetrics and gynecology should properly be combined and also put on a full-time basis. Finally, Flexner also recommended that the best medical school in America train fewer students. He wanted to see total enrollment at Hopkins shrunk to 250. No one would be overstrained by having to do too much teaching.[21]

Osler in Oxford heard of Flexner's Hopkins report through Howard Kelly, who saw himself as one of its principal targets. Over the years, as the fees he charged in practice had come under attack, Kelly had transferred many of his patients and much of his time and attention to his private hospital. He was extremely prosperous and admitted he had somewhat neglected his Hopkins work. The other main target, Kelly reported, was Barker, who since 1905 had established a standard of living that a fixed salary could not possibly support, and had completely reversed his position since his 1902 manifesto.

As a Christian philanthropist, Howard Kelly had given away about three times his total Johns Hopkins income and hardly considered himself contaminated by greed. He was incensed that Flexner was proposing 'a system of peonage similar to nothing else in the world' for the announced purpose of counteracting money making. He tried to argue these points at a meeting of the Hopkins faculty, only to be challenged by Superintendent Hurd for some of the high fees he had charged in the past.

As Hopkins staff thought about the implications of moving to a salaried basis, as the force of Flexner's attack on the clinicians struck home, and as an early and more frankly personal draft of his report got into circulation, the institution was engulfed in meetings, gossip, bitterness, and intrigue. Kelly was sure that the new dean, the obstetrician J. Whitridge Williams, was behind the plan to unite obstretrics with gynecology. Otherwise, he told Osler, there were several forces at work:

> I fear the praise Flexner got for his report on the Med. Schools made him overconfident in his own judgment ... My men and many of the young men feel that Mall is at the bottom of most of the troubles, but I can't see it. They all realize that Howell & Abel are simply guided by principle. Welch they tie up as being led by the nose by Williams. [President] Remsen is watching & not committed ... Dr. Hurd is impossible, irritable & petulant to the last degree ... Well, this is only *canserne* & not complaining, we are really all very serene (aequanimitas?) and stirred up to work all the harder.

Kelly was not serene at all. By his sixth letter in a month to Osler on the subject, he had worked himself into a rage about Welch's and Williams's lack of consultation (Flexner had not met with either Kelly or Barker), about Flexner's brutal criticisms, and about a situation in which they had all become dependent on outside men with money.

> Dr. Welch's dogma that individuals do not count in adjusting important business problems smacks very much of the Guggenheims as I have met them in the smelters of Mexico, and calls up a picture of the train of suicides which followed Rockefeller's early days as he was building up the Standard Oil monopoly. If we could see all the little white stones which mark the graves for which the Rockefeller and the Carnegie interests have been responsible, I wonder if the mountainsides would not look as if a snowstorm had struck them. Meyer [the newly appointed professor of psychiatry, who opposed the scheme on principle] whispered in my ear recently that he was appalled that the Standard Oil was acquiring such a larger interest in our activities. Abel said the same a few years ago ...
>
> There is a strong undertone of criticism of Welch and Halsted, asking very pertinently what original work they themselves have done.[22]

Osler had made so many statements over the years supporting scientific medicine, research, duty, and, in his youth, the desirability of having full-time teachers of medicine, that in the beginning he was quoted on both sides of the Hopkins full-time debate. Knowing none of the details of Flexner's report, he was not at first opposed to the principle of the plan. If they gave the full-time clinicians liberal salaries of $15,000 to $20,000, he told Welch, and were careful that the hospital itself did not try to make big money from its clinicians' work with patients, 'I would be strongly in favour of it.' On the other hand, it would be ruinous to try to pay $7,500 salaries, for the institution would not be able to hold its good men.

He was sensitive to any implication in any of the discussions that he had used his Hopkins position to make money. 'I did not find it hard to spend every cent of the income I made from patients in the 16 years I was in the Hospital,' Osler told Welch, 'and of course a good deal of that went in a sort of legitimate advertising of the Hospital, just such as you have done so much in the exercise of hospitality.' No one at Hopkins, not even Mall, ever did accuse Osler of mercenary motives or neglect of duty, though perhaps some thought it. At least one physician in Toronto, during a discussion of Johns Hopkins as a model for the Toronto General Hospital, offered sharp comment on the Hopkins system:

> As to Johns Hopkins, what has it done? It made Osler a professor in England – gave him a handsome, magnificent position. It has given Dr. Kelly, in another department, a magnificent private hospital from which he gets enormous fees, one of them being $10,000 the other day for an operation on the life of a railway magnate. That is what Johns Hopkins is doing. It is putting those men into positions in which they are able to remunerate themselves very, very handsomely; and then when they begin to get such handsome remuneration the work begins to fall off, and it is deputed, left to assistants, although nominally under their headship. The assistants are greedy for fees, and greedy for the surplus that flows over from the rich man's table.[23]

The more Osler thought about the Hopkins full-time proposals, the less he liked them: 'It is an experiment I would like very much to see tried, but not at the Johns Hopkins first. It might have been different if we had started so.' He could not see how the heads of department could be cut off from active practice (a conclusion which the critical Toronto group also reached). From his own experience, he knew that members of the hospital board would be the very first people wanting private consultations. His best early statement of his views was a May 1911 letter to Barker:

> There are a great many points in favour. It would be a great thing for the country to have teachers and investigators at the Hospitals who were relieved entirely from the cares of private practice. It is a very hard thing to serve two masters. On the other hand it would put a man off a good deal from association with his colleagues, and from what is with many men, it certainly was with me, a most interesting part of one's work – the contact with all sorts and conditions of people in all sorts of places. The

one plan makes a better physician, but the other is likely to develop a stronger man.

Then there is the financial question. It is not a bad thing for a Faculty to have a few men in it who have money to spend, in the way for instance that Kelly has done. Had we started on the suggested plan we could not have made anything like the same impression on the profession. The Trustees have, and I think Dr. Hurd has too, an exaggerated idea of the large fortunes made by the clinical men (I left all my clinical earnings in the US. Ask BOH [Miss Humpton] where they went. I took nothing away except text-book earnings not all of them! which included what I got for the house). The salary that I have heard suggested, $7,500, would of course be impossible. I do not see how you and Thayer could possibly get along with less than double that amount. I am afraid too the tendency would be to make the Hospital more and more a centre for private patients, who should of course be charged large fees ... A dozen appendicitis cases would pay a salary.[24]

Osler might have been content with writing critical private letters to his friends, but the Hopkins president, Ira Remsen, having heard from Welch of his waffling, sent him Flexner's document and other memoranda in the hope of bringing him onside. It had the reverse effect. Osler read Flexner's report as a brutal and ignorant attack on his staff, his principles, and his sense of professionalism. He realized that its criticisms were personal slurs on Kelly, Cushing, Thayer, Finney, Bloodgood, Cullen, and probably himself, among others. Its recommendations he saw as an attempt to impose on clinical medicine attitudes to research and life he had seen practiced by men like Halsted, a drug addict, and Franklin Mall, a narrow, crabbed doctrinaire. On September 1, 1911, Osler sent a fourteen-page printed letter to Remsen, all the Johns Hopkins University and Hospital trustees, Flexner, Hurd, and the administrators and professors of the medical school.

He began by condemning Flexner's 'very feeble grasp of the clinical situation at the Johns Hopkins Hospital' and offering a spirited defense against untrue statements about 'the very men who have done as much, or more, than any others to build up the reputation of the school and to advance the best interests of the profession':

It is not too much to say that these men have done scientific work of a
standard equal to that of the highest of any laboratory men connected with
the University; and in addition work which in practical import, in the translation of Science into the Art, no pure laboratory men could have done. To
speak as Mr. Flexner does of these men as blocking the line and preventing
the complete development of a race or school ... certainly is not true. Take
away the share of the reputation of the Johns Hopkins Medical School ...
contributed from the clinical side, and by the junior staff, and you have it,
in comparison, poor indeed!

Osler judged that the Hopkins record was in fact 'more brilliant from the
clinical than the laboratory side.' Flexner was both unfair and ignorant,
and 'gross injustice is done to the men who have made the Johns Hopkins
Clinical School.'

Osler vigorously defended his own approach to private practice – never
before 2 PM – but did reproach himself for having interrupted his hospital
work for some of the long-distance calls. He said that the hospital and
university owed an immense debt of gratitude to one of its prosperous surgeons: 'I do not believe the history of medicine presents a parallel to the
munificence of our colleague Kelly to his clinic.' Under Kelly's guidance
the clinic became 'the Mecca for surgeons from all parts of the world,' and
Flexner's proposal to merge it with obstetrics flowed solely from 'the fullness of his ignorance.'

As for the full-time scheme, Osler saw the head of a university clinic as
having to be much more than a hands-on researcher. That might suffice in
designated research institutes,

but only a very narrow view regards the Director of a University clinic as
chiefly an agent for research. He stands for other things of equal importance. In life, in work, in word, and in deed he is an exemplar to the young
men about him, students and assistants. 'Cabined, cribbed, confined' within
the four walls of a hospital, practising the fugitive and cloistered virtues of a
clinical monk, how shall he, forsooth, train men for a race the dust and heat
of which he knows nothing and – this is a possibility! – cares less? I cannot

imagine anything more subversive to the highest ideal of a *clinical* school than to hand over young men who are to be our best practitioners to a group of teachers who are *ex officio* out of touch with the conditions under which these young men will live ...

The attempt would, I believe defeat itself. Those best fitted as teachers in the medical schools, the men with larger outlook, would soon kick over the traces and leave the positions to the quiet student-recluses, keen at research, but as little fitted to train medical students for the hurly-burly of life as I would be to direct your laboratory.

I cannot bear to think that any successor of mine should grow up deprived of those delightful associations which I enjoyed with the profession and the public ... A great gap would be left in the education of a clinical teacher who had not known that inner life of the public which we meet in our ministry of health ...

The danger would be of the evolution throughout the country of a set of clinical prigs, the boundary of whose horizon would be the laboratory, and whose only human interest was research, forgetful of the wider claims of a clinical professor as a trainer of the young, a leader in the multiform activities of the profession, an interpreter of science to his generation, and a counselor in public and in private of the people, in whose interests after all the school exists.

Osler had no illusions about universities, like men, being for sale — as they had all seen, years before, on the matter of women students. But in Flexner's proposal, he concluded,

We chance the sacrifice of something that is really vital, the existence of a great clinical school organically united with the profession and with the public. These are some of the reasons why I am opposed to the plan as likely to spell ruin to the type of school I have always felt the Hospital should be and which we have tried to make it – a place of refuge for the sick poor of the city – a place where the best that is known is taught to a group of the best students – a place where new thought is materialized in research – a school where men are encouraged to base the art upon the science of medicine – a fountain to which teachers in every subject would come for inspiration – a place with a hearty welcome to every practitioner who seeks help – a consulting centre for the whole country.

His last thought was that there might be some way to 'divert the ardent souls who wish to be whole-time clinical professors from the medical school in which they are not at home to the Research Institutes to which they properly belong.'[25]

Osler's intervention in Hopkins affairs was like a respected former politician coming out of retirement to denounce a successor's policies, as Theodore Roosevelt was doing with William Howard Taft at exactly that time in the United States, and as Margaret Thatcher in England and Pierre Elliott Trudeau in Canada would do many years later. But Osler had more moral authority in his profession than any of these had in theirs, and he happened to have his actual successor on his side, for Lewellys Barker had concluded that he could not afford to give up his private practice and would resign first.

W.H. Howell, the idealistic physiologist and former dean, who was hurt by what he considered to be Osler's denigration of Hopkins' record of laboratory research, tried to fight back in an eloquent letter of disagreement. But Welch, a canny politician who, with Mall, was using Flexner more or less as a cat's paw, saw the writing on the wall. He now saw how difficult the matter was, he wrote Osler, and was still considering what to do. Suddenly nothing happened – Hopkins did not ask for the grant from the Rockefellers, the Rockefellers did not offer it, and life went on. Other American medical men and institutions joined the debate. Osler added a few cents' worth in private letters, citing physiologists as a group of laboratory men who had fallen out of touch, and returning most tellingly to his experience at Johns Hopkins: 'What I dread is to have a class of clinicians growing up and out of touch, and necessarily out of sympathy with the profession and with the public. This would be nothing short of a calamity. There are always men of the quiet type like Halsted, who practically live the secluded life; to have a whole Faculty made up of Halsteds would be a very good thing for science, but a very bad thing for the profession.'[26] It seemed that Osler's intervention had killed full-time at Johns Hopkins, and ended the battle before any real damage could be done.

For Osler, controversies about health care and medical education were wars fought on two fronts. If his Hopkins friends, acting in the name of science and research, were about to push the revolution too far, his British friends often seemed far too conservative, much in need of prodding to enter the twentieth century. Many British hospitals still had nonexistent laboratory facilities, poor relations with the local profession, no teaching traditions, and no involvement with paying patients. London's too-numerous hospital medical schools still tended to be weak in science teaching, and their clinical work suffered badly from fragmentation, lack of organization, and separation from university affiliation. Everyone in England put too much emphasis on formal examinations, and – a view he published anonymously – 'the Royal Colleges are oligarchies which have lost touch with their licentiates and members ... a stumbling-block in the way of higher medical education.'[27]

So when Osler spoke for British consumption, as he did in several published addresses and in testimony to Lord Haldane's Commission on University Education in London, he sounded like a progressive American reformer, holding up 'St Johns Hopkins' as a model of excellence – even though to some of the Americans at Hopkins his slams at the full-time system would seem like grumpy John Bull Toryism. To the Haldane commission he recommended adopting the best of German and American practice in the creation of 'hospital units,' organized and run by the university, in the leading teaching hospitals.

Sometimes Osler took on British reactionaries and American doctrinaires in the same address. In Glasgow in November 1911, for example, he urged clinicians to spend time in the Royal Infirmary's new pathological institute because laboratories were the wave of the future and every clinician needed to know 'the priceless lessons of the dead house.' Then, obviously thinking of Hopkins, he warned against spending too much time in autopsy room or laboratory:

There are so many seeking the bubble reputation at the eye-piece and the test-tube, it is well for young men to remember that no bubble is so iridescent or floats longer than that blown by the successful teacher. A man who is not fond of students and who does not suffer their foibles gladly misses the greatest zest in life; and the teacher who wraps himself in the cloak of his researches, and lives apart from the bright spirits of the coming generation, is very apt to find his garment the shirt of Nessus.[28]

(The shirt of Nessus was impregnated with poisoned blood. Meant to be protective, it burned the wearer's flesh, driving him to suicide.)

Osler was backing and filling, trying to find a middle way of acting his age, of being an elder statesman still active in the struggle while slipping gracefully towards retirement. After the 1908 revision of his textbook, for example, he corresponded with Barker and others about passing on the authorship and having it gradually become a Johns Hopkins textbook of medicine. Then he changed his mind, and while he enlisted McCrae's help for a major revision in 1912, giving him credit on the title page, he still did much of the work himself. 'The new edition is very exacting and Reggie is working so hard at it,' Grace wrote in the spring of 1912. 'I think he is determined to let the Medical World know he is not living in retirement over here.'[29] In 1912–13 he served a term as president of the British Hospitals Association, trying to persuade hospital administrators to modernize.

No star of the medical world was more visible than Oxford's Osler at the Seventeenth International Medical Congress in London in the summer of 1913. Seven thousand delegates attended medicine's equivalent of the modern Olympic Games – a royal opening, glittering receptions, magnificent dinners, fêtes, excursions, and conversaziones, scholarly events, even a soupçon of spice provided by a suffragette demonstration. Sir William and Lady Osler took a whole floor of Brown's Hotel for the duration of the congress and entertained every day at meals. One night they had 196 dinner guests at the Royal Automobile Club (an exclusive establishment in the elite age of motoring). 'We have had a deuce of a business with this congress & only just escaped alive,' Osler wrote from their recovery holiday in Scotland.[30]

Osler's search for a medical middle way was evident in a splendid meditation he gave to the Glasgow Southern Medical Society in 1912 on the
problem of blood pressure. Fear of high blood pressure readings had now
replaced the bogey of bad urine tests, he argued, causing needless worry
and anxiety among patients 'hipped' on the subject of their blood pressure.
Images of Egyptian pumping stations and irrigation systems jostled with
his steam engine and motor car metaphors as he advised taking high blood
pressure readings seriously (even venesecting in certain hypertensive cri-
ses) while realizing that no drugs were particularly satisfactory. Adjusting
the system – reducing the fuel, slowing the pace, weeding the irrigation
channels – was the best response. The advent of a new image in his prose
suggests that Sir William had himself just changed his shaving habits: 'Of
a dozen blades of a Gillette safety razor, all identical in appearance and in
fineness of edge, some may be used for weeks, even months; others may
have to be cast aside in a few days. So it is with man ... the personal equation has always to be considered.'[31]

Here is the up-to-date Dr Osler, changing the 'Faith Healing' heading
of his text to 'Psychotherapy' in the 1912 revision and exchanging correspondence with an old acquaintance from the days when they both studied
cerebral palsy, Sigmund Freud. We do not know what they wrote to one
another, but in 1910, apparently taking certain Freudian ideas seriously,
Osler began systematically recording his dreams. Carefully and wisely. He
made no attempt to interpret the meaning of his dreams and generally
decided they were 'crazy.' (Pity the modern biographer, who has to agree
that dream data is virtually unusable and cannot spin out elaborate, fanci-
ful interpretations.) At best, he saw psychoanalysis as another kind of faith
healing. The fact that Osler sent a patient to Freud in 1911, in Freud's
disciples' eyes a sign of recognition, could have meant anything.[32] Osler
might have been getting rid of another of the tiresome group he called
'omphalites,' patients whose woes (vide Henry James) centered mostly on
their obsession with their navels.

He continued to publish a few case studies, and the calls for consultation would never end. But more of his time was spent trying to understand
backward, extending his friendship with the immortal dead. In 1912 he

organized a History of Medicine Section of the Royal Society of Medicine. The next year he became president of the Bibliographical Society. The formal reason for his 1913 trip to America was to give the Silliman Lectures at Yale on the historical evolution of modern medicine. Many of the changes in the eighth edition of his text involved expanding the sections on the history of disease. Even his dream recording may have been rooted as much in Aesculapian antecedents – the gods were said to send cures in sleep – as in Freudian psychiatry.

Intellectually, Osler had become deeply influenced by the classical revival of the second half of the nineteenth century, particularly the wave of Hellenism that glorified (and sanitized) everything about the culture of ancient Greece. A student of the Greek philosophers, as translated and celebrated by Oxford's Benjamin Jowett, a close and sympathetic reader of the aesthetic neoclassicism of Walter Pater's *Marius the Epicurean*, he became even more philhellenized at Oxford. His Silliman and other lectures at the beginning of the twentieth century's second decade featured an optimistic celebration of ancient Greece's worship of man, the body, and nature, contrasting so sharply with Israel's quest for God and righteousness. His Silliman Lectures effectively started with Greek medicine and ended in a celebration of the wonderful achievements of nineteenth-century scientific medicine. Osler had anticipated the argument in a 1910 secular sermon to 2,500 listeners at the University of Edinburgh entitled 'Man's Redemption of Man': Greece gives rise to the scientific spirit, and by modern times, with the help of men such as Darwin, medical scientists are able to redeem humanity from pain, fever, and plague. Darwin had caused us to stop thinking of Paradise Lost and look forward to Paradise Regained. Thanks to 'the new socialism of Science,' Osler concluded in 'Man's Redemption of Man,'

> The outlook for the world as represented by Mary and John and Jennie and Tom has never been so hopeful. There is no place for despondency or despair. As for the dour dyspeptics in mind and morals who sit croaking like ravens – let them come into the arena, let them wrestle for their flesh and blood against the principalities and powers represented by bad air and worse

houses, by drink and disease, by needless pain, and by the loss annually to
the state of thousands of valuable lives – let them fight for the day when a
man's life shall be more precious than gold. Now, alas! the cheapness of life
is every day's tragedy.[33]

Osler still traveled to see private patients. When he was not taking the
train to London, he was likely to be in a motor car, driven by his chauffeur.
One day an important rural consultation was jeopardized by a cracked
cylinder head and, at the chauffeur's recommendation, a young Oxford
mechanic named William Morris worked through the night patching it
together. Soon Morris became the Osler family's pet automobile surgeon.
When the car would not start, the cry went out, 'Send for Willy.' In turn,
Morris sent for William Osler when he was overcome by neurasthenia and
ulcers. Morris eventually built a great automobile business and, as Lord
Nuffield, became Oxford medicine's most generous benefactor, partly in
memory of Osler.[34]

Osler also saw private patients in a consulting room at 13 Norham Gardens. Some came a very long way for his advice. On September 29, 1913,
two of them met on his doorstep and recognized one another. They both
lived in Winnipeg, Manitoba. Each had traveled four thousand miles to
consult with Dr Osler.

A few weeks later, Osler spoke to the students' Abernethian Society at
St Bartholomew's Hospital, London, giving a sweeping survey, largely
autobiographical, of the evolution of clinical medicine in his lifetime. He
went into great detail describing his teaching at Hopkins, with its emphasis on the student as 'the pivot around which the machine works,' and he
ended with a forecast that if research became too dominant, the researchers would become that set of 'clinical prigs' he had warned Hopkins against.
'At the same time let me freely confess that I mistrust my own judgement,
as this is a problem for young men and for the future.' He told the students
that his own life had been spent socializing with his professional brethren,
and he stayed around after his talk doing just that. Decades later the sub-

stance of his talk had been long forgotten, but not Sir William's joining in the songs around the piano and his having asked the boys to sing the ribald verses.[35]

There were new boys in Oxford arriving to be initiated into medicine and life. The only books that Wilder Penfield, a Rhodes scholar from Princeton, brought to England with him were the seven volumes of *Osler's Modern Medicine*. He soon got to know Osler, as did another Rhodes man at Christ Church, who recalled:

> A few days after my first term began he came around to my rooms in the Meadow Buildings, said that he was Dr. Osler and had just dropped in to see if I was getting started all right, that he had an office in the Old Library Building and would be glad to give me any help that he might render, that if I had no engagements for next Sunday afternoon to drop in at his house for tea.
>
> Think of the Regius Professor of Medicine at Oxford, and a man as busy as Dr. Osler was, finding time to call on an average 'fresher' and welcome him in such a kindly, humane way! And those Sunday afternoon teas at his house, with what pleasure I recall them! Often Dr. Osler would come out to the door himself, greet you with a slap on the back, put his arm around your shoulders and lead you into the reception room and introduce you to students, professors, and distinguished men and women from the ends of the earth.[36]

Another Princetonian Rhodesian, Wilburt C. Davison, first met the regius professor in 1913 when he rang the doorbell to ask him about doing two years of medicine in one. Osler told Davison it was a silly idea, but he could go ahead if he wanted to. He invited Davison in, told Grace that another American colt trying to buck tradition had arrived, and had him sit down to tea. Once, when Osler was advising Davison to spend time in other places, the green American thought he was recommending a visit to a Paris nightclub with the strange name 'Sore bun.'[37]

As in Baltimore, the students were welcomed as family and exposed to the pretty Canadian girls who would break their hearts. Sunday afternoon

teas became the regular drop-in occasions, but from time to time the old
Saturday night dinners were recreated. When Osler decided to give a course
of lectures in the history of medicine, for example, nine students signed up:

> He gave only two or three lectures during the year, but what a 'feast' they
> were! We would receive a notice giving the subject of the lecture and the
> time appointed, and each notice would be accompanied by an invitation to
> dinner The lecture would be preceded by a nine course dinner, the dishes
> cleared away, cigars and cigarettes passed around, and while we all remained
> seated around the table Dr. Osler would proceed to give the lecture in an
> informal manner and conversational tone. Rare old books and pictures would
> be passed around.

Sometimes Osler met a student in a different venue: when one Oxonian
asked for an appointment to submit his MD thesis, the professor replied
that it would be most convenient to rendezvous in London for tea at the
Royal Automobile Club:

> When we met at the club, the Regius was accompanied by a Canadian
> physician and his wife, to whom he was showing the sights of the metropo-
> lis. The club's guest room was not yet opened; so we went to a fashionable
> teashop in St. James's Street. And there, amidst the tinkle of teacups, the
> buzz of light conversation, and the strains of 'The Merry Widow' waltz, Sir
> William turned over the pages of my thesis and discussed the Pel-Ebstein
> syndrome with me. A few months later, he presented me for the degree.
> There were two candidates ... We lunched with Osler beforehand, and he
> took us in his car to the Sheldonian Theatre for the ceremony. Thus he
> gave up his time to his students, to make it one of the most pleasant of
> memorable days in their lives.[38]

The black sheep of the Osler family, brother Frank, appeared in England at
the end of 1913. Willie had not seen his brother, who had lived mostly in

British Columbia, for thirty years. Frank and his wife Belle were house guests at Norham Gardens over Christmas. Frank was a heavy drinker, somewhat Falstaffian, and his wife's conversation was difficult to endure, but everyone observed the proprieties. The brothers had a remarkable physical resemblance.

Early in 1914 Osler lost two very old friends when Lord Strathcona died in London and Weir Mitchell died in Philadelphia. Osler was a pallbearer for Strathcona, whose rise from the Canadian wilderness through Montreal to the haunts of the British aristocracy had anticipated his own. Mitchell, the grand old man of American medicine, had been yet another of Osler's surrogate fathers. 'Of no man I have known are Walter Savage Landor's words more true: "I warmed both hands before the fire of life,"' Osler wrote about him in an obituary. Mitchell had gone off at eighty-four, still clear headed, 'with a minimum of that "cold gradation of decay" through which so many of us have to pass.'[39]

Revere, as always, was the light of Osler's life. He could never bear the child's suffering when he was sick or bring himself to discipline the boy when he was naughty, leaving it to Grace. As late-life parents of an only child, Willie and Grace worried about Revere as though he were the only boy ever to grow up in the world. There were special schools, special tutors, and probably more gentle exhortations than Revere ever wanted to hear. In near despair in 1910, the Oslers thought they would have to assure their unintellectual son a living as a gentleman farmer. In fact Revere was about to blossom. At puberty he shot up in height, began to be interested in arts and crafts, developed perfect manners, and fished and read, read and fished. After a year of special tutoring to bring up his Greek and Latin, he managed to pass the matriculation exam for Oxford on his second attempt and entered Christ Church in the autumn of 1914.

Revere's closest male friend from his school days, John Slessor (who later became a marshal of the Royal Air Force) remembered 'Tommy' as a beautiful lad who lived in the happiest household he ever knew – and in one of the happiest towns, Slessor added in his memoirs: glorious Oxford, where horses wore straw hats in summer, an Italian organ grinder and his monkey played in the Bardwell Road, and muffin men still plied the streets;

where young men in shorts and sweaters, great scarves around their necks, walked and cycled from college to athletic field, played cricket and tennis, sat down to tea and crumpets, and admired the girls in their long dresses with the tight waists.[40]

Since Revere was not scientifically inclined, Osler had decided that the great collection of medical books he was building would go to McGill University after his death. The idea spurred him into more systematic purchasing, and brother E.B. gave £1,000 to further the collection of incunabula. In the spring and summer of 1914 Osler was beginning to work out the principles he would use in making a catalogue of the collection.

'Wonderful spring, and a great deal going on of one sort and another,' he wrote towards the end of April. He was buying books, trying to arrange for repairs to the tomb of Avicenna, the paramount Arab physician, and was fresh from giving a talk, to the Jewish Historical Society of England, on Israel and medicine. In it, he praised Jewish medical achievements, past and present, admiring the careers of so many of his friends and the way their community honored the profession.[41] A few weeks earlier, he had been one of the organizers of a London dinner to honor the new American surgeon-general, General W.C. Gorgas, who had led the campaigns against yellow fever and malaria in Cuba and during the building of the Panama Canal. On many occasions Osler celebrated that American initiative as a sterling gift to humanity and an indication of the benign consequences that could flow from the white race's involvement in the tropics. He was of course enthusiastic about expanding the study of tropical medicine in London, the center of the greatest empire the world had ever known.

Medical politics, high and low, haunted him. A fraudulent use of his name to endorse a home medical encyclopedia got Osler embroiled in a dispute with the Royal College of Physicians, the out-of-touch oligarchy. When the college bureaucracy behaved foolishly, Olser uncharacteristically and imperiously lost his temper and submitted his resignation. There had to be delicate, high-level negotiations, with appropriate apologies, to persuade the regius professor to reconsider. Over at the Royal Society of Medicine, its genial secretary wrote that they would all be shocked and appalled if Osler violated tradition by declining the honor of election to its presidency: 'It is your clear duty to accept, and for duty's sake you must not refuse,' to which Osler replied, 'Awfully sorry ... It is not my job. I need not go into reasons. It is good of you to think of me.'[42] Osler also turned down an invitation to stand for the University of Oxford's seat in Parliament, which both Conservatives and Liberals urged on him, promising that he would be unopposed. 'I was not even tempted. No new job at my time of life, thank you!'[43]

Meanwhile, the Johns Hopkins full-time issue heated up and boiled over. After two years of inaction – but under mounting pressure from Mall, Williams, and a new hospital superintendent – Welch went ahead in the autumn of 1913 and rammed through the faculty a request to the Rockefeller people for money to implement full-time clinical chairs. Barker, who had a high standard of living, a handicapped child, and invalid relatives to support, refused to go full-time at a total salary of $10,000, or even $15,000. Thayer refused to take his place. In the spring of 1914 a forty-two-year-old New York medical blue-blood, Theodore C. Janeway, signed on as the first full-time professor of medicine at Johns Hopkins.

Osler was deeply angry at Johns Hopkins's treatment of his successor. He let everyone know it, including the most villainous player, Franklin Mall, in about the strongest language he ever used in correspondence. 'What an anomaly to make conditions which can not be accepted by the best clinicians in the country,' Osler wrote Mall in April. 'Personally I think Barker has been treated d— badly. Neither the faculty nor the Trustees has the right at this stage of the game to change the conditions of tenure of his office. Neither morally nor legally – I feel very sore about the whole business.' There is no evidence that Mall replied.[44]

A similar struggle at Harvard was having a very different outcome as its medical stars, led by Dean Christian and the now-transplanted Harvey Cushing, resisted Rockefeller full-time *dirigisme*; eventually the university, in a demonstration of principle and courage rare in any era, turned its back on a major donation. The Harvardians had decided that the Hopkins plan would probably be unworkable as well as unjust, and compromised by allowing their staff to have a limited in-house private practice and the income it generated – what came to be called 'geographical' full-time. Osler thought this was a much sounder course of action and recalled that William Pepper had talked about just such a development twenty years earlier.[45]

After Janeway's appointment – a good one in the circumstances, Osler thought – the men at Hopkins all tried to put the bitterness behind them and get on with making the new experiment work. Howard Kelly was bitter but philosophical, not least because he had diverted most of his patients away from Hopkins and in any case had become obsessed with the use of radium to treat cancer. Halsted, who had long since cut back on his private practice, changed his mind about fees and used the full-time fight to get a higher salary and more help; his wife was left to regret the financial hardships they suffered as their income shrank. Thayer and Barker, both ambivalent idealists, could console themselves with their high reputations and extensive practices. They also found solace in poetry. 'As far as Thayer and I are concerned,' Barker wrote Osler, 'I am reminded of the two lines from Wordsworth, "The witless shepherd that persists to drive / A flock that thirsts not, to a pool disliked." '[46]

No one had been more eloquent than Osler on the general virtue of burying the past, ignoring the future, and getting on with daily business. To students at Yale in 1913 he had given what became one of his most reprinted sermons, 'A Way of Life,' on his philosophy of living in 'day-tight compartments,' an analogy drawn from water-tight bulkheads on steamships (and, he noted, used in spite of the *Titanic*'s fate). One of the ways Osler had compartmentalized his life was to take no more than a passing interest in nonmedical current events. He went on with his busy round in the spring and summer of 1914 paying no attention to the political machinations of the European powers. The only turmoil he noticed that year was the trouble the British were having in northern Ireland, where civil war was a real possibility. Who had any patience left for the Irish? 'I wish they would tow the island into the mid-Atlantic & let the Orange & Green fight it out between them.'[47]

There were splendid ceremonies at Cambridge on June 9, 1914, at the opening of the new physiological laboratories, with honorary degrees for Osler and many other luminaries. On June 16 he saw professionally on the same day the son of the king and a son of the prime minister (and in May he had seen the prime minister's wife). On July 8 he gave a speech on tuberculosis, at Leeds, warning of the need to take action against 'the Angel of the White Scourge.' The Oslers enjoyed a week's family holiday in the fen country, chauffeured in their new Renault, and a visit to Thomas Browne's Norwich. On July 12 Osler turned sixty-five and apparently ignored the occasion. There was a dinner at Oxford on July 16, at the Persian Society in London on July 17, the Bibliographical Society meeting in Cambridge, and more events to come: 'I am shockingly full of engagements.'[48]

Osler insisted that Grace and Revere sail for America without him on July 31 so that the boy would have extra time to visit relatives. Grace noticed how important it was to him that Revere get to know the Oslers. Willie was to join them in September to take part in Johns Hopkins Hospital's twenty-fifth anniversary celebrations. Now he was off to Aberdeen for the British Medical Association meeting, where he summed up a discussion of artificial pneumothorax and proposed the health of the BMA's president at the banquet. A visiting contingent of Austrian doctors missed that dinner because they were 'recalled.' The Britishers who noticed their absence thought it had something to do with a war in the Balkans. They had all been too busy that week to bother with the newspapers. On July 31 Osler went on to the isle of Colonsay to visit the Strathcona/Howard clan. He was still there on Monday, August 3, when news came that a great war was about to begin.

All the Youth and Glory of the Country

The Oslers had paid little attention to assassinations in the Balkans, ultimatums, mobilizations, and declarations of war by Austria, Russia, and Germany. It hardly seemed possible that Britain would be sucked in. Then German troops began marching across Belgium, violating the country's guaranteed neutrality. Suddenly, incredibly, on Tuesday, August 4, 1914, the British Empire went to war.

Grace and Revere were literally at sea, heading for Canada aboard the *Calgarian*. Willie found himself stranded at Colonsay off the west coast of Scotland because all the telegraph lines and trains had been commandeered for military purposes. He could not get south until the end of the week. In London he met up with his brother Edmund, who was already engaged in war finance, and he spent the early days of August helping organize Canadian offers of medical help and doing what he could to contact friends, including William Welch, who were scrambling to leave the continent. A nephew of Grace's who slipped across the Channel to England found himself promptly arrested as a German spy; Osler arranged his release.

On the other side of the ocean, Grace and Revere landed in Quebec, had frantic visits with relatives and friends who rushed up to see them, and on August 13 sailed for England on the *Calgarian*'s return voyage. The ship was now painted black and traveled blacked-out at night for fear of submarines. The possibility that Revere and Grace might stay in Canada or the neutral United States during the war was not considered.

Weeping wives and mothers saw recruits onto the same train that Grace and Revere took for Oxford. When they reached Norham Gardens on August 22, tea was ready on the terrace, and the garden was a mass of roses and snapdragons. 'It was hard to understand why we had rushed back,' Grace wrote. She did see a change in her husband: 'The strangest part of all to me is the absolute seriousness of Dr. Osler. I have never seen him thus since he came first to the University of Penn in 1884.' She also saw the changes in Oxford. Soldiers were billeted in the colleges; the Examination Schools building was being converted into a huge fully-equipped hospital and the college infirmaries into supporting units. Women were volunteering for Red Cross service – within days Grace became chairman of a workroom set up in the museum to make hospital garments. The sleepy village of Ewelme, where the Oslers went to church on their first Sunday together again, had already sent thirty men to war. There were hardly any male voices in the choir.

At sixty-five, the regius professor was not expected to do more than help from the sidelines. He was an honorary colonel of the Oxfordshire militia and was soon in demand as a consultant to some of the private hospitals set up by philanthropic Canadians and Americans. He procured a lieutenant-colonel's uniform which he sometimes wore on hospital visits, but he never held formal rank or served on active duty.

'The nations are still in the nursery stage, squabbling & fighting like children,' he wrote of the situation on August 6, and looked ahead to 'the tragedies that are inevitable.' Everything he knew about armies and war suggested that disease would kill as many soldiers as fighting, bacilli would be more deadly than bullets. So he began alerting the public and the authorities to the need for preventive public-health measures, especially use of the new vaccine against typhoid fever. He hoped it would be possible for the new treatment for syphilis that had emerged from Germany, Paul Ehrlich's 'Salvarsan,' to be manufactured in neutral America.[1]

Revere, aged eighteen, was about to start his undergraduate years at Christ Church. On his next birthday, December 28, he would become eligible to enlist. Although he had taken basic military training at Winchester, he had no interest in or enthusiasm for war. 'Revere meditates and is very quiet,' his mother wrote from Oxford in August. With nothing to do in a college town preparing for war, Revere and Jack Slessor rented Canadian canoes and paddled up the Thames, fishing, swimming in the nude, enjoying the last idyll of their youth.[2]

'Never have I seen in England such wonderful weather as we are having now,' Grace wrote at the end of August. 'Clear, fresh and sunny, day after day. It seems almost mockery when everyone is so depressed and worried.' The battles in France soon became desperate, massive, and very deadly. In sun-drenched Oxford, Grace sat down on September 3 with the first published casualty lists, the university calendar, and *Who's Who*. 'Poor Hallie – her Ronnie's brother was killed – Victor Brooke, a splendid South Africa hero – Lord Abermarle's son – Arnold Keppel – whom Revere knew at Quidenham, an old man but cousin of the Rector. If I was not busy I should *yell* – because I can't stop it (War). The mockery of it all – Glorious weather, roses – carnations, everything rampant ... I almost wish I was in a hideous place – it seems so useless to look on a lovely garden when one's friends are suffering.'[3]

Willie knew the casualties would come. What he was not prepared for, what shocked and horrified him and most men and women of good will in the Allied countries, was the deliberate German destruction of the medieval Belgian university town of Louvain, apparently in reprisal for civilian resistance. A great university library, with its special collections of medieval manuscripts and incunabula, was turned to ashes. 'Willie too listless to talk – except German atrocities,' Grace wrote. 'Since the destruction of Louvain town & University he is willing to believe anything.' Louvain convinced him that the war would have to end in defeat of 'the cursed militarism of Germany,' a view from which he would never waver. The Oslers began organizing support for refugee professors from Louvain, a special Oxford cause, and for the eventual restoration of the university and its library.[4]

Osler's liberal optimism, his Victorian inclination towards faith in
progress, and his internationalism all crumbled in the teeth of German
militarism and its consequences. Grace could hardly believe the change in
him: 'Poor dear Reggie can't go to church – he says he can't endure the
prayers and hymns ... The attitude W.O. is in seems more unreal than
anything else – he allows everyone to abuse the Germans and even says
vicious things himself of the Kaiser. He is sending letters and books to
President Wilson and all the prominent men – about Germany's lying attitude. It is really extraordinary to hear him. We have seven Louvain people
in the house.'[5]

The personal horror was the prospect of Revere going off to war. Despite Revere's pacific nature – he hated the thought of killing – and despite
his American birth and maternal lineage, the boy felt the same call to duty
that was attracting the flower of British youth to volunteer for Lord
Kitchener's armies. Although he was underage, he apparently considered
chucking Oxford and somehow getting into war work. 'Willie was opposed
to his joining anything at once,' Grace wrote in mid-September. 'So it is
decided for him to come to Christ Church. They are to wear uniform – do
lectures – no games – form the new company of Officers Training Corps
and work hard at that. Arthur Howard is doing the same ... I try not to
think we have prevented Revere going into active work at once – but he is
so young and so inexperienced it seemed unnecessarily cruel for Willie and
this OTC training will be much better for the future.'[6] In October Grace
helped Revere move into his rooms at Christ Church, supplying linen from
home and some family pieces of silver that Featherstone Osler had had at
Cambridge. 'He is not doing what he thought would have been better –
but has not complained once – only said, "I will do what Dad thinks best
and train here this term."' His dad remembered to put Revere on the waiting list for membership in the Athenaeum club.

A few days into Revere's first term, Grace wondered if there would be
any 'next term.' There were not seventy undergraduates at Christ Church.
Grace could not stand the Sunday services either. 'I have had the blues today
like sin and wonder what will become of us all.'[7] The idea of going home to
America was not discussed; there would not even be visits during the war.

Their son took daily military drill literally right outside their doors, in the parks. Grace, who turned sixty that year, worked as hard as she ever had in her life, managing the ladies' workroom and arranging for accommodation and support for Belgian professors and their families. She raised thousands of dollars through her American connections, including a major grant from the Rockefeller Foundation to put the 'Louvainites' to work doing research. Willie visited military camps and hospitals, lecturing on public health, urging vaccination for typhoid, and combating the ignorance of those 'sons of Belial,' the antivaccinationists. He carried on with his regular clinics at the Radcliffe Infirmary and with a smattering of private patients. The Oslers' social life ground to a halt: 'It is so extraodinary – no calls – no dinners, no theatre – nothing,' Grace wrote Marjorie Futcher in October. 'Dad said yesterday – "I shall not dress or dine out during the war." He dines in College Sunday night – and Revere brings men for supper & I try not to mention war ... What shall we do if it goes on long?'[8]

Osler's work with military hospitals settled down into three primary attachments. He was Physician-in-Chief at the Queen's Canadian Military Hospital at Shorncliffe, a consultant to the American women's auxiliary hospital at Paignton, and agreed to serve as head physician to the Canadian Red Cross hospital that was being built on Nancy and Waldorf Astor's tennis courts at their great estate, Cliveden, near Taplow. The Oslers had known the Astors socially since their arrival in England. Osler had first treated Nancy Astor, a woman of boundless vitality and ambition, at Johns Hopkins in 1894 when she was fifteen-year-old Nancy Langhorne, daughter of a nouveau riche Virginian.[9] When the British army declined the offer of Cliveden as a hospital site, the Astors had offered it to the Canadians.

Grace soon began worrying about her husband's commitments. She drew the line at having refugees stay in their house for any length of time: 'It is too trying for Willie and he must be protected in every way – all the horrors and war-talk nearly kill him and he often looks ill and worried.'[10] He resisted becoming obsessed with daily war news, but his casual reading was the memoirs of one of Napoleon's medical officers.

The wounded who began arriving in England that autumn were not as disease-ridden as Napoleon's soldiers, or as Osler had expected. His predictions of the likely ravages of ill health on armies were a simple reading from past experience without considering the triumphs of modern medicine and public health. In fact sanitary science and the practice of asepsis were delivering the healthiest troops ever to go into battle. Typhoid, or enteric fever, which had been declining sharply even before the development of a vaccine, did not become a problem on the Western Front. Even high-velocity rifle bullets created relatively clean wounds and seemed almost self-sterilizing, Osler observed. He was astonished at how rifle bullets could pass through the head, chest, or abdomen without doing serious damage. Shrapnel was another matter altogether:

> This is an artillery war in which shrapnel does the damage, tearing flesh, breaking bones, and always causing jagged, irregular wounds. And here comes in the great tragedy – sepsis everywhere, unavoidable sepsis! ... within twelve to twenty-four hours the ragged open wounds have become infected from the clothing or the soil. The surgeons are back in the pre-Listerian days and have wards filled with septic wounds. I have seen sights that remind me of student days at the Montreal General Hospital when all the compound fractures suppurated, and we dressers really had to dress wounds ... The wound of shell and shrapnel is a terrible affair, and infection is well-nigh inevitable.

It was Grace, writing to America, who totaled the wounded into a sense of the human cost: 'Every morning we read of friends being mown down, all the youth and glory of the country, the young men we have known up here; and our only boy training in the park under our eyes – except that I can't look. Work is the only salvation.'[11]

Revere would not wear his uniform home. When he saw his father in uniform for the first time, he was visibly upset. Grace poured out her frustrations – at her age, at being a woman, at being a prisoner of the war – in long letters to her sister, Susan Chapin:

> I wish I could go some where & curse & swear & pound something hard.

Oh – it requires more equanimity than I have to behave myself during *War* ... I probably *like wounds & Hospitals* more than any untrained person there but I am frightened to death of the administrator & keep away. I find it takes too much out of one to talk to the men & hear their stories except occasionally & I am *determined* to hold out and be ready for darker days than we have had – Every night Willie says 'The worst is yet to come' and he must not find me enfeebled.

Every morning Willie donned his old red golf jacket and sat down to write letters – letters to American friends, letters to Canadian relatives and friends, letters to the War Office trying to help make arrangements for relatives and friends – 'a perfect avalanche of correspondence,' he com-plained. By the winter of 1914–15 the 'Open Arms' was as busy as ever, as friends and relatives and strangers who wanted to consult or pay courtesy calls on Dr Osler began pouring in. Many were with the thirty thousand soldiers of the Canadian Expeditionary Force, now in training on Salisbury Plain (Canada had automatically gone to war as part of the Empire). Bel-gian professors wives' were underfoot, too, as Grace turned the living room into a Christmas sewing room for the manufacture of clothing and special presents for Canadian boys, for Belgians ('these people dress so differently underneath that it involves much conversation'), and for anyone the good ladies could befriend.[12]

Archie Malloch, the good-natured son of an old physician friend from Hamilton, arrived fresh from his medical training that autumn and be-came a favorite guest at 13 Norham Gardens between hospital assignments. His journal is an important window on wartime life with the Oslers. Tom McCrae's physician brother, Jack, who had trained for a time at Hopkins, had fought with Canadian troops in the South African War, and then practiced and taught in Montreal, had joined up in his forties as a regular officer in the Canadian Army. He often came over from camp to cadge socks for his men and enjoy Osler hospitality. A nephew and great-nephew came for Christmas, as did two Canadian Tuppers and the Ramsay Wrights, the Toronto academic friends who had retired to Oxford. Vanloads of cloth-ing arrived from the United States, and barrels of apples from Canada. On

Christmas Day 1914 surgeons in the hospitals carved turkeys for the wounded. The Oslers went to church at Ewelme in the morning, gave out Christmas dinners to the old men at the almshouse, and visited the Radcliffe Infirmary and other Oxford hospitals in the afternoon. Grace distributed 325 presents. 'These New England women are full of vitality,' Osler wrote to a New England woman friend. Altogether they were struggling through the winter in fairly good spirits. 'We see too much of the tragedies to make life very happy,' he added.[13]

Revere continued to blossom intellectually, developing a fine taste in literature, a dose of his father's bibliomania, and a great interest in the visual arts, including a knack for sketching which his father must have envied. Osler's letters now invariably included comments on Revere's love of books, their congenial tastes and temperaments, their good times together. For Christmas 1914 he gave Revere a perfect first edition of Izaak Walton's life of George Herbert, 'uncut, unsoiled and just as it left the hands of the printer.'[14] Revere had a happy Christmas at home with the extended family and opportunities to fish on the Thames. Willie decided to change his will so that some of his books might pass to his son. He could not bring himself to think about the 'great question,' as Grace put it, facing the lad after his birthday.

Revere was not yet much of a soldier, despite his drilling in the Officers' Training Corps. He was judged too young and inexperienced to become an officer, in fact had so little heart for it all that even his mother wondered how he could ever become a fighter. But Revere wanted to do his bit and decided that he would not have a next term at Christ Church. He toyed with the idea of running off to India with a territorial regiment or of finding some kind of medical work; then decided to enlist as a private in the Universities Public School Regiment, take basic training, and hope to jump to a good regiment as an officer. He confided in his mother, talking 'wisely, oh so wisely with me,' she wrote. 'He simply can't talk with Willie,' at least on that matter.

On January 5, 1915, Revere brought home his books and his grandfather's silver from Christ Church. 'His lovely room must be dismantled,' Grace wrote to sister Sue. 'What a strange fate after our fear that he might never get in!' Grace's heart was breaking for both her men. 'With you to look up to,' she told her sister, 'and the women I was brought up among I shall do my utmost to hold out and have a cheerful face for the poor dear unselfish angel who is just breaking his heart over giving up his boy to this awful risk.'[15]

Grace had mentioned Revere's interest in the possibility of doing medical work to Bill Francis, who happened to be involved in the McGill Faculty of Medicine's plan to staff a hospital unit for service in France. Francis mentioned to Dean F.S. Birkett, commanding officer of the outfit, that Osler's son might be interested in serving with them. Osler was already helping McGill cut British red tape to have its plans expedited. Revere was about to enlist as a common soldier when a cable arrived from Birkett in Canada asking him to join them as Birkett's private orderly. He would not be a combatant, but he would obviously be serving. Mother, father, and son agreed to take this route. Until the Canadians arrived, Revere would work as assistant quartermaster at the Canadian Red Cross's Duchess of Connaught Hospital at Cliveden.[16]

The character of the Western Front was established in 1915: immobile armies dug into trenches from the Swiss border to the English Channel; massive build-ups of men, artillery, and supplies; vast, vicious battles to gain a few hundred yards of devastated earth; casualties mounting from the tens to the hundreds of thousands and higher; over the battlefields, an everyday stench of death and futility and the wreckage of a generation's highest ideals; noble patriotism giving way to hatred and war-weariness. What Canadian Prime Minister Robert Borden called 'the suicide of civilization.'

From their leafy street in the city of dreaming spires, the Oslers tried to convince neutral Americans that if Britain were to fall, the United States would be next. Many of their American friends were bellicose anglophiles who needed little persuasion. Harvey Cushing, for example, was impatient for an opportunity to put his skills to use. He became one of the organizers of a Harvard medical unit that sailed in the spring of 1915 to do a stint at a special Ambulance Hospital in Paris, created and staffed by Americans. The Oslers were very disappointed, 'ashamed' Grace said, that Johns Hopkins did not organize a similar unit, though they made no public fuss about it.[17] Perhaps the considerable German population of Baltimore was a factor. Perhaps the Germanophilia of Mall, Halsted, Abel, and others on the Hopkins staff came into play.

To his German friends in America, such as the physician and book collector Arnold Klebs, Osler tried to remain cordial: 'We need not talk war.' Despite his early rage at German atrocities, Osler never became a bitter Germanophobe. In the winter of 1914–15 he looked into some of the atrocity stories more fully and decided they had been hugely exaggerated. 'It is a hopeless job to think of getting any truth between the two sides,' he told Klebs. 'I wish they would hang a few of the editors.' Osler talked of an intellectual gulf opening between Britain and Germany that might not be bridged for generations. He never doubted the rightness of the Allied cause, and declined to prolong a correspondence with a pacifist doctor who argued that he had gone back on his internationalist preachings.[18] Like virtually all of the internationalists of his generation, including practically everyone in the socialist movement, he had. Yet he was much more tolerant than brother Edmund, back in Canada, who led a largely successful witch-hunt to oust German professors from the University of Toronto. In 1916 William wrote to the *Times* opposing the cry for reprisal air raids against German civilians.

The doctor in Willie found the medical side of the war intriguing. The campaign against typhoid fever continued to work well. But the Canadian troops training on Salisbury Plain endured a horrible soggy winter – Osler had not seen such mud since his boyhood days in the Canadian bush – culminating in an outbreak of cerebrospinal meningitis. As one of the world's experts on the disease, Osler was consulted frequently. He shared the concern that a new serum treatment for meningitis appeared to be useless, but advised, rightly, that the meningococcus, although extremely malignant, is not easily transmitted. With reasonable precautions the case rate would continue to be low and there was no need for undue alarm. He tutored British doctors on treating frostbite, a condition seldom seen in peacetime in that climate but now almost epidemic in the camps and trenches. And he thought overuse of tobacco and the strain of trench life was producing many cases of 'the old-fashioned irritable heart' which DaCosta had first observed in the American Civil War. He once amused troops at Shorncliffe by lighting up a cigarette at the end of a lecture on the evils of smoking.[19]

As the fighting increased in the spring of 1915, Osler began to see men in much worse shape – nervous wrecks with extreme symptoms of neurasthenia, hysteria, and paraplegia apparently caused by 'shell shock.' 'The truth is, the trenches have been a veritable hell,' he told readers of the *Journal of the American Medical Association*, 'and it is not surprising that a good many of the men show signs of severe nervous shock.' At Norham Gardens the Oslers learned more of the hell of the fighting when Jack McCrae came back from France on leave and told them about the second battle of Ypres, at which the Germans first used poison gas. 'I am *glad* and *sorry* you did not hear him,' Grace wrote her sister. 'He looked thin and worn ... 31 days in the trenches with eight days' rest ... His clothes were awful ... The nerve strain he says is beyond any sensation possible to describe. When they had to stand on the roadside waiting for orders and saw the French Colonials and civilians rushing away from the gas when it was first turned on, he says it was Hades absolutely; and they stood fast ... I felt sick when he left Monday night.'[20]

Most of his friends thought Jack McCrae never recovered from second Ypres. In the midst of the fighting, the literary doctor-soldier had found time to scribble a few lines of verse. Months later, *Punch* published 'In Flanders Fields,' and it became the most famous poem written about the Great War, the most famous poem ever written by a physician. McCrae was transferred to the McGill medical unit, No. 3 Canadian General Hospital (McGill), which arrived in Britain late that spring and soon proceeded to France. Its staff of more than three hundred doctors, nurses, and students included Bill Francis, Campbell Howard, and, of course, Revere, who had been restless and a bit conscience-stricken doing cushy work in the quartermaster's office at Cliveden, interrupted by lunches with the Astors.

One old McGill man never got to see the unit off. T. Wesley Mills, Osler's one-time classmate and assistant, and his successor in pathology, had retired to London with his wife. Osler had helped arrange a pension. On February 13 Mrs Mills was telling her husband a joke over breakfast when his heart failed and he fell dead. Since Mills had designated Osler as his executor, she called Oxford for help. Osler was away, and it became another of Grace's wifely duties to run up to London and arrange for Mills's cremation. Willie wrote a thoughtful obituary notice for the *Canadian Medical Association Journal* reflecting on Mills's 'curious lack of capacity for happiness' and evident disappointment after having striven so hard for success in life. 'It is the careless sinner who goes a-whistling and working through life caring not for what the world thinks, who gets more than his due,' he added, surely thinking of himself. He arranged special help from McGill for Mills's widow.[21]

By the spring of 1915, with wounded men pouring back into Britain and the new hospitals in full operation, Osler was professionally as busy as ever. He visited the Cliveden hospital every Monday, went to Shorncliffe every ten days and to Paignton once a fortnight. In between, there had to be time for his private consultations (his total income stayed roughly constant in the early war years, though a higher percentage of it came from investments), as well as for Oxford duties, other hospital visits and war work, and family. 'One of the busiest ten days I ever had,' he noted in his diary for April 29 – May 8, 1915:

Harrogate on the 29th, interesting case of chronic jaundice. Leeds, Friday, saw Teale and the hospital; back in the evening. On Sat. General Jones of the Canadian [Medical] Contingent spent the day here & went over the local hospitals ... Sunday, Cheltenham to see a case of hematuria. In eve went to London so as to be able to leave early Monday for Woking to see young Wilkes with septic pneumonia following a fracture. While there a telegram to see Mrs. Burns in London. Saw her in p.m. went up again Tues.

a.m. In p.m. went to Cliveden to see medical cases at Canadian hospital. Wed. London again. Thurs. London. Friday London [for visits to Mrs. Burns], and in p.m. Chatham where I lectured to 1500 soldiers. Dinner in Eve by Med. officers of the Garrison. Saturday a.m. saw the Fort Pitt Hospital; made rounds with the young doctors. P.m. went to Bromley to inspect new Canadian Convalescent Hospital.

I traveled 1260 miles which reminded me of old American days & made £519.[22]

Osler neglected to mention that on Thursday, May 6, he welcomed Harvey Cushing for a quick visit, then had to go out in the night to break the news to a colleague of the death of his son. While he was gone, Cushing and Grace and Susan Chapin sat up 'talking the sort of gossip of the war to which W.O. will never listen, for he hears all he can bear during the day.' On Saturday, May 8, they all heard of the torpedoing of the *Lusitania*, with heavy loss of civilian lives. Cushing's Atlantic route home the next day was through waters littered with bodies and wreckage.[23]

Despite Grace's constant worrying about him, Osler stayed healthy and fit. Instead of giving in to age, as he had often enough prescribed, he had decided not to notice it. In 1913 he had defined his new attitude: 'One of two things happens after sixty, when old age takes a fellow by the hand. Either the rascal takes charge as general factotum, and you are in his grip body and soul; or you take him by the neck at the first encounter, and after a good shaking make him go your way.' Young physicians still had trouble keeping up with Osler when he was on the move. Archie Malloch always found a day with him in London extremely strenuous. Osler read medical journals as he traveled, going through a dozen articles to most people's one; he ran up stairs two at a time (three at a time when he was going up to the Bodleian Library). In London Malloch would follow him from Paddington station to Guy's to the British Museum to Quaritch the book dealer, to the Bibliographical Society, and back to Paddington for the Oxford train, on which Osler would again read while Malloch struggled to stay awake.[24]

On other London trips Osler would see patients at their homes or hotels. On April 27, for example, he saw three patients in town, one of whom was the Foreign Secretary, Sir Edward Grey. Grey's eyesight was endangered by pigmentary retinitis, and he was desperately doctor-shopping in hope of positive suggestions. The prime minister had suggested consulting Osler. 'Bad outlook,' Osler noted in his daybook and undoubtedly reinforced his colleagues' warnings to Grey that he had to rest his eyes. In 1914 Grey may never have uttered the famous phrase about the lamps going out all over Europe; but now, for him, they were. Grey ignored his doctors' advice and kept on with the burdens of office, wearing dark glasses.[25]

On May 28, 1915, the Oslers completed ten years in England. 'Extraordinarily happy years,' Willie noted in his daybook:

> Everyone as kind & considerate as could be wished. Grace has been happy and the boy has thriven ... It is a curious thing that with much more leisure literary output has been much less than in the previous decade. With less practice I have saved us much in 10 years, more in fact, than in 40 years of previous practice. I left America with about $3600 [income] from investments which I have increased to above $10,000. I have got a good deal of education & have made a great collection of books for my old school at McGill. I have not done much in the profession here, but I have done three useful things or, better, helped to: 1) the Association of British Physicians; 2) the Quarterly Journal of Medicine; 3) the Historical Section of the Roy. Soc. Medicine ...
>
> From the profession at large I have had the kindest treatment. Altogether it has been the most successful experiment. I have kept very well. I have not had any such sub-sternal threatenings as I used to have in Baltimore. I had one attack of renal colic, the 2nd in 12 years. It has been a great comfort not to live a life of such strain. The one thing I miss is the active teaching and the close association with students & a large group of young doctors; but I console myself with the thirty-one years of strenuous work I had in Canada & in the United States.[26]

The day before he wrote this entry, they saw Revere off to join the McGill unit. A few weeks later the Oslers went to Southampton to see the whole McGill hospital off for France.

Then nothing much happened. The main theater of British fighting in the summer of 1915 was in far-off Turkey, where the Dardenelles campaign ground towards bloody failure. In France the surplus of hospital beds was well ahead of the attrition rate, and the eager medical workers found themselves with nothing to do. The McGill unit set up its thousand-bed hospital along with other units in a medical tent city on a windswept plain near the French coast, at Dannes-Camiers, and twiddled their thumbs in idleness. One of the unit's first patients remarked on being distinctly overtreated. As he was helped out of the ambulance, he recalled, 'the Colonel took my hand, then three lieutenant-colonels took my pulse, four majors hurried to take my temperature, and some blighter took my watch.'[27] Revere sent home for his bicycle and went fishing on his days off.

Grace found the first full wartime summer depressing. She was rattled by constant visitors: Chattie's son Norman convalescing from a wound (his melancholy humming got on her nerves); brother-in-law Frank Osler, taking a water cure for his drinking problem, who was sweet enough but whose wife Belle was a 'queer coot'; and her own relative-by-marriage, Adèle Chapin, a flighty socialite determined to set up her own private hospital. Grace also participated in an endless round of fundraising teas, flag days, and 'Belgianizing.' The able-bodied male servants had gone off to war; it was not yet hard to replace them, though the new chauffeur, an invalid, had a tendency to get lost. Grace often chafed at not having had to suffer any serious hardships: 'When I think how little personal discomfort I am enduring – none in fact – I feel ashamed – but I can't offer my stalwart form for a target.' On the first anniversary of the declaration of war, which Grace thought should be a 'sacred day,' Willie insisted that they attend the wedding of a daughter of Walter Hines Page, the American ambassador. It was a glittering Anglo-American affair; the guests included Prime Minister H.H. Asquith, Sir Edward Grey (looking very good), Henry James, and John Singer Sargent.

Then it was back to dutiful war entertaining: 'Yesterday the Car fetched 5 nurses from Cliveden for luncheon – Such flighty creatures – three of them – apparently over here for *flirtations* only. I hope the McGill Nurses leave Revere alone – of course it is human Nature.' Better flightiness and flirtation than being obsessed by the war. When the Oslers stayed at the country house of Lady Wantage to meet the Archbishop of York, they came away exhausted. 'There were about 12 people and all talked about the War – horrors and mistakes – Willie looked a ghost and could not divert any one. No more visits for me.'[28]

Osler visited France one week in September 1915, his only wartime crossing. The McGill hospital was one of seven medical units clumped together on the Picardy coast. Looking at the scene from nearby downs, Osler was struck by the peacefulness of the white tents gleaming in the evening sun, a few figures in white and khaki flitting about, the occasional lorry driving by. In an Old Testament mood those days, Osler was reminded 'of the description of the tents of Israel pitched in Moab and putting Balaam and Balak to sore perplexity.' He inspected all the hospitals, saw incoming wounded arrive, including the son of a prominent politician, 'shot thro' the chest ... a sad business but the nurses & doctors seemed to know their work.' 'All the interesting and obscure cases were shown him as in the old days in Baltimore,' Campbell Howard remembered, 'and as of yore we received his simple, concise and invaluable advice, and the patient, the cheery smile and the word of encouragement.' He slept in a tent for the first time in forty years – 'a bit breezy, & cold & cramped but snug enough – considering.'.

Revere was serving as assistant quartermaster. There was time for father and son, along with Bill Francis and Campbell Howard, to go off sightseeing – to the old inn at Montreuil, where Laurence Sterne had rested on the first night of his *Sentimental Journey* – and to lunch at a quiet *estaminet*. Osler had not thought he would be allowed to visit the front, but on another day a point was stretched for him, and Jack McCrae took him on a long day's drive just behind the lines. They may have visited the sites from McCrae's poem, where poppies were blowing among row on row of crosses:

> Stationary balloons, aeroplanes, soldiers, camps, billets in farms, brigades of artillery on march – such a scene! ... we saw the bombardment of aeroplanes by the German aircraft guns ... 122 puff-balls could be counted against the clouds, many seemed so close, but the aeroplane sailed about taking the usual daily observations. It was a great sight the most wonderful I have seen.

Miles & miles of motor lorries line the roads waiting to go up in the eve. The whole country is alive with troops. The peasants are hard at work getting in their crops, even between the lines of trenches. Col. McCrae has been fighting all thro the district and took us to several spots on which his battery was stationed. Everywhere great squares of graves – marked with the names of the men of the Regiments.[29]

Osler had been reliving his childhood horror at bloody tales of Israelite slaughter. Back in England, he began a major address on 'Science and War' by suggesting that Jeremiah would say, 'The world is drunken and the nations are mad.' Mankind had not progressed. 'In what a fool's paradise many of us have been living ...' There had been so much apparent progress during the past century, he observed that 'some of us had indulged the fond hope that in the power man had gained over nature had arisen possibilities for intellectual and social development such as to control collectively the morals and emotions, so that the nations would not learn war any more. We were foolish enough to think that where Christianity had failed Science might succeed ... We overlooked the fact that beneath a skin-deep civilization were the same old elemental passions ready to burst forth.'

What could he say now about science, whose rise had been so important in the nineteenth century? Such bitter fruit: 'In two ways science is the best friend war has ever had; it has made slaughter possible on a scale never dreamt of before, and it has enormously increased man's capacity to maim and to disable his fellow man ... This is the day of Nisroch, Chief of Ordnance to Satan in the great war of heaven ... Never since the primal tragedy, when man first shed man's blood, has there been such a carnival of carnage as that which science has made possible during the past year.'

Cushing had told Osler that the sufferings of some of the victims of German gas were beyond all belief. When Osler examined sections of the lungs of gassed soldiers, the fissures and fractures of the alveoli were unlike anything he had ever seen. About the time of his visit to France, he had a rare dream that seemed to mean something. He retold it in 'Science and War':

Explorers in Central Africa had accidentally opened a vein of deadly radium which flowed slowly but imperceptibly like an unseen lava over the surface of the earth, killing by the exhalation of an irrespirable gas. It had crossed the Mediterranean, swept through Europe, and had reached England. Convocation had been summoned by the Chancellor and the members of the University in academic cap and gown awaited the end of all things. On came the irresistible and deadly vapour, swept down the ranks, reached me, and I awoke – gasping for breath.[30]

Osler tried to temper disillusionment with an account of how medical science was saving soldiers' lives through public health and well-organized treatment of the wounded. He paid tribute to scientists such as Paul Ehrlich, a recent casualty of the war, and tried to counter his own foreboding that the war would mean the death of international science for at least a generation. The attempt to sustain optimism was flat as he forced a conclusion: 'This old earth has rarely had a worse year than that through which we have just passed. Men's hearts are failing for fear ... Let us not despair.' After what he had seen in France, Osler privately wondered if the war would ever end.[31]

For Revere there was not enough war, not enough to do at the McGill hospital. After the September-October intake of wounded from the Battle of Loos, the unit was underemployed. Its beautiful marquee tents, a gift to the cause from India, leaked in heavy rain – their cotton ropes shrank and the pegs pulled away – and they blew to tatters in autumn gales. By the end of October the McGill hospital staff shivered in a sea of mud – damp, cold, and patientless. Revere's conscience was bothering him, and he began talking about changing to something more active, such as duty with a field ambulance unit. By now friends of his would have been falling in battle. He must have been asking himself what it would be like after the war to be known to have sat it out behind the lines in a job obtained by family pull. 'I would sacrifice anything to know the boy's Conscience was at rest,' Grace wrote her sister. 'I am so weary rolling about the bed thinking about his worries ... Poor Willie – simply won't or can't talk about it. And I can't talk to other people.'[32]

By mid-November the McGill tents were no longer fit for patients. The hospital was closed down, some of its staff dispersed, and the rest, including Revere, were dropped down a wartime well of neglect. 'I am still with No. 3 which nearly a month ago ceased to be a hospital and which has since become a turbid mud hole, rank with unrest and discontent,' the boy wrote with soldierly literary flare:

> The red-hatted authorities must have forgotten us ... 30 officers, 250 men and 70 nurses have for five weeks sat in cold and draughty tents with the mud oozing through the floors and the rain dripping from the roof, without a thing to do but fight the wind and the rain and stoke the smoking stinking braziers ... Over all, in my eyes at any rate, a mist of impenetrable gloom seems to hang ... We all sit round the oil-can every day. Sometimes someone goes away for the day, sometimes someone writes a letter and usually two or three couples are playing cards with a pile of sous in front of them.[33]

Trying to get the War Office to ease McGill's plight was only one of Osler's burdens back in England. He was on the road three or four days of the week now. He saw the former Canadian prime minister, his old patient Sir Charles Tupper, fifteen times before the statesman's death in 1915 at ninety-four. The round of travels, inspections, and consultations was punctuated more and more often by news of friends losing one son, sometimes two. 'The loss among our friends is shocking – Shafer, Moore, Rolleston, Garrod, Handford, Herringham & others have all lost boys.' Rudyard Kipling's son, not yet nineteen, was missing in action. Harvey Cushing later described Osler as a kind of 'Consoler-General' among his circle – though in fact the stiff-lipped parents did a remarkable job of keeping up appearances. But even the prime minister of Great Britain, four of whose five sons were in khaki, was buckling under the strain of the war and a deteriorating political situation. Both Asquith, suffering from serious exhaustion, and his wife consulted Osler at the end of October. 'A. has been wretched & Mrs. A. He has a hard team to drive.'[34] Eventually the team threw Asquith over, replacing him with David Lloyd George.

When Grace was not tossing and turning at night about Revere, she was worrying about Willie. 'Everyone says W.O. looks well, but why he is not worn out I do not know.' The correspondence burden alone was horrendous – in days of penny postage and 240 pence to the pound, the Oslers bought five pounds worth of stamps at a time.

> The thing that wearies me, and him too but he won't say so, is the continual strain of talking. Every day for weeks there has been an extra person at lunch – someone wanting something. Today a female doctor from Boston, who came for a letter to a Swiss doctor as she is going to work in Zurich. Yesterday it was a Canadian nurse wanting a job. Tomorrow it will be a parson wanting to go to France, and Friday it will be all the Harvard Unit at luncheon in Christ Church Hall and tea here at 4.30. The demands on him never stop.[35]

His relaxation was his library and the grand cataloging project he had designed. Norham Gardens was overflowing in every nook and cranny – upwards of seven thousand books and manuscripts relating to medicine, and several thousand other books that were not part of his basic library. Osler knew it would be a tragedy if his library was broken up, perhaps sold by auction, after his death. So it was to be willed to McGill – not Johns Hopkins, which had the Surgeon-General's Library in Washington close at hand. By 1914 Osler was devoting most of his spare time to arranging and annotating the collection.

After consulting with librarian friends, he had made a somewhat quirky decision to organize and catalog his library in eight sections:

- Prima: works that made up a biographical-bibliographical account of the evolution of science, including medicine
- Secunda: secondary works on the same themes

- Litteraria: literary works written by or about physicians
- Historica: books on medical history
- Biographica: lives
- Bibliographica: books about books
- Incunabula: books from the dawn of printing
- Manuscripts.

Innumerable decisions had to be made. Which book would go where? Too bad that the 'Death, Heaven, and Hell' section on the bookshelves would be broken up. The catalog of the whole, or *Bibliotheca Osleriana*, was to be *raisonée*, or descriptive. So what should be said about each author? About a work's provenance? About its contribution? About its ongoing relevance? About its printing history? What were the gaps in the collection? How could they be filled? All the while that Osler was organizing and cataloging, he kept on buying at auctions and sales, from other catalogs and through friends: 'What are the good Scotch Novels depicting the Doctors life? Ask your Scotch friends' ... 'In your leisure moments look out for any of James Gregory's big controversial pamphlets.' When he awoke in the night, he mentally drafted introductions to the sections of the catalog.[36]

Osler wrote notes about books and authors on index cards and in the works themselves. He had so much to do and so little time that he only scratched the surface of his collection. Even so, he left behind:

- Judgments on authors: 'Theophrastus is even to-day a living and not a dead botanist'; 'I hesitated a long time whether or not to put Averroes in Bibliotheca Prima'; Malthus's '"Essay" is a great book, full of good things. Did ever any one suffer so cruelly and so unjustly in reputation!'
- Unusual anecdotes: 'Garrick wrote on Hill the well-known epigram: "For physic and farces his equal there scarce is / His farces are physic, his physic a farce is."'
- Book auction adventures: The time he inadvertently commissioned two dealers to go after the same set of Galen and wound up bidding against himself.
- Conscience prickings about the Marischal College mark on his edition of Copernicus.

- Personal reminiscences: 'I only saw Darwin once ...'
- Exhortations: 'Glasgow has been slow in doing justice to the memory of her most distinguished medical graduate. There remains a plain duty.'
- Oddities: His Yorkshire patient who remembered being treated by a urine doctor, a descendant of the seventeenth-century 'piss-prophets.'
- Osler on doctors in literature: 'Would that Lydgate existed only in fiction'; 'I love Dr. Thorne for his theory as to the happiness of children – "he argued that the principal duty which a parent owed to a child was to make him happy." Wise man!'[37]

If Osler had lived to finish his notes, the catalog of his library would have been as readable and personal and charming as his textbook. The catch was that being a true collector he would not have considered the library or the catalog finished so long as he lived. He never did get around to having a personal bookplate designed. His student friends could not believe their good fortune at being called in when Dr Osler had his annual 'shed,' giving away surplus.

The British workmanship that had gone into installing the furnace at 13 Norham Gardens almost caused the destruction of the library on November 11, 1915. Grace was awakened at 3.30 AM by the smell of smoke, went downstairs, and found their dining room on fire. The servants dithered while Willie and Revere, who was home on leave, struggled with wet towels over their mouths to rescue priceless incunabula and manuscripts from the smoke-filled room over the dining room. Oxford's firefighters arrived twenty-three minutes after the call: 'Good morning, have you a fire?' they asked at the door. The flames almost broke through before being brought under control. The only seriously damaged book was the dictionary that was kept in the dining room for mealtime reference. After the tumult had ended, Willie went back to bed. Grace supervised weeks of clean-up and repairs.[38]

Osler was laid up over Christmas 1915 with another of his respiratory infections, what Grace called 'an influenzary cold.' She made him stay in bed, steam his throat, and take a tonic. Canadian friends sent ninety-eight barrels of apples for her to distribute. On Christmas Day she helped with the turkey dinners at one of the Oxford hospitals. The plum puddings had just been lit when a convoy of wounded arrived and had to be settled in. Grace helped feed some of the men: 'I was delighted because I was able to really help.' 'Horrid year full of worry and sorrows,' Osler summed up at the end of 1915, appending a list of friends who had lost sons. Still, he was staunchly bellicose: 'The country is going strong. Hit any man on the head for me who says "peace"!'[39]

'Oxford is deserted – only Rhodes scholars & invalids,' Osler wrote in February. The buildup to undreamed-of levels of war was obvious that spring. More troops were billeted in the colleges; every morning in March the 30th Fusiliers, headquartered in the divinity school, marched to the music of their band up Norham Gardens to drill in the parks. At night the city was blacked out for fear of bombing raids by German zeppelins. 'The world here is making dark blinds,' Grace wrote.[40]

Even though there were many empty hospital beds in Oxford, new ones kept being added. The Oslers helped with one convalescent, their Rhodes scholar friend Wilder Penfield, who had broken a leg when the ship taking him to do Red Cross work in France had been torpedoed. When he was landed in Dover, Penfield found flowers waiting. 'The first ever,' he noted in his diary. 'They came from Lady Osler. I can hardly understand all their kind attention.' Penfield was taken into the family to recuperate. He remembered 13 Norham Gardens as 'a defiantly cheerful citadel devoted to hospitality,' with Grace carrying the load of management, and he recorded an incident with children: 'Two little kiddies came in to see "William" as they call Sir William, the other day, and, to amuse them, he took them up to a second storey porch which overlooks the garden and from there he threw water down on Lytle and Davison, who had come to see me. Then, when Lytle put up a lady's umbrella, which lay there, he poured a whole pitcher of water full on him, while the kiddies screamed with delight.'[41]

In February Penfield had heard Osler give a talk about his life to the American Club at Oxford and had found a role model: 'He said, at the end, that his rule had been to like and sympathize with everyone. That's his creed, I think. He is the least sentimental and the most helpful man I've ever seen – and the most lovable. You may believe that he is stimulating to me, too, and is on something of a pedestal. If I were not so dumb, I should have the nerve to hope and dream I might follow in his footsteps.' (In the attempt to do that, the young American must have been mortified as he botched his first autopsy, while Osler watched. 'Splendid! Splendid!' Osler exclaimed. 'It is always better to do a thing wrong the first time.')[42]

The soldiers soon left Oxford, heading for France. In mid-April 1916, all officers' leave was canceled. 'One trembles to think there may be a horrible repetition of last year's fighting,' Grace wrote. 'I saw three men in a row in the Hospital the other day & not one leg left of the six.' Grace remarked on the women conductors on the London buses, the women serving in the dining room at Brown's Hotel, the women gardeners on the estates at Cliveden and Blenheim, and the legless and armless men she saw in Bond Street.[43] Patriotic men had answered the call from all corners of the Empire. The Canadian volunteers included literally dozens of Oslers. Adding in Francis and Bath connections, many of them English, some fifty men of the extended family would go into battle.

Revere, too, had had enough of medical service. His attempt to transfer to a field ambulance unit had been snarled in red tape, so he decided to become a combatant and join the artillery. 'Long association with Jack McCrae has made him a bit bloodthirsty,' his father wrote. It took several months of intense string-pulling to get Revere out of the McGill unit and back into the British army, during which he was able to spend many weeks at Norham Gardens. He was continuing to develop as a young man of literary taste, a wonderful companion to his father, and was also in a homo-erotic stage in his warm friendship with an American school chum, Bob Emmons. At the end of one of Revere's leaves, his mother described how 'he & his Dad were glued to old books all the time he was here and reading to each other every evening, Bob joining in – sitting on the arm of Revere's chair with his arm around him. He is just like a man in love with a girl – Revere seems years older than Bob.' On one of the occasions when Revere's troop train was pulling out of Oxford, he pulled an edition of Keats from his hip pocket and waved it at his doting father on the platform. While

Revere was training to fight, Bob Emmons went off to France to drive an ambulance.[44]

'Aunt Grace, for Heaven's sake keep Revere back if you can as long as possible,' an Osler nephew, Campbell Gwyn, told her. Gwyn was one of only two officers in his regiment who had got through the fighting at St Eloi without being killed or wounded. Grace wrote to America about these awful things one beautiful day in May when she had gone with Willie to Stow-on-the-Wold. She went walking in the fields while he saw a patient:

> I have been sound asleep in a field under a white May-bush, with daisies, buttercups, clover, forget-me-nots and many others under my feet. Such a fine view across the Cotswolds with Kingham and Chipping Norton in the distance ... The day is too superb. I believe my condition of mind is peculiar; I almost resent the glory of the country and the blue sky when I think of the horrors across the Channel and the misery in the hearts everywhere. I believe it is easier to bear when the clouds are gray and the rain coming down ...
>
> Campbell Gwyn ... looked years older and seems so weary ... Campbell told me that for 3 miles in front of the trenches he had just come from he did not believe there was an inch you could put your finger where there were not bits of shell – buried in the ground ... Campbell says huge guns are coming all the time, and not yet used; preparing for the future. Isn't it ghastly to speak of the 'future'?

One afternoon Grace visited seven Oxford acquaintances in an hour. The toll of their boys was two killed, two wounded, one a prisoner, seven more serving in France. 'I tottered home and wondered what fate was in store for the Oslers.'[45]

The fate began less than three weeks later during feinting and skirmishing before the start of the great Somme offensive. Ralph Osler, Frank and Belle's only son, was wounded near Ypres and operated on, but died of peritonitis. Whatever his father's shortcomings, everyone had liked Ralph, and Edmund had treated him like a son. 'Of course this is the beginning and we shall all have our turn,' Grace wrote. Old Canadian friends, the

George Wrongs, lost their son in the carnage of July 1, the official beginning of the Battle of the Somme, a day of 60,000 Empire casualties. Other Oxford men disappeared. By July 4 the Oxford hospitals were full. For a time, at least, the armies had advanced, and of course the newspapers were trumpeting victory upon victory. 'Everyone is hopeful,' Grace wrote, 'but the tragedies are so awful one can't rejoice.' Even before the Somme she had found Sundays depressing – 'for I can think only of the happy days and rows of happy men now killed or maimed, coming in for Tea.'[46]

Willie kept busy all that spring with private consultations, hospital work, organizing a Shakespeare exhibition at the Bodleian (at which he gave a charming opening address), planning postwar summer schools in the history of science, and always puttering with his books. In April he agreed to serve on a royal commission examining university education in Wales, and often went over there. Grace fretted about his travels, his health, his own fretting, even his lack of fretting. During Oxford's zeppelin scare, she reported, he 'stays calmly in bed and refuses to have books packed or anything done. I have wanted to get him away – he has a bad cold & looks badly.'[47]

After Ralph Osler's death, Grace wanted to console Frank and Belle at Norham Gardens but thought it might upset Willie: 'She would drive Uncle crazy and he is growing rather worried & miserable as troubles come near home,' Grace told Bill Francis. 'And Revere's training is bringing him daily nearer the Murderous Mess ... How I long to be happy once more!!!!" When they visited Revere in training near Newcastle, he would not let his mother see the barracks and told her his fellow volunteers were 'without ideals or sympathy.' Grace found him full of 'horribly morbid ideas about the wickedness of war.' Parents and son visited Durham Cathedral, which had a splendid library, although many of the books had been put away for fear of air attacks. 'He has made up his mind to go through with the horrid business & take his chances,' Willie wrote of Revere. 'The war has been a terrible mental shock to many sensitive young fellows. It is bad enough for hardened old sinners like myself.'[48]

Revere's need for training spared him through the blood-drenched summer of 1916. As Willie 'rampaged' and 'careered' about, inspecting hospitals, rushing from deathbed to deathbed, scribbling obituaries of old friends and notes of condolence about friends' sons, Grace's despair was almost total. 'The Casualty lists are so horrible now it makes one ill to look in the papers and one's friends are in trouble in every direction ... So many of the very best are being taken – it seems all so wicked and useless.' In September the prime minister's brilliant son, Raymond Asquith, was killed on the Somme. 'Still the young died,' Edith Wharton would write in her Great War novel, *A Son at the Front*. 'Wherever Campton went, he met elderly faces, known and unknown, disfigured by grief, shrunken with renunciation. And still the months wore on without result.'[49]

In the summer of 1916 Osler became enmeshed in a Canadian controversy whose comic opera overtones would have made it amusing had not so many careers and reputations and, indirectly, soldiers' lives been at stake. The Canadian forces in the Great War fought as part of the British army, under British command. In England there were complex Anglo-Canadian arrangements governing troop accommodation, training, and hospital and medical services. Sometimes the situation bordered on the chaotic as a particularly aggressive and dubiously competent Canadian Minister of Militia and Defense in Ottawa, Sir Sam Hughes, acted as though he personally was in charge of everything to do with every Canadian soldier.

The Canadian medical units, including military and volunteer hospitals, were administered by the Canadian Army Medical Corps, which was responsible jointly to the British Army Medical Service and the Canadian minister of militia. From the beginning of the war, the Canadian and British medical services had effectively merged their efforts, making good use of Anglo-Canadians such as Osler as linchpins. Canadian hospitals in Britain treated wounded soldiers of any nationality; wounded Canadians were treated wherever they could best be accommodated. The system worked efficiently and without significant friction, save perhaps for the unhappy Canadians staffing empty hospitals with the British force on a backwater Balkan beachhead in Salonika. It was also known that the

Canadian Director of Medical Services, Major General G.C. Jones, who had been a political appointment of a previous Liberal government, was *non grata* with the passionate Conservative, Sam Hughes.

In the summer of 1916 Hughes commissioned an ambitious and self-important Toronto surgeon, Herbert Bruce, who had no significant military experience, to make a special inspection of the Canadian medical services in Britain. Bruce and a panel of semi-qualified cronies careered around England, collecting grievances in a fairly obvious witch-hunt aimed at bringing down Jones. Such an investigation was utterly irregular, contrary to British military law and custom, and, in the view of the British Director-General of the Army Medical Service, 'contrary to every sentiment which upright men possess.'[50] Senior medical men became alarmed. Osler heard about the situation, knew Bruce from transatlantic crossing days, and wrote him asking if Jones would be given the equivalent of due process. Osler was furious when he received an impertinent, noncommital reply. Jones, fearing for his career and wanting a private life, persuaded Osler not to resign his Canadian consultantships in protest against the whole arrangement.

The mess worsened when Bruce submitted his report in September and it was leaked to the press. It seemed a damning indictment of the Canadian medical services for failing to treat Canadian boys in Canadian hospitals, for allowing Canadians to convalesce in poorly equipped British volunteer hospitals, and for being staffed with an unduly large number of drunkards, dope addicts, and incompetents. Hughes dismissed Jones and appointed Herbert Bruce as his replacement. 'Really nothing more Gilbertesque has ever happened in the profession,' Osler wrote afterwards. 'A group of a man's subordinates set in judgement on his work, turn him out and take on his job.' He had tried hard to stop the dismissal, cabling Canada's prime minister, R.L. Borden, that he would resign and make the issues of principle public. When Jones went anyway – Borden had more on his mind than a complicated doctors' dispute – Osler did resign, but at Jones's request did not go public with details.

Bruce was utterly incompetent and was reviled by the Canadian medical establishment. But Osler found himself handicapped and was distracted by the fact that Bruce's inquiry had uncovered serious corruption in the hospital Osler was most closely associated with, the Canadian Red Cross establishment on the Astor estate at Taplow. Its chief administrator, one Gorrell, whom the Oslers had criticized for his coarseness but admired for his competence, turned out to have been trading in Red Cross supplies on the black market. Back home in Canada, civilians had purchased socks and then found in the toes notes for soldiers from the patriotic women who had knitted them. Bruce and his party had caught Gorrell with a special cash box in his office. Rumors also swirled around Cliveden that Gorrell had been having an affair with the head nurse, Edith Campbell, whose grandfather had taught Osler at McGill. Under a cloud, Campbell was transferred to another hospital. Entirely innocent, she was bitterly angry, claiming she was being victimized by certain staff members she had reported for drunkenness and by a vindictive Nancy Astor, who had the habit of interfering in everything and with everybody. The Oslers went to bat for Edith, trying to clear her reputation and have her reinstated.

'The worst wars are not all in the trenches!' Edith Campbell remarked to Osler. Sam Hughes had raved 'that he would not have d—d Sr Wm. Osler's intermeddling,' a colleague reported.[51] Herbert Bruce made to Osler the most impolite remark in all his surviving correspondence – that his attitude from the beginning had been 'entirely uncalled for and improper.' 'Uncle will not allow the CAMC to be mentioned,' Grace told Bill Francis. 'There is but one opinion as far as I have heard and every one raging. Uncle has resigned as consultant to all the Canadian Hospitals. Bruce says "Osler – is an able fellow." That sounds like Walt Whitman.'[52]

There would have been more resignations and appeals to the imperial government had not a *deus ex machina* suddenly intervened in the person of the Canadian prime minister, who in early November forced Sam Hughes to resign. The doctors thought the CAMC affair and their protests had caused the firing, but in fact Hughes had been a festering thorn in Borden's side from the beginning of the war, had destroyed all his credibility in one scandalous mess after another, and would probably have been axed even without the Bruce mess. As Osler noted, the erratic minister whom many, including Borden, considered mentally imbalanced, had, like Haman in the Old Testament, finally hanged himself. He characterized Hughes in his letters as a 'bombastic bounder' and an 'unspeakable bounder,' and wondered if his problem was related to general paresis (the final stage of syphilis).[53] A new investigation, which Osler declined to head, repudiated most of the Bruce report. Jones was reinstated, Matron Campbell's name was cleared, and Gorrell, before he could come to trial, committed suicide.

Never having enjoyed conflict or controversy at the best of times, Osler found this Canadian medical circus deeply troubling. Grace had never seen him so upset: 'The C.A.M.C. business nearly killed him with shame and annoyance.' He lost weight and, Cushing thought, verged on a rare bout of depression.[54] Osler did not bother to dignify with comment the extreme medical chauvinism of the Hughes-Bruce report's idea of segregating Canadians in Canadian-care institutions. Apart from being absurdly impractical, expensive, and both unnecessary and unwanted in 1916, it was a recrudescence of the health-care nationalism he had fought all his life. During the months of his resignation he missed his weekly visits to Cliveden.

More deaths, breakdowns, anguished parents, the never-ending stream of visitors and supplicants. 'Every corner of the world seems upside down,' Grace wrote her sister. 'How can I write of the war? The more I hear the worse it seems & the more I see of these poor sufferers the more miserable I am. What it will be in another year I cannot imagine.' While Willie was away, she entertained Frank and Belle Osler. Belle could not stop talking about their lost son. And now in October it was at last Revere's turn to go to the front: 'Oh – Bill. Whoever could have thought such a misfortune could have befallen us? Can we be called on to give him up? I try to be brave about it but when I look at Uncle who has given his life for others' benefit, it seems too cruel.' Willie was phlegmatic: 'We shall be terribly anxious of course, but the cause is worth any sacrifice.'[55]

For all his dislike of war, Revere was relieved finally to be in the thick of it, two months before his twenty-first birthday. 'Thank God I am here at last,' he told his parents. But his description of what he saw, as a lieutenant in Battery A, 59th Brigade, Royal Field Artillery, somewhere in France, would not have lifted their spirits:

> All the country for miles is torn with shells and furrowed with old trenches. I have not seen a live tree or a blade of green grass for weeks. Mud every-where, stinking brown mud with puddles of water in every shell hole, and along every empty trench the wreckage of the battles, old rifles, bombs, all kinds of equipment, steel helmets, numberless unburied dead, which lie as they fell, some singly, others in rows, showing that they died in a charge, caught under a barrage or by a machine gun. Very little attempt has been made to bury them, and now some of them are becoming mere skeletons. One Canadian infantry officer lies in a shell hole propped up against the mud, his hands hanging quite naturally by his side, and his head is bowed just enough to give him the appearance of sleep. His face is placid, and looks so peaceful and undisturbed by all this commotion that we can scarcely help envying him. Others are not so pleasant to pass by, but I must not talk of it anymore, it is not a cheerful subject.[56]

Revere was seeing the Somme battlefield after four months of fighting, a million casualties, and no significant ground gained. They did manage to bury most of the Canadian dead, but German skeletons were left to be picked clean by rats. For the most part, Revere's letters to his parents were not quite as gloomy as his surroundings. He liked his comrades and thought his battery had a good atmosphere. He asked the family to stop sending books, as he had no time to read more.

Now every telegram that arrived at Norham Gardens was opened with frightful anticipation. William was often away in Wales, hearing testimony about the future of medical education there and buttering up opinion to go in his direction – towards a Welsh national university in Cardiff, not local schools with only Welsh brains. The university should have the best brains it could find, Osler told a Welsh audience, 'because the best brains of the country were not one whit too good for Wales.' Professionally, he still found the war work interesting – there was something new every day – 'but I get very tired of the wounded & of sepsis.' 'Every month of the past two years seems a year in itself,' he said to another correspondent, '– and the end is not in sight. There will be an appalling mass of battered humanity to be taken care of. Without any big battle the wounded continue to pour in. We have 1500 beds here – always full.' He later wrote that he never saw a wounded soldier without thinking of his son.[57]

His annual December cold turned into bronchial pneumonia and for two weeks he was sicker than he had been for fifteen years, with fever and a very bad hacking cough. 'Heroin controlled it a little,' he noted in his daybook. The other William of 13 Norham Gardens, the much-beloved butler, who had joined the army, also had pneumonia. He died that month in a military hospital. 'Every one is so depressed and melancholy it is enough to keep one weeping,' Grace wrote. She thought the CAMC mess had contributed to her husband's illness: 'If I could just once tell Dr. Bruce what I think of him I should be happier.'[58]

'We are all busy wringing the neck of Wilson's Peace Dove,' Osler wrote bellicosely on Christmas Eve 1916. He managed to dress and appear on Christmas Day. The house was full of guests as usual, 'but of course our hearts are empty with Revere away.' Revere's unit fired shells all day and into the night on Christmas eve. Their senior sergeant was killed by a German shell. On the twenty-fifth they had an enormous dinner, with real glasses and a real tablecloth, and a plum pudding from Norham Gardens. 'I never knew how much I loved you all and Oxford before now,' Revere wrote to his dad just after Christmas and just before his birthday.

'You have been everything that a father could wish, a dear good laddie,' Willie wrote to Revere on his twenty-first birthday at the end of 1916. 'And it is not often I am sure that father and son have been so happy together.' He and Grace had put aside some £6,500, which they were now transferring to Revere's name so that after the war he would have an income that at least would get him through college. 'It is always so much better for a fellow to have his own money, when possible. Many, many happy returns of the day and I hope when this tyranny is overpast we may have more happy days together – you and I and Muz.'[59]

Grace's widowed sister, Susan Chapin, arrived suddenly in England to-wards the end of 1916 to help out at Norham Gardens. 'I find them both looking well and seeming well,' she reported back to America. 'WO shows the wear & tear of these experiences somewhat – is thinner & whiter – but I am surprised that they do not show it more – They are very externally plucky about Revere ... Grace tries to direct conversation from painful details & they all dwell on other interests as much as possible.' A bit shaken by his illness, Willie was 'on his good behaviour,' according to Grace, and sticking fairly close to home. 'Drinks *Stout*, and is sleeping well.' The ra-tioning of food, especially meat, took a little getting used to, but Osler opined that the British people could easily tighten their belts. When would all the resources of rich America finally be applied to the war? the family wondered. 'When I think of America being left unmolested and glorying in being out of it – I feel raging mad – & am so mortified,' Grace wrote at the end of January 1917. Woodrow Wilson had been re-elected on the record of having kept his country out of the war and was now calling on the nations to accept 'Peace without Victory.' Grace had to turn away from conversations about America's policies, and she had stopped writing to American friends who criticized England. Sue joked about being a 'marooned American.'[60]

Osler did not write much now about war medicine, saving himself for a few major addresses. But in a case that reached Oxford from the south of France he had found a rare parasite, a specimen of *Anobium hirtum*. He wrote up its activities for publication and commissioned a special set of illustrations from an artist at the British Museum. In his long career he had seen only two living examples. These parasites were bookworms, preyers on volumes. The Bodleian Library housed many victims of their ravages – though not, Osler added, any that showed signs of recent attack. In another idle moment he wrote an account of the Athenaeum club's membership election – the blackballing process, the members' horror of 'any suspicion of bad breeding or poor morals,' and the reasons why one of the late King Edward VII's old cronies had been rejected.

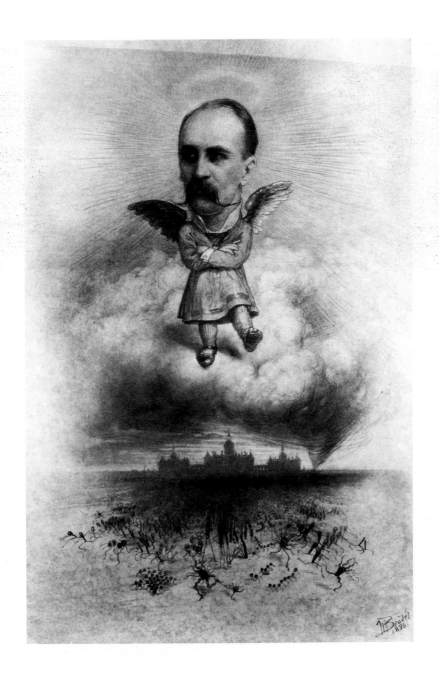

Canonized in his lifetime. 'The Saint' by Max Brödel, 1896.
Note the fleeing microbes.

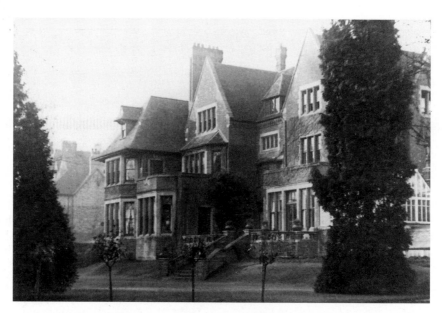

Thirteen Norham Gardens, Oxford. The Oslers' 'Open Arms.'

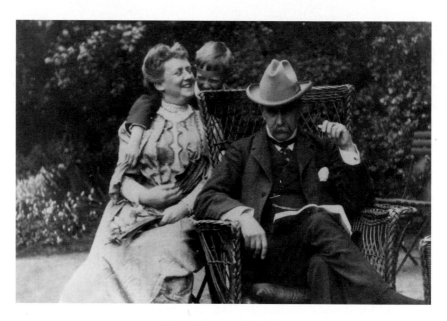

The Oslers in Oxford.

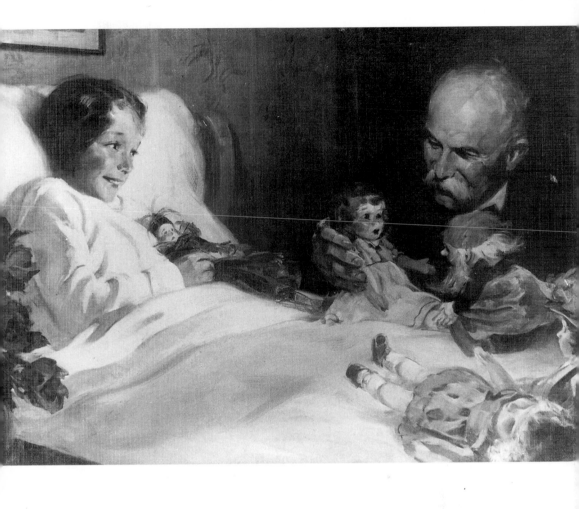

The children's doctor. He found them more interesting than adults.

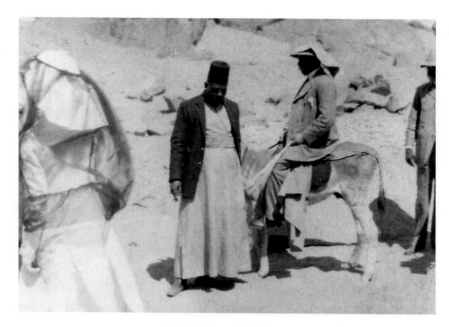

Donkey riding. Egypt, 1911.

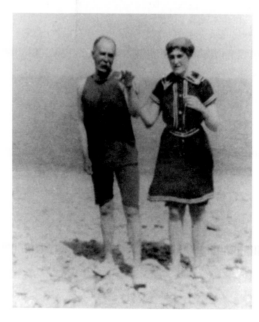

Cavorting on a beach in Wales with a niece, Amy Gwyn, 1911.

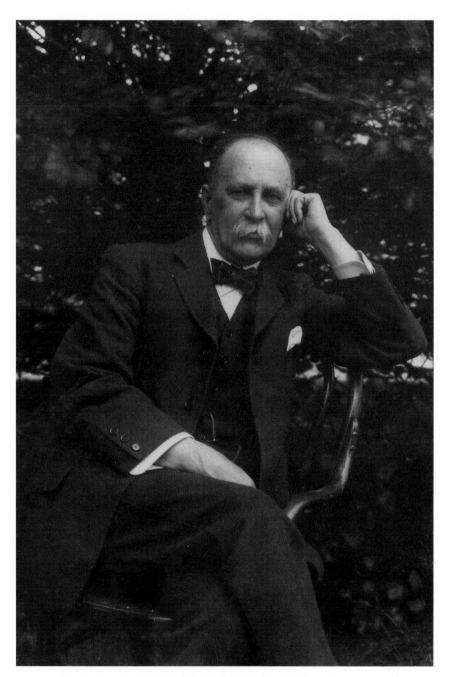

Sir William Osler, age 63, 1912.

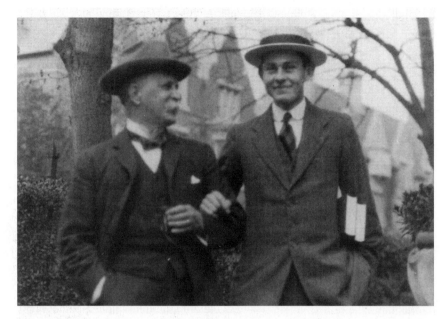

Father and son, peace.

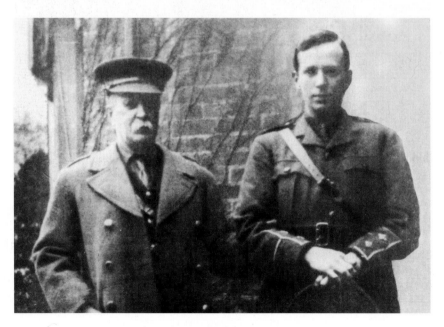

Father and son, war.

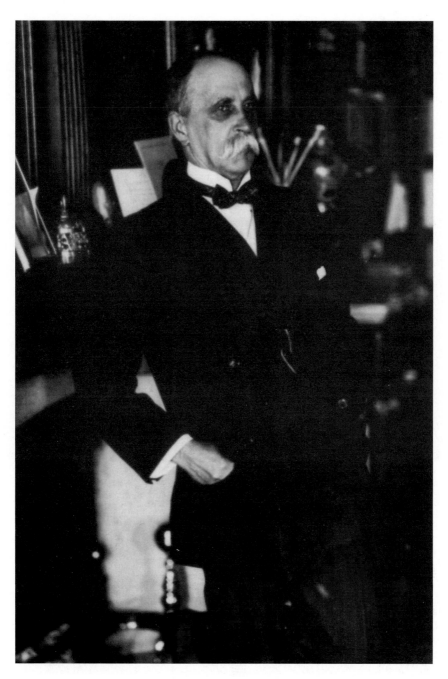

The last picture, 1919.

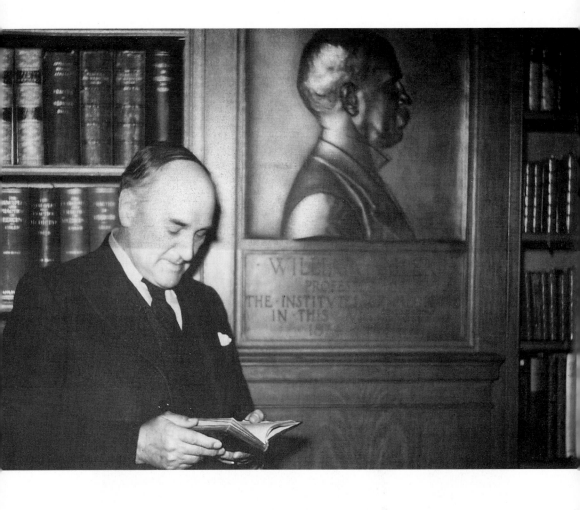

W.W. Francis, High Priest of Oslerolatry.

During the months of Revere's absence young Archie Malloch had become the latest surrogate son of the Osler household, his bookish interest in medical history a delight to the aging collector. Malloch's father was one of several Canadians who made sure the Osler table would always have maple sugar in abundance to replace rationed sweets. Osler grated it onto his morning porridge. British bureaucrats would have stopped packages labeled 'sugar' but let 'maple' go through.[61]

They worried constantly about Revere, whose battery was in action all that winter. But anxiety had become the normal state, and though the war showed no sign of ending, the good news was that Germany's submarine warfare was pushing the United States towards coming in. When it finally happened early in April, the Osler household was 'wildly excited,' Willie wrote. Returning from London, he 'found the front porch bedecked with the Union Jack & Stars and Stripes, & the Revere girls dancing with joy.' And then there was a week of terrible anxiety, 'the first unhappy Easter of my life,' when no mail arrived from Revere during yet another major battle. On that Easter weekend the Canadian Corps had the greatest victory in the country's young history, storming Vimy Ridge. A few days later the Oslers learned that Charlotte's boy, Campbell Gwyn, had been killed in the assault:

> Dearest Sister. This will be a hard blow for you to bear – the first of your children to be taken ... to give up a dear fellow like Campbell is heartbreaking ... what a splendid officer he was. He was a born soldier & knew his job thoroughly ... We are steeling our hearts against the possible blow to us, as Revere's Battery is in the thick of this fight ... Keep up your heart dear – he has died in a good cause.

Grace never expected to see Revere again. 'I have almost *stopped praying*,' she wrote on hearing of Campbell Gwyn's death. 'It seems so useless.'[62]

The only peacetime diseases that continued to ravage all the armies throughout the Great War were gonorrhea and syphilis. Osler made 'The Anti-

Venereal Campaign' the subject of his Oration to the Medical Society of London in mid-May. For the second time he changed the designation of Bunyan's 'Captain of the Men of Death.' Now, he said, it had become syphilis. Osler had compiled statistics on the alarming prevalence of venereal disease in the Canadian and British forces. He knew far more than most about the insidiousness of the spirochete – in Sigmund's phrase, 'the worm that never dieth' – and its ability to cover its tracks in causing death by other causes. He lent all his authority to the new campaign to be truthful about VD, educate the public, overcome the stigma, and hope that good sense would ultimately prevail 'against the most formidable enemy of the race – an enemy entrenched behind the strongest of human passions, and the deepest of social prejudices.' He told his audience about the illustration that used to hang over the mantel in Rev. W.A. Johnson's library in Weston, Ontario. It was a depiction of Christ saying, 'He that is without sin among you, let him first cast a stone at her.' At least the new honesty about venereal disease would mean that sinners might be given Christian treatment.[63]

Despite his parents' forebodings, Revere had not been scratched in six months of fighting. Only his mail had been occasionally held up, making it all the more difficult for a soldier on the Western Front to stay in the hunt for good books from the dealers' catalogs. When he came home for his first leave in May, his father was astonished to find that the boy had become a man: 'You never saw such a burly looking fellow – so grown & filled out, with hands like a navvie & a face weather-beaten like leather. He has literally been in the open since October & physically it has done him no end of good. He is in very good spirits & has had a wonderful experience, as his brigade was the first to cross the advanced trenches beyond Arras ... His nerves are A.1 but it has been a hard experience & it is not easy to get him to talk much.' Revere looked good in the mustache he had grown – 'no Oslerian droop to it,' Grace observed. 'It broke my heart to look at him & to think I may never see him again – One stroke and all may be over.'

While Revere enjoyed ten days of fishing and books and good times with his parents, they endured his leave with a secret sorrow, not telling him until the last day that a close friend, Billie Wright, had been killed in action.[64]

'There is no romance left about this war to any who have been [there],' Sue Chapin wrote Kate Cushing from Norham Gardens. American troops were on their way. 'It is simply sickening to hear of all the young Americans coming to be slaughtered & maimed,' Grace wrote Harvey Cushing early in July. Cushing was with one of the first American medical units to arrive and now was again operating in France. Early in August Grace and Sue went up to London to see a great parade of American soldiers. They stood on the curb across from the American embassy and wept hard.[65]

Willie conducted the annual examination sessions at Oxford, helped put the Welsh royal commission report to bed that summer (they had done an important piece of spadework that would eventually lead to the founding of the Welsh National School of Medicine, for which Osler helped raise money to endow a chair),[66] and he then went off with Grace for a week at Swanage, where they had been so happy with Revere when he was a little boy. Osler prepared a major talk about the future of librarianship, the desirability of creating 'Professors of Books.'

Revere continued to see action. First the battle of Messines Ridge, when the earth shook for miles as the British blew up German lines with mines. Then their guns were part of the tremendous barrage, audible in England, that began the summer offensive in Belgium known as the Battle of Passchendaele. Days of rain turned the attack into a bloody, sodden fiasco. Revere wrote that it was like the Somme all over again: 'Miles and miles of desolation and shell holes, filth and rubbish of every description lying all around. There is scarcely a trench left, and nearly all the dugouts have been blown in ... yet here we are, sitting quite cheerfully, Williams playing his guitar and Capt. Hunt singing, Eldeston reading, and I writing. What brutes we are! I must stop before I depress you.'

'Poor W.O. is almost a skeleton and keeps busy every moment,' Grace wrote, 'but sometimes can't sleep and it makes one very anxious.'[67] Yet for all his worries and his exhaustion with and hatred of the war, Osler never varied in his commitment to the cause, no matter what the cost. In a short article for Christmas 1917, he wrote of the 'call for silent sacrifice, of time, of habits, of comforts, of friends, and of those dearer than life itself.'[68] Terribly hard sentiments, no longer shared with conviction by Grace. After once making a fool of herself by telling wounded men she hoped they would recover in time to march into Berlin – they just laughed at her – she had come round to hoping that the men she loved would suffer merciful wounds that would keep them from combat as long as possible.

Revere himself, like most of the soldiers, hoped he might get a 'blighty,' a wound that would get him back to England.

Aug. 5

Dear Dad:

... I am determined to get P.W.C. (fever without cause) and go to the hospital. What annoys one so much is, that in spite of being soaking wet for four days and nights, I feel, if possible, rather better than usual, and show not the least sign of becoming a casualty.

Aug. 6th. It is fine at last and the land is fairly steaming in the sun ... There is so much to do here – so many little worries and troubles, especially as the Sgt. Major is on leave, that I am in a state of chronic agitation, though I try to keep – outwardly at least – a certain degree of equanimity. We are having a very strenuous time getting ammunition to the battery ... We have 25 horses out of action from wounds of various kinds, mostly caused by barbed wire and sharp stakes or pieces of tin, which are submerged in the mud and invisible. We have to take 50 boxes up tomorrow morning at dawn, and I fear it will be the end of some of the poor beasts. Good night.

On August 23 Revere wrote to his parents that he had been laid up in the mess for a couple of days with a whiff of poison gas, but not enough to send him home. 'I wish it was a little worse,' his mother wrote to Malloch on August 28. Two days earlier she had written a Canadian relative that 'the anxiety is intense. One must keep busy every moment or one would go mad.' The boy was scheduled for leave in another three weeks, and they were planning another seaside idyll in Swanage. In the meantime Grace was also trying to tell Harvey Cushing of Revere's whereabouts so they could get together, and she got a wire off to the surgeon on the morning of the twenty-ninth. 'How awful you would feel if you saw him with a bad head wound,' she had written Cushing earlier.[69]

Revere's unit was in Belgium, not far from Ypres. On Wednesday, August 29, they were trying to move their guns forward onto a ridge. At 4.30 on that quiet afternoon they were bridging a shellhole when suddenly a German 4.2-inch shell burst about five yards away. Nine men were killed or wounded. Revere took shrapnel in his chest, abdomen, and thigh. His comrades got him into a nearby gun pit as more shells rained down; they did what they could to dress his wounds and sent him back on a stretcher. After being carried almost two miles to a dressing station, the heavily-morphinized soldier was placed on a narrow-gauge ammunition railway and moved to a field ambulance; a motorized ambulance then took him to a casualty clearing station, where he arrived about 8:30. 'Thank heavens. This will take me home,' the boy said to one of his attendants. He was conscious, but in shock and bleeding internally.

The American surgeons who happened to be at Casualty Clearing Station 47, Dosinghem, got a message off to Harvey Cushing at a base hospital not far away. An ambulance took Cushing through pouring rain and dark to Dosinghem. Revere was almost pulseless, probably hopeless, but still able to mutter a few words of greeting. G.W. Crile, another outstanding American surgeon, arrived with primitive blood-transfusion equipment. They gave Revere blood, and about midnight two surgeons from New York, William Darrach and George Brewer, operated, while Cushing kept track of the pulse. They closed two perforations in Revere's large bowel and managed to stop the bleeding. Crile gave him another transfusion from one of his more lightly wounded comrades. Before blood-typing, the transfusions probably did no good. 'He appeared to rally, regained his pulse and did very well for about five hours – sleeping most of the time,' Cushing wrote Susan Chapin the next day. 'The end was quite sudden with no struggle. I saw him several times before and after the operation: asked him if he had any messages. He probably did not quite understand and I did not press it. He showed no anxiety – merely wanted to have the operation over.'

They buried Revere right away, without extraordinary ceremony. Cushing cut a button from the boy's tunic. Otherwise there were no grand gestures, no copy of Keats in the grave with him. 'There are some things about these burials in hot weather that don't bear repeating,' Cushing told his wife. He described the scene:

> A soggy Flanders field beside a little oak grove to the rear of the Dosinghem group – an overcast, windy, autumnal day – the long rows of simple wooden crosses – the new ditches half full of water being dug by Chinese coolies wearing tin helmets – the boy wrapped in an army blanket and covered by a weather-worn Union Jack, carried on their shoulders by four slipping stretcher-bearers. A strange scene – the great-great-grandson of Paul Revere under a British flag, and awaiting him a group of some six or eight American Army medical officers – saddened with thoughts of his father ... The Padre recited the usual service – the bugler gave the 'Last Post' – and we went about our duties. Plot 4, Row F.[70]

Back in Oxford, William and Grace began another day of worrying, letter writing, and hosting visitors. Their Isaac had been sacrificed, but the news had not yet come.

TWELVE

Never Use a Crutch

Osler had seen three patients on Thursday, August 30, and written several letters. He was in his library reading articles on asthma, thinking about the next edition of his text, when at 4.15 PM a telegram arrived from Cushing, advising that Revere was dangerously, though not hopelessly wounded. Osler sent Benning with the car to bring Grace, who was making social calls. She knew the reason right away. Osler phoned the War Office and asked permission to rush to France, but was advised to await further word. Grace and William had their bags packed and were waiting to leave when at 8.30 the call came to say Revere was dead.[1]

There was nothing to do. Bodies were not brought home from wars until the Americans began to do it in Vietnam in the 1960s. Revere had already been buried. There would be no memorial service – too many soldiers had died and were dying every day. The practice of public mourning – wearing black, staying in seclusion, using black-bordered stationery – had largely disappeared by 1917. Almost everyone the Oslers knew had lost sons or were worried about sons at the front. Revere's number had come up, the Oslers' turn had come, and life had to go on. The parents put flowers in their boy's room. On Friday a Swiss doctor friend who had not heard the news arrived for lunch at Norham Gardens. They talked of Clemenceau and the Empress Eugénie, and the visitor only learned of Revere's death on the way to the station. On Monday,

September 3, Osler went to Cliveden for his weekly hospital rounds. He got through them, but at lunch with Nancy Astor broke down and sobbed.²

One of the Oslers' surrogate children – Willie had encouraged her to call him Dad – Marjorie Howard Futcher, received two letters that combine to give a remarkable portrait of William and Grace as they met the great tragedy of their lives. The first was from Bill Francis, who had rushed over from France and wrote Marjorie on September 1:

> I was prepared to find them prostrate – but not they. After the first hugging and sobbing on my neck, there were no more tears till bedtime, except a stray one here and there, or when poor Dad would turn toward the fire with one hand on the mantle & head bowed. Apart from this everything seems much the same externally as before. All through dinner there was the same keen interest in everything & everybody's little doings, the same playfulness from Dad, without any painful evidence of its being forced. Telegrams arriving every minute, opened & read & commented on, and 'Got enough pennies for all those boys, Bateman?'
>
> They can even laugh naturally – But there is no avoidance of Revere's name or of conjectures as to how and when he was wounded – how he happened to be brought to 47 C.C.S., next to Harvey's ...
>
> After dinner innumerable letters are answered till mail time. Then Dad sits in his chair cutting the pages of a new book, reading it and manifestly taking it in, commenting upon it to me, in the same old way, and handing it to me when he is finished, and I get a shock when I find that it is printed in German.
>
> Then upstairs in what used to be your room. Here Muz brings out some particularly amusing letters of R's for me to read, and she laughs again over his quaint gentle humour, and only as she puts away the letters and fondles the little leather case, her face turns sad and her eyes moist. Never a word have I heard against the war, not a murmur at the cruelty of it all, or the infinite pathos of the sacrifice ... Oh my dear, it is all the sublimest courage. They save their tears for the night, but they face an empty world bravely.

On September 2, Grace told Marjorie what it was really like:

Oh – Marjorie Marjorie – Our boy has gone – gone – buried in that dank
ground in Belgium and we can never see or hear him on earth. I thought I
was ready – I've been waiting 11 months – but I could never be ready to bear
it with what is called 'Christian resignation' – it does not seem to me God
has much to do with these times and when people say 'God needed these
young lives for some good purpose' I say nothing because the God I have
faith in would not use such means. I could bear it for myself – Any amount,
for my poor feeble Self – but I can't bear it for this angelic man who has
given his whole life to humanity and now has lost his joy & pride. His
wonderful *mental* companion his loving son – It is heart breaking to hear
him sobbing hour after hour and never to see the boy again. We have had
three awful nights – Dear – dear Docci O he bluffs it during the day – and
has been to see his friends – but oh – the darkness – and the thought of our
dear boy – in Belgium – Belgium and we not there.[3]

They had lived with the anticipation so long that the news was almost
a release, what Grace called an 'awful relaxation.' Osler told her sister Sue
that he had known the moment would come from the day the war began.
Grace had written Revere every Saturday night for nine years. Now nothing. 'Oh Kate, dear Kate,' she wrote to Cushing's wife. 'My darling fair
baby has gone – just laid in that wet, cold Belgium. But thank God for two
things – your Harvey was with him and he has gone to a peaceful spot. I
feel sure of that – And we are rather old and may go too very soon – we
hope so ... Thank God your boy is so young. It is the most awful feeling to
see them go and to know he will be killed – nearly all the good ones are –
Day after day the same news comes – our friends on every side – sometimes
two or three sons killed.'[4]

(Nine years later, Kate and Harvey Cushing's firstborn, William, died in
a motor car crash in Connecticut. Cushing heard the news on the morning
of a day he had a difficult operation scheduled. He went ahead with it,
telling his staff of the death later.)

As details came back from the front, the fantastic coincidence of Cushing having been present to attend to Revere was a true comfort. At least the Oslers knew how their boy had died and that everything possible had been done to save his life and that he had had a decent burial. He was not missing in action or rotting in a shell hole in No Man's Land or literally blown to bits. There was comfort, too, in the letters from the officers of Battery A saying that Revere had been a cheerful, hardworking soldier, 'a most charming and courteous gentleman,' who had always done his duties, repugnant as he found them, and at one time had been recommended for a medal, the Military Cross. 'I hope I have not said too much,' his commanding officer wrote, 'but I feel my mother would like to hear any good about me when I get killed.'[5]

William and Grace decided to go ahead with the Swanage vacation they had planned to take with Revere. Now, Grace said, it would be a time of freshening 'before facing life with the lights out.' Before, during, and after the Swanage trip, hundreds of letters and notes of condolence arrived and were answered. Osler's replies were variations on a letter he wrote the night he got the news: 'We have been preparing for the blow. I felt sure the fates would hit me through him. I have escaped all these years without a great sorrow, and have had so much in life, so much more, really, than I have deserved that I have all along felt we could not escape. No father ever had a more congenial son, and I had never to say a cross word to him. Poor Grace! it hits her hard; but we are both going to be brave, and take up what is left of life as though he were with us.'[6]

Osler told Halsted and other correspondents that others had suffered worse, and both parents wrote that they would carry on, trying to bury the pain with work and service. They took Sue Chapin and two little boys from the Max Müller family with them to Swanage. Osler played with the boys on the beach when he was not writing letters. Sister Sue found the Oslers' suffering heartrending, but marveled at the nobility of their spirit. 'Sir William seems to be shrinking away,' she wrote Cushing, 'but I believe he will pull up soon.' Gradually he did – sleeping better, though still alarming Grace with bouts of weeping. 'He looks to me as though his vitality was being sucked out by grief,' she wrote from Swanage.[7] They stopped at a hospital on their way home to visit one of Revere's battery-mates who had survived the deadly shell.

Back in Oxford their life went on. As was said often in those days, they kept the flag flying. Osler busied himself with official duties, consultations, work on his library, and textbook revision. 'We are taking the only medicines for sorrow – time & hard work.' Osler was not immobilized by his grief or by depression, though some nights continued to be bad. Often he slept well, and while he was bone-thin, his appetite stayed good. The flow of visitors to Norham Gardens resumed, including many more Americans. Sue Chapin moved to London to work with the American Red Cross but usually came back on weekends. 'I seem to have more than ever to do and foolishly tried to answer personally all the letters of sympathy,' Grace told Archie Malloch. 'I have finished about 1500.' The sympathy letters gave her little comfort. The worst were the ones with long religious observations: 'Perhaps I am unnatural. One cannot – at least I cannot glory in the loss of the boy even for such a cause.' On one of his trips to London, Osler went to the Athenaeum club and wrote 'Dead' beside Revere's name on its waiting list.[8]

The first Christmas after a death in the family is usually the hardest. Grace considered suggesting they go away, but the house was dry, warm, and comfortable and there was nowhere better to go: 'Everywhere the Christmases grow sadder & sadder. Hardly a house untouched by grief and disappointment.' They filled 13 Norham Gardens with guests – a nephew, two wounded friends, Tom Futcher, and sister Sue, plus fourteen American doctors to supper on Christmas Day. Grace served chicken salad and real apple pie and cheese. 'We got through all right,' she wrote, 'although I really feared my dear Man would faint at the supper table he was so ghastly.' Revere's kit arrived from France on the day before he would have celebrated his twenty-second birthday. Grace could not bear to open it. 'It seems the end of everything.'[9]

Death was everywhere. An American doctor's son training to be a pilot spent a lovely Sunday at Norham Gardens and was killed in a flying accident within the week. His best friend, who stayed with the Oslers to get over the loss, was sent to France and never came back. As well, the old colleagues in America were passing away: James Tyson from Philadelphia days; and Franklin Mall, in Osler's view 'a terrible loss' to Hopkins. There was worse news from Baltimore: Theodore Janeway, Barker's replacement, whose service as Hopkins' first full-time professor had turned him into a desperately unhappy opponent of the full-time system and helped destroy his health, died at age forty-five. Over in France, Jack McCrae, doctor, soldier, and poet, never the same after the fighting at Ypres, died in February 1918 from pneumonia and meningitis. Members of the McGill unit scoured the countryside for poppies in winter to scatter on McCrae's grave. Osler's literary output during these years of war and aging ran heavily to obituaries. Grace wrote:

> Marjorie I sometimes like *to Swear* and stamp my feet over this cursed war & the wreckage it has done. If you could hear our darling sobbing & sighing at night – it would break your heart. He often says to me – when I kiss him good night – & put my hand on his thin face 'I am well knocked out & I doubt if I see it through.' It drives me nearly frantic. He takes good care of himself but I am terrified of pneumonia. I want to get him to Cornwall when it is warm enough ... We are a miserable broken hearted pair.[10]

With their only natural son gone, Grace and Willie turned to 'all our other dear children,' as he put it, for consolation.[11] These included Bill Francis, Archie Malloch, Palmer Howard's children and grandchildren, and most other young folk who came into their orbit. His special friends in 1918 were two Canadian girls, eight-year-old Nadine Harty and her five-year-old sister Betty, whose mother, a distant relative, was living in Oxford while their father fought. William and Grace's letters contain many references to the delightful Harty children and the good times he was having with them. As well, Betty Harty, whose first marriage was to an Osler, lived to share her memories of William Osler with me some eighty years later, the last survivor of all those mentioned in these pages whose paths had crossed his.

Betty Harty Osler Nelles told me of going for walks in Christ Church Meadow with Sir William in 1918 and of his telling her about the flowers and grasses and trees. She would 'burble' back at him, she remembered, her complete innocence and her ignorance of Revere's death making her a perfect companion. She would crawl around under the table in his library and he would ask her to sit on his feet to help keep them warm. One day when he found her digging in the garden he set in to help dig to China. After a while the hole got deep, and he said it would be best if they waited till the war ended and took an airplane to China. When the children wanted to go to the pantomime, Osler led them in rain dances and chants; it always seemed to rain.

When cakes arrived from America, Osler would tell the little girls that the black magic spell had to be removed before they could be eaten, which required cutting out a square piece from the very center. When the children worried about grown-ups' reactions to such antics, Osler would say, 'Who cares about the grown-ups?' Betty still believed in magic and fairies and was a perfect foil for Osler's stories. Sister Nadine was more skeptical but also fell under his spell. 'I think he can see right through our heads,' Nadine said to Betty.

A baby girl went missing in England, and Osler invented the saga of the kidnapped Popkins infant, holding the Harty children spellbound for days with stories of sightings of baby Popkins in far-flung corners of the Empire. He brought the story to a happy ending by borrowing a mother and her baby to stage a Popkins reunion before the delighted children. He told them ghost stories, did card tricks and gave them maple sugar, told them that even girls could grow up to be doctors if they worked hard enough, and promised Betty that when she left England she could have the rabbit from the statue of Peter Pan in Kensington Gardens. The children never thought of him as a grown-up but as one of their own. And Osler remarked diplomatically to an adult, a college fellow, that children were 'the only people in life worth talking to except an occasional College fellow.'[12]

In early March 1918, Cushing was able to visit Oxford on leave. He found the 'Open Arms' full with a motley assortment of guests and visitors:

Sir William though a shadow of his former self sails through these interruptions as though they were the very things he cordially longed for. But any-

one can see that his desk is piled high with unopened and unanswered letters ... There are books and papers everywhere. We slipped away at six and
he made a round of visits on people with children – his many darlings who
find things in his pockets and cuddle about him while he tells another chapter
of some imaginary tale before they go to bed – all over in ten minutes and
he flits to the next, where there is the sound of a desperate pillow-fight and
great hilarity at the head of the stairs.

Grace talked with Cushing about the months of dread while awaiting news
of Revere. 'I think Sir William could not speak,' she told the surgeon afterwards. 'He could not trust himself.' Osler quietly showed his protégé Revere's
book acquisitions list, including the titles he had ordered from the trenches.[13]
    The sorrow and worry did not soon lift. In the spring the launching of a
great German offensive 'depressed him dreadfully,' Grace wrote. On All
Fool's Day 1918 Grace told Bill Francis of her longing for it all to have
been a bad joke. 'We are still at it – and it is all true – hearts & homes
desolated, dread and anxiety everywhere. It all seems so hopeless & useless. One can't believe the world was so wicked that it had to be reproved
in this way. I can never believe that. When I see a *nearly* saintly person like
WO – wrecked & heart-broken – & hear him sighing & sobbing his heart
out at night – I find myself rebelling & almost unforgiving.'[14]

His travels, practice, income, and writing declined in 1918 to about those
of a normally busy consultant. He still had to go to Wales to advance the
cause of a national medical school, and also received a stream of Welsh
visitors to Oxford seeking advice. He turned down another offer of the
presidency of the Royal Society of Medicine and an offer of the presidency
of the Medical Society of London. But he accepted the presidency of the
Classical Association, which went every other year to a distinguished
nonclassicist. Osler was the first physician to serve.
    There were always patients to see, including a particularly hectic round
of consultations at the end of March 1918. Fees were welcome to help pay

the high and rising taxes being levied to help pay for the war. Osler's rounds had expanded in 1917 to include visits to a special hospital for the study of heart disease, located first in Hampstead then in Colchester, where he was one of the consultants. He published very little, but his professional interest was not waning. The heart work brought together pioneering American and British cardiologists, and featured special studies of functional heart disorders, what Osler had written about years earlier as 'irritable heart.' In war it was a hot topic, related to the problem of the dysfunctional or neurasthenic or 'shell-shocked' soldier.[15] Osler also took a keen interest in the early work of younger colleagues on varieties of encephalitis, or sleeping-sickness, and carefully followed the research on 'p.u.o.,' or trench fever; the doctors finally realized that lice were the pathogen carriers.

His work with the functionally impaired centered on the case of sapper 'C' at Cliveden, a man who had been disabled by typhoid fever in 1916 and then become completely immobilized with 'typhoid spine.' They could find nothing organically wrong with the soldier – Osler had several sets of x-rays done – but the slightest touch caused him excruciating pain. Many observers were convinced he was hopelessly paralyzed. Osler insisted he would recover, but in eight months there was no progress. A disgusted resident, Jonathan Meakins, who was convinced the man was malingering, persuaded Osler to transfer him to the National Hospital at Queen Square, London, where new methods of treatment of nervous diseases were being used.

Sapper 'C' was taken off in an ambulance at six in the morning. At ten that night Meakins had a call from Osler, who had received a telegram from London: 'The SOB is walking.' A Canadian doctor, L.R. Yealland, reported that it was an interesting case, which had required ten minutes of treatment. Osler chalked it up as 'a regular Lourdes miracle' and gave one of his last published clinical lectures on his long history of being puzzled by the typhoid spine syndrome. Yealland's wizardry had been to tell the patient that his case was simple, that stimulation by an electric current would immediately cure him, then apply the current, and tell the patient to get up and walk.[16] It was medical faith-healing, reminiscent of some of the cures at St Johns Hopkins.

'We have not (fortunately) much time to think,' Osler told Campbell Howard in the spring of 1918. He said little about the war in his letters and played little part in public life, except for an April 1918 letter to the *Times*, suggesting that Ireland would live for years under the 'curse of Meroz' if it did not do its part in the fighting. Could American Irish Catholics bring the people of their homeland to its senses?[17]

His interest in the future of his profession remained as strong as ever. In May he published a blistering letter to the president of the Royal College of Surgeons attacking 'the rottenness' of its system of fellowship examinations, with its very high failure rate. He characterized the process as 'a reproach alike to teachers and examiners, and worst of all a cruel perversion of mental values to the student.'[18] He was becoming involved in plans to improve postgraduate medical education in London after the war, with the hope of making it a mecca for the American students who surely would no longer be Germany-bound. And he endorsed strengthening the state's presence in medicine. While he had said little about the coming of national health insurance to Britain in 1911 (he never directly concerned himself with the problem of payment for health care), Osler never had any qualms about state support for medical education or research. Now the war was leading to an escalation of the government's involvement in almost all areas of life. Speaking on 'Research and the State' in 1918, Osler argued that the 'invincible prejudice against State aid' in the profession was 'an academic obsession, peculiarly insular and Anglican.' He hoped there would be a strong Ministry of Health backed by a united profession after the war that would reconstruct British medical schools, rearrange the curriculum, and reorganize training in the London hosptals.[19]

When his thoughts turned to the long-term future of medicine in Canada, in a September address to the Medical Society of the Canadian Army Medical Corps, he reasserted his North American individualism. A complete scheme of state medicine might eventually work in Britain, he allowed, but 'personally I do not see that in Canada it would be a feasible thing if any Ministry organised the taking over both the Health and the Disease of the entire community, and offered a service which would minister to both the health and the sickness of the entirely community.' He believed that preventive and public-health work would be much more important in the future, and hoped to see better coverage of Canadian rural districts with traveling clinics and nurses and better maternity centers. All of this could be done

> without interfering with the independence of the practitioner nor with the development of the individual doctor. Personally I am afraid that even under the most favourable circumstances if the general practitioners were made State officials no matter how carefully graded the services would be, there would be that absence of competition and that sense of independence which after all is the most important factor in a man's individuality in his professional career ...
>
> I really do not think that any of the Provinces of Canada would ever be likely to have a complete State control of the profession. I do not believe it would be good for the profession or good for the Public. I think the profession must stand on the individual work of the Doctors ... I have had experience of men who have practised on the cross roads who were specialists in humanity and the best practitioners whom I have ever known and they owed everything not to training but to the individual natural ability that rests in every one of you. (Cheers).[20]

Osler reminisced about the old days in Canada in this and other talks and often around the dinner table, as old men do. He was beginning to pack his portmanteau, as he put it, to be ready for death.[21] After the period of intense mourning for Revere, he gradually brought himself to sort the boy's books and disperse his money, and began to plan a memorial gift to Johns Hopkins. He had set up a modest trust fund for the three Francis children, Bea, Gwen, and Bill, whom he had loved and supported all their lives. The cataloguing, annotating, pruning, and enlarging of his library went on endlessly.

Osler wrote an autobiographical essay on the making of his library. Otherwise, and consistent with the way he had always lived, he chose not to live in the past by writing significant memoirs or reminiscences. For a compulsive writer with a sense of history – who at this time was encouraging Frank Shepherd to put his memories on paper – it was a staunchly forward-looking stance. All that Osler, the Carlylean apostle of day-at-a-time living, did was to jot down a full record of one day's activity. Here is how Osler spent August 1, 1918:

> Breakfast with Major Strong of the U.S. Army, who is staying with us while his Trench Fever Report is going through the Oxford Press.
>
> 9 a.m., motored to station, stopping on the way to leave Mrs. Brock & Muriel (who had just come to Oxford) some flowers.
>
> At Paddington Dr. M's car met me; first to 44 Mile End Road to see a case of big spleen with remarkable symptoms. Then to see a Mrs. B. with polycythemia & the most extraordinary spleen I have ever encountered ... I had seen her 24 years before. Then to see a Mrs. D. with Hodgkin's disease – external & internal & now pressure on the bronchi.
>
> Tube to Piccadilly Circus; called on Evelyn Harty & the children at the Carlton. Went on to the Canadian Club luncheon for Sir Robert Borden; sat between Gen. Goodwin & Prof. Adami.
>
> 3 p.m. to the American Ambassador & discussed his plans [that night, Walter Hines Page wrote his letter of resignation, citing health reasons].
>
> 4 to the tailor's sending on the way a box of cigarettes to one of my specials & a 'cargo' [of sweets] to two other war girls. Then to a meeting of the editors of the *Quarterly Journal of Medicine*.
>
> 5.45 American Women's War Hospital to see two cases – obscure dropsy & a pleurisy with effusion, & a case of transposition of viscera.
>
> Caught the 6.50. Dinner at 8.30. At 9 saw a remarkable case of Polio-encephalitis in a man just brought from France.[22]

Possibly the cigarettes went to W.J. McGregor, an American physician who had been posted with the British forces and was now in a London hospital recovering from a double amputation. Osler visited McGregor often and they talked intimately, though never about Revere. Osler gave the patient advice about facing the future which he never forgot. 'McGregor,' Osler said, 'Never use a crutch.'[23]

It is not clear whether Osler recognized how often he relied on Grace as his crutch. Life at Norham Gardens revolved around her ability and willingness to organize the household, a much greater burden now that servants and good food were both in short supply and Grace had to live every day with sorrow. We do not have a record of a day in Grace's life, but here she is writing to Archie Malloch on June 11, 1918:

> The stream is growing into a wide river of Americans. It pours down on Saturday about 3.03 & 6 p.m. Females too – Norman [Gwyn] is having visits from his relations & has to show the town. I am rushed*er* than ever – for the food business has to be personally supervised and although I hear Sir William saying 'Oh – its no trouble at all' – I find it no easy matter. I can pull through I believe – although sometimes the hole in my heart seems to let much courage out & saps one's vitality. I long for some one to *swear* for me.

And to Malloch's father, back in Canada, a month later:

> The Maple Syrup arrived safely and is such a comfort – You can't imagine what a blessing it is for puddings etc. Not having cream or much sugar the things are rather tasteless and need much encouragement. Sir William is so thin. I try to get in as much sugar as possible. He really has a good appetite but does not gain. He says it is a *broken heart* so I fear I cannot help that. Every few weeks he gets very downhearted and overtired but then pulls up. He gets so tremedously involved in work it is almost impossible to stop him.
>
> With Americans pouring into England our responsibilities increase. At this moment I have my bag packed ready to go to Lincoln – We have heard that young Howard Kelly is injured at an aviation camp & if he needs me I shall be off. I am very strong and have told all my friends who have sons in England that I will go if needed when the boys are in Hospital.[24]

American troop trains passed through Oxford, taking the men from entry at Liverpool to exit for France at Southampton. The Oslers would go down to the station and talk to the soldiers as their trains paused. As Cushing wrote, 'They fathered and mothered, without end, the young soldier-children of their old American friends.' Grace thought anyone they particularly loved was bound to be killed. They took bitter consolation in the thought that Revere was well out of it.[25]

Grace was often desperate for solitude. In the summer of 1918 she longed to escape to the Highlands, alone or with her sister, rather than go with William to another resort hotel where they would always be talking with friends and she would never have a moment to herself. 'I must go where I can lie on my back or stomach on the downs or moors & sleep or cry as I like.' She finally decided that she could not leave Willie, in precarious health, with the anniversary of Revere's death approaching. So she joined him for a week at the Red Lion Inn at Lyme Regis – along with a Toronto niece and her two children, the Harty mother and daughters, the Wright mother and three daughters, the Ogilvies with two more children, and a Boston war widow with a two-year-old. Grace thought she would go mad – 'they all bellowed' – and they cut short the visit. It was a relief to get back to cool and peaceful Oxford – 'and I can be as miserable as I want & not make an effort.' Even Osler's books were failing him as a consolation. 'Docci O would break your heart – Sometimes he has to leave the room or table suddenly when he begins to talk of his book collection or library – There seems no use in it now.'[26]

In late summer, as the German armies finally began to weaken on the Western Front, Osler and his colleagues found themselves fighting an epidemic caused by a virulent form of influenza, sometimes called influenzal pneumonia (and called 'flugrip' by Osler when talking to a child). Osler escaped the the flu himself in 1918. But millions on the home front, young and old, did not. The doctors were not sure whether influenza was caused by bacteria or some other still undetectable microbe – though it hardly mattered, for they had neither vaccine nor treatment. Osler turned down an invitation to speak at a meeting on the subject, saying he was too busy treating patients, many from doctors' families, and had nothing special to say anyway. 'I have been seeing such tragedies,' he wrote of the flu epidemic.[27] From the autumn of 1918, we have a last description of Osler at the bedside, supplied by the mother of a little girl:

> He usually entered the sick room as a little goblin ... and instantly turned the sick room into fairyland – talking fairy language with us about the dolls, flowers, birds & the behaviour of the weather ... The most exquisite moment came one cold raw November morning – when he brought out from inside his coat a beautiful red rose carefully wrapped up in paper & told little Janet how he had watched this last rose of summer growing in his garden & how the rose had called out to him as he passed by to take her along with him to see his little lassie ... That morning we all had a fairy tea party ... Sir William talking to the rose, his little lassie & her Mother – in a most exquisite way & presently he slipped out of the room, just as mysteriously as he entered it, all crouched down on his heels.[28]

Janet McDougall died on November 14, three days after the end of the Great War. The last of Osler's friends to lose a son in battle was his old classmate and colleague from McGill, Frank Shepherd. On October 11 Osler wrote Shepherd a note of sympathy, going on to mention the toll of war: 'Of the twenty members of the College Club in London, 15 of us have lost sons, & some like poor Garrod two; another friend has lost all three. It is particularly hard to have these tragedies happen to us towards the end of our lives, & when Fortune in other respects has been so kind.' In the last days of the war the British had been preparing to bomb Berlin. Osler, who had protested such acts in 1916, now would have applauded. 'Two years changed me into an ordinary barbarian,' he later recalled.[29]

There is no mention of the November 11, 1918, armistice in his or Grace's letters. He probably spent the day seeing wounded soldiers and flu patients. The strain had told on him. 'My bolt is shot,' he remarked on November 14, declining a request to take on a new duty. On November 16, Warfield Longcope, who in a few years would assume Osler's position at Hopkins, visited Oxford. The town was very quiet, and 13 Norham Gardens was very chilly, with most of its rooms closed because coal rationing made it impossible to use the furnace. Only the library and the dining room were being used downstairs. 'In the library, Sir William stood in front of the mantel, his back to a miserable little fire in the grate, trying to warm his hands. All the buoyancy and gaiety and the engaging wave of the hand had disappeared. The wonderful chief had shrunken to a little old gentleman.'[30]

Grace had thought it would be harder to bear the loss of their son when peace came. In December she wrote home to an old friend describing her feelings about the first weeks:

> What a sad world it has been and is – Even now it is strange that even in all the rejoicing tears are flowing – Even the soldiers do not seem very gay and the homecoming men are so weary, they can hardly stumble along ... It is very strange here – no training in the Parks – no flying over head. The calm is very oppressive after four years of noise. I can hardly imagine what it must be at the front. I was in the Hospital today and nearly cried at what I saw – cases of fractured femur with terrible wounds – One American boy with both legs off and one arm – poor chap only been twenty minutes in the front line – no complaint – just as cheery as possible. It is astonishing what they do to the legs – they put the stumps onto pegs now – made of papier maché – very softly padded – after the leg is quite well they put on the real leg – one hears men talking about their legs – getting them etc as though they were new hats ...
>
> We have escaped influenza – thus far – Sir William has been Angelic about taking care of himself. These are hard days for us, but one must welcome boys back and rejoice with parents who have their treasures safe in their homes once more ... Perhaps next summer you will be coming over to see the wrecked France and wrecked Oslers.[31]

The men headed home and the hospitals gradually shut down. Everyone came to Oxford to say goodbye. 'Portions of the Canadian & American Armies seemed to have demobilized in this house,' Grace wrote. Osler threw off a cold at the beginning of the Christmas season, but Grace reported him in low spirits. 'He has been in the mood he gets every few months when it seems as though the burden was too heavy to bear.' The only relief to the desolation of Christmas Day, Bill Francis remembered, was Frank Osler getting drunk and very amusing.[32]

In 1919 the Oslers put the war, Revere's death, and old age behind them and got on with their good life in Oxford. When Harvey Cushing came in January to say goodbye, he found everything 'very much like old times': 'Sir Wm. in his old form and having regained his weight – full of books and the house with a succession of people ... They are certainly wonders – the Os.' Cushing dined with Osler at high table at Christ Church, the resumption of formal college dinners after a three-year break. 'The war is surely over.' The one change in tradition was the advent of smoking in the Common Room, a change some attributed, perhaps jokingly, to Osler.[33]

The whole world seemed to be passing through the 'Open Arms' that winter, Cushing observed – even the Oxford birds flying in to get the crumbs at tea, and someone joked about the day a dirigible had landed unannounced. All of Cushing's Harvard unit were fed and tea'ed and on the sabbath went to the Radcliffe Infirmary to see Osler give a 'Sunday School' class on the wards. In the afternoon the house thronged with men in uniform, Rhodes scholars, nurses, stranded Americans, relatives, and distinguished scientists, including C.S. Sherrington and Sir Almroth Wright. Wright had been one of George Bernard Shaw's prime satirical targets in *The Doctor's Dilemma*. 'Wright and Osler – could there be a greater contrast?' Cushing mused. 'The professional cynic and the professional optimist.'[34]

The optimist chided a Rhodes scholar who said his brother had been too shy to come to tea. Osler said the house was a 'School for Shyness.' Rose Johnson, a frequent guest in these years, remembered how Osler would 'torment the most shy, stiff & reserved of bachelor dons about imaginary love-affairs in a room full of strange people too & get away with it, where any other man in the world would have [been] mortally offended.' Her turn came one day when a petticoat broke and she stuffed it in a purse, but he spied it, and 'with a whoop of pleasure he dashed around the corner into the midst of his guests dragging me with one hand & waving his spectacular flag with the other.'[35]

Osler had a smart new secretary, was getting special help from the British Museum with his library of medical incunabula (now the best collection in the kingdom, he reckoned), and had just completed organizing the book collection he intended to donate to Johns Hopkins University in honor of Revere. Supported by an Osler gift of $35,000 – the money they had set aside for Revere – the books were to form the library of an undergraduate Tudor and Stuart Club (modeled after Yale's Elizabethan Club). The books included first editions of Milton, Shelley, Keats, Donne, *Gulliver's Travels*, much Izaak Walton material, and a special collection of Walt Whitman's magazine, articles, and other ephemera that Osler had purchased from a British 'Waltite.' Osler suggested that Cushing's bedtime reading on his visit should be Whitman's 'Memoranda during the Civil War.'[36]

Osler excitedly added to his library in the early months of 1919 several of Pasteur's original articles and an Assyrian cuneiform tablet from about 700 BC. The tablet was a fragment of a medical text, apparently plundered from German excavations at Assur. 'Humph,' Grace commented, 'it looks like a piece of Scotch short-cake.' Osler now had his books organized into the categories he planned to use in the catalogue, and he had a fair bit of indexing done, but he told Fielding Garrison that there were at least five years of annotating ahead, 'a race between the Catalogue and Pallida Mors.' To Bill Francis he estimated that he needed 'ten more years of not too senile leisure' to round out his library and finish his catalogue. Francis, who was in and out of Oxford constantly, later challenged the view that Osler's spirit had collapsed after Revere's death: 'Sir Wm. and Lady O. "carried on" exactly as before. Nobody could have borne such a loss more bravely. "The old spirit" was NOT "gone," and it is doing them both a rank injustice to say so.'[37]

In a gesture fraught with symbolism, of events past and to come, Osler, in the absence of the house staff at the end of January 1919, went to the Radcliffe Infirmary's dead house and did the autopsy on a forty-three-year-old male victim of influenzal pneumonia complicated by spinal meningitis. He wrote the case up for publication in the *Lancet*. He published an article that winter in the *British Medical Journal* on the severe anemias of pregnancy. And he wrote the *BMJ* about the case of a septuagenarian doctor who had survived a quarter-century of severe aortic insufficiency. Fanatical bicycling and morphine addiction had kept the man going. Osler ended the narrative with a characteristic flourish: 'Perhaps the case illustrates the truth of the clinical axiom of my friend, Dr. Ellis of Elkton, Md. – "Hippocrates rusticus" Weir Mitchell used to call him – Opium alone retards the progress of a chronic disease.' For all of Osler's belief in natural therapy, it had not occurred to him that the bicycling had done the man more good than the opiates.[38]

He had his presidential address to the Classical Association coming up that spring and also had agreed to give a lecture in the autumn about his old patient, Walt Whitman. He took a leadership role in two organizations aimed at fostering postgraduate medical studies by Americans in London. He was continuing to serve term after term as president of the Bibliographical Society and was working with Charles Singer and his wife to foster the history of medicine and science at Oxford, with special emphasis on summer schools. He turned down yet another feeler about standing for the Oxford seat in Parliament but was delighted to be elected to England's most exclusive dining club, 'The Club,' founded by Dr Johnson and Joshua Reynolds in 1764. Its thirty members, the cream of the cream, met fortnightly in London. In discussion at the British Medical Association's spring meeting, Osler gave a 'pithy' talk advocating tough preventive measures against venereal disease and at another session strongly endorsed a protest against antivivisectionist legislation. He loved dogs, he said, but loved his fellow man more. Osler continued to see one or two patients a day. He wanted to get on with his prewar project to restore the tomb of Avicenna.

Grace saw the pattern of overcommitment and overwork developing and seems to have felt he was losing the ability to organize his time and work productively. She drew the line when he began talking about going to a Red Cross conference at Cannes. She reminded him of his overdue obligations, and herself wrote to one of the organizers:

You can't imagine what this winter has been with people – all the American hospital staffs breaking up in or near London have poured down here; and Canadians as well. It has been the greatest pleasure but it has been impossible to get steadily at any work ... Perhaps you will understand. I am very anxious that Sir William should not be over-tired; the strain of the four years and the tragic end and sorrow have told upon him. I am confident that with caution he should live to a good old age and I want to spare him all unnecessary effort, for the good of mankind.

Early in 1919 Osler's friend and colleague Archibald Garrod lost a third son to wartime injuries. In the aftermath of the conflagration, Osler showed little interest in monuments to the glorious dead. He was less interested in – and in fact was contemptuous of – the spiritualist revival in England, which largely reflected the pathetic efforts of parents to contact the souls of their boys buried in Flanders fields. Grace was very interested in the tending of Revere's grave, and in later years she visited it several times. After Osler set up the private memorial at Hopkins, and as time began to heal, the references to his son in his letters became less immediate and sorrowful. He had always believed in memorializing and immortalizing the glorious medical dead, but on at least one occasion he seemed to want to let the war dead alone while the world looked to the future; when the people of Oxford were considering a war memorial, Osler urged that they should 'put every halfpenny you get into decent houses for the poor.'[39]

May 1919: 'Never has Oxford been more wonderful – never,' Grace writes. Everything is in bloom. 'The streets and parks, to say nothing of the town and river, look as though Nature had gone mad.' Classics professors and teachers from all over the kingdom are pouring into Oxford for the meeting of the Classical Association.

Osler begins the meeting with his presidential address. He speaks from the black oak pulpit of the divinity school, wearing his scarlet gown, 'looking mediaevel and wonderful' Grace thinks. His subject is 'The Old

Humanities and the New Science.' Despite his opening levities, he is a sombre speaker, meditating on the foolishness of their prewar optimism ('How full we were of the pride of life!'), on the barbarism they all succumbed to during the war, and on the tragedy of that most classically and scientifically learned of all nations, Germany. The bulk of his address is a plea to bridge the gap between the humanities and the sciences, for students of classics to learn about classical science and for scientists to combat their parlous overspecialization. 'Paraphrasing Mark Twain's comment upon Christian Science, the so-called Humanists have not enough Science, and Science sadly lacks the Humanities.' Osler says he hesitates to try to describe a new humanized philosophy of science, 'since like Dr. Johnson's friend, Oliver Edwards, I have never succeeded in mastering philosophy – "cheerfulness was always breaking in."' He ends on an optimistic note, comparing postwar society to bodies made stronger after fighting off infections, and quoting Hippocrates on the need for 'philanthropia and philotechnia,' the love of mankind and the love of work.

Osler is not the first speaker to call for a reunion of science and the humanities, and certainly will not be the last. It is not his best speech, but there is nothing wrong with it; it will be another generation before C.P. Snow, in a famous essay, turns the need to bridge the two cultures into a cultural cliché. Osler is a very rare physician to give such a talk and to have demonstrated in passing an encyclopedic knowledge of both the cultures. The very fact that William Osler chose to give this speech at this time makes it a great success. William Welch, over on a visit, pronounces it 'Osler at his very best' – but what else would Welch say? Before and after the speech, classicists take in the special displays of ancient scientific instruments and books that Osler has arranged – ever since the presentation of his MD thesis at McGill, he has favored the show-and-tell method.

Grace has some two hundred classicists to tea at 13 Norham Gardens. She has given in and hired a caterer: 'Everything was very nice indeed except the waitresses who were dressed in bright green! and no caps! But it was a glorious afternoon and everyone outside.' The next day she is only an ornament at a reception at the Ashmolean Museum and is able to slip off by herself and think about it all. Everyone has been congratulating her on her husband's remarkable knowledge, and the speech seemed to disprove the fears she and Sue had had since the beginning of 1917 that he was going downhill. 'I thought it was a pity that so wise a doctor-man had shown so little wisdom in selecting so big a jackass for a wife. However, perhaps with his hospitable inclinations his house might not have been as comfortably arranged for guests had he selected an intelligent, artistic, *sloppy* wife; that's my one consolation.'[40]

Another month and a somewhat chilly day in Oxford, and this delightful woman is hostess for the visit of the United States Army's General George Pershing, along with Herbert Hoover, chief of American relief operations in war-torn Europe. They are to receive honorary degrees at Oxford's Encaenia, or convocation, which is ending its wartime hiatus with an act of homage to the great Allied warriors. The visitors arrive with their aides in big U.S. Army cars. Grace has a fire going in the drawing room and sandwiches, coffee, and drinks ready. Nancy Astor drops in before the ceremony, kisses George Pershing, and asks him to dance. 'We dressed the degree people up in scarlet gowns with velvet hats, and all went down in cars.' The procession and the ceremony at the Sheldonian Theatre are marvelous, of course, though the use of Latin throughout disconcerts many of the American visitors. Grace most enjoys the luncheon afterwards at All Souls. 'Fancy my astonishment when I found I was to be taken in by Sir Douglas Haig & sat next him & Admiral Beatty on my right – Joffre directly opposite and Gen. Pershing. I felt I really must be the *British Isles* I was so well protected.'

Grace tells Sir Douglas Haig of the soldierly valor of the young friend who is tending the wine at the luncheon, and when Haig speaks to him he nearly cries; and Grace, full of memory, does. In the version of these ceremonies Harvey Cushing published in the first Osler biography, he found it tactful to omit Grace's account of the master of Balliol mistaking Nancy Astor for Mrs Asquith. He also omitted Grace's comments on the chancellor's wife, a much younger and very modern American socialite: 'Defend me from Lady Curzon. She was really indecent – She had a black silk Stockinette chemise shaped garment on – low necked & short sleeved ... no belt or string at the waist. Two strings of enormous pearls – & a floppy hat with a fringe of uncurled feathers dangling in her eyes & her painted face showing between. We all really nearly perished.' Later in the day Grace tucks Pershing and his aides in for a nap at the 'Open Arms.' In the evening the men all go over to Christ Church to dine and then motor off to London. 'So that's all; such a business.'[41]

Nearing his seventieth birthday, Osler's web of interests stretched from Canada to Austria as he reached out to people whose views he had opposed. Professionally, the full-time experiment that was causing all sorts of problems at Johns Hopkins – Osler knew it and still opposed it – was also being implemented with Canadian philanthropists' money at the University of Toronto. Osler generously threw a special luncheon for all the professors of medicine in the United Kingdom to meet Toronto's Duncan Graham, the first full-time professor of medicine in the British Empire.

It had been several years since anyone had honored the German medical scientists whose devotion to their calling and support from the state had given birth to full-time research and so impressed the young Osler. Their empires were in ruins and some of them were literally starving in the chaos of the first postwar winter. Osler wrote to a European friend inquiring about conditions in Austria, and when he learned how serious the hardship was, he became an early and constant supporter of Allied relief efforts. Herbert Hoover was deeply worried about the European situation when he visited Oxford in June. Osler's former student, Alice Hamilton, came to Norham Gardens about the same time as part of a Quaker mission to give aid to Germans. Worrying that Revere's death might have left Osler bitter, she found him very concerned about German children and happy to give her letters of introduction.[42] He was also serving on a committee to restock the university library in Louvain, Belgium.

The friends who had idolized Osler years before in America and the friends he had made in England then and since prepared handsome tributes for his seventieth birthday. The most elaborate was a two-volume collection of essays, what the Germans call a *Festschrift*, in his honor, which was to have more than 150 contributors. It was a too ambitious gesture, especially with Welch as the chair of the committee, and was not ready in time for July 12, 1919. The group at Johns Hopkins, *sans* Welch, did man-

age to get out a special issue of the *Johns Hopkins Hospital Bulletin*, with a
score of papers and poems about Osler in the early years there and a bibliography of some 730 of his publications. Other journals had special articles
and editorials; Casey A. Wood and Fielding Garrison dedicated *A Physician's
Anthology of English and American Poetry* to Osler; and a flood of telegrams
and mail and gifts poured into Norham Gardens. Osler was struck by the
sepulchral overtones of it all. 'They are pouring oleo-margarine over the
Septuquitarian!' he told Mabel Purefoy FitzGerald. 'Did you see the JHH
Bulletin. Pity I had not died – fine obituary flavor.'[43]

At a small dinner party in London hosted by eighty-five-year-old Clifford
Allbutt, Osler's friends gave him a dummy copy of the *Festschrift* and paid
the appropriate tributes. Osler had trouble with his composure as he read a
prepared speech, mainly about the good fortune of his life, and with a concluding thanks to Grace. 'Loving our profession, and believing ardently in
its future, I have been content to live in and for it.' The list of contributors
to the volumes reminded him of his 'vagrant career,' he said: 'Many cities,
many men. Truly with Ulysses I may say, "I am a part of all that I have
met."'[44]

Completing three score and ten years, Osler began to cough at the birthday dinner, and on the train back to Oxford Grace knew he was coming
down with another bronchial infection. He called it 'an anaphylactic birthday bronchial shock.' The attack was severe but short. He was in bed for a
week, and one day at tea with Grace and Malloch joked about how much
better if would have been 'if the fever and pneumococcus had taken me off.
How dramatic and what a relief to all those young fellows who have just
written my obituary notices in the JHH Bull.'[45]

He pulled out of this bout fairly quickly and began dispatching his birthday thank-you notes, plus a letter to the *Times* suggesting that the American experiment in prohibition would not be good for Britain. His favorite
comment about his and other successful men's longevity was that it had
been a good innings. To one of the Hopkins reminiscers he mentioned his
surprise at having lasted as long as he had, 'for I must have driven the

machine hard in those early days. Still, I did not drink & have no spirochaetes.' People who saw him towards the end of July thought he was in good form. Malloch remembered seeing him 'getting up from the break-fast table with his red golf jacket flying out behind and a spoonful of por-ridge in his hand as he ran after two gleeful small boys around the tennis court – but his aim was not correct, and the porridge struck the trousers of a nephew standing by in uniform.' An American doctor came to tea the day before the Oslers left for a long summer holiday – he was the last of 1,600 American visitors to whom the Oslers had given tea since the begin-ning of the war – and he recalled that 'age had dealt kindly with Osler ... The black mustache had changed to gray, but otherwise the last fifteen years seemed to have passed unnoticed. In the old-time twinkle of the eye, the winning smile and the elastic, boyish activity, we saw the Dr. Osler his American friends had always known.'[46]

The six-week holiday on the Isle of Jersey was a splendid summer idyll, a throwback to all the good times by the sea before the war – except, of course, for Revere's absence. They had rented a pink cottage – privacy for Grace – overlooking St Brelade's Bay and glorious beach. 'This is a won-derful spot – such rocks & sea, beats Bar Harbor & not a soul to speak to!' Osler enthused to a Boston friend.[47] Despite Grace's misgivings, Osler was healthy enough after the first week to venture into the water, and soon both Oslers were bathing every day at noon. He drank stout and ate lob-ster, put on weight, became 'as brown as a Cornishman can,' and skipped and drew medical diagrams on the beach, played with puppy dogs, turned cartwheels, and stood on his head in the water. 'You should see Grace gawalloping in the sea!' He made friends with a little French girl who went for walks with him, and he visited Oxford students at an archeological dig and called them the 'Cro-Magnon girls.' 'I was never so lazy in my life,' Grace wrote.[48]

In the evenings he read the poetry of Walt Whitman and worked on the lecture about his poet-patient which he planned to give in the fall. Whitman's poems were beginning to grow on him. Osler was not sure how he was going to treat the question-mark about Whitman's sexuality. Whitman's fervent disciple Dr R.M. Bucke had always resented the sugges-tion of homosexuality, and Osler did not think he could deal with the issue before a mixed audience. Personally he was inclined to acknowledge in Whitman 'a male passion which is not base, i.e. physical.' Coincidently, while he was working on Whitman in Jersey, his old pacifist correspondent, A.A. Warden, mentioned to him the similarity of his notion of equanimity to Whitman's lines:

> Me imperturbe, standing at ease in Nature,
> Master of all, or mistress of all – aplomb in the midst of irrational things, ...
> Me, wherever my life is lived, O to be self-balanced for contingencies!
> O to confront night, storms, hunger, ridicule, accidents, rebuffs, as the trees
> and animals do.[49]

Before, during, and after his holiday, Osler worked to do a good turn for McGill medicine as the faculty neared its hundredth anniversary. The organization of McGill's medical and surgical clinics had lagged behind both Johns Hopkins and the University of Toronto, partly because of friction between the university, the Montreal General Hospital, and the Royal Victoria Hospital. Osler outlined to Dean Birkett an approach he should take towards instilling both new spirit and new organization at McGill. As part of his proposals Osler suggested that the professors of medicine and surgery be 'whole-time ... or, if thought wiser, largely so.' In view of the troubles Hopkins was experiencing with full-time (no one would take the chair; Thayer was serving *pro tem*), this appears to have been an unusual change of heart. Osler may have felt that the job of modernizing clinical instruction in Montreal and bolstering McGill's research potential would take a man's complete energies. It was also probably a necessary condition of getting the very large Rockefeller grant Osler suggested McGill solicit – he wrote both Welch and John D. Rockefeller, Jr, urging them to stretch a point about donations outside the United States and help his alma mater. He sent off a blizzard of letters to key people in Montreal urging support for the reforms and talking about how hospitals were becoming 'great institutions for the study and prevention of disease, and laboratories of social service.' 'I hope something may come of it,' he wrote about the Montrealers. 'They need stirring up a bit.'[50]

'I am feeling much happier about Willie,' Grace told her sister towards the end of August. 'He must never again get so muddled with work – and of course people will not come in such shoals.' By the end of the holiday Osler had regained all of the 21 pounds he had lost during the war, weighed in at 154 pounds, and felt unusually fit. Back in harness, as men who had grown up with horses and buggies liked to say, perhaps eager to cover the costs of his holiday, he responded to a request for a consultation in Glasgow. On September 23, accompanied by three doctors, he saw Mrs Fulton Martin, who had 'one of those remarkable Erythema cases (all sorts of skin lesions and for three months on and off consolidation of both lower lobes).' We have no idea what Osler said or prescribed. His bill for the consultation was £525, probably based on the common British travel fee for consulting of a guinea (21 shillings) a mile. The bill was paid.[51]

Osler went on to Edinburgh to see old friends and talk with medical people about future research grants he would have a hand in doling out, having agreed to serve on the first government grants committee. Dr Lovell Gulland, with whom he stayed, was surprised to find 'how little the war and his son's death had changed him outwardly. He was as cheerful and jolly as ever, and as enthusiastic.' The only problem was that he seemed more interested in Gulland's four-year-old grandson than in any of the physicians. The boy called him Willie Mosler. One afternoon Gulland's wife found Osler and the child playing bears in the nursery, 'with Osler easily the most active and infantile of the two!'[52]

A national railway strike was imminent and Gulland urged Osler to postpone his overnight trip home. Osler had brushed aside inconveniences many times in his travels, as had his father in the Canadian forests, and decided to push on anyway. He left Edinburgh on a Friday evening and on Saturday morning woke up to find himself stranded at Newcastle, 250 miles from home. A doctor friend managed to get him a car and driver. Osler knew he should not overtire himself, but the weather was good and he was well wrapped; so he traveled on, stopping for a few hours sleep in an old inn. When he finally got home on Sunday, September 29, after a strenuous two-day journey, he was coughing again.[53]

It started slowly. On Monday and Tuesday he saw a patient, a Miss Husband, a doctor's daughter. But mostly he stayed in bed, nursing the cold, or perhaps the flu – we will never know exactly what bug had struck him. He canceled appointments (the Whitman lecture would never be given or finished), writing to one correspondent on October 6 that bronchitis had left his tubing very sensitive. To another he observed that having carried the pneumococcus for a great many years, 'I must get my resistance heightened.' 'This attack is not as bad as July,' Grace wrote to Archie Malloch on the seventh, 'but I am very worried & disappointed. He was so well.'[54]

He would be up for a while, sit in the sun, then start coughing and take to bed. On the twelfth Grace found him feeling sorry for himself and depressed. He told her he would be an old man with chronic bronchitis. 'I trust it will pass quickly this time,' she wrote. Oxford was enveloped in the tail end of the influenza pandemic that season. There was even talk of postponing the term. Grace noted the arrival of the first postwar crop of Rhodes scholars, with their wives and babies. 'All will have bronchitis I am sure.' Grace and all the servants at Norham Gardens had colds. Aspirin stopped hers, she thought.[55]

On October 13 Osler's temperature rose to 102.5, and for five days he was wretched, tossing and groaning, overcome with paroxysms of coughing, too weak to get out of bed, and haunted by bad dreams, including one of being captured and put on trial by Bolsheviks. A.G. Gibson attended him, assisted by William Collier; Grace summoned Malloch from London and hired a special nursing sister. All sorts of treatments were tried, including poultices; only opium or morphine gave him relief. Depressed and worried, Osler told Grace on the fourteenth that he would not pull through. Then he rallied, and on October 19 wrote a delightful letter to his sister-in-law, Sue Chapin, who was back in America:

> Help! help! sister Sue! and several times over you must have heard my *cri de coeur* ... sent across the waters. Why should I have had to wait for a 70th birthday to get practical knowledge of all varieties of Pelvic (Crown) Derby?

I knew nothing of bedpans! nobody had ever lectured to me on their variety
& uses – Is there a special course at Harvard on them? and in the US are you
allowed private ones like railroad cars? Have they the variety combining all
the advantages of a cradle and an incubator; and I hear that different cities
have different rituals, and that at some Hospitals – like the Brigham – it is
not a ritual but a true cult.

As for things called *Water Bottles* – they never told me the use of these
highly ornamental & artistic bits. My Septuagen. committee has sent apologies for not including articles on them in the birthday volume. Altogether
I have had a — — of a time ... There is nothing I do not know of the
varieties & vagaries of coughs & coughing – the outcome is far away. Shunt
the whole pharmacopoeia, except opium. It alone in some form does the
job. What a comfort it has been! Poor Sister! Worried to death of course.
For two days I felt very ill & exhausted by the paroxysms.[56]

The fever subsided, but the cough lingered, and he was very weak, sitting up only a few hours a day. When he did not take 'dope,' he woke up in
the night and hacked for hours in paroxysms that sometimes reminded
him of whooping cough. He had probably been hit by the influenza virus,
but viruses could not yet be identified. From the beginning there was probably secondary bacterial infection in his lungs. He told his Hopkins friends
(it is not clear whether he was guessing or had had tests) that the organisms involved were 'No 3 Pneumococcus and M. catarrhalis,' and he informed another correspondent that he was suffering from 'one of those low
broncho-pneumonias so common after influenza.' Malloch wrote to Cushing
at the end of October saying that Osler 'had rather a rotten time of it but
there was never any danger ... His good spirits are returning and he is reading a lot to himself. His appetite is very good ... All will now be well.' The
patient himself had resumed firing off notes and letters. 'It is a nuisance to
be knocked out in this way, but think of my innings!'[57]

About 11 PM on November 7, Osler suddenly felt on his right side 'a stab
& then fireworks, pain on coughing & deep breath.' It was acute pleurisy.
The infection had spread to the membranes around his lungs, inflaming
them and causing adhesions. Twelve hours later, 'a bout arrived which ripped

all pleural attachments to smithereens, & with it the pain.' Now he be-came deeply pessimistic. When Grace spoke to him on the seventh about convalescing on the Riviera, he told her he preferred to go to Heaven from his own bed. 'I wish he did not know so much,' she told Malloch. The next day was worse; Osler told her he was bound for Golders Green, the London crematorium. 'It seems too tragic Archie. Everything he said in the begin-ning is coming true & whatever he says always does come true – so how can I ever hope for anything but a fatal ending?'[58]

He felt and could hear the rubbing of his infected pleura. Gibson found in his sputum Pfeiffer's bacillus, *Hemophilus influenzae*, which often accom-panied and was still often thought to be the cause of influenza. On Bill Francis's urging, Osler's old friend, Sir William Hale-White came down from London, examined him, and pronounced a favorable outlook. Osler was buoyed, and seemed to pick up and settle into a reasonably pleasant convalescence. He read constantly – 'How I should have liked to get drunk with Charles Lamb'[59] – and managed to write a review of a biography of Victor Horsley. On November 11, 'Silence Day,' he observed with Grace the two minutes when all England was quiet. 'A[unt] G[race] called me up to the sick room and we listened for the 11 o'clock signal,' Bill Francis told Marjorie Futcher. 'When it came A.G. knelt across the bed and cried si-lently while "Dear Dad" lay back with his eyes closed & his hand on her head.' The patient was able to make jokes to his doctors, telling Gibson that the only thing wrong with him was a bed sore. He wrote Sir John MacAlister that he was making 'pleasant excursions from one side of the bed to the other' and 'enjoying life immensely,' adding, 'It is not likely that I shall ever get up again!' MacAlister assumed he was on his deathbed and rushed down from London on the next train. Osler urged Malloch to come – 'if only to see the bacilli. The Sputa have a vivid look.'[60]

Osler had been bedridden for almost two months, and towards the end of November it became obvious that he was weakening. On November 22 he was still telling Frank Shepherd and others that time would heal him: 'I should be furious if I did not see dear Revere's library in good order and my own catalogue ready for the printers before my call comes – but this seems greedy after the good innings I have been given.' Grace found him reciting

Tennyson's 'Tithonus,' the lament of an immortal warrior turning into a wizened old man. He knew that septuagenarians with pneumonia following influenza often did not recover – usually did not recover. He could not complain: 'Except in one particular I have had nothing but butter & honey.'[61]

Through the last week in November Osler continued to write cards and notes. Some were still optimistic; others had a tone of farewell. In one letter he looked ambiguously towards eternity: 'The confounded thing drags on in an unpleasant way,' he told Mabel Brewster, 'and in one's 71st year the harbour is not far off. And such a happy voyage! & such dear companions all the way! And the future does not worry. It would be nice to find Isaac there, with his friend Izaak Walton & others, but who knows.' One day he was dressed and had his picture taken in front of his fireplace, surely in someone's expectation that he might not pull through. He looks ghastly. His sockets are shrunken and discolored, those of a corpse, but the eyes still burn, perhaps with vitality, perhaps with fever.

Time was failing to heal Osler's body – it no longer had the strength to throw off the infection. The doctors were optimistic, but Grace did not believe them. 'The medical men think there is no serious change,' she wrote on November 27. 'Stopping morphine tonight – giving atropine. Want him in a chair tomorrow. They say "Very slow recovery." Perhaps they know but *he* knows better.'[62]

A second nurse was hired for night duty at 13 Norham Gardens. At some point an oxygen inhaler was brought in. No one suggested moving Osler to a hospital; in England hospitals were still the resort only of the destitute. Everyone knew that his infection could be spreading. Empyema might be developing as pus accumulated in the pleural cavity; abscesses might be forming in the lungs. No one seems to have asked if a chest x-ray would do a better job of tracking Osler's problems than the doctors' hands, ears, and stethoscopes. Osler himself did not ask for one – though in the 1916 edition of *Principles and Practice* he had commented on the value of x-rays in diagnosing pleurisy.

He did think his infection must be spreading and that pus must be accumulating, probably in his pleural cavity. If the bacteria could not be killed, it was possible and desirable to drain off festering pools of pus with hollow needles. Archie Malloch thought Osler wanted to be 'needled,' and urged it on the other doctors. Hale-White came from London again and conferred with Gibson and Collier. A very high white-cell count suggested a more serious condition than they had realized. The doctors agreed to try the needling, or thoracentesis. Malloch came down from London with a syringe and needles, and so did Sir Thomas Horder, distinguished physician to the royal family and a consultant of last resort. When they told Osler they would be going in, he quipped, 'Nurse and I were going to do it ourselves some day before breakfast.'[63]

On December 5 Osler was given a local anesthetic, and Horder inserted a needle into the pleural cavity on his right side, draining off about fourteen ounces of turbid yellow fluid, in which Gibson found *Hemophilus influenzae*. Osler afterwards told Malloch that it was worth it to live to be seventy and have an exploratory puncture done so painlessly. When he also said, 'I know I'm going, since you have begun to make a pin-cushion of my back,' Malloch did not think he was just joking. When Malloch tried to reassure him the next day, he said, 'Archie you lunatic: I've been watching this case for two months and I'm sorry I shall not see the post mortem.'

He was too weak to read or write letters but dictated his will and gave instructions about his books, his autopsy, and the disposition of his brain. He began to have periods of drowsiness and disorientation. His pulse increased and he worried that his heart would fail in one of his coughing spasms. Digitalis was prescribed, along with heavy doses of morphine or opium. One of his nurses, Edith Edwards, remembered him as a model patient, never complaining, still concerned about Grace. Grace and the others took turns reading to him, most often from Walter Pater's *Marius the Epicurean*. A few special visitors were allowed in, including Nancy Astor, Bob Emmons, Bill Francis, and Sue Chapin, who had arrived from America. It was generally known that he was gravely ill. Nurse Edwards remembered that the only treatment he objected to was mixtures of drugs. 'Why spoil a wonderful drug like opium by mixing it with inferior things,' he would say to her.

Every morning Osler would talk to a portrait of little Muriel Howard that he kept by his bed. In the evening, after being given his hypo, he liked to recite – sometimes with nurse's help – lines from Poe's 'For Annie':

> And I rest so composedly
> Now, in my bed,
> That any beholder
> Might fancy me dead,
> Might start at beholding me
> Thinking me dead.

There was always a plate of lemon slices beside him, Edwards recalled. 'When he was lying apparently too ill to move he would quietly reach out his hand for a piece which would alight with unerring aim on Lady Astor's or my head.'[64]

Osler's experience as a physician with forms of pneumonia had always been frustrating. He had virtually thrown up his hands, rationalizing it as the old man's friend. His pessimism in his own case – he told Grace there was never but the one ending – is understandable. But it did not translate into a desire to die. No one intimated that Osler gave up the fight or wanted to die. The idea of, say, a mercifully high dose of morphine was never hinted at. The notion that Osler was dying of a broken heart from mourning Revere is not supported by the evidence. On December 8 he muttered that if he pulled through he would write up his case from the patient's standpoint. On the eleventh he appreciated the arrival of a new addition to his library, a volume with some of the original papers on anesthesia. He told Malloch to write in the book, 'All things come to them who wait but it was a pretty close shave this time!'

Horder aspirated him again on the fourteenth, drawing off about a pint of fairly clear fluid. Horder was optimistic, but Osler's white-cell count was higher still and Malloch wanted more probes. On December 17 Grace told a Canadian niece:

> I cannot give my *own* opinion as I am entirely influenced by what Uncle tells me and has from the time he became so very ill. It seems as though the

infection wavered up & down and each time it gets very bad it reduces his strength that much. We have had Sir Thomas Horder from London twice and he has aspirated drawing off fluid each time. The cough is less but his pulse very irregular. I can only hope & pray his wonderful vitality is sufficient to fight these beasts. The doctors thinx [*sic*] so but they do not know as much as he does.[65]

Horder probed further with extra-long needles on December 21, entering the lung and drawing off foul-smelling and bloody pus. 'You've got it, my boy,' he remembered Osler saying to him – but we now know that the foul smell was probably a sign of further invasion by anaerobic bacteria.[66] Osler's lungs were clearly abscessing and the doctors agreed to go in surgically the next day to try to get better drainage. For once coming close to resignation, Osler was not without a last quotation: 'I feel as Franklin said, "I've gone so far across the river – it is too far to go back and have it all over again."' 'Think of an operation for empyema at 70,' he whispered to Grace.

Sir Charles Gordon-Watson, a leading surgeon from Bart's, arrived with a colleague and an anesthetist on the morning of the twenty-second. The operation was done at 13 Norham Gardens in Osler's bedroom. Gordon-Watson cut away some four inches of Osler's right ninth rib,[67] opened his pleural cavity, and drained off 10-12 ounces of blood-stained, stinking fluid. He put in a tube and a gauze wick for drainage. Osler stood the operation well, and the doctors judged it a success.

When the drainage tube pulled loose for some reason the next day, it was not reinserted, perhaps because pus was wicking out anyway. Now Osler did not rally, his fluid levels were low, his white-cell count soaring. He asked for a Christmas Eve reading of Milton's 'Hymn' to Christ's Nativity, which he had always read to Revere, but he could not hear it to the end. On the twenty-seventh he said to Malloch, 'I am not too far gone to know that the "successful operation" has not cleared up everything. There must be some pus in a pocket somewhere – perhaps in the lung.'

Afterwards it was clear that he was right. His right lung had a number of small abscesses; more successful puncture or drainage, even guided by x-rays, probably would not have made a difference in the long run. The quality of the medical treatment Osler got in his last illness can be debated, but probably the debate is irrelevant. Osler could not throw back the several kinds of bacteria that had multiplied in his lungs and probably long since spread to his blood stream. No available medication had the power to kill the bacteria. On November 15 Osler had urged a mechanically inclined friend to get to work on 'a broncho-tracheal street sweeper, worked automatically by the in & expiratory air, aided by the spiral action of the ciliated epithelium,' because the pharmacopaeia offered no relief.[68]

For completeness' sake, or on an outside chance of beating the odds, he perhaps should have been x-rayed weeks earlier, aspirated earlier, operated on in hospital, and had twenty-four-hour medical attendance and better fluid replacement after surgery. Even in 1919, electrocardiograph and blood-pressure readings would have supplied more exact if not sufficient data on his condition. On December 27 Osler was too sick to appreciate the arrival at Norham Gardens of the first copy of his birthday *Festschrift*, which was entitled *Contributions to Medical and Biological Research, Dedicated to Sir William Osler … In Honour of his Seventieth Birthday, July 12, 1919, by His Pupils and Co-Workers*. The two articles in these volumes on the detection of abnormalities in the lung recommended x-ray examination. One American author added that it was much too dangerous to go searching for abscesses with sharp-pointed instruments.[69] If Osler had still lived in Baltimore in 1919, he would have been admitted to Johns Hopkins Hospital at a fairly early stage in his illness and would have been given a higher, more modern standard of care. He might have lived a few weeks longer.

He had a fairly good day on December 28 and on the morning of the twenty-ninth murmured that the outlook was more favorable. Horder came to examine him. The assistant surgeon reopened the wound and cleaned it, hoping to get better drainage. Horder was worried about Osler's high, irregular pulse.

The doctors went downstairs to lunch, leaving Osler with Sister Edwards. Osler suddenly told her he thought he had had an accident about the bedpan. In fact he was hemorrhaging internally, and soon went into shock. The sister brought Horder up, who ordered injections of strychnine, a desperate gesture in those days, now realized to be useless, along with morphine. Osler's dressings were bloody, but they could not find the source of the bleeding. His last words were to Malloch: 'Hold up my head.' They gave the unconscious physician liquids rectally. His pulse faded. Grace gave him oxygen.[70] Death came peacefully, as he had taught that it does to most people, at about 4.30 that afternoon. Sue Chapin, Bill Francis, Malloch, Horder, Gibson, and the two nurses were in the room with Grace when William Osler's life ended.

THIRTEEN

Osler's Afterlife

Full circle. The day after his death, Osler's body lay on a table for post-mortem pathological investigation. It had been his wish, in keeping with his sense of medical tradition, that the attending physician do the autopsy. Osler would also have approved, possibly instructed, that the procedure take place in his home. It is a scene hard for us to imagine – the draining, cutting, sawing, oozing – even doctors remark on how messy and unpleasant the job must have been. Osler had said that he wished he could be present, having taken such a lifelong interest in the case.

A.G. Gibson and an assistant took only ninety minutes to examine the internal organs and remove the brain, which was to go to America. Gibson confirmed the pleurisy, empyema, and abscesses in the lung that everyone had suspected towards the end of the illness. He could not find the source of the hemorrhage that had been the immediate cause of death – possibly something had gone wrong with the surgery or the cleansing of Osler's wound – but the mess in Osler's lower right lung, which was turned to pus by bacterial action, made it evident that the bleeding had been a mercy. At best he might have lingered for a week or two.

Doctor Jeremiah Barondess concludes, as the doctors did in 1919, that Osler's last illness was 'empyema due to *Hemophilus influenzae*, related to bronchopneumonia with multiple abscess formation due to the same organism, all following a viral respiratory infection in an elderly male with multiple prior bronchopulmonary infections ... The initial event may well have been influenza, and the occurrence of the illness near the end of the great pandemic ... supports this proposition.'[1] The autopsy did not show any other lesions in the lungs – the effects, if any, of Osler's smoking habit were not evident. Anaerobic bacteria and other unidentified microbes and anomalies were probably also present. Gibson, who may have had little taste for doing anything but his formal duty with Osler's body, never reported histological findings and probably did not make any microscopic investigations. It has been suggested that these might have shown that the infections over the years had left Osler with chronic bronchiectasis, or dilation of a bronchus, which helps to explain his inability to throw off the final invasion.

He had some atherosclerosis causing narrowing of the anterior branch of the left coronary artery and pinpoints of urates in a kidney, but otherwise was in good shape for a seventy-year old. More circles. If Osler had been able to throw off his bronchial infections, he might have enjoyed his parents' longevity and lived well into his nineties. If he had done so, he might have witnessed the triumphant closing of a chapter in the history of the conquest of bacteria – the discovery of sulfa drugs, penicillin, and other antibiotics. Had such drugs been available to treat him in 1919 – antibiotics frequently clear up similar infections today – he would have lived to celebrate their discovery.

If he had had only three more years, the physician who had hailed the conquest of myxedema by thyroid extract as one of the greatest achievements in medical history, and who had speculated on the possibility of diabetes being similarly defeated through endocrine research, would have seen yet another circle close. Osler would have been transported into ecstasy at the announcement in 1922 of the isolation of the internal secretion of the pancreas and its almost-miraculous effect in bringing starved, dying children back to life and health. He would have been especially thrilled that the near resurrections happened in Canada, at Toronto General Hospital and the University of Toronto. And he would surely have almost claimed paternity – the clinician who started the Toronto research and shared the Nobel Prize for the discovery of insulin was Fred Banting, son of the William Banting who was baptized in Bond Head by Featherstone Osler on the same day in 1849 that he christened his own William. Osler would probably have made jokes about how magically medicated that holy water must have been. In 1923 Lady Osler invited Banting to stay at 13 Norham Gardens. Banting was thrilled to have slept in Osler's bed.

After the autopsy the body lay in a coffin in Osler's room. Osler's favorite copy of Browne's *Religio Medici* rested atop the coffin. Just before midnight on December 31, 1919, Grace and Archie Malloch came in and stood for a moment. 'To think that these two dears have gone and left this big lump behind,' Lady Osler said.[2] The funeral was from Christ Church on the gray wintry afternoon of January 1. The cathedral was filled to overflowing; an unusually high number of the mourners were women. After the reading of the burial service, the congregation sang 'Oh God Our Help in Ages Past' and, in Latin, William and Revere's favorite hymn, Abelard's 'O quanta qualia.' Mendelssohn's Funeral March was played, and the congregation filed out of the cathedral into the soft twilight, in traditional order: University Marshal, choir, chaplains, canons, the Dean, the mourners, the Vice-Chancellor, proctors, the Regius Professor of Physic (Cambridge), representatives of learned societies and medical institutions, members of the university. Grace did not weep. 'I felt a sensation of immense pride,' she wrote a few hours afterwards to William's eldest brother, Featherston Osler, 'and made up my mind to be thankful he had gone in the full mental strength of his career, loved and respected by the world.'[3]

The body remained overnight in the Lady Chapel at Christ Church. Grace and others took comfort in the symbolism of the resting place, near the remains of the Saxon shrine of St Frydeswyde and the tomb and effigy of Robert Burton. In the starlit darkness and then glorious sunrise of the next morning, Archie Malloch accompanied the hearse through the small towns of the English countryside to the crematorium at Golders Green. Grace, Sue Chapin, one other friend, Bill Francis, and Sister Edwards came up from Oxford for the committal service. Frank Osler walked all the way from his London lodgings to be at his brother's cremation. The body was burned. Francis brought the ashes to Oxford, where they were put in the library, then the safe, and then taken to Christ Church to await final disposal.

Telegrams poured in from around the world, and mourners reached deep for superlatives to describe the grand old man of medicine. A Canadian doctor told the *Times* that 'medicine without Osler seemed impossible.' Strong medical men wept at the thought of carrying on without their leader. Herbert Fisher, a British cabinet minister and dining-club companion of Osler's, wrote Grace that 'nobody ever lived who had to such a remarkable degree the gift of making other people feel that life was worth while ... He appeared to those of us who met him in the ordinary transactions of life to be as perfect as it is given human frailty to be.'[4] A correspondent to the *Times* argued that he was 'the greatest physician of history,' and George Adami, long-serving professor of pathology at McGill who had recently become vice-chancellor of the University of Liverpool, elaborated:

> While we admit freely that there have been greater medical men – Harvey, for example, Vesalius, John Hunter, Claude Bernard, Lister, yet, when we pass in review the great physicians, those who by their lives, their practice, their teaching, and their writings, have exercised the greatest influence over the greatest number of their fellows, putting together all those powers which make the complete physician, Osler must be awarded the first place ... Think of those years at Johns Hopkins, when Osler revolutionized the teaching of medicine and of clinical medicine in a community of seventy millions. Think of the influence wielded by his textbook ... There is no physician who during his lifetime has had so profound an influence upon so great a number: no one individual who has done so much to advance the practice of scientific medicine, no one whose personal intimacy with his fellows in the profession has covered so wide an area – Canada, the United States, Great and Greater Britain and the leaders in medicine the world over: no one, in short, who has combined in the same degree the study, practice, and teaching – the science and the art of medicine.[5]

With tears in her eyes in 1997, eighty-five-year-old Elizabeth Harty Osler Nelles told me that she did not remember hearing of Dr Osler's death in 1919. She and her family were back in Canada. What she did remember, she said, was doing Osler's rain dance and his rain chants, but not being able to make it rain. Another obituarist wrote that those who had known Osler 'will look back and remember that for us was the privilege of having seen and felt power without evil – a transcendently beautiful life.'[6]

As Osler had done for his medical heroes, his followers now set out to assure that he would live on in memory. Grace wanted 13 Norham Gardens to go on as it had. 'I wonder if ever a man died and yet lived as our beloved one is doing?' she wrote four months after his death. 'It is simply astounding. People come in here and talk about him as though he would soon walk in. His very atmosphere pervades every place & every friend. No voices are dropped. His jokes are repeated. I think it one of the most remarkable manifestations of human & humane influences I have ever known. We must keep it up. It is keeping me alive.'[7]

Tom McCrae took over the textbook and kept it in print under the authorship of Osler and McCrae. Grace asked Harvey Cushing to write Osler's biography. Cushing had become the world's most famous brain surgeon. His reaction to hearing the news of Osler's death had been to exclaim to Malloch, 'Archie what a beautiful life! Will there ever be another such. Certainly you and I will never know another to compare.'[8] In the middle of a life and career as busy as Osler's had ever been, Cushing set to work with characteristic energy to memorialize the man who was everything he wished he could be. He issued public appeals for Osler correspondence and other memorabilia and by the summer of 1920 had three secretaries at work in Oxford transcribing material. In passing, he arranged to have the medical historian Fielding Garrison revise Osler's old Silliman Lectures for publication as *The Evolution of Modern Medicine*.

Cushing was a relentless, meticulous pursuer of detail, an indefatigable collector of documents, even going behind Lady Osler's back to get at her own letters to her family (though he never opened Osler's 'Inner History of Johns Hopkins' and never knew the truth about Halsted's addiction). He first thought the biography would take a year and be a 'pen sketch' of Osler's life. Instead, he spent five years of summers and spare time – he wrote early in the morning, operated for six or eight hours, and then wrote again in the evenings, chain-smoking as he wrote – and gave birth to an enormous 1,000,000-word manuscript. The Oxford University Press persuaded him to pare it down to about 600,000 words. Cushing's *The Life of Sir William Osler* was published in 1925 in two volumes totaling 1400 pages.

Lytton Strachey had begun to revolutionize the craft of biography in 1918 with his volume of elegant, iconoclastic character studies, *Eminent Victorians*. 'I am a humble surgeon, not a Strachey,' one of the world's least-humble members of one of the world's least-humble professions wrote about his effort.[9] Cushing's *Life* was a plodding, reverential, year-by-year (and sometimes day-by-day) 'life-and-letters' of Osler, exactly the kind of biography Strachey had reacted against. It was dense with half-edited chunks of Osler letters and speeches, and it was tactful on all matters where living people, of whom there were many, might be offended. Grace and others close to Osler had read the manuscript, asked for a few more tactful changes, and pronounced the work perfect.

Cushing's *Osler* was a major critical and popular success. While a few reviewers told the truth about its verbiage – it was twice as long as a recent life of Christ, three times that of the standard biography of Pasteur – Osler's friends, who did most of the reviewing, gloried in every detail and pronounced it a masterpiece, not a word too long, an instant classic in the art of biography. They had a point in knowing that Cushing was not distorting what he had seen in writing lovingly about 'one of the most greatly beloved physicians of all time' and that by often letting Osler speak for himself, Cushing had, literally, made Osler speak again. Even the exacting Baltimore critic H.L. Mencken could say of the biography: 'The curious enchantment that he worked upon all who had any sort of contact with him is visible on every page.' In this sense, despite Grace's forcing him to omit the Brödel drawing of 'The Saint,' Cushing had achieved what one correspondent had told him would be a 'stiff task ... to paint the shimmer of the Oslerian wings!'[10]

The biography sold handsomely in America, a bit less well in Britain, and was honored in 1926 with a Pulitzer Prize, which in those years was awarded for 'the best American biography teaching patriotic and unselfish services to the people, illustrated by an eminent example.' By remarkable coincidence – and as a sign of the impact that the rise of medicine was beginning to have in American life – the Pulitzer Prize in fiction that year went to Sinclair Lewis for his novel glorifying medical research, *Arrowsmith*. Lewis contemptuously turned down the award, which was also to honor wholesome, elevating writing. Cushing wrote friends that he had nothing but contempt for the spirit of Lewis's novel, which had mythologized research and denigrated medical practice. Cushing hoped his Osler biography would be an antidote to *Arrowsmith*.[11]

Cushing tried to convey a sense of Osler's immortality through the final image of his book. As Osler's body lies in the Lady Chapel of Christ Church Cathedral, Cushing imagines it being visited by a procession of spirits, led by Revere, and including all the immortals of medical history, the great medical men of Osler's lifetime, his pupils who had predeceased him, and all the young men who had visited Norham Gardens and been killed in the war. The image was a concession that Osler himself might not have made to faith in spiritual immortality. If Osler had hoped to live on, it would have been through his writing and his books, and through others' memory of him, rather than as one of the disembodied wandering souls that poor Arthur Conan Doyle was spending his dotage trying to detect.

Cushing's books certainly succeeded in preserving the memory of Osler for those who cared to read and keep reading. The other main way his life and work would go on, everyone hoped, would be through his library, the Osler Library. It was willed to McGill, but the catalog was unfinished. Osler's instructions gave Grace complete discretion in the shipping of the books, though he had suggested that the books could go out to Canada and the cataloging be finished later. His advice to McGill was that the books should form the basis of a library that would educate students in the history of medicine and science and be a center for research in those areas. He hoped

McGill would appoint a 'good scholar' as a librarian, but in a postscript to his last wishes about his books he suggested that Bill Francis might be appointed permanent or temporary librarian.[12]

Just before Osler's death, Francis had accepted a position Osler had found for him with the International Red Cross in Geneva. William and Grace had always treated Bill as a son, and over the years Osler had written many letters on his behalf as he drifted, in uncertain health, from practice into medical writing and editing. On the day of Osler's funeral Grace wrote that she was worried about Francis's future. 'He is heart broken – has never known another father.' The whole library business, which Bill knew about – Osler had made him one of his literary executors – would take time to sort itself out. In the meantime, Grace pressed Bill to go to Geneva and make a success of the job there. Experts from the Bodleian Library who had been helping with the cataloging could finish that job. Osler's other literary executor, and by now the family's other main surrogate son, was Archie Malloch. He, too, was moving on, completing his medical education with a view to returning to Canada to practice. Malloch, who married one of Osler's great-nieces, had considered staying in England, he had written Cushing in the autumn of 1919, 'but naturally do not wish to hang on to Sir Wm's coat-tails.'[13]

McGill set up an Osler Library committee. Grace scotched their original plan for a great health sciences library under the Osler name, saying it must be reserved for his collection. The Canadians knew of Osler's suggestion about Francis (which Grace seconded as 'a solution of many difficulties') but decided to offer the Osler librarianship to the Oxford medical historian, Charles Singer. When he turned them down, they decided, late in 1921, to appoint Francis.[14] Francis returned to 13 Norham Gardens at the beginning of 1922, bringing with him the wife and baby daughter he had acquired in Geneva. Grace invited them to stay at the house while Bill tidied up the cataloging and organized the shipping of the books to Canada. She assumed it would all be wrapped up in a few months, certainly no later than the autumn.

A situation then developed that is closer to the stuff of television soap opera than medical biography. By Oslerian standards Bill Francis's work

habits were horrible. He would sleep and breakfast late, take his time getting down to business, get easily distracted, and carry on late into the night,
smoking heavily all the while. Grace soon became appalled at his slow
progress. And she could not get along with Bill's wife, who seemed to be
more at home chatting with the servants in the kitchen than participating
in the social life of Oxford dowagers.

The books did not go out to Canada in 1922, 1923, or 1924. From the
point of view of getting things done, Francis was very nearly the worst of
all possible choices – a stubborn perfectionist, meticulous to an impossible
degree in the hunt for errant commas and quotation marks, who did not
know how to work efficiently or steadily and was periodically immobilized
by migraine headaches and other ailments. He would not accept Grace's
offer to hire professional helpers. When old family friends such as Ramsay
Wright pitched in, and when R.H. Hill of the Bodleian Library continued
to contribute his expertise to a labor of love, Francis alienated them with
his slowness and his habit of redoing all their work.

Outsiders could not believe the slow pace of work on the Osler catalog.
Insiders like Malloch, pleaded with Francis to get on with it, to no avail.
His eighty-one-year-old aunt, Jennette, who was living quietly in Toronto,
urged him not to trespass on Grace's hospitality.[15] Grace became frantic
and began to suspect that a family of conscienceless parasites had invaded
her home, were living off her money, and ruining her twilight years. Her
letters to Malloch, clearly her favorite surrogate son, and to others, became a litany of grievance, pain, and anger: 'Never in my life have I felt so
helpless' ... 'Never could I have expected to find myself in such a plight' ...
'She belongs to a class of woman I have never before met' ... 'He is the
embodiment of selfishness' ... 'He is a moral coward with a sensitive nature
and blessed with a *common wife*' ... 'I am caught in a trap ... I fancy I shall
die in the trap. It is slow torture.'[16] She had increasingly sharp confrontations with Francis and his wife ('I was afraid I would hit him' ... 'I refuse to
be insulted in my own house' ... 'I had a decided talk with Hilda who turned
Billingsgate on me & told me how she & the baby hated me'),[17] and finally
in early 1925 she insisted that they leave her house. She gave them money
to rent their own place. They did, and work on the catalog continued.

Grace had no financial problems. Aside from her own resources, she had inherited property from her husband valued at £15,865.[18] She enjoyed the companionship of her sister, old friends, and members of the Oxford community (though she had little to do with the new regius, Archibald Garrod, whose loss of his three sons in the war gave him sorrow enough of his own), and she enjoyed helping young men who were interested in fostering the spirit they had heard and read so much about. One of the medical students who had known Osler briefly during the war, Geoffrey Keynes (brother of the economist), had become a dedicated bibliographer and was producing the definitive bio-bibliographic work on Sir Thomas Browne, dedicated to Osler; in 1922 Grace and Malloch attended the ceremony in Norwich at which Browne's skull was finally buried. An American Rhodes scholar, John Fulton, who had Oslerian interests, tastes, and energy in full measure, declared himself a latchkeyer and in a few months became one of the household, yet another adopted boy. One of Fulton's friends, Arnold Muirhead, also treasured the hospitality of the 'Open Arms' and later wrote a warm biographical memoir of Grace. In 1923 Sue Chapin moved to Oxford, learned to drive, and bought a car; the two Revere women enjoyed tootling about England in their 'Fordie' while complaining about touring Americans clogging the highways. Grace never went back to the United States; she several times visited Revere's grave and the graves of other young friends in France and Belgium.

Incredibly, Francis fussed with the cataloging through 1925, 1926, and 1927. McGill, which had designed and built a special room for the Osler Library, became increasingly impatient, but now Grace felt trapped by the whole procedure – the Oxford University Press was working with Francis and Hill to publish the catalog, and if the books and the librarian left for Canada before it was finished, the great work might never be done. So Grace, whose health was beginning to deteriorate, let the absurdity continue. Francis sometimes told people that he had never really succeeded at anything in his life and that this was his chance to do something well. Finally, at the beginning of 1928, Francis's wife Hilda also lost patience and told Grace her husband would never finish, that he would spend his life in Oxford at this job if he could get away with it.[19] Grace enlisted support from the people at the Press, who concluded that Francis had the kind of scholarly timidity that would cause him to go on forever. They all conspired to force him to perform. The last index cards and proofs were taken from him while he was still cogitating over commas.[20]

Grace Revere Osler did not live to see Francis finish his life's work. She had developed high blood pressure, had one or more slight strokes, and quietly died in her bed on August 31, 1928. She was seventy-four. No autopsy was done on her as she had said often that she did not want to be 'cut up.' Her funeral service was also at Christ Church Cathedral, filled despite the vacation period, and her body, not cut up, was cremated. William Welch happened to be visiting from America and attended, full of thoughts about the old days. Frank Osler, so physically like his brother that he seemed an apparition, came down from London to pay his respects. Throughout her widowhood, Grace had kept contact with Frank and Belle, who had a sense of restraint and self-respect that kept them from abusing her good will. Some who met Frank in these years were taken aback at the sight of Dr Osler still living.

In the late autumn of 1928 Ramsay Wright and R.H. Hill settled the final details of the catalog without regard to Francis, who had become a nervous wreck, close to a breakdown.[21] Sue Chapin supervised the packing of the eighty-six cases containing about 8,000 books, which were shipped to Canada on the Canadian Pacific liner, *Duchess of Athol*. Valued at £2,000–£3,000 on Osler's death, the library was now insured for £10,000. Many of its single volumes are worth far more than that today. After the books had gone, Susan Chapin closed up the house in Oxford and went home to the United States.

Francis brought William and Grace's ashes to Montreal where they were interred amongst the books. The Osler Library was officially opened in the medical building at McGill on May 29, 1929. The Clarendon Press, Oxford, had published the 786-page *Bibliotheca Osleriana: A Catalogue of Books Illustrating the History of Medicine and Science Collected, Arranged and Annotated by Sir William Osler, Bt., and Bequeathed to McGill University.* W.S. Thayer gave the keynote speech, 'The Heart of the Library,' in which he meditated on the ashes giving life to the books and on the 'immortality which lies in the transmission through generations of the beneficent influence of a noble life.' Cushing, who also attended and was still inclined to spectral imagery, wrote Mabel FitzGerald that the library was beautiful, and 'I am sure the spirit of WO and Tanta Grace will hover about it affectionately.'[22]

There were many other tributes. Over the years Osler plaques, rooms, halls, lectureships, essay contests, cairns, busts, lectureships, medals, and in the Second World War a Liberty ship, were dedicated, most of the commemorations being at the institutions with which he had been associated. Major attempts to raise large sums to honor him with buildings, first in Baltimore while he was alive, then posthumously at Oxford, did not work – in Cushing's view because they were such transparent attempts to trade on his name for fundraising. On the other hand, William Welch told Grace that the Rockefeller announcement of $5 million in support of Canadian medical institutions in December 1919 was largely the result of Osler's campaign in the last few months of his life.[23] In 1924 the Rockefeller Foundation gave McGill $500,000 to implement a university clinic at the Royal Victoria Hospital, the director to be the whole-time professor of medicine.

In the 1920s and afterwards, practically everyone who had known Osler published reminiscences or tributes. Many were prodded to do it by McGill's Maude Abbott, who as editor of the *Bulletin* of the International Association of Medical Museums turned a routine issue into a 633-page *Sir William Osler Memorial Volume*, published in 1926. Abbott spent the rest of her life keeping track of Osler's bibliography and writing about him. She concluded her own autobiographical memoir with a tribute to him 'whose keen interest in my work and broad human sympathy pierced the veil of my youthful shyness with a personal stimulus that aroused my intellect to its most passionate endeavor.'[24]

Many editions were published of the most accessible of Osler's writings, including 'The Student Life,' 'A Way of Life,' *Aequanimitas*, and *An Alabama Student*. At McGill and other centers, and eventually across North

America, it became popular to present incoming and graduating medical students with editions of one or another of Osler's works. Casey Wood, an ophthalmologist who had been Osler's first clinical clerk in Montreal and was introduced to bibliomania by him during a transatlantic crossing, spent his retirement mailing to the Osler Library gifts of books and manuscripts on Hindu and Arabic medicine and ophthalmology collected from the far corners of the world. Harvey Cushing gave McGill the Osler archive he had created while working on *Osler* and encouraged others to provide material too. 'They will help someone some day to write a better, briefer and more accurate biography than I have done.'[25] In 1931 Osler's former neighbor and patient Edith Gittings Reid published a 300-page biography, *The Great Physician*, which was little more than potted Cushing with added adulation. It went through five printings in five months.

In the 1920s and 1930s most of Osler's former colleagues slipped into retirement. Halsted, who was deeply affected by Osler's death, died of complications following gall-bladder surgery in 1922. Howard Kelly left Hopkins in 1919, interested himself in radium, snakes, and religion, and lived into his mid-eighties, dying in 1942. Someone had once said there was a quality of unreality about Kelly.

The grand old man of medicine in the United States had become 'Popsy' Welch. Instead of retiring from Johns Hopkins, Welch became the first director of its School of Hygiene and Public Health in 1920 and its first professor of the history of medicine in 1929. He maintained his position as consummate American medical politician, with a direct line to Rockefeller money, and as godfather to many of the leading lights of American medical research. A genial cigar-smoker to the end of his life, honored in one birthday celebration after another, Welch had gradually put on weight and, with his goatee looked, exactly like a Kentucky colonel about to open a fried chicken stand. In the 1920s and 1930s Welch restlessly wandered around the old European medical centers and spas and the old American amusement parks ('who can tell what daring shoot-the-chutes thrilled the wastrel of eighty-two?' his biographers wonder),[26] trying to relive the good old days. They were mostly gone. There were no more glittering international medical congresses in Paris, Berlin, Vienna, London; only a trickle of

American medical students went off to the old German haunts; even Coney Island and Atlantic City had seen better days. Welch spent much of his time in Europe buying books for the grandiose William H. Welch Medical Library that was erected at Johns Hopkins with Rockefeller money. He also secured an endowment for the Hopkins chair in the history of medicine.

Harvey Cushing and Welch sparred politely to claim Osler's *imprimatur* for their differing views on the full-time system, which was still being hotly contested at many American medical schools. In an otherwise glowing review of *Osler*, Welch pointed out that Cushing had neglected to cite Osler's last letters about McGill, which supported its adoption of full-time professorships. The Rockefeller Institute republished Welch's review, distributing thousands of copies. Cushing was annoyed, not least because he was convinced that Osler had never changed his mind about full-time; he believed that Osler had at worst taken one of his middle-of-the-road, prevaricating positions. This was probably true, and by the end of the 1920s it was probably irrelevant as passions began to cool, the Flexners retired, and doctrinaire attitudes about whole-time faded. A balance of sorts was eventually finally be struck in most institutions, and even Johns Hopkins, whose program in medicine had been crippled for years by the dispute, recovered its equilibrium.

Harvey Cushing, who was often critical of Hopkins through the 1920s, briefly considered succeeding Welch as Professor of the History of Medicine, but chose to retire to Yale instead. When Welch died in 1934, Cushing rejected feelers to write his biography. He happily turned over his Welch files to the chosen biographer, Simon Flexner, but would not have been pleased by Flexner and his son's Arrowsmithian interpretation of Welch and his band of researchers as the men who made the great age of American medicine. Cushing himself, perhaps the most talented, creative, and towering figure in American medicine in the first third of the twentieth century, died in 1939 at the same age as Osler, seventy. When Simon and James Thomas Flexner published *William Henry Welch and the Heroic Age of American Medicine* in 1941, it was left to Bill Francis, the Osler librarian, to protest at their neglect of Osler's contribution to the golden age of Johns Hopkins and American medical progress.[27]

But who would take William W. Francis, the Osler librarian at McGill – correction, he liked to call himself 'Osler's Librarian' – very seriously? The disciples of high achievers tend to be either other high achievers cut from the same cloth – a Harvey Cushing, a Wilder Penfield, a Geoffrey Keynes – or men and women with a void in their lives to be filled. Francis was one of the latter. The effectively fatherless Francis children had adored and worshipped their Uncle Willie. All his life Bill Francis had looked to Osler as a substitute father, had been taken into his home, and had basked and profited from his glory. After being forced to finish the one great work of his life, making an annotated list of Osler's books, Francis settled in to be the keeper of Osler's shrine at McGill.

The Osler Library *was* a shrine, architecturally a cross between a church and a mausoleum. Under Francis's stewardship, it was not so much a place to worship books as a place to worship William Osler – whose ashes lay behind a plaque displaying his effigy, with his favorite books on either side, in an altarlike setting. Francis was not so much a librarian – he had no interest in adding to the collections or subscribing to periodicals or carrying out Osler's interest in making the library a center for research – as he was a high priest of the temple, a keeper of the relics. He liked giving tours, telling stories about Osler, and answering minute bio-bibliographic inquiries. His lectures on the history of medicine began and ended with Osler. He unselfconsciously referred to the library as the 'shrine' and invented little rituals, as in his treatment of a donated edition of Browne's *Religio Medici*: 'I shall "sanctify" it by placing it for a while in the holy of holies with the ashes before it takes its place with the other Brownes on the shelves. Also I am letting the Chief in on this note of appreciation by taking his own fountain pen out of the show-case to sign this letter.'[28]

Francis had brought over a vast array of Osler relics from 13 Norham Gardens, some of which, such as Osler's desk, found their way to the library. Francis kept Osler's old suits, tuxedo, and fur coat, as well as his bed. Unlike Archie Malloch, who had quit medical practice to become the

librarian of the New York Academy of Medicine and had left England so as
not to hang on Osler's coattails, Francis literally wore them.[29]

Osler's book collection was so rich that even Francis's passivity – he
habitually underspent and saw no interest in having his budget increased –
could not dim the library's long-term importance as a center for medical
history. Although Harvey Cushing had given McGill his Osler correspondence, he and two other great medical book collectors, John Fulton and
Arnold Klebs, all Osler devotees, agreed to donate their libraries to Yale,
where they became the basis of another great history of medicine collection. If Francis had had an ounce of enterprise, he would have at least tried
to make the Osler Library the primary repository of rare medical books in
North America.

Instead, he was content to tend the ashes and rummage through the old
books, while censoring the collection. The writings of E.Y. Davis were not
available for perusal or publication; and Francis did not think Osler's quip,
'I am going to retire from active life; I am going to Oxford,' should be
published lest it offend his Oxford friends.[30] So Francis tended the shrine
and gave out extra copies of Osler's offprints as souvenirs for favored pil-
grims and acolytes. There were a number of such people whose lives had
been touched by Osler – or, increasingly, by Cushing's *Osler* – who enjoyed
getting together in Osler clubs to talk about Osler, medical history, books,
and the need for humanism in the practice of medicine. The Osler Club of
London was the most clearly devoted to maintaining the ideal of the physician as a learned, genteel member of the upper reaches of society.[31] A
market in Osleriana began to develop in America and Britain as collectors
became interested in the various editions of his works and in any private
letters that might become available.

The most demonic collector was Esther Rosenkrantz, MD, whom we
last saw as one of Osler's social service workers during her medical studies
at Johns Hopkins. She had practiced in California, taught at the University of California, never married, and by the 1930s had become 'Osler mad'
in her determination to collect all his publications, and more. Rosenkrantz
collected stones from the ruins of the old manse at Tecumseth, a picture of
the old outhouse in which Willie had presumably shat, and bits of ground

on which he had walked. Did Rosenkrantz literally worship the man? Of course. She told Osler's nephew Norman Gwyn (who himself was having charred wood from the manse ruins made into gavels for Osler clubs) that there had been three great men: 'Christ, who gave us love ... Shakespeare, whose gigantic human knowledge was a freak of nature, and WO, who was the combination of them both for his love of mankind and intellectual and gigantic brain.'[32]

Priest and priestess of the Osler cult corresponded often, exchanging texts and relics. To her Bill was 'Saint Francis'; to him she was an 'Osleriolatrix.' Francis teased her about not adding the Osler Liberty ship and Pullman car to her collection.[33] He thrilled her with the gift of Osler's attaché case. An envious Osleriolater (or should it be 'Oslerolater'? they asked themselves), Myron Prinzmetal, had to be content with a broken flask.

Francis was not just playing. His Osler worship was similar to R.M. Bucke's promotion of a Walt Whitman cult years earlier. He suggested that Osler's character best resembled that of 'Christ, with a sense of humour.' In 1949, on the hundredth anniversary of Osler's birth, he wrote Rosenkrantz:

> In the childhood of the world our 'Chief' would have become a demigod and finally a full-fledged god of medicine like his friends Imhotep and Aesculapius. Nowadays, in what sometimes looks like the old age of a possibly-moribund world, his life, his achievements and, above all, his character (whch is perhaps the immortal part of him) are heartening rays of hope. To me, he is nothing less than proof positive of the perfectability of man.[34]

In that generation's memory, Osler could do no wrong. Wilburt C. Davison wrote in 1950 that he and his contemporatories 'cannot write about Osler without going into rhapsodies about him.' Davison, who had gone on from Oxford days to become the founding dean of Duke University's medical school, collected 261 adulatory phrases used in the literature about Osler, ranging from 'abundant learning' to 'zest for work.' But a new generation that did not have these memories knew next to nothing about Osler, Davison admitted. When he spoke about Osler to medical students, their faces would be blank; at best, there would be a vague recollection of a physician famous in the nineteenth century.[35]

As the Osler generation died off, the number of Osler clubs dwindled, the Tudor and Stuart Club at Johns Hopkins University faded away and its library was dismantled, and a pilgrim to Oxford in 1954 found 13 Norham Gardens empty, unkempt, and plaqueless. The Oslers had left it to Oxford as a home for the Regius Professor of Medicine, but Osler's successors had chosen not to use it. After sixteen editions, the great textbook, *The Principles and Practice of Medicine*, was allowed to go out of print in 1947. Osler's Victorian-Edwardian medical and social world seemed ages removed from nuclear energy, the Cold War, the welfare state.

Some Oslerians, and many outsiders, wondered if Osler's reputation had not also been hurt by his followers' adulation. Even Harvey Cushing had been so worried about Osler coming across as a 'plaster saint' in his biography that he had gone out of his way to sharpen conflicts in Osler's life which barely existed. Bill Francis, on the other hand, kept the lid firmly on anything in the Osler Library that might begin to chip the paint on his saint's effigy.

Almost anything. The story was not to be found in the Osler Library, but among the insiders it circulated for many years. It was that the 'baby professor' at McGill in the 1870s and 1880s had not been a celibate workaholic. The legend was that the worldlywise and beautiful British Osler cousins, Marian and possibly Jennette, had tempted all the country-raw Osler boys from the day they arrived in Canada and had slept with several of them. It was whispered that one or perhaps two or even three of the children born to Marian Francis while Willie Osler was constantly in and out of her house in Montreal belonged to Willie Osler. Bill Francis was always the one named in the rumors as Osler's real son, Gwen and Bea as his possible daughters.[36]

All of Willie's close relatives had died – brothers Featherston and E.B. and sister Chattie in the 1920s; brother Frank, the last of Featherstone and Ellen's children, in 1932; and cousin Jennette in her ninety-ninth year in

1938. None of his Osler nephews or nieces had been as close to him as the Francis children, Palmer Howard's children, or Archie Malloch. When a great-niece, Anne Wilkinson, wrote an Osler family history, *Lions in the Way* (1954), she picked up the story of Willie and Marian's affair from Norman Gwyn, one of Chattie's sons. Wilkinson was a sometimes neurotic poet who had a number of affairs of her own in the 1950s, so she had little trouble crediting the sexual tales she heard. She wrote a bit of the story into *Lions in the Way* ('Marian was also loved, particularly by her male cousins') and more into her journals.[37] While no one had the nerve to spell out the gossip in print, it continued to spread widely, evidence that another of those eminent Victorians had been human after all. Having it both ways, some writers implied that Osler's later saintliness had been atonement for a great sorrow, that his cheerfulness masked an underlying melancholia. If Osler appeared to be good, it was really because he had been bad, and if he appeared to be happy, he had really been sad.

There seems to be no truth in the stories of cousinly sexual romping and bonking. I have read thousands of personal letters by, to, and about Osler, the Francises, and the rest of their family circle, and I cannot find the slightest hint that an affair took place between Marian and Willie, or be-tween Marian and anyone but her husband. It would have been almost inconceivably out of character for everyone involved, and I do not believe it could have been covered up in the written documents (and I know how gullible I will appear if these judgments, which are supported by the most knowledgeable Osler descendants, turn out to be wrong). Moreover, nei-ther Bill Francis nor any of his sisters resembled William Osler physically, intellectually, in work habits, or in strength of character. Revere, the real son, on whom Osler singularly doted – none of the surrogates was as deeply loved – was turning into a man with many of his father's characteristics, before his life was snuffed out. Grace did think Bill Francis was very much like his grandfather, Edward Osler.[38]

The story of an Osler-Francis affair may have originated with a disap-pointed suitor of Marian's in the 1860s who then married an Osler. It cer-tainly fed on the love and support Osler gave the neediest Francis children all his life and, through trust funds, for the rest of their lives. He did treat them almost as though they were his own children, just as he also treated the Howard children and, in one way or another, scores of medical students and others. It may have been comforting for Bill and his sisters to think that perhaps their real father was the world-famous doctor they had always loved and revered, rather than the shadowy, unstable man they never knew. After Lytton Strachey, in the age of Freud, modernism, and the shattering of idols generally, it was easier to imagine Victorians as having been sexually undisciplined than it was to come to grips with their creative sexual repression. And the vogue for psychoanalysis spawned a fad for psycho-biography so methodologically sloppy that it could reduce a man's lifetime of cheerfulness to evidence of existential angst. One of Cushing's unpublished judgments about Osler was how extraordinary it was to have lived seventy years without significant depression. Edith Gittings Reid, who also knew the Oslers well, thought neither William nor Grace was at all difficult to understand: 'Their characters were obvious and would have worried psychologists exceedingly because of there being nothing to worry about.'[39]

A new surge of interest in Osler began in the 1960s. Anxiety about high-technology high-cost medicine's tendency to neglect the humanity of patients was growing in many circles. The profession entered a period of political and social insecurity, to which some reacted by looking backwards nostalgically to an Oslerian golden age. The first generation of men and women interested in Osler who had not known him and wanted to do more than wallow in memory and anecdote had come of age. So had medical history as a discipline, and it was difficult to read or write the history of modern medicine without bumping into Osler. Canadians were proud to have given Osler to the world, even if a research-obsessed generation found it hard to understand the fuss about a man who seemed not to have discovered anything. At the Osler Library the Francis regime (he died in 1959) gradually gave way to professionalism, openness, and an interest in furthering historical research.

The Osler revival included an international effort, spearheaded by Lord Walton of Detchant, to refurbish 13 Norham Gardens in Oxford, as well as the erection of more cairns and plaques in Canada, and the ongoing expansion and vitalization of the Osler Library. It almost included the naming of McMaster University's new medical school, in Hamilton, Ontario, after Osler, but the idea was finally vetoed on the ground that he was becoming a cliché. The strong sense of history and tradition at the Johns Hopkins Medical Institutions led to the resurrection in 1968 of *The Principles and Practice of Medicine* as a multi-authored, patient-centered textbook of internal medicine. Most important, in 1970 a group of North American physicians, medical librarians, and historians came together to create the American Osler Society, an exclusive fan club *cum* learned society, devoted to preserving Osler's memory and advancing the values he represented.

The stream of books and articles about Osler, which had never entirely dried up, swelled again, fed annually by presentations at the American Osler Society and in England to the Osler Club of London. In medicine generally, and at Johns Hopkins in particular, Osler continued to be one of the most frequently cited of all dead physicians. He had written and said so much that was quotable on so many subjects (sometimes he could be quoted on both sides of an issue), and he had become for medical students, with their short time-horizon, the man who stood at the beginning of medicine. In this sense Osler assumed the position that Hippocrates and Galen had held in his day. To write the modern history of a disease you might begin by looking up what Osler had said about it in the 1890s.

Even novelists got into the act, as the great Canadian writer Robertson Davies made the hero of his 1994 tale, *The Cunning Man*, a holistic disciple of Osler. Moreover, as Timothy Garton Ash noted in an essay on George Orwell, it is a very select company of writers and thinkers who enjoy the 'double tribute' of having their names made into both adjectives and nouns – Orwell, Marx, Freud, Darwin, Dickens, Tolstoy, Joyce, James.[40] Osler also qualifies, as do Shakespeare and Jesus Christ. He would never have aspired to the apparently unique distinction of also generating a verb, 'oslerize' as a synonym for euthanasia.

Serious students of medical history were still uneasy. Was most of this just another round of boosterism and cultism, Oslerolatry for the 1980s and 1990s? How could the Cushing biography still be taken seriously as the font of Osler scholarship? How could anyone wade through the thickets of Osler's prose, his tangles of quotation and allusion? Wasn't Osler just another medical male chauvinist, who had kicked Gertrude Stein out of Hopkins and made that crack about three sexes? Weren't the Oslerians self-promoting, anachronistic elitists? When would the icon be turned into a real person?[41]

He had been real to practically everyone in the Anglo-American and European medical worlds during one of the most spectacular eras in the advance of medicine. Their love and respect for him was real, as were his achievements. As a young man, he had embraced the medical calling with an ardor comparable to Walt Whitman's embrace of America. All of Osler's life was a love affair with doctoring and doctors. As a microscopist and pathologist he worked on the frontiers of medical science in the 1870s and 1880s. As a hospital clinician and private practitioner he not only joined the elite but soon came to define its standard of excellence. As a medical educator he was the single most important figure in giving American medical students real medical experience, as clinical clerks in hospitals. As teacher, physician, author, and counselor, he was mentor to thousands of students, male and female – those who knew him personally, those who knew him through his textbook, those who read his inspirational essays, and those who sat at the feet of his disciples. Many of them acted, as he had with his mentors, on the Hippocratic vow 'to reckon him who taught me this art equally dear to me as my parents.'

The twentieth century was not kind to the authority of tradition, either in medicine or among generations. As the past lost its hold on the present, ideas of the aged being mentors to the young, parents passing on wisdom to children, anyone looking backwards into history for inspiration, or anyone being inspired by anything, seemed to crumble. Whereas clinical practitioners in Osler's day could still talk across generations about patients' signs and symptoms, the researchers and discoverers of the twentieth century looked relentlessly forward, only to the new.

Ironically, it was the insecure revolutionaries of the 1960s and 1970s, the new female professionals, who reminded everyone of the importance of tradition with their talk of their need for role models. Osler had been an unrivaled role model to medical men and some medical women for about half a century. Even at the end of the millennium, it was likely that the cool veneer of postmodern medical students – everyone had developed aequanimitas and serenity now – sometimes hid a deep need for authority and inspiration and knowledge. In 1997 Dr Charles S. Bryan published a major book in that vein, *Osler: Inspirations from a Great Physician*. I was working on this biography in the Osler library, sitting at Osler's desk, one day in September 1997 when a freshman student at McGill quietly slipped into the inner sanctum and, in an act of secular worship, placed at the foot of the Osler plaque a bouquet of flowers and a card asking for Osler's blessing on his studies.

Will Osler continue to persist – as, say, writers persist, as Whitman has persisted, as Jane Austen and George Eliot, whose world shaped the Osler family before it came to America, have persisted, and as Orwell and Darwin, but not Marx and Freud or most of Osler's medical contemporaries, have persisted? Some very good physician-historians are finding in some of Osler's case studies an understanding of the complexity of clinical conditions ranging from chest pain to pneumonia that later generations have tended to simplify.[42] Others rightly dismiss most of his medical writing as dated, of only historic or very specialized interest. No one today would presume to master as much of medicine as Osler reached and grasped. Neither his historical nor his sermonizing essays, most of which were outstanding in their day, now have much appeal, though Osler will always be well represented in dictionaries of quotations and aphorisms, and he may never be surpassed as English-speaking medicine's most inspirational father-figure, mentor, and role model.

From at least the 1960s, Osler's image was employed by medical humanists in their campaign to temper the profession's faith in scientific medi-

cine. Too often, it seemed, the practice of medicine had become imper-
sonal, with machines and tests taking over the art of diagnosis, and pills
and potions giving a quick fix to patients' suffering. After the antibiotic
revolution, the problems of treating chronic, degenerative, and lifestyle-
induced diseases seemed to cry out for the holistic, patient-centered approach of the later Osler. Perhaps Oslerian idealism and his sense of the
doctor as a gentleperson of culture could be an antidote to the profession's
constitutional weakness for big bucks, flashy cars, and high living.

Fair enough, so long as it was remembered that the real Osler was also a
rigorous disciple of science and the scientific method. He had a delightful
bedside manner and inspired warm feelings of hope and confidence, but he
gave individual patients very little of his time. He charged high fees, came
to be chauffeured around in a flashy car, and regretted that champagne did
not agree with him. Osler saw no reason why the tables of those physicians
who had paid their dues with years of hard work and service should not be
laden with cakes and ale. There was nothing wrong with good men expecting their worth to be recognized.

Modern editions of *The Principles and Practice of Medicine* are far more
patient-centered than Osler's versions ever were, and modern doctors probably spend more time talking to their patients than Osler did. By the end
of the twentieth century, ideas of patient empowerment and autonomy in
clinical practice, as well as patient-centeredness in academic medical education, had gone to lengths that would have astounded Osler. Indeed, sometimes the search for new Oslers in medicine seemed to reflect a desire to
return to the good old days when we automatically deferred to the physician's
authority, looking to our doctors for salvation. Only believe, and the healing begins.

As a young man Osler was caught up in the nineteenth century's crisis
of faith in traditional religion as a path towards salvation. A minister's son
who rejected the supernatural for the natural world, he personified the
creation at the end of the century of a new ministry of health. To the
practice of medicine, medical education, and medical writing, Osler brought
the rich lode of Christian ideas of service, Christian imagery, and biblical
knowledge. He was the high priest of his emerging profession – though not

so much medicine's Pope as its Archbishop of Canterbury. In medicine Osler was an Anglican to the core, an exquisite symbol of the mingling of the great streams of science and art, study and practice.

Was Osler's faith in medicine as the profession that succeeds in saving us from plagues and pain impossibly simple-minded? Events of the twentieth century, beginning with the war that took Revere Osler's life and shattered much of his father's world, spoiled many people's faith in progress. The idea of history as progress is particularly repugnant to many historians. Or perhaps it is only repugnant in theory. I was once on a panel of historians asked to debate the best time in history to be alive. We all instantly agreed on the present. The main reason, we each suggested, is that medical progress ensures a better chance of having a long and healthy life. Osler saw more clearly than many in not abandoning all optimism and hope after the horrors of 1914–18. As the discovery of insulin demonstrated so soon after his death, the war had destroyed only humanity's faith in moral progress, not the capacity for science-based improvement of the human condition.

Osler's foresight about old age was less sound. Still infected by a fatalism learned from studying sclerotic arteries and deteriorating organs in the dead house, he completely missed the possibility of a successful assault on 'fixed period' attitudes to age, achievement, and retirement. This happened spectacularly in the last third of the twentieth century, as octogenarians began running marathons and life expectancy soared. Still, as the twentieth century ended, what might be called a neo-Oslerian push for the recognition of a natural lifespan and acceptance of a pleasant death, through either passive or active euthanasia, was becoming popular, not least as a way of holding the line on medical costs.

If Osler had lived into the age of antibiotics, he might have reconsidered his views on aging and the fixed period. After he went to Oxford he made few concessions to age in his own life. He was so conscious of the stages of life, of life and time passing, because he realized, I think, how short it all is. For his Christian parents, life went on forever. Once Osler had abandoned faith in immortality, he knew the terrible brevity of the period fixed by the capacities of the human body. When William James marveled at Osler's energy and interests, Osler is said to have told James that he was fearfully conscious of time, that it was the only commodity he wished he could buy much of, because there was so much he could do with it.[43] If there was any undertone of sadness in a happy and wonderfully successful life, it flowed from Osler's understanding that there is no final escape from the oblivion of the grave and the dead house.

He did escape intellectually, moving backwards and forwards through history and communing with the dead through reading and memory and acts of commemoration. In the world of the living, he used time to the fullest, not as a driven workaholic but taking the good of every hour, never wasting one. Osler did not fear death, but he understood the shortness and precariousness of life. He was determined to have a good innings. In fact, he had a spectacular game. He rose from a parsonage on the fringes of the wilderness to become one of the transmitters of the heritage of the Old World to the New, to retirement as one of the ornaments of Oxford at the height of the Empire's glory. His Canadian balance of British culture and American energy, a product of the same template as his Anglicanism, made him at home in both worlds, out of place in neither. Above all, he was at home in medicine, which knew no national boundaries. His special satisfaction and enduring example came in the quest and camaradie of healing, struggling to realize the gospel of helping to make it possible for men and women and children to have more time and less pain. This was and is a life well lived.

Osler's body ends as ashes by his books and as a specimen in a museum. His brain was carried to Philadelphia by Tom McCrae and deposited at the Wistar Institute of Anatomy and Biology.[44] In scientists' first love affair with neurology, during the 1880s, they had believed that brain morphology and intellectual capacity were probably related. If the brains of criminals could be studied productively, so could the brains of honest men of distinction. As a founding member of the Wistar Institute, and in the blush of that enthusiasm, Osler had agreed to bequeath his brain for study.

By the 1920s these simplistic theories had been largely discredited and this field of neurological investigation had become a backwater. Cushing, for example, took no interest in Osler's brain. It took nine years before a worker at the Wistar Institute got around to publishing a comparative study of Osler's and two other scholars' brains, concluding that his was well developed, well nourished, and therefore favorably set for functional activity. Nothing more was learned, and the brain, packed in formaldehyde-soaked cotton, sat year after year in its jar in Philadelphia.

In 1959 Wilder Penfield, by then the world-famous director of the Montreal Neurological Institute, was enticed into giving a lecture at the Wistar Institute by an offer to lend him Osler's brain for study. Penfield took the brain to Montreal, where it was subjected to histological examination, again with no findings of any importance, and returned to Philadelphia.

In the 1980s it was realized that parts of Osler's brain totaling 163 grams in weight were missing. The loss apparently occurred during the Montreal excursion, though there were stories that over the years certain Oslerians who visited the Wistar Institute had been allowed to take away bits of the brain as a souvenir. In 1987 the brain was moved to the Mutter Museum at the College of Physicians of Philadelphia. Two years later a jar containing six sections of Osler's brain was offered at an auction. The curators of the Mutter raised $1,000 from Oslerians and friends of the museum to buy back the missing sections, which were reunited with the somewhat dilapidated whole. Some slides of Osler brain tissue escaped custodial purview and were bought by a second-hand book dealer. As well, the tip of the occipital lobe was missing. Some Oslerians were certain they had seen it in a jar in Esther Rosenkrantz's collection, which had been willed to the University of California at San Francisco. This was denied.

At the end of the century Osler's brain, his last pathological specimen, rested at the Mutter Museum, less the 3.6 grams apparently in private collections. It was usually kept on the table Osler had used to do autopsies in the Blockley morgue in the 1880s. Soon it would be returned to the Wistar Institute. Some neurologists believe that with the blossoming of molecular biology it may become feasible to learn something of value from such preserved tissues – not to mention the possibility of cloning! Future studies of Osler's DNA might contribute to future books about his character. If that happens, the progress of scientific medicine will have affected even the art of biography.

Notes and Sources

William Osler, his family, and many of his friends wrote letters the way later generations use the telephone and electronic mail. Osler probably wrote at least a thousand letters, cards, and notes a year – upwards of fifty thousand during his lifetime. Perhaps twenty thousand of these survive in collections around the world, mostly in North America and Great Britain. In the early 1920s Harvey Cushing assembled what is still the largest collection of Osler correspondence as part of his preparation to write the official biography, his *Life of Sir William Osler* (referred to in the notes as 'Cushing'). Cushing then gave almost all of his Osler materials to the Osler Library at McGill University. Catalogued there as the Cushing Papers (CPOL), this collection has been my single most importance source, not least because it also includes all of Cushing's other research acquisitions (including extensive correspondence with people who knew and remembered Osler), his notes, and his various drafts of the biography.

Over the years the Osler Library received many other donations of Osler letters, some of them originals that Cushing had copied, others that he never saw. These form the Osler Library's basic collection of Osler Papers (OPOL), and they have been supplemented there by a number of other collections, such as the Archibald Malloch Papers, which contain hundreds of letters from Lady Osler, and the W.W. Francis Papers (FPOL), which when sifted produce many nuggets of Osleriana. The Osler Library, which should always be the depository of choice for Osler material, also holds Osler's daybooks, notebooks, private patient records, drafts of published and unpublished articles, and the other riches of his library, much of it catalogued in the *Bibliotheca Osleriana* (BO). The CPOL contain transcripts of many of Grace Revere Osler's letters, the originals of which have disappeared, which Cushing obtained surreptitiously and could not use in the biography. Harvey Cushing's own vast collection of papers at Yale University Library (CPY) contains much correspondence about Osler and the biography, as well as Cushing's diaries, and his letters from his early years at Johns Hopkins.

After a fire in Dundas, Ontario, destroyed much of the Osler family correspondence, William and Featherston organized the remaining family journals and several hundred letters into five bound volumes that now comprise the important Osler Family Papers in the Public Archives of Ontario (OFPOA), in Toronto. Another small but rich collection of family material is at the Thomas Fisher Rare Book Library, University of Toronto (OPUT).

The Chesney Archives of the Johns Hopkins Medical Institutions has its own significant collection of Osler Papers (OPJH), including important patient records from hospital practice. The Chesney's collections of Welch Papers, Barker Papers, Halsted Papers, Mall Papers, Abel Papers, as well as its collections of institutional records, were extremely important. I investigated small collections of other Osler or Osler-related manuscript material, some very useful, some redundant, and some trivial, in a score of other repositories, ranging from the Huntington Library in California to the College of Physicians of Philadelphia to the Bodleian Library in Oxford, and in several private collections. The single most useful small collections were the archives of the Osler Club of London, held at the Royal College of Physicians, and the Dorothy Reed Mendenhall Papers at Smith College, Northampton, Mass. All archival sources are cited in the notes.

There are now 1628 entries in the authoritative bibliography of Osler's publications, compiled by Richard L. Golden and Charles G. Roland: *Sir William Osler: An Annotated Bibliography with Illustrations* (San Francisco: Norman Publishing, 1988), and Richard L. Golden, *Addenda to: Sir William Osler An Annotated Bibliography with Illustrations* (Huntington, New York: privately issued, 1997). My notes simplify the bibliographers' authoritative entries, often citing the most readily available sources of Osler articles, particularly the collections of his essays: *Aequanimitas, With Other Addresses to Medical Students, Nurses and Practitioners of Medicine*, expanded 2nd edition (Philadelphia: Blakiston's, 1922); *An Alabama Student and Other Biographical Essays* (London: Oxford University Press, 1908); and *Selected Writings of Sir William Osler* (London: Oxford University Press, 1951).

There are listings for 1588 books and articles about Osler in Earl F. Nation, Charles G. Roland, and John P. McGovern, eds., *An Annotated Checklist of Osleriana* (Kent State University Press, 1976) and Earl F. Nation, *An Up-Dated Checklist of Osleriana* (privately published, 1988). Osler scholarship continues to expand and is best sampled in the two volumes of selected transactions of the American Osler Society: Jeremiah A. Barondess, John P. McGovern, and Charles G. Roland, eds., *The Persisting Osler* (Baltimore: University Park Press, 1985), and Barondess and Roland, eds., *The Persisting Osler, 2* (Malabar, Florida: Krieger, 1994). The most important of the earlier collections of tributes and reminiscences is *The Sir William Osler Memorial Volume*, Bulletin 9 of the International Association of Medical Museums (Montreal, 1926), edited by Maude Abbott.

A very large number of other primary and secondary sources have been consulted and, where useful, are cited appropriately in the notes.

ABBREVIATIONS

Aequanimitas	William Osler, *Aequanimitas, With Other Addresses to Medical Students, Nurses and Practitioners of Medicine*, 2nd edn., with additional addresses (Philadelphia: Blakiston's, 1922).
Alabama Student	William Osler, *An Alabama Student and Other Biographical Essays* (London: Oxford University Press, 1908)
AM	Archibald Malloch
Autobiographical Notes	'Sir William Osler's Autobiographical Notes,' edited and introduced by E.H. Bensley and Donald G. Bates, *Bulletin of the History of Medicine* 50 (1976), 596–618; ms. in Osler Library.
BHM	*Bulletin of the History of Medicine*
BMJ	*British Medical Journal*
BO	*Bibliotheca Osleriana* (originally published 1929; reprint edition, Montreal: Osler Library, 1969). Italicized references (*BO*) are to the text of the catalogue.
Chesney, *Johns Hopkins*	Alan M. Chesney, *The Johns Hopkins Hospital and the Johns Hopkins University School of Medicine: A Chronicle*, 3 vols. (Baltimore: Johns Hopkins University Press, 1943, 1958, 1963).
CMAJ	*Canadian Medical Association Journal*
CMSJ	*Canada Medical and Surgical Journal*
Continual Remembrance	Howard L. Holley, ed., *A Continual Remembrance: Letters from Sir William Osler to His Friend Ned Milburn, 1865–1919* (Springfield, Ill.: Charles C. Thomas, 1968)
CPOL	Cushing Papers, Osler Library, McGill University
CPY	Cushing Papers, Yale University Library
Cushing	Harvey Cushing, *The Life of Sir William Osler*, 2 vols. (Oxford: Clarendon Press, 1925)
EO	Ellen Free Pickton Osler
FLO	Featherstone Lake Osler
FPOL	W.W. Francis Papers, Osler Library, McGill University
GRO	Grace Revere Osler
HC	Harvey Cushing
HVO	Leonard Weistrop, ed., *H.V.O.: The Life and Letters of Dr. Henry Vining Ogden, 1857–1931* (Milwaukee: Milwaukee Academy of Medicine Press, 1986)
Inner History	William Osler, 'The Inner History of the Johns Hopkins Hospital,' edited and introduced by Donald G. Bates and E.H. Bensley, *Johns Hopkins Medical Journal* 125 (1969), 184–94; ms in Osler Library.

JAMA	*Journal of the American Medical Association*
JH	Johns Hopkins Medical Institutions (Alan M. Chesney Archives)
JHM	*Journal of the History of Medicine*
NEJM	*New England Journal of Medicine*
NYPL	New York Public Library
OFPOA	Osler Family Papers, Public Archives of Ontario, Toronto
OL	Osler Library, McGill University
OPJH	Osler Papers, Chesney Archives, Johns Hopkins Medical Institutions
OPOL	Osler Papers, Osler Library, McGill
OPUT	Osler Papers, Thomas Fisher Rare Book Library, University of Toronto
Osler Memorial	Maude Abbott, ed., *The Sir William Osler Memorial Volume*, Bulletin 9 of the International Association of Medical Museums (Montreal, 1926)
Persisting Osler	Jeremiah A. Barondess, John P. McGovern, and Charles G. Roland, eds., *The Persisting Osler* (Baltimore: University Park Press, 1985); Barondess and Roland, eds., *The Persisting Osler, 2* (Malabar, Fla: Krieger, 1994)
PPM	William Osler, *The Principles and Practice of Medicine* (New York: D. Appleton & Co., various editions)
Records	*Records of the Lives of Ellen Free Pickton and Featherstone Lake Osler* (Oxford: privately printed, 1915)
Selected Writings	*Selected Writings of Sir William Osler* (London: Oxford University Press, 1951)
WO	William Osler
WWF	William Willoughby Francis

NOTES

The sources of all direct quotations and other significant facts and incidents are noted. Articles whose authorship is not given are by Osler. For manuscript sources enough detail is provided to locate material with the help of standard finding aids. Unless otherwise indicated, letters cited from the Cushing Papers at the Osler Library (CPOL) are from the chronological file corresponding to their date. References to the Cushing Papers at Yale (CPY) have either a microfilm reel and page number, or, if a single number is given, it is to a folder in the collection. Readers with queries about any notes or sources should contact the author at the University of Toronto or refer to the master manuscripts of this book deposited in the Osler Library.

Preface: On Doing an Osler Autopsy

1 Lawrence J. Rhea, 'Osler and Pathology,' *Osler Memorial*, 13; Welch review of Cushing's *Osler*, CPY, 124:39.
2 See, for example, Charles G. Roland, 'On the Need for a New Biography of Sir William Osler,' in Jeremiah A. Barondess and Charles G. Roland, eds., *The Persisting Osler, 2: Selected Transactions of the American Osler Society, 1981–1990* (Malabar, Fla: Krieger, 1994), 73–84. The two *Persisting Osler* volumes are the most useful compendiums of recent Osler scholarship and hagiography.
3 Walt Whitman, 'Preface,' *Leaves of Grass*.

1: English Gentlemen with American Energy

1 Hubert Cole, *Things for the Surgeon: A History of the Resurrection Men* (London: Heinemann, 1964), 39; Ed Osler Jr to J. Cornish, 14 June 1816, OPOL.
2 Ed Osler Jr to J. Cornish, 14 June 1816, OPOL.
3 Ed Osler Jr to J. Cornish, 8 July 1816, 28 Mar. 1817, OPOL.
4 Ed Osler Jr to J. Cornish, 6 Sept. 1816, OPOL.
5 See Ruth Richardson, *Death, Dissection and the Destitute* (London: Routledge and Kegan Paul, 1988).
6 Ed Osler Jr to Ed Osler Sr, 26 Feb. 1818, 20 Aug. 1819, OPOL.
7 Ed Osler Sr to Featherstone Lake Osler (FLO), 21 Sept. 1831, OFPOA.
8 Ed Osler Sr to FLO, 22 June, 17 May 1831, OFPOA.
9 Notes on Edward Osler by Jennette Osler, OL, BO7603; W.W. Francis (WWF) to L.L. Mackall, 21 Apr. 1932, FPOL, 8.
10 Capt. Powell to Ed Osler Sr, 20 Mar. 1820, OFPOA, 2.
11 Ed Osler Sr to FLO, 20 July 1831, OFPOA, 2.
12 'First Journal of Featherstone Osler, 1828–1830,' in *Records of the Lives of Ellen Free Pickton and Featherstone Lake Osler* (Oxford: Oxford University Press for private circulation, 1915).
13 FLO to Sam Osler, 5 Feb. 1828, OFPOA; *Records*, 45.
14 Rev. Edward Lake to 'My Dear Sir,' 18 Nov. 1829, OFPOA, 5:33.
15 *Records*, 22–3; FLO to Ed Osler Sr, 2 Apr. 1828, 14 June 1831, OFPOA, 2.
16 FLO to Ed Osler Sr, 19 Apr. 1831, OFPOA, 2.
17 Anne Wilkinson, *Lions in the Way: A Discursive History of the Oslers* (Toronto: Macmillan, 1956), 15; *Records*, 23–4. The circumstantial evidence supporting Wilkinson's conclusion that the ship Osler described in his memoirs must have been the *Beagle* is compelling.
18 Ed Lake to Ed Osler Sr, 2 Apr. 1830, OFPOA, 5.
19 FLO to Ed Osler Sr, 15 May 1831; FLO to 'My Dear Sister,' 15 May 1829, OFPOA, 2.
20 Ed Lake to FLO, 2 Dec. 1831, OFPOA, 5:34; FLO draft letter, 1832, OFPOA, 2:64.

21 FLO to Henrietta, 10 Nov. 1832, OFPOA, 2:65.

22 FLO to his mother, 6 Feb. 1833, OFPOA, 2.

23 *Records*, 24.

24 'Sketch of the Early Life of Mrs. Featherstone Osler ... Jotted Down by ... Miss Jennette Osler,' in *Records*, 1–20.

25 'Early Life of Mrs. Osler'; *Records*, 25.

26 *Records*, 25, 16.

27 Documents re FLO and the church, OFPOA, 3; *Records*, 240.

28 *Records*, 240.

29 Ibid., 118.

30 Ibid., 124.

31 Ibid., 250.

32 Ibid., 18, 256.

33 Penciled notes by FLO on his trip from Quebec to Toronto, OFPOA, MU2298, 2:1:A.

34 FLO to Francis Procter, 12 July 1837, OFPOA, 2:103.

35 FLO to his mother, 15 Jan. 1838, OFPOA, 2:77; *Records*, 144–5.

36 *Records*, 191, 156; 'Notes taken by Mrs. A.E. Williamson, read ... 14 Dec. 1912,' CPOL, 59.

37 *Records*, 133–4.

38 Ibid., 133–4, 163.

39 Ibid., 170–3.

40 Ibid., 201.

41 FLO to Francis Procter, 27 July 1838, OFPOA, 2:107.

42 EO to Mrs Procter, 1 Jan. 1841; EO to FLO, 27 June 1843, OFPOA, 4.

43 *Records*, 32–5, but the picnic is misdated.

44 FLO to Francis Procter, 26 Oct. 1837, OFPOA, 2:104.

45 *Records*, 41.

46 Ibid., 169.

47 William Westfall, 'The Divinity 150 Project,' unpublished manuscript in possession of the author.

48 FLO to EO, 13 May 1843, OFPOA, 2.

49 FLO to Hugh Richardson, 21 June 1854, Ontario Archives, MU2112, 'Interesting Correspondence between a Minister of the Church of England and a Layman of the Methodist Church.'

50 FLO to Edward Osler, 12 Feb. 1840, OPUT.

51 Curtis Fahey, *In His Name: The Anglican Experience in Upper Canada, 1791–1845* (Ottawa: Carleton University Press, 1991), 259; John Toronto to Septimus Ramsey, 30 April 1840, OFPOA, 3:41; W.R. Farquhar to Edward Osler, 17 March 1804, OFPOA, 3:24.

52 Following an error in FLO's autobiographical sketch, Cushing (1:13) misdates this visit as 1841 and places it in Ellen's company.

53 FLO to F. Procter, 6 Feb. 1840, OFPOA, 2:112.

54 Ellen (Nellie) Osler to Jennette Osler, 12 Jan. 1868, OPUT; FLO to Edward Osler, 12 Feb. 1840, OPUT; FLO to his mother, 8 Mar. 1851, OFPOA, 2:98.

55 FLO to EO, 13 May 1843, OFPOA, 90; FLO to his mother, 8 Mar. 1851, OFPOA, 2:98.

56 FLO to 'My dear sister,' 19 Mar. 1840; Jennette Osler to her mother, Nov. 6, 1866, OPUT.

57 EO to her mother and sisters, 19 June 1843, OFPOA, 4.

58 Ms. of 'A Way of Life,' WO pencilled notes, OL, BO7654.

59 Ibid.

60 B.B. Osler to Featherston (Fen) Osler, 20 Oct. 1854, OFPOA, Loose Correspondence

61 Ms. of 'A Way of Life,' WO penciled notes, OL, BO7654.

62 'Pathological Institute of a General Hospital,' *Glasgow Medical Journal*, Nov. 1911.

63 B.B. Osler to Fen Osler and EO to Fen Osler, 13 Mar. 1856, OFPOA, Loose Correspondence.

64 'The School of Physic, Dublin,' in WO, *Men and Books* (Durham, N.C.: Sacrum Press, 1987), 29.

65 *Science and War* (Oxford: Oxford University Press, 1915), 5; 'Oration on the Opening of the New Building of the Medical and Chirurgical Faculty of the State of Maryland, 13 May 1909,' *Bulletin of the Medical and Chirurgical Faculty of Maryland*, June 1909, 248–59; WWF note, CPOL, 42; Henry Hurd to HC, 6 May 1920, CPOL, 59.

66 Dundas *True Banner*, 2 June 1864, CPOL, 59, and files of the Dundas, Ontario, Public Library; Wilkinson, *Lions*, 120.

67 Draft of an address for the Medical School branch of the YMCA, 4 Oct. 1898, anecdote in crossed-out material, OL, BO7664.

68 FLO to mother, 8 Mar. 1851, OFPOA, 2:98; FLO to Fen, 28 Apr. 1857, OFPOA, Loose Correspondence.

69 WO, 'Home-Bred Malaria,' *Lancet*, 20 Oct. 1917, 621; EO to Fen, 1 and 20 May 1855; 24 June, 16 Nov. 1856, OFPOA, 4.

70 'Elisha Bartlett,' in *Alabama Student*, 108; Elizabeth Osler to Jennette Osler, 8 Dec. 1880, OPUT; WO commonplace book, OL, BO7665(iii).

71 EO to WO, Oct. [1865], OFPOA, 4; 'Intensive Work in School Science,' *Nature*, 13 Jan. 1916, 554.

72 Milburn to HC, 8 Apr. 1920, CPOL, 59/9; WO to Milburn, 13 July, 1 Aug., 17 Oct. 1865, in Howard L. Holley, ed., *A Continual Remembrance: Letters from Sir William Osler to His Friend Ned Milburn 1865–1919* (Springfield, Ill.: Charles C. Thomas, 1968), 13–16; Canon Jarvis to Arthur Jukes Johnson, 4 Jan. 1921, CPOL, 61/32.

73 'A Way of Life,' 1913, *Selected Writings*, 239; WO to Ned Milburn, 28 Feb., 24 Jan. 1866, *Continual Remembrance*, 23, 21.

74 Jennette Osler 1866 travel diary, OPUT; Jennette Osler to Charlotte and Wm Henry Osler, 18 Sept. 1866, OPUT.

75 Jennette Osler to her parents, 6 Nov. 1866, and to her mother, 4 Feb. 1867, OPUT.

76 Jennette Osler to her parents, 6 Nov. 1866, OPUT.

77 Jennette Osler to Mamma & WH, 21 May 1867, OPUT; WO to Jennette Osler, 25 May 1867, CPOL, 63/11. For discussion of the myth of the Osler cousins as bewitching sirens, see below, pp. 494–6.

2: Learning to See: Student Years

1 WO to Ned Milburn, 28 Feb. 1866, *Continual Remembrance*, 22–3.

2 Ibid.; EO to WO, 25 Feb. 1867, CPOL, 63/7.

3 Norman Gwyn to HC, 12 Nov. 1920, summarizing newspaper accounts, CPOL 1866.

4 EO to WO, 19 Apr. 1866, CPOL; EO to WO, 10 and 30 May 1866, OFPOA.

5 WO to Jennette Osler, 1 Jan. 1868, OPUT.

6 Nellie Osler to WO, Sept. 1866, CPOL, Letters to WO, 1940 file (following 1919 file); Rev. Canon Jarvis to Arthur Jukes Johnson, 4 Jan. 1921, CPOL 1866; Richard L. Golden, 'Sir William Osler's Angina Pectoris and Other Disorders,' *American Journal of Cardiology*, 60 (July 1987), 175.

7 F.K. Dalton, 'The Reverend William Arthur Johnson,' *Journal of the Canadian Church Historical Society*, 8, no. 1 (Mar. 1966), 2–15; *Canadian Churchman*, 12 June 1902; Carl Berger, *Science, God, and Nature in Victorian Canada* (Toronto: University of Toronto Press, 1983), 9; James H. Cassedy, 'The Microscope in American Medical Science,' *Isis*, 1976, 76–97.

8 W.A. Johnson field book, entry 505, CPOL 1866; WO, 'The Collecting of a Library,' *BO*, xxi.

9 WO to Jennette Osler, 25 May 1867, CPOL.

10 'Intensive Work in School Science,' *Nature*, 13 Jan. 1916, 554.

11 Jennette Osler to Mother, 17 July 1867; Nellie Osler to Jennette, 7 Aug. 1867, OPUT; WO, 'On Canadian Fresh-Water Polyzoa,' *Canadian Naturalist* 10, no. 7 (1883), 399.

12 Jennette Osler to parents, 8 Nov. 1866, OPUT; *A Continual Remembrance*, ch. 5; T.A. Reed, *A History of Trinity College Toronto* (Toronto, 1952), ch. 4.

13 WO notes on ms. of 'A Way of Life,' OL, BO7654; 'Intensive Work in School Science,' *Nature*, 13 Jan. 1916, 554.

14 Norman B. Gwyn, 'The Early Life of Sir William Osler, His Cultural and Scientific Training, *Oster Memorial*, 141n.

15 WO to Jennette Osler, 1 Jan. 1868; Nellie Osler to Jennette Osler, 12 Jan., 17 June 1868, OPUT.

16 'The Collecting of a Library,' *BO*, xxii; The Master-Word in Medicine,' *Aequanimitas*, 371.

17 *Religio Medici*, Everyman's Library edn. (London: J.M. Dent, 1906), 17, 18, 26.

18 Nellie Osler to Jennette Osler, 17 June 1868, OPUT.

19 Rev. Canon Arthur Jarvis, to HC, 18 July 1921, CPY, 547; Jarvis to Arthur Jukes

Johnson, 4 Jan. 1921, CPOL 1866; GRO note on WO's reminiscences, June 1919, CPOL 1868.

20 Richard H. Shryock, *The Development of Modern Medicine* (New York: Knopf, 1947; facsimile, New York: Hafner, 1969), 157; Edward C. Atwater, 'Internal Medicine,' in Ronald L. Numbers, ed., *The Education of American Physicians: Historical Essays* (Berkeley: University of California Press, 1980), 143–74; also Charles E. Rosenberg, 'The Therapeutic Revolution,' in Morris J. Vogel and Charles E. Rosenberg, eds., *The Therapeutic Revolution* (Philadelphia: University of Pennsylvania Press, 1979), 3–25; John Harley Warner, *The Therapeutic Perspective* (Cambridge, Mass.: Harvard University Press, 1986; WO, *The Evolution of Modern Medicine*. (New Haven: Yale University Press, 1923).

21 'Currents and Counter-Currents in Medical Science,' in O.W. Holmes, *Medical Essays, 1842–1882* (Boston: Houghton, Mifflin, 1883), 203.

22 Fred C. Shattuck, 'Address to the Aesculapian Society, January 1920,' *Boston Medical and Surgical Journal*, 28 July 1921, 105.

23 W.G. Cosbie, *The Toronto General Hospital 1819–1965* (Toronto: Macmillan, 1975), 71–81.

24 J. Beattie Crozier, *My Inner Life: Being a Chapter in Personal Evolution and Autobiography* (London: Longmans, 1898), 225, 227.

25 WO notebook, OL, BO7666(b); 'Specialism in the General Hospital,' *American Journal of Insanity* 69, no. 5 (1913), 847; 'The Master-Word in Medicine,' *Aequanimitas*, 368–9.

26 *Hardwicke's Science-Gossip*, 1 Feb. 1869, 44.

27 WO Notebook, 211, OL, BO7666(c); 'Trichina Spiralis,' *Canadian Journal of Medical Science* 1 (1976), 134–5, 175–6; 'Canadian Diatomaceae,' *Canadian Naturalist* 5 (June 1870), 142–51; Dr Albert Macdonald memoir of WO, CPOL 1868.

28 Dr Albert Macdonald, Dr John Standish memoirs of WO, CPOL 1868; Cushing, 1:25–6; HC corres. with Ned Milburn, CPY, 562.

29 'The Future of the Medical Profession in Canada,' 9 Sept. 1918, OL, BO7668, mss of unpublished papers; on Evans, see BO2547; Jean Ware and Hugh Hunt, *The Several Lives of a Victorian Vet* (London: Bachman and Turner, 1979), 99.

30 Obituary, James Graham, *BMJ*, 29 July 1899, 317.

31 'Master-Word in Medicine,' *Aequanimitas*, 371; 'The Collecting of a Library,' BO, xxii; WO draft of BO Introduction, CPOL, 35.

32 'Master-Word in Medicine,' *Aequanimitas*, 370; WO, 'James Bovell, M.D.,' *Canadian Journal of Medical Science* 5 (April 1880), 114–15; C.E. Dolman, 'The Reverend James Bovell, M.D., 1817–1880,' in G.F.G. Stanley, ed., *Pioneers of Canadian Science* (Toronto: University of Toronto Press, 1966).

33 'The Natural Method of Teaching the Subject of Medicine,' JAMA, 15 June 1901, 1673.

34 'Master-Word in Medicine,' *Aequanimitas*, 371; FLO to Lizzie, 6 Oct. 1870, OFPOA, 2:100; Mark E. Silverman, 'James Bovell: A Remarkable Nineteenth-Century Physician and the Forgotten Mentor of William Osler,' CMAJ 148 (1993), 953–7.

35 Kenneth M. Ludmerer, *Learning to Heal: The Development of American Medical Education* (New York: Basic Books, 1985), 48; for McGill, see Joseph Hanaway and Richard Cruess, *McGill Medicine*, vol. 1: *The First Half Century, 1829–1885* (Montreal: McGill-Queen's University Press, 1996).

36 For conditions at McGill and the MGH, see Francis J. Shepherd, *Reminiscences of Student Days and Dissecting Room* (Montreal: privately printed, 1919); W.B. Howell, *F.J. Shepherd – Surgeon: His Life and Times* (Toronto: Dent, 1934); WO on lecture notes, BO7598.

37 F.J. Shepherd, 'Yesterday and To-Day,' an address to the undergraduates' medical society, June 1898, *Montreal Medical Journal*, Apr. 1899, 7; Howell, *F.J. Shepherd*, 24.

38 WO, 'The Medical Clinic: A Retrospect and a Forecast,' *BMJ*, 3 Jan. 1914, 10–16; Shepherd, *Reminiscences*, 5–6.

39 WO notebook, OL, BO7666d; Shepherd, *Reminiscences*, 12; Edward Bensley, 'Palmer Howard,' *Dictionary of Canadian Biography*, 11:428–9; Medico-Chirurgical Society of Montreal, *Minutes*, 5 Nov. 1870, OL, cited in FPOL, WWF to CD Parfitt, 28 July 1940.

40 Osler, 'The Medical Clinic,' *BMJ*, 3 Jan. 1914, 10–16.

41 Jennette Osler to EO, 16 Jan. 1871, CPOL.

42 WO, *Introductory Lecture on the Opening of the Forty-Fifth Session of the Medical Faculty McGill University, Oct 1, 1877* (Montreal, 1877), 10–11; 'University of Trinity College Medical Examination, April 1871,' *Canada Lancet* 3 (1870–1), 374, 381.

43 ('Benj') to Charlotte Osler ('Chattie'), 6 July 1871, CPOL; 'A Way of Life,' *Selected Writings*, 239; crossed-out material in WO draft address for the Medical School branch of the YMCA, 4 Oct. 1898, OL, BO7664 (I).

44 'Hospital Reports,' *Canada Medical Journal* 8 (Sept. 1871), 107ff.

45 WO, 'The Student Life,' *Aequanimitas*, 441; 'The Collecting of a Library,' *BO*, xxiii; WO obituary of Howard, *Medical News* 54 (1889), 383; WO memorandum book, OL, BO7665(viii), 'B.'

46 'A Way of Life,' *Selected Writings*, 239–40 (WO slightly misquotes Carlyle); WO, 'Samuel Wilks,' in WO, *Men and Books* (Durham, N.C.: Sacrum Press, 1987), 5.

47 WO to Jennette Osler, 22 Oct. 1871, CPOL; WO, 'Samuel Wilks,' in WO, *Men and Books*, 5; Montreal *Gazette*, 28 Oct. 1871; Shepherd, *Reminiscences*, 7; WO, 'After Twenty-Five Years,' *Aequanimitas*, 212; Malloch Journal notes, 15 Nov. 1914, CPOL; WO to Adam H. Wright, 19 Sept. 1911, AW note, CPOL.

48 B.N. Wales, 'Recollections of Sir William Osler during His Graduation Year at McGill,' CPY, 607; personal notes of Adam H. Wright, CPOL 1868.

49 'Collecting of a Library,' *BO*, xxiv; 'Osler's Autobiographical Address to the American Club, Oxford, 12 Feb. 1916,' OL, 8303, 1916 folder; Cushing 1:85; the ms, 'Case Reports and Autopsy Reports,' OL, BO7664 (I), seems to contain draft pages from the thesis and gives the autopsies as twenty.

50 'Annual Convocation of McGill University,' *Canada Medical Journal* 8 (1871–2),

472–3; McGill version of the Hippocratic oath in WO, 'The Lessons of Greek Medicine,' unpublished lecture, 27 May 1910, OL, BO7664(iii).

51 W.A. Johnson to James B. Johnson, 9 Dec. 1874, CPOL, 90:28; also Norman B. Gwyn, ed., 'The Letters of a Devoted Father to an Unresponsive Son,' *BHM* 7 (1939), 335–51.

52 Archie Malloch Journal, 23 July 1917, CPOL; WO notebook, OL, BO7666(n).

53 WO to Jennette Osler, 7 Sept. 1872, OPUT; Thomas McCrae, 'The Influence of Pathology on the Clinical Medicine of William Osler,' *Osler Memorial*, 38; WO review of *Supplement to the Catalogue of the Pathological Museum* ... in *American Journal of Medical Science* 84 (1882), 229–30.

54 Palmer Howard to WO, 25 Oct. 1872; WO draft to Howard, undated, prob. 7 Nov. 1872, CPOL.

55 Wm. Dawson to WO, 28 Nov. 1872; Geo. W. Campbell to WO, 29 Nov. 1872; Palmer Howard to WO, 6 Dec. 1872, CPOL.

56 Scrap torn from WO to Jennette Osler, c. Jan. 1873, CPOL. In Cushing, 1:372–3, a differently worded fragment of this is misdated ten years later.

57 WO notebook, OL, BO7666(k); WO, 'The Medical Clinic,' *BMJ*, 3 Jan. 1914, 10–16; 'London Correspondence,' *CMSJ* 1 (1872–3), 548–51. Limit of surgery: 'The Growth of Truth,' *Selected Writings*, 208.

58 WO draft to Palmer Howard, c. 7 Nov. 1872, CPOL; WO notebook, 'Short Notes on a Course of Practical Physiology by Dr. Burdon-Sanderson at University College, London, 1872–73,' OL, BO7666(i).; WO remarks on J.F. Payne, *BMJ*, 26 Nov. 1910, 1751; 'On the Action of Certain Reagents, Atropia, Physostigma and Curare on the Colourless Blood-Corpuscles,' *Quarterly Journal of Microscopical Science*, n.s. 1873, 307–9.

59 'An Account of Certain Organisms Occurring in the Liquor Sanguinis,' *Proceedings of the Royal Society*, 18 June 1874, 391–9; WO notebook, OL, BO7665(i); C. Lockard Conley, 'Osler as an Experimental Hematologist,' *Persisting Osler*, 169–72; Alastair H.T. Robb-Smith, 'Why the Platelets Were Discovered,' *British Journal of Haematology* 13 (1967), 618–37; Robb-Smith, 'Osler's Influence on Haematology,' *Blood Cells* 7 (1981), 513–33. Howard, in *CMSJ* 2 (1873–4), 208.

60 'The Library School in the College' (Aberdeen: Aberdeen University Press, 1917; reprinted from *The Library Association Record*, Aug.–Sept. 1917), 23.

61 'The Collecting of a Library,' *BO*, xxiv; John Brown, *Horae Subsecivae: Locke and Sydenham with Other Occasional Papers* (Edinburgh: Thomas Constable, 1858), xi; BO4396.

62 Terrie Marie Romano, 'Making Medicine Scientific: John Burdon Sanderson and the Culture of Victorian Science' (Yale University, PhD dissertation, 1993), 267. The story was told by J.J. Abel; others have told similar stories of other researchers; WO to Jennette Osler, 16 Dec. 1872, CPOL.

63 WO to Chattie, 16 Apr. 1874, CPOL; on Darwin, Cushing 1:118, citing a note in an unidentified book in the OL; WO to Jennette Osler, 9 Nov. 1872, OPUT.

64 WO to Jennette Osler, 16 Jan. 1873, CPOL; WO, 'Sir Thomas Browne,' *Alabama Student*, 271.

65 WO, 'Berlin Correspondence,' *CMSJ* 2 (Nov. 1873), 231–3, 308–15; 'The Medical Clinic' *BMJ*, 3 Jan. 1914, 10–16, fragmentary notes, WO to Chattie, 23 Nov. 1873, CPOL.

66 WO, 'Correspondence,' *CMSJ* 2 (Mar. 1874), 451.

67 'The Making of a Library,' *BO* xxiv; 'Berlin Correspondence,' *CMSJ* 2 (1873), 311.

68 Ilza Veith, 'Sir William Osler, Acupuncturist,' *Persisting Osler*, 129; WO, 'Ephemerides,' *Montreal Medical Journal* 23 (1894–5), 879; WO to Chattie, 23 Nov. 1873, CPOL.

69 N.B. Gwyn to HC, 21 May 1920, CPOL 1874; Palmer Howard to WO, 6 July 1874, CPOL.

3: The Baby Professor

1 Dr Hiram Vineberg to HC, 17 Feb. 1926, CPY, 121:240–2; Marian Osborne, 'Recollections of Sir William Osler,' *Osler Memorial*, 171–4; 'Student Reminiscences: Montreal Period,' *Osler Memorial*, 175–84; WO, 'After Twenty-Five Years,' *Aequanimitas*, 201–2.

2 Ibid.; account book, OL, BO7668.

3 'Valedictory Address to the Graduates ... March 31, 1875,' *CMSJ* 3 (1874–5), 433–8.

4 Minutes of the Medical Faculty, 5 April 1875; McGill Archives, RG38, 1; Cushing, 1:130n.

5 WO daybook, 1874, OL, BO7668 (contains both expenses and income).

6 WO, 'Haemorrhagic Small-Pox,' *CMSJ* 5 (1877), 289–304, reprinted in WO, *Clinical Notes on Small-Pox* (Montreal, 1877); 'Copy of a Letter from Dr. Osler' (to the Nevilles), CPOL 1875; 'Valedictory Address to the Graduates in Medicine and Surgery, McGill University ... 31st March, 1875,' *CMSJ* 3 (1874–5), 433–8.

7 WO, 'Haemorrhagic Small-Pox,' *CMSJ* 5 (1877), 304; WO, *Clinical Notes on Small-Pox*; 'Commencement Address,' Johns Hopkins Nurses' Training School, 7 May 1913, *Johns Hopkins Hospital Nurses' Alumnae Magazine* 12 (1913), 73; OL, BO7665(x), notes labeled 'Religio Studentis.'

8 Jennette Osler to EO, [26] Dec. 1875, CPOL; 'Case of Scarlatina miliaris,' *CMSJ* 4 (1875), 49–54.

9 WO to Arthur Jarvis, Jan. 1876, Cushing, 1:143. See also William B. Spaulding, 'William Osler's Experiences with Smallpox,' *Persisting Osler*, 2:269–79.

10 'Introductory Remarks, to, and Synopsis of, Practical Course on Institutes of Medicine,' *CMSJ* 4 (1875), 202–7; 'The Growth of a Profession,' *CMSJ* 14 (Oct. 1885), 150.

11 WO, '"On the Practical Teaching of Morbid Anatomy," the Introductory Lecture of the Course in Demonstrative Pathology,' McGill, 5 Oct. [prob. 1878], OL, BO7664, unpublished papers, 1; *Introductory Lecture on the Opening of the Forty-Fifth Session of*

the Medical Faculty, McGill University, 1 Oct. 1877 (Montreal, 1877), 14; Casey Wood reminiscence, *Osler Memorial,* 178.

12 'On the Pathology of Miner's Lung,' *CMSJ* 4 (1875–6), 145–68; minutes of the Medico-Chirurgical Society of Montreal, OL; Alvin Rodin, *Oslerian Pathology: An Assessment and Annotated Atlas of Museum Specimens* (Lawrence, Kans.: Coronado Press, 1981); Geo. A. Armstrong reminiscence, *Osler Memorial,* 176.

13 Edward J.A. Rogers to HC, 8 Dec. 1920, CPY, 592.

14 Clipping re address to Cardiff Medical Society, 20 June 1916. CPOL.

15 'Notes of the Second Demonstration in the Morbid Anatomy Course in McGill College,' reported by J.R.B. Howard, *Canadian Journal of Medical Science* 6 (1881), 351–3.

16 Beth M. Belkin and Francis A. Neelon, 'The Art of Observation: William Osler and the Method of Zadig,' *Archives of Internal Medicine* 116 (1992), 863–6; F.J. Sladen, 'Osler as Clinician,' *North Carolina Medical Journal* 10 (1949), 607–10; Rufus Cole, 'Dr. Osler: Scientist and Teacher,' *Archives of Internal Medicine* 84 (1949), 54–63.

17 Lauder Brunton to Fielding Garrison, in Garrison, 'Physician's Letters,' in *Contributions to Medical and Biological Research, Dedicated to Sir William Osler … In Honour of his Seventieth Birthday, July 12, 1919, by His Pupils and Co-Workers,* 2 vols. (New York: Paul Hoeber, 1919), 716; *CMSJ* 7 (Feb. 1879), 329–35.

18 William Boyman Howell, *F.J. Shepherd: Surgeon* (Toronto: Dent, 1934), 79; D.J. Gibb Wishart reminiscence, *Osler Memorial,* 177.

19 *Introductory Lecture on the Opening of the Forty-Fifth Session of the Medical Faculty McGill University, 1 Oct. 1877* (Montreal, 1877), 12.

20 'Harvard School of Medicine,' *Canadian Journal of Medical Science* 2 (1877), 274–6; Joseph Hanaway and Richard Cruess, *McGill Medicine,* vol. 1 (Montreal: McGill-Queen's University Press, 1996); 'Brief Description of the New Physiological Laboratories, McGill College,' *CMSJ* 9 (1880–1), 198–201.

21 Notes from Bowditch family, CPY, 80:170.

22 D.A. Murphy, quoted in Leon Z. Saunders, 'From Osler to Olafson: The Evolution of Veterinary Pathology in North America,' *Persisting Osler,* 2:313–54. See also P.M. Teigen, 'William Osler and Comparative Medicine,' *Canadian Veterinary Journal* 25 (1984), 400–5.

23 Lisa Wilkinson, *Animals and Disease: An Introduction to the History of Comparative Medicine* (Cambridge: Cambridge University Press, 1992).

24 'Verminous Bronchitis in Dogs,' *Veterinarian* 50 (1877), 387–97; Teigen, 'William Osler and Comparative Medicine'; Thomas W.M. Cameron, 'Sir William Osler, Parasitologist,' *CMAJ* 30 (1934), 553–6.

25 WO to JO, 23 Jan. 1878, OPUT and CPOL; 'On the Pathology of the So-Called Pig Typhoid,' *Veterinary Journal,* June 1878.

26 *Introductory Lecture … Oct. 1, 1877;* 'The Medical Library in Post-Graduate Work,' *BMJ* (1909), 925–8; Malloch Journal notes, 15 Nov. 1914, CPOL.

27 Edmund J.A. Rogers, 'Personal Reminiscences of the Earlier Years of Sir William Osler,' *Osler Memorial*, 163–70.

28 A.H.T. Robb-Smith, 'Did Sir William Have Carcinoma of the Lung?' *Chest* 66 (Dec. 1974), 712–16, and 67 (Jan. 1975), 82–7.

29 Jennette Osler to EO, 26 Dec. 1875, CPOL.

30 WO to Marian Francis, July 1877; Edith Wendell to HC, undated (1920–21), CPOL 1877; draft ms of 'Life,' CPOL (ch 8, 15), WO to Miss Greenough, 28 Aug. 1878.

31 Daybook, 1877, OL, BO7668; A.K. Haywood to HC, 12 May 1920, CPOL 1878.

32 'The Medical Clinic: A Retrospect and Forecast,' *BMJ* 1 (1914), 10–16; George Savage to HC, 'Obituary of Sir William Osler,' CPY, 594.

33 Cushing, 1:177; CPOL 1878; minutes of the Medico-Chirurgical Society of Montreal, 8 June 1877, OL; PPM, 1st edn, 282; 'Osler, Peter Redpath, and Acupuncture,' OL *Newsletter* 16 (June 1974); Ilza Veith, 'Sir William Osler, Acupuncturist,' *Persisting Osler*, 125–9 (misses the Hingston reference).

34 H.E. MacDermot, *A History of the Montreal General Hospital* (Montreal, 1950); Anna C. Maxwell, 'Struggles of the Pioneers,' *American Journal of Nursing* 21 (1920–1), 320–9. WO, 'Commencement Address' to the nurses of the Johns Hopkins Training School, 7 May 1913, *Johns Hopkins Hospital Nurses' Alumnae Magazine* 12 (1913), 79.

35 BO1629; 'Internal Medicine as a Vocation,' *Aequanimitas*, 142.

36 Minutes of the Faculty of Medicine, 21 Apr. 1880, McGill Archives, RG38, 1.

37 Daybook, 1874, OL, BO7668; WO, 'Professor Wesley Mills,' *CMAJ* 5 (1915), 338–41.

38 'On the Advantages of a Trace of Albumin and a Few Tube Casts in the Urine of Certain Men above Fifty Years of Age,' *New York Medical Journal* 74 (Nov. 1901), 949–50; WO, 'The Right Hon. Sir Charles Tupper, Bart.' *Lancet* 2 (1915), 1049–50; T.J. Murray, 'Serving Two Masters: The Relationship between Sir Charles Tupper and Sir William Osler,' paper delivered to the American Osler Society, 1993.

39 Marian Osborne, 'Recollections of Sir William Osler,' in *Osler Memorial*, 171; also, Jennette Osler response to HC questionnaire, CPOL 1875.

40 Jennette Osler to HC, 26 Aug. 1921, CPY, 1092; ms of Marian Osborne's 'Recollections,' Kelen Collection, privately held.

41 Norman B. Gwyn, 'Some Details of Osler's Early Life as Collected by a Near Relation,' *North Carolina Medical Journal* 10, no. 9 (Sept. 1949), 494–6.

42 Shepherd speech, *Dinner to Dr. William Osler, May 2, 1905, Waldorf-Astoria, New York* (privately printed, 1905); eggs and salt: cited in Esmé Wingfield-Stratford, *The Victorian Sunset* (London: Routledge, 1932), 78; Percy Bath Francis to Marian Francis, 4 May 1882, Kelen Collection, privately held; ms of Kinghorn lecture, 'Osler,' 31 Jan. 1951, OPOL, folio box.

43 Mrs Hayter Reed to HC, 6 Oct. 1925, CPY, 121:5–9.

44 G. Cantlie to H.V. Ogden, 27 Dec. 1883; WO to Ogden, 23 Dec. 1883, in *HVO*:

The Life & Letters of Dr. Henry Vining Ogden, 1857–1931 (Milwaukee: Milwaukee Academy of Medicine, 1986), 53–5, 236.

45 Charles Roland, ed., 'Sir William Osler's Dreams and Nightmares,' *Persisting Osler*, 58–9.

46 *PPM*, 1st edn, 180.

47 Joseph Pratt, *A Year with Osler* (Baltimore: Johns Hopkins University Press, 1949), xii.

48 Casey A. Wood reminiscence, *Osler Memorial*, 178.

49 WO, *Summer Session Clinics. 1882, Delivered in the Montreal General Hospital* (Montreal: Printed for a Committee of the Students, 1882), 1.

50 David I. Macht, 'Osler's Prescriptions and Materia Medica,' *Transactions of the American Therapeutic Society* 35 (1936), 69–85.

51 'Clinical Remarks on the Nephritis of Pregnancy,' *Canadian Practitioner* 8 (1883), 137; WO to Jennette Osler, Jan. 1877, CPOL.

52 Howell, *F.J. Shepherd: Surgeon*, 121.

53 *Summer Session Clinics. 1882.* 3, 4.

54 *Summer Session Clinics. 1882*, 2:13

55 'The Cold-Bath Treatment of Typhoid Fever,' *Medical News*, 3 Dec. 1892, 628.

56 *Summer Session Clinics. 1882*, 4:34.

57 R.B. Bean, ed., *Sir William Osler: Aphorisms from his Bedside Teachings and Writings* (New York: Schuman, 1950), 23; Sheldon Stephens to Mother, 28 Dec. 1884, McCord Museum, McGill University, G.W. Stephens Papers, box 1, 10.

58 *Summer Session Clinics. 1882*, 3, 4.

59 'American Association for the Advancement of Science,' *CMSJ* 8 (1879–80), 63–8.

60 WO and A.W. Clement, 'An Investigation into the Parasites in the Pork Supply of Montreal,' *CMSJ* (Jan. 1883); WO and Clement, 'Cestode Tuberculosis: A Successful Experiment in Producing it in the Calf,' *American Veterinary Review*, April 1882; WO, 'On Echinococcus Disease in America,' *American Journal of Medical Science* 84 (1882), 475–80; Review of Catalogue of the Pennsylvania Hospital Museum, *American Journal of Medical Science* 84 (1882), 229–30; 'Report on Pictou Cattle Disease Investigations,' by Professor Wm. Osler, Canada, *Sessional Papers, 1883.* no. 14, part 36, 289–93; 'Official Account of the Typhoid Outbreaks at Lennoxville,' *CMSJ* 9 (1880–1), 436–45.

61 'On Certain Parasites in the Blood of the Frog,' *Canadian Naturalist* 10, no. 7 (1883), 406–10; 'The Third Corpuscle of the Blood,' *Medical News*, 29 Dec. 1883, 701–2.

62 'The Reserves of Life,' *St Mary's Hospital Gazette*, 6 Nov. 1907; WO unsigned review, *CMSJ* 7 (1878–9), 409.

63 Proceedings of Medico-Chirurgical Society of Montreal, 25 July 1880, *CMSJ* 8 (1879–80), 16–17; 'Canada Medical Association,' *Canadian Medical Record* 7 (1878–9), 329–36; WO, 'Catalogue of a Series of Specimens Illustrative of the

Morbid Anatomy of the Brain and Spinal Cord,' exhibited at Ottawa, Sept. 1880, by William Osler, *CMSJ* 9 (1880–1), 106; 'Case of Medullary Neuroma of the Brain,' *Journal of Anatomy and Surgery* 15 (1881), 217–25. 'Three Cases of Brain Disease,' *CMSJ* 8 (1880), 295–304; 'Cases of Insular Sclerosis,' *CMSJ* 9 (1880–1), 1–11.

64 'On the Brains of Criminals,' *CMSJ* 10 (1881–2), 383–98; also 'Report on the Brains of Richards and O'Rourke,' *CMSJ* 11 (1882–3), 461–6.

65 H.V. Ogden ms, 'The Murderer's Brain,' CPOL 1881.

66 Francis J. Shepherd, *Reminiscences of Student Days and Dissecting Room* (Montreal, 1919); WO to Shepherd, 11 Jan. 1919, OPOL, 7; 'Clinical Remarks on a Case of Hodgkin's Disease,' *CMSJ* 11 (1882–3), 712–17.

67 *HVO: The Life and Letters of H.V. Ogden*, 17–18; WO, 'A Backwood Physiologist,' *Alabama Student*, 167–8.

68 WO ms., 'The Future of the Medical Profession in Canada,' 9 Sept. 1918, OL, BO7664 (IV).

69 *HVO: The Life and Letters of H.V. Ogden*, 18–19.

70 Osborne, 'Recollections of Sir William Osler,' *Osler Memorial*, 172–3; Dr J. Herbert Darey to HC, 29 Jan. 1922, CPY, 520.

71 Osborne, 'Recollections,' *Osler Memorial*, 172; ms. of Marian Osborne, 'Reminiscences,' Kelen Collection, privately held; 'EYD' memo, CPOL 1884.

72 'Professional Notes ...' ms OL, BO7641. See William D. Tigertt, 'An Annotated Life of Egerton Yorrick Davis, M.D., an Intimate of Sir William Osler,' *JHM* 38 (1983): 259–97.

73 Malloch Journal, 26 July 1919, CPOL.

74 Thomas D. Brock, *Robert Koch: A Life in Medicine and Bacteriology* (Science Tech/Springer Verlag, 1988), 114; for Tupper, see note 38 above, 'On the Advantages of a Trace of Alumin.'

75 WO, 'The International Medical Congress,' *CMSJ* 10 (Sept. 1881), 121–5.

76 'On the University Question,' *CMSJ* 12 (Jan. 1884), 373–4; 'McGill University,' *CMSJ* 10 (May 1884), 631–4.

77 Minutes of the Faculty of Medicine, 1882–3, McGill Archives, RG38, 1; Hanaway and Cruess, *McGill Medicine*, 1:96–7; Shepherd, *Reminiscences*, 9, 10.

78 R.F. Ruttan, A. Schmidt reminiscences, *Osler Memorial*, 182, 183.

79 Malloch Journal, 26 July 1919, CPOL.

80 R.H. Fitz to James Tyson, 30 June 1884, CPOL.

81 Banquet report, *Medical News*, 18 Oct. 1884, 445; Richard L. Golden, 'Reginald H. Fitz, Appendictis, and the Osler Connection: A Discursive Review,' *Surgery* 118, (1995), 504–9.

82 'After Twenty-Five Years,' *Aequanimitas*, 203; WO to W.G. MacCallum, 24 July 1919, CPOL.

83 'After Twenty-Five Years,' *Aequanimitas*, 204.

84 Dr Wm M. Donald to HC, 21 July 1922, CPY, 521.

85 Cushing, 1:215–16.

4: The Best Men: Philadelphia

1 'Rudolf Virchow: The Man and the Student,' remarks at the Virchow celebration, Johns Hopkins, 13 Oct. 1891, *Boston Medical and Surgical Journal* 125 (1891), 425–7.

2 'Letters from Berlin,' *CMSJ* 12 (1883–4), 721–8.

3 'Notes of a Visit to European Medical Centres,' *Archives of Medicine* (N.Y), 12 (1884), 170–81; 'Letter from Berlin,' *CMSJ* 12 (1883–4), 582–5.

4 'Rudolf Virchow: The Man and the Student,' remarks at the Virchow celebration, Johns Hopkins, 13 Oct. 1891, *Boston Medical and Surgical Journal* 125 (1891), 425–7.

5 'Letters from Berlin,' *CMSJ* 12 (1883–4), 721–8; 'Notes of a Visit to European Medical Centres,' *Archives of Medicine* (N.Y), 12 (1884), 170–81.

6 Cushing, 1:199.

7 Cf. Thomas D. Brock, *Robert Koch: A Life in Medicine and Bacteriology* (Science Tech/ Springer-Verlag, 1988), 169.

8 'Notes of a Visit'; WO to George Ross, 10 June 1884, CPOL; WO to H.V. Ogden, 18 June 1884, CPOL.

9 'Letter from Leipzig,' *CMSJ* 13 (1884–5), 18–22.

10 'Notes of a Visit'; WO to H.V. Ogden, 1 Aug. 1884, CPOL.

11 Ernest Earnest, *S. Weir Mitchell, Novelist and Physician* (Philadelphia: University of Pennsylvania Press, 1950), 211; *PPM*, 1st edn, 223.

12 George W. Corner, *Two Centuries of Medicine: A History of the School of Medicine, University of Pennsylvania* (Philadelphia: Lippincott, 1965), 168.

13 Howard Kelly, 'Osler as I knew Him in Philadelphia and in the Hopkins,' in *Sir William Osler: Brief Tributes …* (Baltimore, 1920; reprinted from *JHH Bulletin*, 1919), 107.

14 'Statement Obtained from Dr Minis Hays,' CPOL 1884 (which differs considerably from the version published in Cushing, 1:220–1); HC note, 'In 1881 …' CPOL 1881.

15 Francis H. Shepherd, 'The Osler Oration,' *CMAJ* 21, no. 2, (1929), 131–7.

16 WO to H.V. Ogden, 1 Aug. 1884, *HVO: The Life and Letters of Henry Vining Ogden*, 58; WO to Shepherd, 19 June 1884, CPOL; 'Osler's autobiographical address to the American Club, Oxford, 12 Feb. 1916, OL, 8303; draft of WO to Tyson, 17 June 1884, OL, BO7665(ii).

17 Mitchell 1884 travel diary, College of Physicians of Philadelophia, mss 2/0241-03, Weir Mitchell Papers, 12; WO, ms obit. of Weir Mitchell, CPOL 1914; 'L'Envoi,' *Aequanimitas*, 470.

18 R.H. Fitz to Tyson, 30 June 1884; Sanderson, Bastian, Flint to Tyson, Aug. 1884, CPOL; W.R. Gowers to Weir Mitchell, 14 July 1884, CPY, 121:398.

19 S. Weir Mitchell circular letter, 17 Aug. 1884, University of Pennsylvania Archives, U. of Penn. General Files, 1884.

20 Minutes of the Faculty of Medicine, 24 June 1884, McGill Archives, RG38, 1; Palmer Howard to WO, undated, CPY, 121:399.

21 Board of Trustees, Minutes, 7 Oct. 1884, University of Pennsylvania Archives; A. Schmidt reminiscence, *Osler Memorial*, 183; Montreal *Gazette*, 14 Nov. 1884.

22 H.A. Hare, 'William Osler as a Clinician and Teacher,' *Transactions, College of Physicians of Philadelphia*, 3rd ser., 42 (1920), 131–9; WO notes and draft articles on voices and accents, commonplace book, OL, BO7665(viii); WO unpublished papers, vol. 5, OL, BO7664; Wm. T. Sharpless to Dr S.M. Hamill, 2 Nov. 1921, CPOL 1885.

23 WO ms, 'Univ. of Penn ... 1885,' OL, BO7664 (II); Hare, 'Sir William Osler as a Clinician and Teacher.'

24 Thomas Hubbard to HC, 25 July 1925, CPOL, 57; Hare, 'Sir William Osler as a Clinician and Teacher.'

25 Cushing, 1:234; Dock, 'Dr. William Osler in Philadelphia,' *Osler Memorial*, 209; WO commonplace book, notes on 'Voices,' OL, BO7665(viii).

26 WO to Dr Geo Wilkins, 1 Nov. 1884, OL *Newsletter* 85 (June 1997).

27 Cushing, 1:284–5; HC to Alfred Stengel, 17 Apr., 26 May 1926, CPY, 84:60ff; Alfred Stengel to HC, 23 Apr., 10 May 1926, CPY, 121:276–9; HC to A.C. Abbott, 21 May 1925, CPY, 498; A.C. Abbott to HC, 20, 22 May 1925, CPY, 120:640–8.

28 HC notes, CPOL, 188; copy of unsigned Pepper story in Maude Abbott Papers, OL, 438/30; WO, 'William Pepper,' in *Alabama Student*, 227.

29 Corner, *Two Centuries of Medicine*, esp. 161; on the campus and labs in 1884, see J.J. Abel to Mary Abel, 1, 5, 8 June 1884, JH, John J. Abel Papers, 63; Hare, 'Sir William Osler as a Clinician and Teacher'; H.C. Wood to John S. Billings, 12 Jan. 1894, NYPL, Billings Papers; WO to HP Bowditch, 20 June 1886, Harvard Medical School, Countway Library, HMS c. 5.2.

30 George Dock, 'Dr. William Osler in Philadelphia' *Osler Memorial*, 208–11.

31 Memo of Dr Samuel McClintock Hamill, written for HC, Sept. 1921, CPOL 1886; WO, 'On the Treatment of Pleurisy with Effusion by Hay's Method,' *Medical News*, 11 Dec. 1886, 645–6; PPM, 1st edn, 211.

32 Richard L. Golden, 'Sir William Osler and the Anatomical Tubercle,' *Journal of American Academy of Dermatology* 16 (1987), 1071–4; WO, 'Clinical Memoranda,' *Montreal Medical Journal*, 17 (1888–9), 418–19.

33 W.G. MacCallum, 'Osler at Blockley,' *BHM* 10 (1941), 78; A.A. Bliss, *Blockley Days: Memories and Impressions of a Resident Physician, 1883–1884* (Philadelphia, 1916), 17–18.

34 Memo of Dr Samuel McClintock Hamill, written for HC, Sept. 1921, CPOL 1886; Truman G. Schnabel, 'William Osler at the Philadelphia Hospital,' *Medical Life* 41 (1934), 75–88; M. Howard Fussell reminiscences, E.B. Krumbhaar file, CPY, 553.

35 Earnest, *S. Weir Mitchell*, 91.

36 John L. Rothrock to Marian Hague Rea, *BHM* 10 (1941), 94–5.

37 Randall C. Rosenberger, 'Blockley Post House,' *BHM* 10 (1941), 84–8.

38 W.W. Keen to WO, 12 July 1916, 27 Nov. 1910, OL, 153 (BO3106); G.E. Erikson, 'Sir William Osler and William Williams Keen,' OL *Newsletter* 11 (Oct. 1972).

39 WO ms, 'Walt Whitman. An Anniversary Address with Personal Reminiscences,' OL, BO7660; Philip W. Leon, *Walt Whitman and Sir William Osler: A Poet and His Physician* (Toronto: ECW Press, 1995). Leon also prints all of Whitman's comments on Osler, as recorded in Horace Traubel's, *With Walt Whitman in Camden*, 7 vols. (1953–92), but misses Osler's 31 Jan. 1888 note; also Harold D. Barnshaw, 'Walt Whitman's Physicians in Camden,' *Transactions, College of Physicians of Philadelphia*, 4th ser., 31 (1964), 227–30.

40 Whitman, cited in Leon, *Whitman and Osler*, 30; WO to H.V. Ogden, undated [misdated 1884], HVO: *The Life and Letters of Henry V. Ogden*, 239.

41 WO, 'Walt Whitman ...' OL, BO7660.

42 Horace Traubel notes, 3 July, 5 Oct., 3 Dec. 1988, cited in Leon, *Whitman and Osler*, 182, 185.

43 Medico-Chirurgical Society of Montreal, Minutes, 16 Feb. 1877, OL; 'Vaginismus,' *Medical News*, 13 Dec. 1884, 673; 'Extrauterine Pregnancy Changed to Intrauterine Pregnancy by Electricity,' *Medical News*, 6 Mar. 1886, 279.

44 Francis H. Shepherd, 'The Osler Oration,' *CMAJ*, 21, no. 2 (1929), 131–7; 'Aequanimitas,' *Aequanimitas*, 11.

45 'The Goulstonian Lectures on Malignant Endocarditis,' delivered at the Royal College of Physicians of London, March 1885 (London, 1885); Raymond D. Pruitt, 'William Osler and his Goulstonian Lectures on Malignant Endocarditis,' *Mayo Clinic Proceedings* 57 (Jan. 1982), 4–9.

46 'The Growth of a Profession,' *CMSJ* 14 (Oct. 1885), 129–55; 'The Model Hospital,' *Canadian Journal of Medical Science* 6 (1881), 154–6.

47 Ibid.; W.S. Middleton, 'William Osler and the Blockley Dead House,' *Journal of Oklahoma State Medical Association*, 69, no. 9 (Sept. 1976), 387–97.

48 WO to Geo. Wilkins, 1 Nov. 1884, OL *Newsletter* 85 (June 1997); Marian Francis to Jennette Osler, 'Sunday evening,' OPUT.

49 *Medical News*, 4 July 1885, 27 ff.; Hays, Pepper, corres., John S. Billings Papers, NYPL, reel 9; A. McGehee Harvey, *The Association of American Physicians, 1886–1986: A Century of Progress in Medical Science* (Baltimore: The Association, 1986).

50 Harvey, *The Association of American Physicians*, 24, 26, 48, 49; William Welch to Emma Welch Walcott, 25 June 1886, Welch Papers, JH, 69; Hobart A. Hare, 'William Osler as a Teacher and Clinician in Philadelphia,' *Osler Memorial*, 216.

51 'Discussion,' *Transactions of the Association of American Physicians*, 18 June 1886, 96; WO, 'The Malarial Germ of Laveran,' *Medical News*, 4 Sept. 1886, 265; 'An Address on the Haematozoa of Malaria,' *BMJ*, 12 Mar. 1887, 557–62.

52 *PPM*, 1st edn, 128; 'On Phagocytes,' *Medical News*, 13, 20 Apr. 1889, 393–6, 421–5.

53 'On the General Etiology and Symptoms of Chorea,' *Medical News*, 15, 22 Oct. 1887, 437–41, 465–70; 'Chorea' (unsigned WO editorial), *Medical News*, 21 Nov. 1885, 574–5; 'The Cardiac Relations of Chorea,' *American Journal of Medical Science*, (1887), 371–86.

54 *The Cerebral Palsies of Children* (Philadelphia, 1889); Freud ref. in WO to Harry

Thomas, 30 May 1911, CPOL; Freud, *Infantile Cerebral Paralysis* (1897; translated and republished, Coral Gables, Fla.: University of Miami Press, 1968).

55 'Puerperal Anaemia, and Its Treatment with Arsenic,' *Boston Medical and Surgical Journal*, 18 Nov. 1888, 454–5; 'On the Use of Arsenic in Certain Forms of Anaemia,' *Therapeutic Gazette*, 3rd ser. (Nov. 1886), 741–6.

56 *PPM*, 1st edn, 113; 'Diseases of the Blood and Blood-Glandular System,' in William Pepper, ed., *A System of Practical Medicine by American Authors* (Philadelphia: Lea Bros., 1885), 3:882–950; 'Note on Nitro-Glycerine in Epilepsy,' *Journal of Nervous and Mental Disease* 15 (1888), 38–9; 'Antifebrin,' *Therapeutic Gazette*, 3rd ser. (Mar. 1887), 163–7.

57 'The Treatment of Pneumonia,' *Medical News*, 11 Dec. 1886, 660–1; 'The Cold Bath in Typhoid Fever,' *Medical News*, 2 Jan. 1886, 13–14; 'Rectal Injections of Gas in the Treatment of Phthis,' *Medical News*, 2 Apr. 1887, 377.

58 'The Treatment of Typhoid Fever,' *Medical News*, 24 Dec. 1887, 739–40.

59 'Rectal Injections of Gas,' *Medical News*, 29 Jan. 1887, 127–8; *PPM*, 1st edn, 118; HC draft ms. of 'Life,' CPOL, ch. 11, 32.

60 'Liebermeister on the Treatment of Pneumonia,' 'Typhoid Fever at the Cincinnati Hospital' *Medical News*, 21 April 1888, 437–9; 'The Cartwright Lectures on Fever,' *Medical News*, 26 May 1888, 578–9.

61 'The Mortality of Pneumonia,' *Lancet*, 17 Nov. 1888, 983, reporting WO in *University Medical Magazine*, Phil., no. 2; 'The Treatment of Pneumonia,' *Medical News*, 11 Dec. 1886, 660.

62 'The Treatment of Pneumonia in the Philadelphia Hospitals,' *Medical News*, 5 Mar. 1887, 260–3; 'Treatment of Typhoid Fever in the Philadelphia Hospitals,' *Medical News*, 10 Dec. 1887, 676–80.

63 Richard L. Golden, 'Reginald H. Fitz, Apprendictis, and the Osler Connection: A Discursive Review,' *Surgery* 118 (1995), 504–9; W.R. Riddell, 'A Story about William Osler,' *Medical Record* 158 (1945), 22.

64 WO, 'On the Symptoms of Chronic Obstruction of the Common Bile Duct by Gallstones,' *Annals of Surgery* 11 (1890), 161–85; 'A Clinical Lecture on the Ball-Valve Gall-Stone in the Common Duct,' *Lancet*, 15 May 1897.

65 Howard Kelly, 'Osler as I Knew Him in Philadelphia,' *Osler Memorial*, 260.

66 'The Irritable Heart of Civil Life,' CMSJ (1887), 617–19; Charles F. Wooley, 'From Irritable Heart to Mitral Valve Prolapse: The Osler Connection,' *American Journal of Cardiology*, 53 (March 1984), 871–4; Charles Mercer, Clinical Notes from the University of Pennsylvania, 1887–1890, Coll. of Phys. of Phil., mss 2/0150–01 Acc. 1989–105–05, 71–2.

67 J.P. Crozier Griffith to HC, 8 Sept. 1921, CPY, 534.

68 'The Weir Mitchell Treatment,' *Medical News*, 1 May 1886, 491–2; 'Notes and Comments,' CMSJ 16 (1887–8), 447–8.

69 Commonplace book, OL, BO7665 (viii), 'W.'

70 'The Collecting of a Library, BO, xxvii.

71 Noticed by Felix Cunha, *Osler as a Gastroenterologist* (San Francisco, 1948), 30.

72 George Dock, 'Doctor Osler's Use of Time,' *Archives of Internal Medicine* 84 (1949), 51–3.

73 WO ms, 'The Writing of a Textbook,' in WO's copy of *PPM*, 1st edn, OL.

74 See correspondence in OL, 153 (BO5928); affidavits, OL, 537, folio box 17; correspondence in CPOL 1886; the discovery of 'Railway Winnie' in FPOL, Minish file; C.B. Farrar, 'Osler's Story of "The Baby on the Track,"' *CMAJ*, 28 Mar. 1964, 781–4.

75 EO to Chattie, 28 June, 7 Apr., 15 July 1887; EO to WO, 20 Apr. 1887, 14 Sept. [no year given], OFPOA, 4.

76 EO to Chattie, 28 June 1887, 9 Nov. 1886, OFPOA, 4; Anne Wilkinson, *Lions in the Way* (Toronto: Macmillan, 1956), 249, 172–3.

77 WO's letters to the Francis children, more than 180, are in the Francis files, OPOL.

78 WO to Mullin, 8 Nov. 1886 (orig. in Osler-Mullin corres., Hamilton, Ont., Academy of Medicine), CPOL 1886; Minutes of the Faculty of Medicine, 11 Oct. 1886, University of Pennsylvania Archives.

79 Marian Francis to HVO, 3 Oct. 1887, *HVO: The Life and Letters of H.V. Ogden*, 64–5; HC note of remarks by GRO, CPOL 1888.

80 WO obit. of John S. Billings, *BMJ*, 22 Mar. 1913, 641–2.

81 King to Billings, 30 Sept. 1888, NYPL, Billings Papers, reel 11; WO daybook, 1888, OL, BO7668.

82 GRO to HC, Sept. 1922, CPOL 1889.

83 'Aequanimitas,' in *Aequanimitas*, 3–11; Robert Austrian, 'Concerning Osler and Agnew: A Note on Historical Discrepancies,' *Persisting Osler*, 2:121–6; H.P. Bowditch to his wife, 6 May 1889, CPOL 1890.

5: Starting at Johns Hopkins

1 Johns Hopkins to Francis T. King, et al., 10 Mar. 1873, cited in Alan M. Chesney, *The Johns Hopkins Hospital and the Johns Hopkins University School of Medicine: A Chronicle* (Baltimore: Johns Hopkins University Press, 1943), 1:13.

2 Chesney, *Hopkins*, 1:30.

3 HC memo, 23 Jan. 1908, of Welch reminiscing about his youth, CPY, 123:708–10; quotation from Simon Flexner and James Thomas Flexner, *William Henry Welch and the Heroic Age of American Medicine* (Baltimore: Johns Hopkins University Press, 1941), 110.

4 Flexner and Flexner, *Welch*, 128, 131–3.

5 Francis T. King to J.S. Billings, (JSB) 13 Feb. 1887, Billings Papers, NYPL.

6 Lauder Brunton to JSB, 24 July 1893, Billings Papers, NYPL.

7 WO to JSB, 5 July 1888, King to JSB, 5 July, Welch to JSB, 7 July, King to JSB, 25 July 1888, Billings Papers, NYPL.

8 W.H. Welch to Emma Welch Walcott, 23 Oct. 1888, JH, Welch Papers, 69.

9 Ellen Osler to WO, 4 Oct. 1888, OFPOA, 2.

10 King to JSB, 4 July 1888, Billings Papers, NYPL; Gert H. Brieger, 'The Original Plans for the Johns Hopkins Hospital and Their Historical Significance,' *BHM* 49 (1965), 518–28.

11 Francis J. King to JSB, 17 Mar. 1889, Billings Papers, NYPL; WO, 'The Inner History of the Johns Hopkins Hospital,' *Johns Hopkins Medical Journal* 125 (1969), 184–94.

12 Francis J. King to JSB, 29, 31 Jan. 1889, and Gilman to JSB, 13 Feb. 1889, Billings Papers, NYPL; WO, 'The Medical Clinic: A Retrospect and a Forecast,' *BMJ*, 3 Jan. 1914; WO to E. Schäfer, 17 Apr. 1890, CPOL.

13 WO report to the Medical Board, 30 Jan. 1890, Medical Board minutes, JH, RG2, series c.

14 King to JSB, 29 Jan. 1889, Billings Papers, NYPL.

15 H.A. Lafleur, 'Early Days at the Johns Hopkins Hospital with Dr. Osler,' *Osler Memorial*, 268–72; H.L. Mencken, *Happy Days, 1880–1892* (1936; reprint, Baltimore: Johns Hopkins University Press, 1996), 153–4, 284–96.

16 A.M. Harvey et al., *A Model of Its Kind: A Centennial History of Medicine at Johns Hopkins* (Baltimore: Johns Hopkins University Press, 1989) 1:25; H.A. Lafleur, 'Early Days at the Johns Hopkins Hospital,' *Osler Memorial*, 269; W.H. Welch to Franklin Mall, 17 Aug. 1889, Mall Papers, JH, 3.

17 W.T. Councilman, 'Osler in the Early Days at the Johns Hopkins Hospital,' *Boston Medical and Surgical Journal* 182 (Apr. 1920), 341–5.

18 John Fulton Diaries, 28 Aug. 1927, Sterling Library, Yale.

19 H.A. Lafleur, 'Early Days at the Johns Hopkins Hospital,' *Osler Memorial*, 268; Councilman, 'Osler in the Early Days at the Johns Hopkins Hospital,' *Boston Medical and Surgical Journal* 182 (Apr. 1920), 341–5; Lewellys Barker, *Time and the Physician* (New York: Putnam's, 1942), 100.

20 Francis, quoted in Cushing, 1:319–20.

21 Ramsay Wright to HC, 22 Mar. 1921, CPOL 1890; E.A. Sharpey-Schäfer to HC, 8 June 1920, CPY, 48:434; WO, 'Letters to My House Physicians,' *New York Medical Journal* 52 (1890), 81–2, 163–4, 191–2, 274–5, 333–4.

22 T.D. Brock, *Robert Koch: A Life in Medicine and Bacteriology* (Madison, Wis.: Science Tech, 1988), 196; Welch to William W. Welch, 12 Aug. 1890, Welch Papers, JH, 68.

23 WO, 'On the Value of Laveran's Organisms in the Diagnosis of Malaria,' *JHH Bulletin* 1 (Dec. 1889), 11; 'Two Cases of Pernicious Malaria,' *JHH Bulletin* 18 (Dec. 1891), 161–2.

24 WO to J.H. Musser, 26 Mar. 1890, CPOL.

25 H.A. Lafleur, 'Early Days at the Johns Hopkins Hospital with Dr. Osler,' *Osler Memorial*, 271; WO, 'Preliminary Note on Koch's Method of Treatment of Tuberculosis,' *JHH Bulletin* 9 (Dec. 1890), 108; 'Report on the Koch Treatment in Tuberculosis,' *JHH Bulletin* 10 (Jan. 1891), 7–15; WO to JSB, 17 Dec. 1890, Billings Papers,

NYPL; WO, 'Tuberculous Pleurisy,' *Boston Medical and Surgical Journal* 129 (1893), 53–7, 81–5, 109–14, 134–8.

26 WO to H.V. Ogden, 12 Oct. 1892, CPOL.

27 Appleton files, OPOL, 11; WO account, BO3544.

28 WO account, BO3544; Hunter Robb to HC, 29 Apr. 1920, CPY, folder 529; Cushing, 1:358.

29 Lyman Powell, 'William Osler and Old Age,' *New York Times*, 4 Jan. 1920.

30 WO to Jennette Osler, undated, prob. 1891, OPUT; WO to H.V. Ogden, 2 Nov. 1891, CPOL.

31 *PPM*, 1st edn, 984; Welch to HC, 8 Aug. 1922, CPY, 123:1016–23.

32 See A. McGehee Harvey and Victor A. McKusick, eds., *Osler's Textbook Revisited* (New York: Appleton-Century-Crofts, 1967).

33 I am not convinced by Faith Wallis's ingenious argument in 'The Literary Styles of Sir William Osler,' OL *Newsletter* 51 (Feb. 1986). Wallis suggests that Osler's 'paratactic' style derives from his Christian heritage and gives *Principles and Practice* its prophetic tone. In fact, the more deliberately priestly and prophetic Osler became, the more ornate or 'hypotactic' his prose. The voice of his text was honed, not in delivering revelations or prophecies but as a judgemental voice in the dead house, telling and totaling the ravages of disease and the condition of the deceased; Charles S. Bryan, 'Osler, Lyman, and Page: A Tale of Three Texts,' *Annals of Internal Medicine* 116, no. 12 (June 1992), 1021–4.

34 *PPM*, 1st edn, 359, 686, 950, 967, 337.

35 Robert J. Miciotto, 'Carl Rokitansky: A Reassessment of the Hematohumoral Theory of Disease,' *BHM* 52 (1978), 183–99; Steven J. Peitzman, 'Osler's Treatment of Bright's Disease,' paper read to the American Osler Society, Apr. 1997.

36 *PPM*, 1st edn, 492, 479, 475, 421, 422.

37 Ibid., 530, 549, 882, 569, 588, 472, 495, 926, 84, 282, 820, 963.

38 David I. Macht, 'Osler's Prescriptions and Material Medica,' *Transactions of the American Therapeutic Society* 35 (1936), 69–85.

39 *PPM*, 1st edn, 76, 276, 320, 529, 866, 928.

40 'Recent Advances in Medicine,' *Science*, 27 Mar. 1891, 170–1.

41 Ibid; 'On Specialism,' *Medical News*, 14 May 1892, 542–5; 'Lectures on the Diagnosis of Abdominal Tumours,' *New York Medical Journal*, 3 Feb. 1894, 129.

42 *PPM*, 1st edn, 473, 482, 439, 906.

43 Ibid., 35, 252.

44 Appleton Sales Statement, 1 Feb. 1894, OPOL, 11; note on flyleaf, WO copy of *PPM*, 2nd edn, OL, BO3545; Paul J. Edelson, 'Adopting Osler's *Principles*: Medical Textbooks in American Medical Schools, 1891–1906,' *BHM* 68 (1994), 67–84.

45 AM to HC, 13 June 1920, CPY, 37:454; Cushing, 1:357–8.

46 'Notes Written in January–March 1929 [about GRO] by Archie Malloch,' OPOL, folio box; Arnold Muirhead, *Grace Revere Osler, a Brief Memoir*. (Oxford: Oxford University Press, for private circulation, 1931).

47 'Notes Concerning Lady Osler,' 2–5 Aug. 1928, Arnold Muirhead/Lady Osler Papers, Osler Club of London, England, Archives, vol. 3; J.C. DaCosta, 'Character Sketch of Professor Samuel W. Gross,' *Selections from the Papers and Speeches of John Chalmers DaCosta* (Philadelphia: W.B. Saunders, 1931), 220–7; John Fulton, 'Grace Revere Osler: Her Influence on Men of Medicine,' *BHM* 32 (1949), 341–51.

48 WO to J.C. Wilson, 'Sunday,' CPY, reel 80, folder 519, Clarendon Press file; HC note of Wilson's recollections, CPOL 1892; HC to Alfred Stengel, 26 Apr. 1926, CPY, 84:600; HC's embellishment of the story (Cushing 1:362) cost him Wilson's friendship.

49 EO to Chattie, 29 Apr. 1892, OFPOA, 4; WO to Lafleur, 24 May 1892, OPOL, 5; Welch to Emma Welch Walcott, 21 June 1892, Welch Papers, JH, 69.

50 J.J. Abel to Mary Abel, June 1892, Abel Papers, JH, 63.

51 Ramsay Wright to HC, 22 Mar. 1921, CPOL 1890; 'Letters to My House Physicians,' 21 May 1890, in *Selected Writings*, 162; 'Teacher and Student,' *Aequanimitas*, 32.

52 Carole Haber, *Beyond Sixty-Five: The Dilemma of Old Age in America's Past* (Cambridge: Cambridge University Press, 1983).

53 'Teacher and Student,' *Aequanimitas*, 32; Richard Golden, 'Lyman Powell, William Osler, and Oliver Wendell Holmes,' *OL Newsletter* 72 (Feb. 1993).

54 'Recent Advances in Medicine,' *Science*, 27 Mar. 1891, 170–1; 'Doctor and Nurse,' *Aequanimitas*, 14–20; Helen E. Marshall, *Mary Adelaide Nutting: Pioneer of Modern Nursing* (Baltimore: Johns Hopkins University Press, 1972), 48.

55 'Remarks on Specialism,' *Medical News*, 14 May 1892, 542–4.

56 'Teacher and Student,' *Aequanimitas*, 42; 'Physic and Physicians as Depicted in Plato,' *Aequanimitas*, 49.

57 Cushing, 1:364; WO to H.A. Lafleur, 18 Feb. 1893; WO to John A. Mullin, Feb. 1893, CPOL.

58 D.C. Gilman to the Executive Committee, Johns Hopkins University Board of Trustees, 9 Nov. 1888, in Johns Hopkins University School of Medicine, Founding Documents – The Opening of the School of Medicine, the Women's Medical Fund and Related Materials, JH, RG1, series b. This discussion also draws on Chesney, *Johns Hopkins*, vol. 1; Mary R. Walsh, *Doctors Wanted: No Women Need Apply: Sexual Barriers in the Medical Profession, 1835–1975* (New Haven: Yale University Press, 1977); Regina Sanchez-Moran, *Sympathy and Science: Women Physicians in American Medicine* (New York: Oxford University Press, 1985); Helen Lefkotwitz Horowitz, *The Power and Passion of M. Carey Thomas* (New York: Knopf, 1994).

59 Mary Gwinn Hodder to Logan Pearsall Smith, early 1938, School of Medicine, Founding Documents ... The Womens Medical Fund and Related Materials, JH, RG1, series b.

60 Flexner and Flexner, *Welch*, 217; Welch to F.P. Mall, 7 Nov. 1891, Mall Papers, JH.

61 Henry Hurd to D.C. Gilman, 15 Aug. 1890, Welch Papers, JH, Hurd file; Hurd to the Board of Trustees, 11 Mar., 11 May 1891, Johns Hopkins Hospital Board of Trustees, Supporting Documents, JH; W.T. Councilman, 'Osler in the Early Days at

the Johns Hopkins Hospital,' *Boston Medical and Surgical Journal* 182 (Apr. 1920), 344; Hurd to the Board of Trustees, 11 Oct. 1892.

62 Lilian Welsh, *Reminiscences of Forty Years in Baltimore* (Baltimore: Norman Remington, 1925), 40–1.

63 WO to Lafleur, 12 Jan. 1893, CPOL; Henry M. Thomas, 'Some Memories of the Development of the Medical School and Osler's Advent, *JHH Bulletin* 30 (1919), 185–9.

64 Minutes, Johns Hopkins Hospital Board of Trustees, 11 Oct. 1892, JH; King to JSB, 29 and 16 June 1891, Billings Papers, NYPL.

65 WO to Lafleur, 12 Jan. 1893, CPOL. Cushing chose, wrongly I think, to draw upon a 1921 reminiscence by Welch in attributing this quip to Osler.

66 Chesney, *Johns Hopkins*, 1:221.

67 Helen Lefkowitz Horowitz, *The Power and Passion of M. Carey Thomas* (New York: Knopf, 1994), 228–32.

68 WO to Ira Remsen, 'Whole-Time Clinical Professors,' 1 Sept. 1911 (privately printed, Oxford University Press), OL, BO7651.

69 Welch to F.P. Mall, 4 Mar. 1893, Mall Papers, JH; WO to J.J. Abel, 26 Mar. 1892, 2 Mar. 1893, Abel Papers, JH, 43.

70 Welch to Mall, 24 Apr. 1893, Mall Papers, JH; WO to Edward Schäfer, 3 Oct. 1893, CPOL; W. Bruce Fye, 'H. Newell Martin: A Remarkable Career Destroyed by Neurasthenia and Alcoholism,' *JHM* 40, no. 2 (Apr. 1985), 133–66.

6: We All Worship Him

1 Percy Hookman, 'A Comparison of the Writings of Sir William Osler and His Exemplar, Sir Thomas Browne,' *Bulletin of the New York Academy of Medicine* 72 (1995), 136–50.

2 Chesney, *Johns Hopkins*, 2:12–15; Florence R. Sabin, *Franklin Paine Mall: The Story of a Mind* (Baltimore: Johns Hopkins University Press, 1934), 123–9.

3 Sabin, *Mall*, 138–41, 154–6.

4 Brenda Wineapple, *Sister Brother: Gertrude and Leo Stein* (New York. Putnam's, 1996), 123; A.M. Harvey et al., *A Model of Its Kind* (Baltimore: Johns Hopkins University Press, 1989), 162; Florence Sabin interview with Wm. Welch, 9 Dec. 1933, Welch Papers, JH, 178; Mall to G. Minot, 10 Nov. 1899, Florence Sabin Papers, American Philosophical Society, Philadelphia, Mall Bio. files, Notes no. 9.

5 Welch to Emma Welch Walcott, 18 Apr. 1895, Welch Papers, JH, 69; Fielding Garrison to HC, 29 Mar. 1920, CPY, 81:535.

6 Aloofness and student recollection: D.R. Mendenhall Memoirs, Mendenhall Papers, Sophia Smith Collection, Smith College, 3, E, 25; Simon Flexner and James Thomas Flexner, *William Henry Welch and the Heroic Age of American Medicine* (Baltimore: Johns Hopkins University Press, 1941), 162, 170; Osler and Pithotomists, CPOL 1896; Hugh Young, *A Surgeon's Autobiography* (New York: Harcourt Brace, 1940), 65.

7 Donald G. Bates and Edward H. Bensley, eds., 'The Inner History of the Johns Hopkins Hospital' (by William Osler), *Johns Hopkins Medical Journal* 125 (1969), 184–94.

8 Mays, in Grace Crile, ed., *George Crile: An Autobiography* (New York: Lippincott, 1947), 115; D. Eugene Strandness, Jr, 'Osler and His Thoughts for Us in 1991,' *American Journal of Surgery* 162 (Aug. 1991), 99.

9 Curt Proskauer, 'Development and Use of the Rubber Glove in Surgery and Gynecology,' *JHM* 13 (1958), 373–81; J.M.T. Finney to George M. Smith, 1 Dec. 1937, cited in John F. Fulton, *Harvey Cushing* (Springfield, Ill.: Thomas, 1946), 237–8.

10 Thayer, 'The Chief,' *NEJM* 207 (1932), 13, 563–70. On Halsted, see also Sherwin B. Nuland, *Doctors: The Biography of Medicine* (New York: Knopf, 1988), ch. 13; W.G. MacCallum, *William Stewart Halsted, Surgeon* (Baltimore: Johns Hopkins University Press, 1930); Samuel James Crowe, *Halsted of Johns Hopkins* (Springfield, Ill.: Charles C. Thomas, 1957); Ralph Colp, Jr, 'Notes on Dr. William S. Halsted,' *Bulletin of the New York Academy of Medicine*, ser. 2, 60, no. 9 (Nov. 1984), 876–87.

11 Charles A. Fecher, ed., *The Diary of H.L. Mencken* (New York: Knopf, 1989), 10; J.M.T. Finney, *A Surgeon's Life* (New York: Putnam's, 1940), 102; JHH Board of Trustees, Minutes, Apr. 14 1891, JH; Finney, *A Surgeon's Life*, 318.

12 Finney, *A Surgeon's Life*, 294–5, 292.

13 Chesney, *Johns Hopkins*, 2:38, 81–3; JHH Board of Trustees, Minutes, 10 Dec. 1895 – 10 Mar. 1896, JH; Welch to Mall, 11 Jan. 1896, Mall Papers, JH, 3.

14 Chesney, *Johns Hopkins*, 2:82; Finney, *A Surgeon's Life*, 287–9; 'Shifting Dullness': Peter D. Olch, 'William S. Halsted: The Antithesis of William Osler,' *Persisting Osler*, 202; Archibald Malloch, *Short Years: The Life and Letters of John Bruce MacCallum, MD, 1876–1906* (Chicago: Normandie House, 1938), 78.

15 Osler 'Inner History;' HC to Kate Crowell, 21 Aug. 1898, CPY, 17, 495; Audrey W. Davis, *Dr. Kelly of Hopkins: Surgeon, Scientist, Christian.* (Baltimore: Johns Hopkins University Press, 1959); Willard E. Goodwin, 'William Osler and Howard A. Kelly: "Physicians, Medical Historians, Friends,"' *BHM* 20 (1946), 611–52; Mendenhall Memoirs, Smith, 3, E, 55.

16 Jeannie Albert Brown, *Doctor Tom Brown Memories* (New York: Richard R. Smith, 1949), 17; George W. Corner, *The Seven Ages of a Medical Scientist: An Autobiography* (Philadelphia: University of Pennsylvania Press, 1981), 113. Fulton, *Cushing*, 681

17 Mendenhall Memoirs, Smith, 3, E, 25ff; Chesney, *Johns Hopkins*, 2:83; Wineapple, *Sister Brother: Gertrude and Leo Stein*, 124, 141.

18 Dr Henry Christian to Dr E.K. Marshall, 9 July 1950, Abel Papers, JH, 131; Paul D. Lamson, 'John Jacob Abel: A Portrait,' *JHH Bulletin* 68 (1941), 155; also John Parascandola, *The Development of American Pharmacology: John J. Abel and the Shaping of a Discipline* (Baltimore: Johns Hopkins University Press, 1992).

19 Mall to L.F. Barker, 29 June 1897, Barker Papers, JH.

20 J.B. MacCallum to 'Home,' April 1899, quoted in Malloch, *Short Years*, 78.

21 'The Natural Method of Teaching the Subject of Medicine,' *JAMA* 26 (1901).

22 Rufus Cole, 'Dr Osler: Scientist and Teacher,' *Archives of Internal Medicine* 84 (1949), 54–63; W.G. MacCallum, 'A Student's Impression of Osler,' *CMAJ* (Osler Memorial Number), July 1920, 47–50; Joseph H. Pratt, *A Year with Osler: 1896–1897: Notes Taken at His Clinics in the Johns Hopkins Hospital* (Baltimore: Johns Hopkins University Press, 1949), 2–3, 75, 102, 123, 101, 140.

23 Henry A. Christian, 'Osler: Recollections of an Undergraduate Medical Student at Johns Hopkins,' *Archives of Internal Medicine* 84 (1949), 77–83.

24 Finney, *A Surgeon's Life*, 278n; Mendenhall Memoirs, Smith, 3, E, 47.

25 Richard L. Golden, ed., *Oslerian Verse* (Montreal: Osler Library, McGill University, 1992), 78–9.

26 George Blumer, 'Random Recollections of Sir William Osler in the Early Nineties,' *Osler Memorial*, 306–8; W.T. Longcope, 'Random Recollections of William Osler,' *Archives of Internal Medicine* 84 (1949), 93–103; Henry A. Christian, 'Osler: Recollections of an Undergraduate Medical Student at Johns Hopkins,' *Archives of Internal Medicine* 84 (1949), 77–83; WO, 'The Natural Method of Teaching the Subject of Medicine,' *JAMA* 26 (1901), 1673–9.

27 D.R. Mendenhall Memoirs, Smith, 3, F, I, 13; W.T. Longcope, 'Random Recollections of William Osler,' *Archives of Internal Medicine*, 84 (1949), 93–103.

28 Charles Bardeen to HC, 13 Jan. 1924, CPY, 505; J.H. Pratt, *A Year with Osler*, 172–3; WO, 'Leprosy in the United States, with the Report of a Case,' *JHH Bull.*, 9 (Mar. 1898), 47–9.

29 Watson S. Rankin, 'Reminiscences of Osler,' *JAMA* 210 (1949), 2240.

30 Lawrason Brown, 'Reminiscences,' *Osler Memorial*, 442–3; D.R. Mendenhall Memoirs, Smith, 3, E, 54.

31 Frank J. Sladen, 'Sir William Osler: The Indispensable Man in Medicine,' *Alexander Blain Hospital Bulletin* 9 (1950), 172–85; matrimony, W.S. Thayer to HC, 18 Dec. 1922, CPY, 123:430–1; for the excellence of the medical services, see Walter Baumgartner to Gustav Baumgartner, 12 Jan. 1902, Baumgartner Collection, Washington University, St Louis; Pat Nixon to Olive Read, 29 Jan. 1906, Pat Nixon Papers, Trinity University, San Antonio, Texas.

32 Francis H. Shepherd, 'The Osler Oration,' *CMAJ* 21 (1929), 131–7.

33 Alice Hamilton, *Exploring the Dangerous Trades: The Autobiography of Alice Hamilton, MD* (Boston: Little Brown, 1943), 53; Edith Gittings Reid, *The Great Physician* (London: Oxford, 1931), 157.

34 H.A. Hare to HC, 29 June 1925, CPOL, 57; D.R. Mendenhall Memoirs, Smith, 3, E, 33; Student Records, Examination Results, 1895–1905, JH.

35 WO to H.V. Ogden, undated [c. Aug. 1893], CPOL 1893; WO, Montreal *Gazette*, 1 Jan. 1914, cited in Faith Wallis, 'Piety and Prejudice,' *CMAJ* 156 (1997), 1549–51.

36 Augusta Tucker, *Miss Susie Slagle's* (New York: Harper, 1939; repub. Baltimore: Johns Hopkins University Press, 1987); John Sedgwick Billings to Katharine Hammond, 11 Mar. 1894, 14 Nov. 1893, Hammond-Bryan-Cumming Papers, University of South Carolina.

37 See the expression of this view in Sarah Orne Jewett, *A Country Doctor* (Boston: Houghton Mifflin, 1884), and Osler's comment on it in BO5003.

38 D.R. Mendenhall Memoirs, Smith, 3, E, 8.

39 'Nurse and Patient,' *Aequanimitas*, 155–66; Hamilton, *Exploring the Dangerous Trades*, 52.

40 Nixon Papers, Pat Nixon to Olive Read, 29 Sept. 1906, Pat Nixon Papers, Trinity University, San Antonio, Texas; Gerald Weissman 'Against *Aequanimitas*,' in Weissmann, *The Woods Hold Cantata: Essays on Science and Society* (New York: Dodd Mead, 1985), 211–22.

41 D.R. Mendenhall Memoirs, Smith, 3, E, 8ff.

42 Esther Rosencrantz to John R. Fulton, 22 Oct. 1947, Esther Rosencrantz Papers, University of California at San Francisco Health Sciences Library, 150, file 2055; Esther Rosenkrantz to WWF, 25 Nov. 1941, FPOL; Wineapple, *Sister Brother: Gertrude and Leo Stein*, 131; Mendenhall Memoirs, Smith 3, E, 8, 51.

43 T. McCrae to HC, 4 Feb. 1901, CPY, 36:819; D.R. Mendenhall Memoirs, Smith, 3, F, I, 1–12, 18–21 and 3, E, 8.

44 Lillian Welsh, *Reminiscences of Thirty Years in Baltimore* (Baltimore: Norman, Remington, 1925), 44, 41; Hamilton, *Exploring the Dangerous Trades*, 52; Cone, 'Making Ward-Rounds with Dr Osler,' *Osler Memorial*, 320; Flexner and Flexner, *Welch*, 230.

45 John L. Graner, 'Osler and His Students: The "Sweet Pea" Episode,' *Diabetes Care* 17 (1994), 1547–8; WWF to Esther Rosencrantz, 21 Nov. 1941, FPOL.

46 Gene Nakajima, 'Gertrude Stein's Medical Education and Her Evolving Feminism,' ms in Student Records, Stein file, JH; Advisory Board of the Medical Faculty, Minutes, 5 June 1901, JH; Office of the Registrar, Record of Examinations, June–Dec. 1901, JH; aphorism cited in A.H.T. Robb-Smith, 'Osler's Influence on Haematology,' *Blood Cells* 7 (1981), 523; Stein's Hopkins experiences are also recounted in Wineapple, *Sister Brother: Gertrude and Leo Stein*; James R. Mellow, *Charmed Circle: Gertrude Stein and Company* (New York: Praeger, 1974); and Linda Wagner-Martin, *'Favored Strangers': Gertrude Stein and Her Family* (New Brunswick, N.J.: Rutgers, 1995).

47 L.F. Barker, *Time and the Physician* (New York: Putnam, 1942), 97.

48 Charles Burr, Morris Lewis recollections, *Osler Memorial*, 225, 228; Judith Robinson, *Tom Cullen of Baltimore* (New York: Oxford University Press, 1949), 93–4.

49 James F. Mitchell, 'Memories of Dr Halsted,' *Surgery* 32 (1952), 451–60.

50 Elizabeth Thies to HC, 10 May 1920; Frieda Thies to HC, 2 Aug. 1920, CPY, 602; Jeannie Albert Brown, *Doctor Tom Brown Memories* (New York: Richard R. Smith, 1949), 14.

51 Mabel Southard to HC, 25 May 1920, CPY, 595; Rachel Bonner to HC, 9 Apr. 1921, CPY, 507; Elizabeth Thies to HC, 10 May 1920, CPY, 602.

52 'The Hospital as a College,' *Aequanimitas*, 331–2, 342.

53 Malloch, *Short Years*, 126.

54 Rufus Cole, 'Perfectionism in Medicine,' *JHH Bulletin* 79 (1946), 190–201.

55 EO to Lizzie, 21 Feb., 7 Mar. 1895; EO to WO, 19 Jan. 1891, OFPOA, 4; Anne Wilkinson, *Lions in the Way* (Toronto: Macmillan, 1956), 203.

56 WO to E. Schäfer, 1 Jan. 1896, CPOL; GRO to Mother, 3 Jan. 1896, CPOL, 58; HC to Father, 6 Dec. 1903, CPY, reel 16.

57 W.G. MacCallum, 'A Student's Impression of Osler,' *CMAJ* Osler Memorial Number), July 1920, 47–50; Jas. W. Walker to HC, 7 Apr. 1920, CPY, 607.

58 GRO to H.V. Ogden, 14 June 1895, CPOL 58; WO to [?], CPOL, 1897 (Cushing, 1:463–4).

59 GRO income: 'Sir William Osler's Autobiographical Notes,' ed. E.H. Bensley and D.G. Bates, *BHM* 50 (1976), 596–618; Arnold Muirhead, *Grace Revere Osler, a Brief Memoir* (Oxford: Oxford University Press, 1931 for private circulation, 1931). Sue Woolley notes about Lady Osler, 24 Mar. 1929, Muirhead Papers, Osler Club, London; WWF to Seymour Thomas, 20 Dec. 1934, FPOL; 'The Student Life,' *Aequanimitas*, 439; 'The Linacre, Harvey, and Sydenham Triptych,' OL *Newsletter* 23 (Oct. 1976).

60 Gittings Reid, *The Great Physician*, 133.

61 *Aequanimitas*, 139.

62 'On the Association of Enormous Heart Hypertrophy, Chronic Proliferative Peritonitis, and Recurring Ascites, with Adherent Pericardium,' *Archives of Pediatrics* (NY), 13 (1896), 1–10; 'The Ball-Valve Gall-Stone in the common Duct,' *Lancet*, 15 May 1897, 1319–23.

63 'On Sporadic Cretinism in America,' *American Journal of the Medical Sciences*, 106 (Nov. 1893), 503–18; PPM, 2nd edn, 756; 'Sporadic Cretinism in America,' *American Journal of the Medical Sciences*, 114 (Oct. 1897), 378–401.

64 PPM, 2nd edn, 749; 3rd edn, 842; 'Addison's Disease, *Medical Bulletin* (Philadelphia), 18 (1896), 81–4; 'On Six Cases of Addison's Disease,' *Internal Medicine Magazine* 5 (Feb. 1896), 3–11; Clark T. Sawin, 'Osler as Mirror: The Treatment of Addison's Disease with Adrenal Extract in the 1890s,' paper to the American Osler Society, May 1995.

65 'The Study of the Fevers of the South,' *JAMA* 26 (1896), 999–1004.

66 'The Diagnosis of Malarial Fever,' *Medical News* 70 (Mar. 6, 1897), 289–92.

67 'Studies in Typhoid Fever, II. The Treatment of Typhoid Fever,' *JHH Reports* 4, (1894), 3; 'Studies in Typhoid Fever: III, Five Years' Experience with the Cold Bath Treatment,' *JHH Reports* 5 (1895), 325; 'The Cold-Bath Treatment of Typhoid Fever,' *Medical News* 61 (1892), 628–31.

68 'Note on Arsenical Neuritis following the Use of Fowler's Solution,' *Montreal Medical Journal* 21 (1893), 721–4; 'The Study of the Fevers of the South,' *JAMA* 26 (1896), 1002.

69 *The Problem of Typhoid Fever in the United States*, address to the Medical Society of the State of New York, 1 Feb. 1899, pamph. (Baltimore, 1899); 'Typhoid Fever in Baltimore,' *JHH Reports* 4 (1894–5), 159–67.

70 'The Function of a State Medical Society,' *Maryland Medical Journal* 37 (1897), 73–7; 'Sporadic Cretinism in America,' *American Journal of the Medical Sciences* 114 (1897), 388.

71 *PPM*, 2nd edn, 308, 1077, 872, 316.

72 'Teaching and Thinking,' *Aequanimitas*, 124; 'The Fevers of the South,' *JAMA* 26 (1896), 1004.

73 AM to HC, 21 Aug. 1921, CPY, 37:532.

74 Baltimore *American*, 1 Apr. 1905, OPJH, 2.

75 Katharine Hammond to her mother, Oct. 1893, Hammond-Bryan-Cummings Papers, University of South Carolina; Sandra F. McRae, 'Leaders in American Medicine: William Osler and the "Canadian Club" in Medicine at Johns Hopkins,' unpub. research paper, 1987; WWF to B.C. MacLean, 13 Nov. 1951, FPOL; WO to Tom Futcher, 20 July 1919, Futcher Papers, OL.

76 For insight into Hopkins's Canadian connection, see Sandra F. McRae, 'The "Scientific Spirit" in Medicine at the University of Toronto, 1880–1910' (PhD thesis, University of Toronto, 1987), esp. ch. 5.

77 EO to Chattie, 17 July 1895, OFPOA, 4.

78 WO to Ed Schäfer, 1 Jan. 1896, CPOL; WO to H.V. Ogden, 17 Jan. 1895, CPOL; WO to Ed Schäfer, 6 Feb. 1900, CPOL; WO to L.F. Barker, '14th' [Aug. 1914], Barker Papers, JH, 5.

79 Halsted to HC, 7 Dec. 1895, CPY, 27:921; Edward F. Cushing to HC, 6 July 1895, CPY, 15:243; HC to Father, 15 Oct. 1896, CPY, reel 16.

80 HC memo on Halsted, Jan. 1925, CPY, 114:676.

81 Ibid., 678; the standard biography is John F. Fulton, *Harvey Cushing* (Springfield, Ill.: Thomas, 1946); for the German duelist, see J.F. Mitchell, 'Memories of Dr Halsted,' *Surgery* 32 (1952), 451–60.

82 HC to Kate Crowell, 15 Mar. 1898, CPY, 17:343; HC to Father, Oct. 1897, CPY, reel 16; Samuel Clark Harvey, 'The Story of Harvey Cushing's Appendix,' *Surgery* 32 (1952), 501–14.

83 HC memo on Halsted, Jan. 1925, CPY, reel 114; shirts: Willis D. Gatch, 'My Experiences with Dr Halsted,' *Surgery* 32 (1952), 466–8; HC to Mother, 20 Feb. 1898, CPY, 15:3; HC to Kate Crowell, 15 Nov. 1898, CPY, 17:630.

84 Excerpt WO to Edward Y. Cushing, 9 Feb. 1899, CPY, 89:700; T. McCrae to HC, 18 Aug. 1899, CPY, 36:797; undated Halsted notes, CPY, 114:716ff; Halsted note in HC to Kate, 29 Apr. 1899, CPY, 17:728.

85 HC to Kate Crowell, 10 July 1900, CPY, 17:838.

86 T. McCrae to HC, 4 Feb. 1901, CPY, 36:819; HC to Kate Crowell, 27 Oct. 1901, CPY, 17:994; CPY, 36:824. Thomas McCrae to HC, 11 June 1901, CPY, 36:824; HC to Father, 18 May 1902, CPY, reel 16.

87 *The Nation and the Tropics*, address delivered in the London School of Tropical Medicine, 26 Oct 1909 (London: Oxford, 1909), 14.

88 F.T. Gates to WO, 13 Apr. 1904, OPOL, 4; also Gates to WO, 4 Mar. 1902, and Gates, *Chapters in My Life* (New York: Free Press, 1977), 181–2.

7: The Great American Doctor

1 Lawrence J. Rhea, 'Student Reminiscence,' *Osler Memorial*, 311.
2 Conversation with A.M. McGehee-Harvey, 22 Feb. 1996.
3 L.F. Barker, 'Osler at Johns Hopkins,' *CMSJ*, 47 (1920), 139; 'Interesting People,' by H.L. Mencken, undated clipping, CPOL 1905, June–Dec. file.
4 Cushing, 1:649.
5 'Ephemerides, 1897,' *Montreal Medical Journal* 25 (1896–7), 645; Lawrason Brown, 'Reminiscences,' *Osler Memorial*, 444.
6 'Ephemerides, 1895,' *Montreal Medical Journal* 23 (1894–5), 518–20.
7 'Ephemerides, 1896,' *Montreal Medical Journal* 24 (1895–6), 890–3.
8 'The Student Life' *Aequanimitas*, 424.
9 W.S. Thayer, 'Reminiscences of Osler in the Early Baltimore Days,' *California and Western Medicine* 31 (1929), 161–8.
10 E.G. Reid, 'A Giver of Life,' in Reid to HC, 20 June 1920, CPY, 590.
11 WO to H.V. Ogden, 13 Jan. 1893, CPOL; BO5314; John Fulton, 'A Day in London,' 12 July 1928, OPOL, folio box; Cushing 1:637; C.B. Farrar, 'I Remember Osler, Psychiatrist,' *American Journal of Psychiatry* 121 (1965), 761–2; Farrer, 'Osler at Johns Hopkins,' *University of Western Ontario Medical Journal* 20 (1950), 127–35.
12 BO5314; T. McCrae, 'Osler and Patient,' *JHH Bulletin* 30 (1919), 201–2.
13 WO to F.L. Shepherd, 30 Jan. 1899, CPOL; Cushing, 1:685; *The Treatment of Disease*, the Address in Medicine before the Ontario Medical Association, Toronto, 3 June 1909 (London, 1909).
14 Undated reminiscence enc. in Mabel Balew [?] to HC, 19 Jan. 1926, CPY, 121:190; E.M. Brockbank to WO, 22 Sept. 1906, CPOL.
15 W.H. Welch to HC, 26 Jan. 1909, CPY, 123:811–12; AM, 'William Osler,' address to Society of Surgeons of New Jersey, 15 May 1946, Malloch Papers, OL; W.S. Thayer, 'The Chief,' *NEJM* 207 (1932), 565.
16 'Notes on Aneurysm,' *JAMA* 38 (1902), 1483–6; 'The Medical Aspects of Carcinoma of the Breast, with a Note on the Spontaneous Disappearance of Secondary Growths,' *American Medicine*, 1 (1901), 17–19, 63–6.
17 'Books and Men,' *Aequanimitas*, 222; JHH, Medical Society meeting, 20 Jan. 1902, *JHH Bulletin*, 135 (1902), 147; D.R. Mendenhall Memoirs, Smith, 3, F, I, 12.
18 Truman Gross Schnabel, 'William Osler at the Philadelphia Hospital,' *Medical Life* 41 (1934), 75–88; WWF to Donald H. Williams, 31 Mar. 1959, FPOL; 'The Home in Its Relation to the Tuberculosis Problem,' *Medical News* 83 (1903), 1105–10; Edward B. Krumbhaar to HC, 7 May 1921, CPY, 553.
19 'Notes on Aneurysm,' *JAMA* 28 (1902), 1483–6.
20 'On the Advantages of a Trace of Albumin and a Few Tube Casts in the Urine of Certain Men above Fifty Years of Age,' *New York Medical Journal* 74 (1901), 949–50; John F. Fulton, *Harvey Cushing* (Springfield, Ill.: Thomas, 1946), 212–16.
21 WO, 'Lectures on Angina Pectoris and Allied States,' *New York Medical Journal* 64 (1896), 177–83, 249–56, 345–50.

22 See W. Bruce Fye, 'The Delayed Diagnosis of Myocardial Infarction: It Took Half a Century!' *Circulation* 72 (1985), 262–71.

23 WO to Dr J. Herbert Darey, 2 Feb. 1905, CPOL.

24 'Draft of Address to the Graduates of the Year 1900 of Johns Hopkins University,' OL, BO7664 (I). Also 'Medicine in the Nineteenth Century,' *Aequanimitas*, 227–76.

25 'Ephemerides,' *Montreal Medical Journal* 23 (1894–5), 877–9; Tom Cullen to HC, 27 Feb. 1922, CPY, 515; Fielding H. Garrison, 'Osler's Place in the History of Medicine,' *Osler Memorial*, 31.

26 JHH Board of Trustees, Minutes, 1 Feb. 1904, JH.

27 'The Faith that Heals, *BMJ* (1910), 1470–2; 'The Home Treatment of Consumption,' *Maryland Medical Journal* 43 (1900), 8–12; 'Medicine in the Nineteenth Century,' *Aequanimitas*, 274; 'Draft of Address to the Graduates of the Year 1900,' OL, BO7664 (I).

28 T. McCrae, 'Osler and Patient,' *JHH Bulletin* 30 (1919), 201–2; Walter Baumgartner to Gustav Baumgartner, 5 Nov. 1901, Baumgartner Collection, Archives, George Washington Medical School, St Louis.

29 JMT Finney, *A Surgeon's Life* (New York: Putnam's, 1940), 282–3.

30 C.E. Newman, 'Osler as a Physician,' *Oslerian Anniversary* (London: Osler Club of London, 1976), 12; 'Remarks on Organization in the Profession ... to the Nottingham Medical Society,' *BMJ*, 4 Feb. 1911, 237–9.

31 Daybooks, OL, BO7668, passim; WO to Thayer, 20 Aug. 1898, CPOL; WO to Lafleur, 28 Mar. 1900, CPOL; W.S. Greenfield to WO, 1 Mar. 1900, CPOL. George T. Harrell's failure to notice the travel time component of Osler's charges is a major weakness in his otherwise good article, 'Osler's Practice,' *Persisting Osler*, 105–23.

32 Thayer, 'Reminiscences of Osler in the Early Baltimore Days,' *California and Western Medicine* 31 (1929), 161–8; WO, 'Inner History.'

33 JHH Board of Trustees, Minute files, Henry Hurd to Board of Trustees, 10 Feb. 1903, JH; Peter D. Olch, 'William S. Halsted and Private Practice: A Re-examination,' *Surgery* 72 (1972), 804–11; WWF remarks to the Halsted Society, 24 Feb. 1955, OL, 153, BO2886; also Peter D. Olch, 'William S. Halsted: The Antithesis of William Osler,' *Persisting Osler*, 199–204.

34 WO to C.F. Martin, 7 Dec. 1903, CPOL; WO to H.V. Ogden, 8 Jan., 4 Jan. 1904, CPOL. Also HVO: *The Life and Letters of H.V. Ogden*, 103, 295–6; WWF to Wm. White, 14 Dec. 1954, FPOL.

35 WO to James B. Johnson, 18 Sept. 1901, CPOL; WO to GRO, 17 Mar. 1911, OL, 8282; Thayer, 'Reminiscences of Osler in the Early Baltimore Days,' *California and Western Medicine* 31 (1929), 161–8; D.R. Mendenhall Memoirs, Smith, 3, F, I, 30.

36 'The Healing of Tuberculosis,' *Climatologist* 2 (1892), 149–53; PPM, 1st edn, 252.

37 JHH Board of Trustees Minutes, 15 Feb. 1898, JH; Charles D. Parfitt, 'Osler's Influence in the War against Tuberculosis,' *CMAJ* 47 (1942), 293; Laennac Society,

JHH Bulletin 11 (1900), 331; Louis Hamman, 'Osler and the Tuberculosis Work of the Hospital,' *JHH Bulletin* 30 (1919), 202–3; students' reports, OPJH, 17.

38 WO-Flick corres., CPOL, 14.

39 GRO to H.B. Jacobs, 17 Aug. 1901, OPJH, 1; Earl F. Nation, 'Osler and Tuberculosis,' *Chest* 64 (1973), 84–7; *PPM*, 4th edn, 108; Jessica M. Robbins, 'Class Struggles in the Tubercular World: Nurses, Patients, and Physicians, 1903–1915,' *BHM* 71 (1997), 412–34.

40 Edith G. Reid, *The Great Physician* (New York: Oxford University Press, 1931), 136–7.

41 C. Allbutt to WO, 27 Jan. 1894, OPOL, 11, 18.8; Robert Hutchison, 'William Osler,' *Quarterly Journal of Medicine* n.s., 18 (1949), 275–7.

42 WO to H.V. Ogden, 25 Oct. 1898, CPOL; 'Autobiographical Notes,' 1898; WO to GRO, 22 July 1898, CPOL.

43 WO to H.V. Ogden, 1 Mar. 1898, CPOL.

44 WO to W.S. Thayer, 12 Aug. 1898; WO to Lafleur, 22 Oct. 1898, CPOL; also HC to Kate Crowell, 16 Sept. 1898, CPY, 554.

45 Cushing, 1:481, 496.

46 W.S. Thayer, 'Reminiscences of Osler in the Early Baltimore Days,' *California and Western Medicine*, 31 (1929), 161–8.

47 W.S. Greenfield to WO, 1 Mar. 1900, CPOL.

48 Cushing, 1:518; WO to Schäfer, 27 Mar. 1900, CPOL; WO to H.V. Ogden, 10 June 1900, CPOL; WWF to B.H. Cleveland, 22 Jan. 1945, FPOL; BO5839.

49 Welch to D.C. Gilman, 27 Mar. 1900, cited in W. Bruce Fye, 'William Osler's Departure from America: The Price of Success,' *NEJM* 320 (1989), 1426 (reprinted in *Persisting Osler 2*); Schäfer to WO, 27 Mar. 1900, W.S. Greenfield to WO, 28 Mar. 1900, CPOL; HC to Kate Crowell, 10 July 1900, CPY, 17:838.

50 GRO to H.V. Ogden, 23 Feb. 1901, CPOL, 58; WO to L.F. Barker, 17 Nov. 1900, Barker Papers, JH.

51 OL, BO7664, ms of unpublished papers, draft of an address for the Medical School branch of the YMCA, 4 Oct. 1898, OL, BO7664 (I).

52 'The Faith that Heals' *BMJ*, 18 June 1910, 1470–2.

53 *PPM*, 2nd edn, 585; 3rd edn, 109.

54 'A Study of Dying. J.H.H., W. Osler,' OL, BO7644; commonplace book, OL, BO7665(iii), 14.

55 HC note on Ingersoll Lectures, CPOL 1904.

56 *Science and Immortality.' The Ingersoll Lecture, 1904* (Boston: Houghton Mifflin, 1904); WWF to Wm Colgate, 5 Sept. 1940, FPOL.

57 C.W. Eliot to HC, 8 Apr. 1920, CPOL 1902; HC memo 'Ingersoll Lecture,' CPOL 1904.

58 'Robert Burton,' *Selected Writings*, 87–8; Felix Cunha, *Osler as a Gastroenterologist* (San Francisco, 1948), 57.

59 'Books and Men,' *Aequanimitas*, 220, 224.

60 Jennifer Connor, 'Purveyors of Medical Knowledge: Physicians, Librarianship, and the Social Transformation of the Medical Library Association,' ms history of MLA, in press.

61 See especially Genevieve Miller, 'In Praise of Amateurs: Medical History in America before Garrison,' *BHM* 47 (1973), 586–615.

62 'The Collecting of a Library,' *BO*, xxviii.

63 WO to Kelly, undated, in Willard E. Goodwin, 'William Osler and Howard A. Kelly,' *BHM* 20 (1946), 624–5; GRO to H.B. Jacobs, 14 July 1901, CPOL, 58; HC to Father, 29 Sept. 1901, 21 May 1903, CPY, reel 16.

64 Thomas Barnes Futcher, 'Sir William Osler, Bart,' *JH Alumni Magazine* 9 (1920–1); 2–8; WO to HC, 25 July 1903, CPOL, 52; BO2278.

65 'Autobiographical Notes'; WO to Shepherd, 18 Oct. 1901, CPOL.

66 'Autobiographical Notes'; Wm Howard Taft to HC, 29 Aug. 1922, CPY, 602; GRO to H.B. Jacobs, 17 June 1902, OPJH.

67 WO to HC, 3 Mar. 1902, CPY, 89:709–10; Walter to Gustav Baumgartner, 12 Oct. 1902, Baumgartner Collection, Archives, Washington University School of Medicine, St Louis.

68 'Chauvinism in Medicine,' *Aequanimitas*, 277–306.

69 'The Master-Word in Medicine,' *Aequanimitas*, 373–4.

70 OPOL 1903 file; 'Autobiographical Notes'; WO to T. McCrae, 24 Nov. 1903, CPOL; HC to Kate Cushing, 21 July 1904, CPY, 17:1293; Fulton, *Cushing*, 228n.

71 'Peyronie's Disease – Strabisme du penis,' *Boston Medical and Surgical Journal* 143 (1903), 245, 485; M.B. Wesson, 'Peyrone's Disease,' *Journal of Urology* 49 (1943), 350–6; A.H.T. Robb-Smith, 'Osler's Sense of Humour,' ms in OL.

72 'Chronic Cynosis with Polycythaemia and Enlarged Spleen: A New Clinical Entity. *American Journal Medical Science*, n.s., 126 (1903), 187–201; A.H.T. Robb-Smith, 'Osler's Influence on Haematology,' *Blood Cells* 7 (1981), 513–33; Maxwell M. Wintrobe, 'Osler's Chronic Cyanotic Polycythemia with Splenomegaly,' *JHH Bulletin* 85 (1949), 75–87.

73 'On the So-called Stoke-Adams Disease,' *Lancet* (1903), 516–24; re BBO: WO to Shepherd, 11 Feb. 1901, CPOL; WO to L.F. Barker, [misdated 17 Nov. 1900], Barker Papers, JH; Norman Gwyn to Esther Rosenkrantz, 7 July 1948, Rosencrantz Collection, University of California at San Francisco, Health Sciences Library; WO on tobacco and pulse from his 'Lectures on Angina Pectoris.' My interest in WO's work on Stokes-Adams disease was stimulated by Charles F. Wooley's 1996 paper to the American Osler Society, 'Osler on Slow Pulse, Stokes-Adams Disease and Sudden Death in Families.'

74 Wm G. MacCallum, 'Osler as a Pathologist,' *JHH Bulletin* 341 (1919), 197–8; Norman Gwyn to Bernard Cohen, 7 Apr. 1937, Archives of the Medical and Chirurgical Faculty of the State of Maryland, box 44, file 1; Rufus Cole, 'Dr Osler: Scientist and Teacher,' *Archives of Internal Medicine*, 84 (1949), 54–63. Also, C.H. Bunting, 'Dr Osler as Pathologist,' *BHM* 32 (1949), 336–40.

75 F.P. Mall to L.F. Barker, 3 Aug., 30 July 1902, 15 Feb. 1905, Barker Papers, JH;
    Florence R. Sabin, *Franklin Mall: The Story of a Mind* (Baltimore: Johns Hopkins
    University Press, 1934), ch. 10.

76 Comments to this effect in Walter Baumgartner's letters to his father from JH,
    Baumgartner Collection, Archives, Washington University School of Medicine,
    St Louis; and in W.S. Thayer's articles in *Osler and Other Papers* (Baltimore: Johns
    Hopkins University Press, 1932).

77 WO to George Dock, undated [Baltimore], OPOL, 3; Florence R. Sabin notes on
    interview with Welch, 9 Dec. 1933, Welch Papers, JH, 178; HC to Dr W.S.
    McCann, 12 Nov. 1925, CPY, 560.

78 John Sedgwick Billings to Katherine Hammond, 6 Sept. 1894, Hammond-Bryan-
    Cumming Papers, University of South Carolina.

79 Full-time file, H.A. Kelly to WO, 3 May 1911, OL, 'Whole-Time Clinical Professors,
    J.H., 1911–14,' BO7651.

80 JHH Board of Trustees, Minutes, 22 Dec. 1898, 13 Mar., 19 June, 19 July 1900,
    11 Mar. 1902, 10 Feb. 1903, JH.

81 WO to Barker, 23 Sept. 1902, Barker Papers, JH.

82 WO, 'Autobiographical Notes,' 1904.

83 WO to Libman, 14 Sept. 1906, CPOL; F.P. Mall to L.F. Barker, 30 Oct. 1901, Barker
    Papers, JH; HC to Kate Cushing, 30 Sept. 1904, CPY, 17:1353.

84 Cushing, 1:680–1; Walter Baumgarten to Gustav Baumgarten, 23 Apr. 1902, Baum-
    garten Papers, Archives, Washington University School of Medicine, St Louis.

8: Leaving America

1   Kate Cushing to H.K. Cushing, 11 Feb. 1904, quoted in John F. Fulton, *Harvey
    Cushing* (Springfield, Ill.: Thomas, 1946), 233; HC memo, 7 Feb. 1904, CPOL; GRO
    to Marjorie Howard, 11 Feb. 1904, Futcher Papers, OL; WO to T.R. Boggs, 18 Feb.
    1904, OPOL, 3; WO to Judge Harlan, 7 Mar. 1904, CPOL.

2   Chesney, *Johns Hopkins*, 2:376–96.

3   Correspondence re regius professorship in CPOL 1904 files, esp. E.W.A. Walker to
    Arthur Thomson, 6 Jan. 1904, and Arthur Thomson to W.C. Bosanquet, 13 Jan. 1904.

4   Charles W. Eliot to F.C. Shattuck, 23 May 1904, CPOL; HC note on 'Ingersoll
    Lecture' memorandum, CPOL 1904; clipping, 29 June 1904, OPOL, 12.

5   Cushing I, 643; J.B. Sanderson to WO, 8 June 1904, CPOL; also Sanderson to WO,
    30 June 1904, CPOL.

6   GRO note in 19 June 1904; WO to Sanderson, 21 June 1904, CPOL.

7   H.D. Rolleston to HC, 17 Sept. 1920, CPY, 59; HC to Kate Cushing, 24 July 1904
    [later misdated 21 July], CPY, reel 17.

8   H.M. Sinclair, 'Some Ups and Downs of Oxford Science,' in Kenneth Dewhurst, ed.,
    Oxford Medicine (London: Sandford Publications, 1970), 9; Cushing, 1:649; HC to
    Kate Cushing, 27 July 1904, CPY, 17:1303–4.

9 Cushing 1:649; WO, 'Autobiographical Notes,' an apparent later addition to the 1904 summary.

10 WO to George Dock, 10 Aug. 1904; WO to Mall, 8 Aug. and Gilman, 8 Aug.; to Abel, 6 Aug.; to Rolleston, 8 Aug.; to James C. Wilson, 10 Aug.; to McCrae, 6 Aug.; to Thayer, 6 Aug.; to Halsted, 6 Aug., all in CPOL 1904; WO to Judge Harlan (chair, Hopkins Board of Trustees), 6 Aug. 1904, OPJH; WO to EO, 6 Aug. 1904, CPOL.

11 GRO to C.N.B. Camac, 1904, in Earl F. Nation and John P. McGovern, eds., *Student and Chief: The Osler–Camac Correspondence* (Pasadena: Castle Press, 1980), 31; GRO to Susan Chapin, 'Friday No Thursday pm,' 1904, CPOL, 58.

12 F.R. Sabin to Mrs Mall, 8 Sept. 1904, Sabin Papers, JH; Welch to WO, 30 Aug. 1904, CPY, 123:615; H.M. Hurd to WO, 14 Aug. 1904, OPOL, Misc. File; S. Weir Mitchell to WO, 14 Aug. 1904, CPY, 121:411; W.S. Thayer, 'The Chief,' *NEJM* 297 (1932), 563–70.

13 Undated article, 'Interesting People,' by H.L. Mencken, CPOL June–Dec. 1905 file; Cushing, 1:655.

14 GRO to HC, 23 Sept. 1904, CPOL, 52; HC to C.N.B. Camac, 2 July 1923, CPY, 516.

15 Mall to Ira Remsen, Mar. 1905, in Chesney, *Johns Hopkins*, 2:436; L.F. Barker, *Time and the Physician* (New York: Putnam's, 1942), 144.

16 HC memo, CPY, 123:620ff.

17 OPOL, 3, WO to Dock, undated from 1 W. Franklin; WO to Dock, Pointe-à-Pic, '14th,' OPOL, 3; Rupert Norton to L.F. Barker, 2 Jan. 1905, Barker Papers, JH; Chesney, *Johns Hopkins*, 2:439.

18 Welch to Ira Remsen, 28 Oct. 1904, Halsted to Remsen, 1 Mar. 1905, Ira Remsen Papers, Eisenhower Library, Johns Hopkins University; Mall to Barker, 1 Jan., 15 Feb. 1905, Barker Papers, JH.

19 WO to T. McCrae, 28 Jan. 1905, CPOL; WO to L.F. Barker, 4 Mar. 1905, Barker Papers, JH; WO to George Dock, 9 June 1905, OL, 476, Dock file.

20 Barker, *Time and the Physician*, 150; Mall to Barker, 4 Mar. 1905, Barker Papers, JH.

21 HC to Father, 25 Oct. 1904, 6 Apr. 1905, CPY, 370; Fulton, *Cushing*, 239.

22 Thomas B. Futcher, 'Dr. Osler's Renal Stones,' *Archives of Internal Medicine*, 84 (1949), 40.

23 'The Student Life,' *Aequanimitas*, 2nd edn, 413–44.

24 'Unity, Peace, and Concord,' *Aequanimitas*, 2nd edn, 447–65; HC to Father, 29 Apr. 1905, CPY, 370.

25 'The Fixed Period,' *Aequanimitas*, 2nd edn, 391–411.

26 Newspaper clipping files, OPJH, 2; Cushing, 1:669.

27 Clipping, 11 July 1908, CPOL; *Finnegan's Wake* (London, 1939), 317; J.B. Lyons, 'Osler and Ireland,' OL *Newsletter* 73 (June 1993); CPY, 106:446ff, clippings; David B. Hogan, 'Sir William Osler: Fixed Terms, Fixed Ideas, and "Fixed Period,"' *Annals of the Royal College of Physicians and Surgeons of Canada* 28 (1995), 25–9; WO, 'Autobiographical Notes.'

28 HC to Father, 25 Feb. 1905, CPY, 370.

29 Thomas R. Cole, *The Journey of Life: A Cultural History of Aging in America* (Cambridge: Cambridge University Press, 1992); William Graebner, *A History of Retirement: The Meaning and Function of an American Institution* (New Haven: Yale University Press, 1980); W. Andrew Achenbaum, *Old Age in the New Land* (Baltimore: Johns Hopkins University Press, 1978); David Hackett Fischer, *Growing Old in America*, expanded edn. (Oxford: Oxford University Press, 1978); Carole Haber, *Beyond Sixty-Five: The Dilemma of Old Age in America's Past* (Cambridge: Cambridge University Press, 1983); Gerald J. Gruman, ed., *The 'Fixed Period' Controversy: Prelude to Ageism* (New York: Arno Press, 1979).

30 Cushing, 1:415; Morris Fishbein, *A History of the American Medical Association, 1847–1947* (Philadelphia: W.B. Saunders, 1947), 170–1.

31 BO4742.

32 *Dinner to Dr William Osler, Previous to His Departure for England ... May 2, 1905* (privately printed pamphlet, n.d.); Richard L. Golden, ed., *Oslerian Verse* (Montreal: Osler Library, 1998), 58–9; WO address, 'L'Envoi,' *Aequanimitas*, 2nd edn, 469–74.

33 CPY, 89:707, HC intro.

9: A Delightful Life and Place

1 WO daybooks, 1905, OL, BO7668; WO to Thayer, 30 May 1905, CPOL; WO to HC, 2 June 1905, CPOL, 52.

2 GRO to Mother, 19 June, 31 May, 8, 9, 15 June 1905, CPOL, 58.

3 GRO to Mother, 23 June, 10 July, 3 Nov., 27 July 1905, CPOL, 58; GRO to HC, 15 July 1905, CPOL, 52.

4 GRO to HC, 15 July 1905, CPOL, 52.

5 WO to W.S. Thayer, Aug. 1905, CPOL; WO to Mrs H.M. Thomas, 25 May 1906, CPOL; also, John F. Fulton, *Harvey Cushing* (Springfield, Ill.: Thomas, 1946), 246, quoting HC to Father, 2 Feb. 1906.

6 GRO to Mother, 25 June, 18 Sept. 1905, CPOL, 58.

7 Ibid., 19 June 1905.

8 Ibid., 6, 18 Aug. 1905.

9 For a historian's view of its deep significance, see John Harley Warner, *Against the Spirit of System: The French Impulse in Nineteenth-Century American Medicine* (Princeton: Princeton University Press, 1998), 363–4.

10 Cushing, 2:25.

11 WO to Weir Mitchell, 18 Nov. 1910, CPOL.

12 GRO to Mother, 10 Nov. 1905, CPOL, 58; WO to H.V. Ogden, 15 Feb. 1910, CPOL.

13 WO to HC, 23 Mar. 1906, CPOL, 52.

14 WO, 'Autobiographical Notes,' 1907; Ellen Osler obit. clippings, OFPOA, 4.

15 'Autobiographical Notes,' 1906; WO to A.B. MacCallum, 12 June 1906; WO to John Hoskin, 31 Dec. 1906, CPOL.

16 'Autobiographical Notes,' 1907.

17 WO to C.P. Howard, 18 Sept. 1905, CPOL; Lloyd Stevenson, 'W.W. Francis,' *BHM* 34 (1960), 373–8.

18 WO to Campbell Howard, 16 Sept. 1897, CPOL. For the Osler-Howard relationship, see R. Palmer Howard, *The Chief: Doctor William Osler* (Canton, Mass.: Science History Publications, 1983), and Palmer H. Futcher, 'The Letters of William Osler to Marjorie Howard,' *Transactions and Studies, College of Physicians of Philadelphia*, 5th ser., 12 (1990), 413–43.

19 WO to Marjorie Howard, 29 Jan. 1907, 21 Aug. 1909, Sept. 1909, in Palmer H. Futcher, 'The Letters of William Osler to Marjorie Howard,' *Transactions and Studies, College of Physicians of Philadelphia*, 5th ser., 12 (1990), 413–43.

20 GRO to Mother, 9 Oct. 1905, 20 Nov. 1905, CPOL, 58.

21 WO to Weir Mitchell, 3 Mar. 1907, CPY, 121:430.

22 WWF ms, 'Showman's Patter,' OL, 213; Alex Sakula, 'Rudyard Kipling, Sir William Osler, and the History of Medicine,' *Kipling Journal*, June 1983, 10–24; WO to HC, 3 Jan. 1908, CPOL, 52.

23 WO to W.S. Thayer, 7 Feb. 1908, CPOL.

24 Cushing, 2:53.

25 Bodleian Library notes, CPOL, 2; BO5443.

26 WO to S. Weir Mitchell, 17 Aug. 1906, OPOL.

27 WO to D.C. Gilman, 28 Dec. 1907, CPOL; WO, *Thomas Linacre* (Cambridge: Cambridge University Press, 1908), 42.

28 Notes removed from BO7648, OL, 153; James Robertson to WO, 25 Oct. 1908, CPOL.

29 WO to HC, 12 July 1906, CPOL, 52.

30 Charles M. Lea to WO, 16 Aug. 1904, OPOL, 12.

31 WO to T. McCrae, 22 Jan. 1908; WO to Maude Abbott, 23 Jan. 1908, CPOL. For Abbott's life, see Douglas Waugh, *Maudie of McGill: Dr Maude Abbott and the Foundations of Heart Surgery* (Toronto: Hannah Institute and Dundurn Press, 1992), and Margaret Gillett, 'The Lonely Heart: Maude E. Abbott,' in G.J. Clifford, ed., *Lone Voyagers: Academic Women in Coeducational Universities, 1870–1937* (New York: Feminist Press at CUNY, NY, 1989); also Maude Abbott, 'Autobiographical Sketch,' *McGill Medical Journal* 28 (1959), 127–52.

32 WO to T. McCrae, 12 May 1908 (re Holmes), CPOL; Richard H. Lampert, 'Osler and His Publishers,' *Transactions, College of Physicians of Philadelphia*, 3rd ser., 5 (1983), 177–90.

33 PPM, 3rd edn, 569.

34 E.C. LeRoy et al., 'A Student's Ode to Osler's Text,' *Persisting Osler*, 2:61–71.

35 By Henry Sigerist; see, Elizabeth Fee and Thedore M. Brown, eds., *Making Medical History: The Life and Times of Henry E. Sigerist* (Baltimore: Johns Hopkins University Press, 1997), 73.

36 *The Growth of Truth as Illustrated in the Discovery of the Circulation of the Blood,*

Harveian Oration, Royal College of Physicians, London, 18 Oct. 1906, pamphlet (London: H. Frowde, 1906; reprinted as 'Harvey and His Discovery,' *Alabama Student*, 295–334).

37 'The Evolution of the Idea of Experiment in Medicine,' *Transactions of the Congress of American Physicians and Surgeons* 7 (1907), 1–8.

38 'Professor Osler on Women Doctors,' *Lancet* 13 July 1907, 131; 'The Reserves of Life,' *St. Mary's Hospital Gazette* 13 (1907), 95–8.

39 'Splenic Polycythaemia with Cyanosis,' *Proceedings, Royal Society of Medicine*, 1 (1907–8), Clinical Section, 41–3; 'On Telangiectasis Circumstripta Universalis,' *JHH Bulletin*, 18 (1907), 401–3; 'On Multiple Hereditary Telangiectases with Recurring Haemorrhages,' *Quarterly Journal of Medicine* 1 (1907), 53–8.

40 'On Ochronosis,' *Quarterly Journal of Medicine* 1 (1908), 199–208; Alexander G. Bearn, *Archibald Garrod and the Individuality of Man* (Oxford: Clarendon Press, 1993).

41 'Chronic Infectious Endocarditis, *Quarterly Journal of Medicine* 2 (1908–9), 219–30; Richard L. Golden and Thomas A. Horrocks, 'William Osler's Views on Malignant Endocarditis from an "Unknown" Report,' *American Journal of Cardiology*, 15 Jan. 1989, 241–3; Warfield T. Longcope, 'Sir William Osler and Bacterial Endocarditis,' *JHH Bulletin* 85 (1949), 1–45.

42 WO and A. Keith, 'Stokes-Adams Disease,' in C. Allbutt and H. Rolleston, eds., *A System of Medicine by Many Writers* (London: Macmillan, 1909), vi, 130–56; Charles F. Wooley and Michael Bliss, 'Osler: Slow Pulse, Stokes-Adams Disease and Sudden Death in Families,' unpublished ms.

43 E.H. Bensley, 'Sir William Osler and Mabel Purefoy FitzGerald,' *OL Newsletter* 27 (1978).

44 Gertrude Jefferson, 'Reminiscences of Sir William Osler,' CPY, 527; Peter H. Schurr, *So That Was Life: A Biography of Sir Geoffrey Jefferson* (London: Royal Society of Medicine Press, 1997).

45 WO to HB Jacobs, 20 Nov. 1908, CPOL.

46 WO to Mabel Brewster, 31 Dec. 1908, CPOL; WO to Weir Mitchell, 20 Nov. 1908, CPY, 121:454; also Charles Coury, 'Sir William Osler and French Medicine,' *Medical History* 11 (1967), 1–14.

47 Lawrason Brown, 'Reminiscenes,' *Osler Memorial*, 447.

48 'Impressions of Paris,' *JAMA* 52 (1909), 701–3, 771–4.

49 Cyril B. Courville, 'Sir William Osler and His Portraits,' *BHM* 32 (1949), 353–77.

50 WO to HC, 8, 11 Feb., 1909, CPOL, 52; GRO to Kate Cushing, 11 Feb. 1909, CPOL, 58; WO note, 17 Feb. 1909, BO7665(v), 51.

51 WO note, 1 Mar. 1909, BO7665(ix); WO to J. Wm. White, 2 Mar. 1909, CPOL.

52 'Note on the Relation of the Capillary Blood-Vessels in Purpura,' *Lancet*, 15 May 1909, 1385–6; WO to A.C. Gibson, undated, OPOL.

53 'Old and New: Oration on the Occasion of the Opening of the New Building ... 13 May 1909,' *Bulletin Medical and Chirurgical Faculty of Maryland* 1 (1908–9), 248–59.

54 WO to H.B. Jacobs, 11 June 1909, CPOL.

55 *The Treatment of Disease: The Address in Medicine before the Ontario Medical Association, 3 June 1909* (London: H. Frowde, 1909); also *BMJ* (1909), 185–9.

56 'Remarks on the Medical Library in Post-Graduate Work,' *BMJ* (1909), 925–8; 'The Collecting of a Library,' *BO*, xxx.

57 WO to HC, 25 Jan. 1910, CPOL, 52; Cushing, 2:211.

58 'A Record Day at Sotheby's,' *BO*, xxxv; WO note, *BO*, 692; Christie's price supplied by W. Bruce Fye.

59 WO to Mabel Brewster, 21 Aug. 1908, 16 Aug. 1910, CPOL.

60 'Autobiographical Notes,' 1908.

61 WO, *The Lumleian Lectures on Angina Pectoris* (London, 1910), reprinted from the *Lancet*, 12, 26 Mar., 9 Apr. 1910, 28.

62 WO to H.B. Jacobs, 25 Jan. 1910, CPOL; WO to HC, 25 Jan. 1910, CPOL, 52; WO to Harry Thomas, 8 Sept. 1910, CPOL; WO to Weir Mitchell, 18 Nov. 1910, CPY, 121:462; AM, 'William Osler,' address 15 May 1946 to Society of Surgeons of New Jersey, AM Papers, OL.

63 WO to GRO, 22 Feb., 13 Feb., 1911, OL, 8282; WO to HC, 22 Feb. 1911, CPOL, 52; WO to H.M. Thomas, 5 Mar. 1911, CPOL.

64 WO to GRO, 1, 16 Mar. 1911, OL, 8282.

65 WO to GRO, 17 Mar. 1911, OL, 8282.

66 WO to GRO, 10 Feb., 26 Mar. 1911, OL, 8282.

67 WO to GRO, 1, 4, 15 Mar. 1911, OL, 8282; GRO to WWF, 20 Feb. 1911, OPOL.

68 WO to GRO, 19 Mar., 15, Feb., 27 Mar., 20 Mar. 1911, OL, 8282.

69 WO to Susan Revere Baker, early 1910, OPOL; WO to Muriel Brock, 31 Mar. 1910, enc. in Brock to HC, 2 July 1921, CPY, 508

70 GRO to H.B. Jacobs, 27 Mar. 1911, OPJH.

10: Sir William

1 WO to WWF, '22nd,' 1911, OPOL; 'Autobiographical Notes,' 1911; HC note of comments by GRO, CPOL 1911; WO to Chattie, 21 June 1911, CPOL; WO to F.C. Shattuck, 4 Sept. 1911, CPOL.

2 GRO to HC, 4 July [1911], CPY, 42:38; HC to GRO, 22 Aug. 1922, CPY, 83, folder 577.

3 Agnes Repplier, *J. William White, M.D.: A Biography* (Boston: Houghton Mifflin, 1919), 132, 162.

4 Wm James to WO, 3 May 1910, OL 163, from BO3075; also published in Ludwig Edelstein, 'William Osler's Philosophy,' *BHM* 20 (July 1946), 27–93.

5 Henry James to Theodora Bonsanquet, 2 Mar. 1910, in Leon Edel, ed., *Henry James Letters* (Cambridge, Mass.: Belknap Press, 1984), 548–9; Henry James (nephew) to HC, 22 Aug. 1923, CPY, 547.

6 WO to J. Wm White, 16 Sept. 1910, CPOL; HC to Henry James (nephew), 25 Aug.

1923, CPY, 547; also Henry D. Janowitz and Adeline R. Tintner, 'An Anglo-American Consultation: Sir William Osler Refers Henry James to Sir James Mackenzie,' *JHM* 43 (1988), 297–308; Leon Edel, *Henry James, 1901–1916: The Master* (Philadelphia: Lippincott, 1972), 443–9.

7 WO, *The Lumleian Lectures on Angina Pectoris* (London, 1910), reprinted from the *Lancet*, 12, 26 Mar., 9 Apr. 1910; Christopher Lawrence, 'Moderns and Ancients: The "New Cardiology" in Britain 1880–1930,' in W.F. Bynum, C. Lawrence, and V. Nutton, eds., *The Emergence of Modern Cardiology* (London: Wellcome Institute, 1985), 1–33; Robert A. Aronowitz, *Making Sense of Illness: Science, Society, and Disease* (Cambridge: Cambridge University Press, 1994), ch. 4: 'From the Patient's Angina Pectoris to the Cardiologist's Coronary Heart Disease.'

8 'Life in the Tropics,' unpub. lecture, c. 1911, OL, BO7664 (III); 'An Address on High Blood Pressure' *BMJ* (1912), 1173–7.

9 W. Bruce Fye, 'The Delayed Diagnosis of Myocardial Infarction: It Took Half a Century!' *Circulation* 72 (1985), 262–71.

10 WO to L.F. Barker, 25 Jan. 1910, CPOL; Robert Hutchison, 'William Osler,' *Quarterly Journal of Medicine*, n.s., 18 (1949), 275–7; Patrick Mallam, 'Billy "O,"' in Kenneth Dewhurst, ed., *Oxford Medicine* (London: Sandford Publications, 1970), 94–9.

11 A.D. Gardner, 'Some Recollections of Sir William Osler at Oxford,' *JAMA* 210 (1969), 2265–7.

12 F.G. Hobson, 'Sir William Osler, Bart.,' in Dewhurst, ed., *Oxford Medicine*, 88–93.

13 WWF to Ralph H. Major, 13 Oct. 1949, FPOL; K.M. Elisabeth Murray, *Caught in the Web of Words: James A.H. Murray and the* Oxford English Dictionary (New Haven: Yale University Press, 1977), 310–12. See also H. Rocke Robertson, 'W.O. and the O.E.D.,' *OL Newsletter* 68 (1991).

14 WO notes copied by HC, CPOL, 2; the originals of these notes are in WO's copy of W.D. Macray, *Annals of the Bodleian Library* (Oxford: Rivington's, 1868), given to the Bodleian Library on condition that it not be available for study during the twentieth century.

15 WWF to Dr E.P. Scarlett, 25 Oct 1941; WWF to AM, 28 May 1952, FPOL; John Trotter, 'Robert Bridges,' in Dewhurst, ed., *Oxford Medicine*, 76–83.

16 WO daybooks, 28 Mar., 22 Oct. 1913, OL, BO7668; GRO note, CPOL 1913.

17 WWF to JHM (Fulton file), 16 Aug. 1955; Tom Cullen to WWF, 21 Oct. 1949, FPOL.

18 WO undated notes, A.G. Gibson file, OPOL; WO to W.C. Rivers, 19 Aug. 1919, Countway Library, BMS c. 92.2.

19 WO daybooks, OL, BO7668; George T. Harrell, 'Osler's Practice,' *Persisting Osler*, 105–23.

20 WO to Lawrason Brown, 9 Nov. 1910, CPOL; Paul W. Harrison to HC, 18 July 1926, CPY, 121:300; Weir Mitchell to Osler, 29 Nov. 1911, CPY, 121:480; George W. Corner, *The Seven Ages of a Medical Scientist: An Autobiography* (Philadelphia:

University of Pennsylvania Press, 1981), 61. Also Jonathan Meakins memoirs (1959), OL, 867/57, box 8, 44.

21 'Report on the Johns Hopkins Medical School, Submitted by Mr Abraham Flexner to Mr Frederick T. Gates ... 1911,' printed as appendix B in Chesney, *Johns Hopkins*, 3:287–309.

22 Kelly to WO, 1, 3, 20, 29 May 1911, OL, BO7651.

23 WO to Wm. Welch, 23 May 1911, in Chesney, *Johns Hopkins*, 3:138; G.F.W. Ross, in 'Meeting of Toronto General Hospital Board on Staff Re-organization with the Permanent Members of the Medical Faculty of the University of Toronto,' 10 Oct. 1907, in J.W. Flavelle Papers, Queen's University Archives, Kingston, Ont., Toronto General Hospital files.

24 WO to H.M. Thomas, 18 Apr. 1911; WO to Barker, 18 May 1911, CPOL.

25 *'Whole-Time Clinical Professors,' A Letter to President Remsen Johns Hopkins University*, pamphlet (Oxford, 1911), printed in full in Chesney, *Johns Hopkins*, 3:176–83.

26 W.H. Howell to WO, 5 Oct. 1911; Welch to WO, 26 Oct. 1911, printed in Chesney, *Johns Hopkins*, 3:184–6; WO to Dock, 30 Oct. 1911, CPOL 1912 file.

27 'London University Reform,' pt. 2, *Quarterly Review*, July 1913, 220–30 (WO scribbled on his copy that he wrote it).

28 'The Pathological Institute of a General Hospital,' address at the Royal Infirmary, 4 Oct. 1911, *Glasgow Medical Journal* 76 (1911), 321–33.

29 WO to L.F. Barker, draft, 25 Jan. 1910, Kelen Collection, privately held; GRO to WWF, 2 Mar. 1912, OPOL.

30 WO to L. Mackall, 20 Aug. 1913, CPOL.

31 'An Address on High Blood Pressure,' *BMJ*, 2 Nov. 1912, 1173–7.

32 Charles G. Roland, ed., 'Sir William Osler's Dreams and Nightmares,' *Persisting Osler*, 45–64; Ernest Jones to Sigmund Freud, 31 Aug. 1911, in R.A. Paskauskas, ed., *The Complete Correspondence of Sigmund Freud and Ernest Jones, 1908–1939* (Cambridge, Mass.: Belknap Press, 1993), 114–15.

33 *Man's Redemption of Man*, pamphlet (London: Constable, 1910); WO, *The Evolution of Modern Medicine* (New Haven: Yale University Press, 1921); on hellenism, see Frank M. Turner, *The Greek Heritage in Victorian Britain* (New Haven: Yale University Press, 1981).

34 A.D. Gardner, 'Some Recollections of Sir William Osler at Oxford,' *JAMA*, 22 Dec. 1969, 2265–7; David Sargant, 'William Osler and William Morris,' in Dewhurst, ed., *Oxford Medicine*, 142.

35 WO, 'The Medical Clinic: A Retrospect and a Forecast,' *BMJ*, 3 Jan. 1914, 10–16; R.E. Barnsley to F.P. Bett, 10 Sept. 1959, Osler Club of London Archive.

36 McD. McLean to HC, 5 Apr. 1920, CPOL, 29.

37 Wilburt C. Davison, 'Sir William Osler: Reminiscences,' *McGill Medical Journal* (1949), 157–89; also John McGovern, 'Wilburt Cornell Davison: Apostle of the Osler Tradition,' *Persisting Osler*, 265–76.

38 McD. McLean to HC, 5 Apr. 1920, CPOL, 29; Sir Arthur S. MacNalty, 'Osler at Oxford,' *Archives of Internal Medicine* 84 (1949), 135–42.

39 WO obit. of Mitchell, *BMJ* (1914), 120–1; WO to J.W. White, Feb. 1914, CPOL.

40 Sir John Slessor, *These Remain: A Personal Anthology* (London: Michael Joseph, 1969), ch. 1.

41 'Israel and Medicine,' *CMAJ* 4 (1914), 729–33.

42 A.M. Cooke, 'William Osler and the Royal College of Physicians of London,' in *Oslerian Anniversary* (London: Osler Club of London, 1976), 1–8; corres. in CPOL, 13, and at the Library of the Royal College of Physicians of London; J.Y.W. MacAlister to WO, 29 May 1914; WO undated reply, CPOL.

43 WO to Mabel Brewster, 10 July 1914, CPOL; WO, 'Autobiographical Notes,' 1914.

44 WO to F.P. Mall, 18 Apr. 1914, Florence Sabin Papers, American Philosophical Society, Philadelphia, Mall biography files, Notes no. 9.

45 WO to Thayer, 14 Jan. 1914, CPOL.

46 Kelly to WO, 26 Nov. 1913, OL, BO7651; Caroline Halsted to Mrs Herbert M. Evans, 1 Nov. 1914, CPY, 114:821–2; L.F. Barker to WO, 8 Apr. 1914, OL, BO7651.

47 WO to HB Jacobs, 23 June 1914, CPOL.

48 'Autobiographical Notes,' 1914; daybook, 1914, OL, BO7668; Cushing, 2:419.

11: All the Youth and Glory of the Country

1 WO to Mabel Brewster, 6 Aug. 1914, CPOL; also WO to H.M. Hurd, 10 Aug. 1914, CPOL; GRO to Susan Chapin, 16, 23, 24, 27 Aug. 1914, CPOL, 55; WO seriousness: GRO to Tom Futcher, 27 Aug. 1914, Futcher Papers, OL; Orville H. Bullitt (the arrested nephew) to Thomas M. Durant, 30 Nov. 1973, OPOL, folio box; WO letter to the *Times*, 27 Aug. 1914.

2 GRO to Susan Chapin, 24, 27, Aug. 1914, CPOL, 55; John Slessor, *These Remain: A Personal Anthology* (London: Michael Joseph, 1969), ch. 1. Slessor misdates the trip.

3 GRO to Susan Chapin, 4 Sept. 1914, CPOL, 55.

4 GRO to Susan Chapin, 1 Sept. 1914, CPOL, 55; WO to Mabel Brewster, 4 Sept. 1914, CPOL.

5 GRO to Susan Chapin, 15 Sept. 1914, CPOL, 55.

6 Ibid.

7 Ibid., 9, 15 Oct. 1914.

8 GRO to Marjorie Futcher ('Dear Child'), 27 Oct. 1914, Futcher Papers, OL.

9 Nancy Astor to HC, 25 Jan. 1921, CPY, 497.

10 GRO to Susan Chapin, 15 Oct. 1914, CPOL, 55.

11 WO, 'Medical Notes on England at War,' *JAMA*, 26 Dec. 1914, 2303–5; GRO to H.V. Ogden, 4 Nov. 1914, CPOL, 55.

12 GRO to Susan Chapin, 12 Nov. 1914, CPOL, 55; WO to Fielding Garrison, 30 Nov. 1914, CPOL; GRO to Susan Chapin, 1 Dec. 1914, CPOL, 55.

13 CPOL, 55, GRO to Susan Chapin, 25 Dec. 1914, CPOL, 55; WO to Mabel Brewster, 14 Dec. 1914, CPOL.

14 Revere Osler to H.B. Jacobs, 27 Dec. 1914, CPOL, 21.

15 GRO to Susan Chapin, 5 Jan. 1915, CPOL, 55; also GRO to WWF, 15 Dec. 1914, OPOL.

16 GRO to WWF, 31 Jan. 1915, OPOL; Revere Osler to HB Jacobs, 20 Mar. 1915, CPOL, 21; GRO to Susan Chapin, 15 Jan. 1915, CPOL, 55.

17 Cushing, 2:503n; WO to S. Whitridge Williams, 16 Dec. 1915, CPOL; GRO to AM, 31 Aug. 1916, OL, 573/1/23; also GRO to Marjorie Futcher, 3 Sept. 1916, Futcher Papers, OL.

18 WO to AC Klebs, 7 Jan. 1915, WO to T. McCrae, 22 Jan. 1915; Dr A.A. Warden to Joseph Leidy, 22 Dec. 1922; Warden to HC, 30 Apr. 1923, CPY, 607.

19 'On Cerebro-Spinal Fever in Camps and Barracks,' *BMJ*, 30 Jan. 1915, 189–90; WO to George Dock, 15 Mar. 1915, CPOL; Donald Armour to HC, 7 Aug. 1921, CPY, 497.

20 'Medical Notes on England at War,' *JAMA* (1915), 679–80, 2001–2; GRO to Susan Chapin, 9 June 1915.

21 GRO note following GRO to WWF, 31 Jan. 1915, OPOL; GRO to Susan Chapin, 13 Feb. 1915, CPOL, 55; WO, 'Professor Wesley Mills,' *CMAJ* 5 (1915), 338–41.

22 Daybook, 8 May 1915, OL, BO7668.

23 John F. Fulton, *Harvey Cushing* (Springfield, Ill.: Thomas, 1946), 401–3.

24 WO obit of 'Robert Fletcher,' in *Men and Books* (Durham, N.C.: Sacrum Press, 1987), 45; AM, 'Sir William Osler at Oxford,' *Osler Memorial*, 363–77.

25 WO daybook, 27 Apr. 1915, OL, BO7668; 'Autobiographical Notes,' 1915; G.M. Trevelyan, *Grey of Fallodon* (Longmans: London, 1937), 271–3, 326–7; Keith Robbins, *Sir Edward Grey* (London: Cassell, 1971), 321.

26 Daybook, 28 May 1915, OL, BO7668.

27 R.C. Fetherstonhaugh, *No. 3 Canadian General Hospital (McGill) 1914–1919* (Montreal: Gazette Printing, 1928), 22.

28 Various GRO letters, spring summer 1915, esp. GRO to Susan Chapin, 2 Mar., 6 Aug., 29 Aug. CPOL, 55.

29 *Science and War: An Address at the University of Leeds Medical School, 1 October 1915*, pamphlet (Oxford: Clarendon Press 1915), 26; A.C.P. Howard, 'Recollections of Sir William Osler's Visit to No. 3 Canadian General Hospital (McGill),' *Osler Memorial*, 419–20; WO to Mabel Brewster, 7 Sept. (mailed later) 1915, CPOL.

30 *Science and War*, pamphlet, 1915.

31 WO to Mabel Brewster, 7 Sept. 1914 (mailed later), CPOL.

32 GRO to Susan Chapin, 9 Nov. 1915, CPOL, 55.

33 Revere Osler to Susan Chapin, 3 Dec. 1915, CPOL, 21.

34 WO to H.M. Thomas, 25 Nov. 1915, CPOL; John Buchan to HC, 8 Oct. 1923, CPY, 508; WO to J. Wm White, 4 Nov. 1915, CPOL.

35 GRO to Susan Chapin, 1 Dec. 1915, CPOL, 55.

36 WO to Mabel FitzGerald, 2 Mar., 26 June 1917, OPOL; AM diary, 18 Dec. 1915, CPOL.

37 BO 263, 494, 1296, 266, 352, 566, 1565, 3024, 2125, 4770, 5526.

38 GRO to Susan Chapin, 13 Nov. 1915, CPOL, 55; WO daybook, 11 Nov. 1915, OL, BO7668.

39 GRO to Susan Chapin, 1, 27 Dec. 1915, CPOL, 55; 'Autobiographical Notes,' 1915; WO to Fielding Garrison, 30 Dec. 1915, CPOL.

40 WO to Leonard Mackall, 7 Feb. 1916, CPOL; GRO to Susan Chapin, 16 Feb. 1916, CPOL, 56.

41 Wilder Penfield, *No Man Alone: A Neurosurgeon's Life* (Boston: Little Brown, 1977), 36–8; Wilder Penfield, 'Sir William Osler,' *University of Western Ontario Medical Journal* 2 (1941), 79–88.

42 Jefferson Lewis, *Something Hidden: A Biography of Wilder Penfield* (New York: Doubleday, 1981), 53–4; Wilder Penfield, 'A Medical Student's Memories of the Regius Professor,' *Osler Memorial*, 386.

43 GRO to Susan Chapin, 16 Apr., 3, 17 May 1916, CPOL, 56.

44 WO to Marjorie Howard Futcher, undated, OL, 893, M82; GRO to Susan Chapin, 13 Mar. 1916, CPOL, 56; HC note on WO to J.W. Churchman, 29 Feb. 1916, CPOL.

45 GRO to Susan Chapin, 26 May 1916, CPOL, 56.

46 GRO to Susan Chapin, 19 June, 23 July 1916, CPOL, 56; GRO to AM, 14 May 1916, OL, 573/1/6/3.

47 GRO to WWF, 3 Apr. 1916, OPOL.

48 OPOL, GRO to WWF, 19 June, 6 July 1916, OPOL; WO to Susan Chapin, 9 July 1916, CPOL.

49 GRO to WWF, 24 Sept. 1916, OPOL; Edith Wharton, *A Son at the Front* (New York: Scribner's, 1923), 372.

50 Sir Alfred Keogh to WO, 6 Sept. 1916, CPOL, 1. For the affair, see the correspondence and memoranda contained in CPOL, folder 1, including W.G. Adami's detailed unpublished account. See also Herbert A. Bruce, *Politics and the C.A.M.C.* (Toronto: William Briggs, 1919); Andrew Macphail, *Official History of the Canadian Forces in the Great War: The Medical Services* (Ottawa: King's Printer, 1925); Robert Craig Brown, *Robert Laird Borden: A Biography*, vol. 2 (Toronto: Macmillan, 1980).

51 Edith Campbell to WO, 30 Dec. 1916; W.G. Adami to WO, 4 Sept. 1916, CPOL, 1.

52 Herbert Bruce to WO, 19 Oct. 1916, CPOL, 1; GRO to WWF, 30 Oct. 1916, OPOL.

53 WO to T. McCrae, 25 Dec. 1916, CPOL.

54 GRO to AM, 19 Nov. 1916, OL, 573/1/26; Cushing, 2:539.

55 GRO to Susan Chapin, 3, 10 Sept. 1916, CPOL, 56; GRO to WWF, 15 Oct. 1916, OPOL; WO to Mabel Brewster, 10 Oct. 1916, CPOL.

56 GRO to WWF, 30 Oct. 1916, OPOL; Revere Osler to Susan Revere, n.d., Futcher Papers, OL. The Futcher Papers contain the best collection of Revere's letters from the front.

57 John Cule, 'Sir William Osler and his Welsh connections,' *Postgraduate Medical*

Journal 64 (1988), 568–74; WO to W.S. Thayer, 17 Nov. 1916, CPOL; WO to J. Collins Warren, 4 Dec. 1916, CPOL; WO to Mabel Brewster, 9 Sept. 1917, CPOL.

58 Daybook, Dec. 1916, OL, BO7668; WO to H.B. Jacobs, 23 Dec. 1916, CPOL; GRO to Agnes Gollop, 23 Dec. 1916, OPOL; GRO to Tom Futcher, 10 Dec. 1916, Futcher Papers, OL.

59 WO to T.B. Futcher, 24 Dec. 1916, Futcher Papers, OL; WO to Mabel Brewster, 25 Dec. 1916, CPOL; Revere Osler to parents, 26, 27 Dec. 1916, CPOL, 21; WO to Revere, 28 Dec. 1916, CPOL.

60 Sue Chapin to Marjorie Futcher, 2 Nov. 1916, Futcher Papers, OL; GRO to WWF, 29 Jan. 1917, OPOL; GRO to Marjorie Futcher, 8 July 1916, Futcher Papers, OL; GRO to AM, 3 Feb. 1917, OL, 573/3/5.

61 WO, 'Illustrations of the Bookworm,' *Bodleian Quarterly Record* 1 (1914–16), 355–7 (reprinted in *Selected Writings*, 250–3); WO memorandum, 'An Election at the Athenaeum,' 12 Mar. 1917, CPOL; Osler/Matthew Family Papers, privately held, GRO to 'AMO' (Annabel Margaret Osler), 4 Nov. 1917.

62 WO to Mabel Brewster, 3, 8 Apr. 1917, CPOL; WO to Charlotte Gwyn, 14 Apr. 1917, CPOL; GRO to Marjorie Futcher, 26 Apr. 1917, Futcher Papers, OL.

63 'The Anti-Venereal Campaign,' *Transactions of the Medical Society of London* 11 (1917), 296–315.

64 WO to Mabel Brewster, 15 May 1917, CPOL; HC undated note, CPOL, 21; GRO to Marjorie Futcher, 21 May 1917, Futcher Papers, OL.

65 GRO to Kate Cushing, 29 May 1917, CPOL; GRO to HC, 3 July 1917, CPOL, 52; WO to Mabel Brewster, 25 Aug. 1917, CPOL.

66 John Cule, 'Sir William Osler and His Welsh Connections,' *Postgraduate Medical Journal* 64 (1988), 568–74.

67 Revere to GRO, 11 June 1917, Futcher Papers, OL; GRO to HC, 19 Aug. 1917, CPOL, 52.

68 *Lloyd's Weekly News*, 24 Dec. 1917.

69 WO to W. Davison, 11 Aug. 1917, CPOL; Revere Osler to WO, 5 Aug. 1917, Futcher Papers, OL; GRO to AM, 28 Aug. 1917, OL, 573/3/10; Osler/Matthews family papers, privately held, GRO to 'AMO' (Annabel Margaret Osler), 26 Aug. 1917; GRO to HC, Sunday, 19 Aug. 1917, CPY, 42:40–2 (HC's published version of this letter, 2:575, is differently worded).

70 HC war diary, 30 Aug. 1917, CPY 110:1306; HC to Susan [Chapin], 30 Aug. 1917, CPY, 18:743; HC to Kate Cushing, 7 Aug. [misdated] 1917, CPY, 17:727; WO to Wm Welch, 6 Sept. 1917; CPY, 123:982. A further collection of letters describing Revere's death is now in the Futcher Papers, OL.

12: Never Use a Crutch

1 WO daybook, Aug.–Sept. 1917, OL, BO7668; WO note, 'The Last Chapter,' CPY, 706; GRO to Marjorie Futcher, 2 Sept. 1917, Futcher Papers, OL.

2 HC notes, CPOL, 1917; Nancy Astor to HC, 25 Jan. 1921, CPOL 1917.

3 WWF to Marjorie Futcher, 1 Sept. 1917, GRO to Marjorie Futcher, 2 Sept. 1917, Futcher Papers, OL.

4 AM journal, 20 Jan. 1918, CPOL. GRO to Kate Cushing, 1 Sept. 1917, CPY, 110:1639–42.

5 Major Vivian A. Batchelor to WO, 1 Sept 1917, Futcher Papers, OL; mother ref. in WO to Mabel Brewster, 30 Sept. 1917, CPOL.

6 GRO to HC, 7 Sept 1917, CPY, 42:87–90; WO to Mabel Brewster, 30 Aug. 1917, CPOL.

7 Sue Chapin to HC, 13 Sept. 1917, CPOL; GRO to Marjorie Futcher, 9 Sept. 1917, Futcher Papers, OL.

8 WO to C.D. Parfitt, 14 Nov. 1917, CPOL; GRO to AM, 11 Dec. 1917, OL, 573/3/12; Arthur Keith to HC, 20 Oct. 1920, CPY, 522.

9 GRO to AM, 16, 27 Dec. 1917, OL, 573/3/14–15; GRO to Marjorie Futcher, 27 Dec. 1917, Futcher Papers, OL.

10 WO to Henry Hurd, 11 Jan. 1918, CPOL; Florence R. Sabin notes on full-time, 4 Feb. 1939, Welch Papers, JH, 178; HC to Kate, 3 Feb. 1918, CPY, 18:848; GRO to Marjorie Futcher, 18 Feb. 1918, Futcher Papers, OL.

11 WO to Campbell and Ottilie Howard, 31 Aug. 1917, CPOL.

12 Interview with Elizabeth Harty Osler Nelles, 25 Feb. 1997; WO to Ernest Barker, 31 Jan. 1919, CPOL.

13 HC diary, Monday, 4 Mar. 1918, CPY, 111:869; GRO to HC, 'Thursday Eve,' CPOL 1918; the original diary does not contain the remark in Cushing, 2:596, 'I could hear him sobbing as he went back up the stairs.'

14 GRO to WWF, 1 Apr. 1918, OPOL.

15 Charles F. Wooley, 'From Irritable Heart to Mitral Valve Prolapse: The Osler Connection,' *American Journal of Cardiology* 53 (1984), 870–4; Joel D. Howell, '"Soldier's Heart": The Redefinition of Heart Disease and Specialty Formation in Early Twentieth-Century Great Britain,' in William Bynum et al., *The Emergence of Modern Cardiology* (London: Wellcome Institute, 1985),

16 Jonathan C. Meakins, 'Memoirs,' OL, 867/57, box 8, 92; WO 'Typhoid Spine,' CMAJ (1918), 490–6; Cushing, 2:589; E.D. Adrian and L.R. Yealland, 'The Treatment of Some Common War Neuroses,' *Lancet*, 9 June 1917, 867–72; Yealland, *Hysterical Disorders of Warfare* (London: Macmillan, 1918), 245–6.

17 WO to CP Howard, 2 Apr. 1918, CPOL; *Times*, 25 Apr. 1918; Cushing, 2:509.

18 WO letter, *Lancet*, 9 May 1918, 715.

19 WO remarks, *Lancet*, 8 June 1918, 804.

20 'The Future of the Medical Profession in Canada,' unpublished address to the Medical Society of the CAMC, Shorncliffe, 9 Sept. 1918, OL, 7664 (IV).

21 AM journal, 7 Feb. 1919, CPOL.

22 WO notes, 1 Aug. 1918, 'An Interesting Day,' OL, 326/40/86.

23 Dr W.J. McGregor to HC, 7 Feb. 1929, CPY, 618.

24 GRO to AM, 11 June 1918, OL, 573/4/22; GRO to Dr Archie Malloch, Sr, 14 July 1918, OL, 573/2/8.

25 Cushing, 2:609; WO to Mabel Brewster, 16 Aug. 1918, CPOL; GRO to AM, 11 July 1918, OL, 573/4/8; GRO to WWF, 'Monday' [1918], OPOL.

26 GRO to AM, 11 July, 24 Aug. 1918, OL, 573/4/8, 573/4/5; GRO to Marjorie Futcher, 6 Sept. 1917, Futcher Papers, OL.

27 WO to Babs Chapin, 3 June 1918, OL, 326/40/75; WO to AM, 14, 31 Oct. 1918, CPOL; WO to AM, 7 Nov. 1918, BO11277; also WO to Geo. Dock, 17 Oct. 1918, Dock Papers, OL, 476.

28 Mrs Wm. McDougall to HC, 19 Oct 1923, CPY, 560.

29 WO to F.J. Shepherd, 11 Oct. 1918, CPOL; 'The Old Humanities and the New Science,' *Selected Writings*, 13.

30 WO to Sir John MacAlister, 14 Nov. 1918, CPOL; Warfield T. Longcope, 'Random Recollections of William Osler,' *Archives of Internal Medicine* 84 (1949), 93–103.

31 GRO to Mary [Jacobs], 5 Dec. 1918, OPJH.

32 GRO to HC, 28 Dec. 1918, CPY, 113:139; GRO to AM, 27 Dec. 1918, OL, 573/4/1; WWF to A.W. Franklin, 27 Dec. 1932, Osler Club of London, Archives.

33 HC diary, 19 Jan. 1919, CPY, 113:88; HC to Kate, 19 Jan. 1919; CPY, 19:3–4.

34 HC diary, 2 Feb. 1919, CPY, 113:124.

35 Ibid.; Rose Johnson to HC, 9 Jan. 1922, CPY, 548.

36 WO to President, Johns Hopkins University, 31 Jan. 1919, CPOL; HC diary, 2 Feb. 1919, CPY, 113:124; George T. Harrell, 'The Osler-Endowed Tudor and Stuart Club,' *Persisting Osler*, 2:161–9.

37 HC diary, 24 Jan. 1919, CPY, 113:92; WO to Fielding Garrison, 18 Mar. 1919, CPOL; WO to Garrison, 18 Mar. 1919, CPOL; WWF 'Address,' in *Harvey Cushing's Seventieth Birthday Party, April 8, 1939* (Springfield, Ill.: Charles C. Thomas, 1939), 21; Francis challenge in Willard E. Goodwin, 'William Osler and Howard A. Kelly,' *BHM* 20 (1946), 650n.

38 'Influenzal Pneumonia,' *Lancet*, 29 Mar. 1919, 501; 'Endurance in Aortic Insufficiency,' *BMJ*, 11 Jan. 1919, 55.

39 GRO to Col. C.P. Strong, 6 Mar. 1919, CPOL; WO to Mayor of Oxford, 1 May 1919, CPOL.

40 GRO to Sue Chapin, 18 May 1919, CPOL, 41; also Welch to HC, 21 Jan. 1920, CPY, 123:969–70.

41 GRO to Sue Chapin, 24 June 1919, CPOL, 41; also GRO to AM, 26 June 1919, OL, 573/5/41; *Times*, 26 June 1919.

42 Alice Hamilton memorandum, CPOL 1919.

43 WO to Mabel FitzGerald, 10 July 1919, OPOL, 3.

44 WO remarks, clipping from *The Hospital*, 19 July 1919, CPOL.

45 WO to J.Y.W. MacAlister, 20 July 1919, CPOL; AM journal, 26 July 1919, CPOL.

46 WO to H.M. Thomas, 20 July 1919, CPOL; AM, 'William Osler,' unpublished address to Society of Surgeons of New Jersey, 15 May 1946, Malloch Papers, OL;

Walter L. Bierring, 'A Day with Dr. Osler in Oxford,' *Archives of Internal Medicine* 84 (1949), 143–8.

47 WO to G. 'Cheyne' [Shattuck] [1919], Countway Library, BMS, misc.

48 WO to Sue Chapin, 22 Aug., 6 Sept. 1919, CPOL; AM to HC, 7 Sept. 1919; CPY, 113:345–8; W.W. Francis memo, 1936, CPOL 1919; GRO to AM, OL, 573/5/30.

49 WO to W.C. Rivers, 19 Aug. 1919, Countway Library, BMS, c. 92.2; A.A. Warden to WO, 24 Aug. 1919, CPOL.

50 WO to Dean Birkett, 29 July 1919, Birkett file, OPOL, 3; WO to Farquhar Robertson, 12 Sept. 1919, CPOL; WO to C.P. Howard, Aug. 1919, CPOL.

51 Fragment, GRO to Sue Chapin, c. 22 Aug. 1915, CPOL, 41; WO to 'Thayer, Mac & Futcher,' 27 Oct. 1919, CPOL; WO daybook, 1919, OL, BO7668.

52 G. Lovatt Gulland to HC, 15 Aug. 1920, CPY, 534.

53 GRO to Sue Chapin, 29 Sept. 1919, CPOL, 41; WO to 'Thayer, Mac & Futcher,' 27 Oct. 1919, CPOL.

54 WO to Sir Harry Reichel, WO to AF Hurst, 6 Oct. 1919, CPOL; GRO to AM, 7 Oct. 1919, OL, 573/5/27.

55 GRO to AM, 12 Oct. 1919, OL, 573/5/25.

56 WO to Mabel Brewster, 29 Oct. 1919, CPOL; extracts from letters of GRO to Mrs Gwyn, CPOL; WO to Susan Chapin, 19 Oct. 1919, CPOL, initial ms, ch. 29, 74.

57 WO to 'Thayer, Mac & Futcher,' 27 Oct. 1919, CPOL; AM to HC, 3 Nov. 1919, CPOL; WO to Mabel Brewster, 29 Oct. 1919, CPOL.

58 WO to BO Humpton, 9 Nov. 1919, CPOL; GRO to AM, 8, 9, Nov. 1919, OL, 573/5/15, 573/5/10.

59 WO to Tom McCrae, 17 Nov. 1919, CPOL; WO to Sir Humphry Rolleston, 5 Nov. 1919, CPOL.

60 HC note, CPOL, 1919; WO to Sue Chapin, 'Silence Day,' 1919, CPOL; WWF to Marjorie Futcher, 11 Nov. 1919, Futcher Papers, OL; WO to AM, 12 [Nov.] 1919, BO11277.

61 WO to F.J. Shepherd, WO to Mabel Brewster, 22 Nov. 1919, CPOL; GRO to AM, 27 Nov. 1919, OL, 573/5/5; WO to Parkes Weber, 25 Nov. 1919, CPOL.

62 WO to Mabel Brewster, 25 Nov. 1919, CPOL; GRO to AM, 27 Nov. 1919, OL, 573/5/3.

63 AM, 'A Narrative of Osler's Last Illness' (Malloch's journal notes, also in CPOL 1919), OL *Newsletter* 47 (Oct. 1984); unless otherwise noted, this is the source of the remaining details and quotes. The standard modern account of the illness is Jeremiah A. Barondess, 'A Case of Empyema: Notes on the Last Illness of Sir William Osler,' *Persisting Osler*, 69–80, which includes the autopsy; it can be supplemented with Harold N. Segall, 'A Commentary on the Last Illness of Sir William Osler,' OL *Newsletter* 50 (Oct. 1985). I am indebted to Dr Barondess and to Dr John Dirks for further advice on these details.

64 HC note on Poe's lines, 'For Annie,' CPY, 89, folder 708; Edith Edwards to HC, 24 Sept. 1920, CPY, 523.

65 GRO to 'AMO' (Annabel Margaret Osler), 17 Dec. 1919, Osler/Matthews family papers, privately held.

66 Horder remarks, 'Recent History of Pneumonia,' Osler Club Symposium, *BMJ* 19 Jan. 1952, 156; anaerobic bacteria: Dr. Charles S. Bryan to author, 1 Nov. 1998.

67 According to the autopsy; Malloch's 'Narrative' says seventh rib.

68 WO to Dear S— 15 Nov. 1919, Library of the Royal College of Surgeons of England, London.

69 Frederick T. Lord, 'Pulmonary Abscess'; C.R. Bardeen, 'Detection of Abnormal Tissues within the Lungs,' in *Contributions to Medical and Biological Research, Dedicated to Sir William Osler ... In Honour of his Seventieth Birthday, July 12, 1919, by His Pupils and Co-Workers*, 2 vols. (New York: Paul Hoeber, 1919), 640–9, 915–17.

70 Sue Chapin to Margaret Revere, 30 Dec. 1919, CPOL.

13: Osler's Afterlife

 1 Jeremiah Barondess, 'A Case of Empyema: Notes on the Last Illness of Sir William Osler,' *Persisting Osler*, 79.

 2 AM journal, 31 Dec. 1919, CPOL.

 3 GRO to Hon. Featherston Osler, 1 Jan. 1920, CPOL, 41.

 4 Herbert Fisher to GRO, 1 Jan. 1920, Osler-Matthews Papers, privately held.

 5 F.R. Fremantle to the *Times*, 2 Jan. 1920; J.G. Adami, 'Sir William Osler: The Last Days,' *Osler Memorial*, 424–5.

 6 Unidentified ms obituary, Los Angeles Country Medical Society Collection, Huntington Library, box 10, Correspondence (Local Historical) file.

 7 GRO to Geo. Dock, 22 Mar. [1920], Marvin Stone collection, privately held.

 8 HC to AM, 29 Dec. 1919, CPY, 37:415.

 9 HC to Dr Joe Collins, 29 Apr. 1925, CPY, 515.

10 Cushing, 2:685; H.L. Mencken, *The American Mercury*, August 1925; Arthur Keith to HC, 4 May 1920, HCY, 82, folder 552.

11 HC to Edgar H. Wells, 12 May 1926, CPY, 608.

12 WO, Memoranda relating to ... Bibliotheca Osleriana, 25 Mar. 1919; WO postscript, 30 July 1919, OL, 326/11/17.

13 WWF to Marjorie Futcher, 11 Nov. 1919, Futcher Papers, OL; GRO to Dr Richard Strong, 1 Jan. 1920, CPOL, 41; AM to HC, 7 Sept. 1919, CPY, 113:345–8.

14 GRO to Maude Abbott, 5 Dec. [prob. 1920], OPOL; Osler Library Committee files, OPOL, 18.

15 AM to HC, 28 Aug. 1923, CPY, 37:632; Jennette Osler to Bill and Hilda Francis, 13 Apr. 1922, Kelen Collection, privately held.

16 GRO to AM, 4 Feb. 1923, OL, 573/9/8; GRO to AM, 25 Feb. 1923, OL, 573/9/12; GRO to AM, 24 Jan. 1924, OL, 573/10/1; GRO to AM, 27 July 1924, OL, 573/10/32; GRO to Mallochites, 30 Nov. 1924, OL, 573/10/52. See also the excerpts from these and other letters in Frederick B. Wagner, *The Twilight Years of Lady Osler* (Canton, Mass.: Science History Publications, 1985).

17 GRO to Kitty Malloch, 22 Feb. 1924, OL, 573/11/3; GRO to AM, 27 Jan. 1924 [1925], OL, 573/12/4; GRO to Mallochs, 23 Feb. 1925, OL, 573/12/9.

18 Clipping, OPOL, 14, 326/36.

19 GRO to AM, 2, 18 Feb. 1926; OL, 573/15/3, 573/15/5; Lloyd Stevenson, 'WW Francis,' *BHM* 34 (1960), 373–8.

20 John Johnson, 'Record of Interview,' Osler Catalogue, 31 Jan. 1928, OPOL, 2, GRO Publishers file; John Fulton to HC, 3 July 1928, CPY, 24:90.

21 John Fulton to Arnold Muirhead, 24 Dec. 1928, John F. Fulton Papers, Yale University Library, 126, folder 1740.

22 'The Heart of a Library,' in W.S. Thayer, *Osler and Other Papers* (Baltimore: Johns Hopkins University Press, 1932), 42–50; HC to Mabel Fitzgerald, 5 Aug. 1929, CPY, 23:286.

23 W.H. Welch to GRO, 3 Feb. 1920, OPOL, 2, GRO Sympathy file.

24 Maude Abbott, 'Autobiographical Sketch,' *McGill Medical Journal*, 28 (1959), 127–52.

25 HC to James C. Wilson, 10 Dec. 1924, CPY, 613.

26 Simon Flexner and James Thomas Flexner, *William Henry Welch and the Golden Age of American Medicine* (Baltimore: Johns Hopkins University Press, 1941), 449.

27 WWF to Simon Flexner, 29 Nov. 1941, FPOL; A.C. Klebs to WWF, 13 Aug. 1942, FPOL.

28 WWF to Dr M. Pierce Rucker, 28 Mar. 1939, FPOL.

29 WWF to Dr W.C. Gibson, 31 Mar. 1955, FPOL; WWF 'At Osler's Shrine,' *Bulletin of the Medical Library Association* 26 (1937), 1–8; Lloyd Stevenson 'W.W. Francis,' *BHM* 34 (1960), 373–8. The best profile of Francis is Faith Wallis, 'W.W. Francis: Scholar and Showman of the Osler Library,' ms article 1995, of which a condensed version was published in the OL *Newsletter* 80 (Oct. 1995) and a longer version in Peter McNally, ed., *Readings in Canadian Library History*, vol. 2 (Ottawa, Canadian Library Association, 1996).

30 WWF to R.B. Bean, 7 Nov. 1931; WWF to Dr J. McKeen Cattell, 13 Mar. 1936, FPOL; also WWF to A.C. Corcoran, 17 Nov. 1942, FPOL.

31 See Joseph W. Lella, 'The Osler Club of London, 1928–38: Young Medical Gentlemen, Their Heroes, Liberal Education, Books, and Other Matters,' *Canadian Bulletin of Medical History* 12 (1995), 313–38.

32 Earl F. Nation, *Esther Rosenkrantz, MD, and Her Collection of Osleriana* (pamphlet, n.p., n.d.); J.F. Fulton to Alfred Franklin, 30 May 1947, Osler Club of London Archives, Muirhead Papers; Esther Rosenkrantz to 'Dear Big Brother' [Norman Gwyn], 1 Dec. 1949, Rosenkrantz Collection, Health Sciences Library, University of California at San Francisco.

33 WWF to J.H. Pratt, 1 June 1951, FPOL.

34 WWF to Gilbert Highet, 26 Jan. 1953, FPOL; WWF to Esther Rosenkrantz, June 1949, FPOL.

35 Wilburt C. Davison, 'Osler's Influence,' *Journal of the Association of American Medical Colleges* 25 (1950), 161–73.

36 In conversations and interviews with Osler and Francis descendants, as well as other
    Osler scholars, I regularly came across versions of this story. The Montreal cardiolo-
    gist Harold N. Segall remembered first hearing it from a member of the Osler family,
    probably Norman Gwyn, in 1929, and there may be an allusion to it in Gwen
    Francis Andras to HC, 10 Jan. 1922, CPY, 497; the view of the randy Osler men is
    spread in WWF to Anne Wilkinson, 10 June 1953, FPOL.

37 Anne Wilkinson, *Lions in the Way* (Toronto: Macmillan, 1956), 143; Anne
    Wilkinson, *The Tightrope Walker: Autobiographical Writings of Anne Wilkinson*
    (Toronto: University of Toronto Press, 1992), 81, 84–5; also various files of the
    Anne Wilkinson Papers, Fisher Rare Book Library, University of Toronto.

38 GRO to AM, 24 Feb. 1924, OL, 573/10/7.

39 HC to Dr Joseph Collins, 29 Apr. 1925, CPY, 515; Edith Gittings Reid, *The Great
    Physician* (New York: Oxford, 1931), 136.

40 Ash, 'Orwell in 1998,' *New York Review of Books*, 22 Oct. 1998.

41 The most vigorous attack was Gerald Weissmann's essay, 'Against *Aequanimitas*,' in
    his *The Woods Hole Contata: Essays on Science and Society* (New York: Dodd, Mead,
    1985); the most thoughtful commentator on the Osler industry was a former Osler
    librarian, Philip Teigen. See Teigen, 'William Osler and Comparative Medicine,'
    Canadian Veterinary Journal 25 (1984), 400–5; 'William Osler's Historiography: A
    Rhetorical Analysis,' *Canadian Bulletin of the History of Medicine* 3 (1986), 31–49;
    'An Apology for Commemorative History: An Essay Review,' *JHM* 51 (1996), 79–
    85; see also Charles G. Roland, 'On the Need for a New Biography of Sir William
    Osler,' *Persisting Osler*, 2:73–84.

42 See, for example, Charles F. Wooley, Elizabeth H. Sparks, Harisios Boudoulas,
    'Aortic Pain,' from the Division of Cardiology, Department of Internal Medicine,
    Ohio State University, 563–89; Steven L. Berk, 'Bacterial Pneumonia in the Elderly:
    The Observations of Sir William Osler in Retrospect,' *Journal of the American
    Geriatric Society* 32 (1984), 683–5; Robert A. Aronowitz, *Making Sense of Illness:
    Science, Society, and Disease* (Cambridge: Cambridge University Press, 1994), ch. 4:
    'From the Patient's Angina Pectoris to the Cardiologist's Coronary Heart Disease.'

43 Related in Felix Cunha, *Osler as a Gastroenterologist* (San Francisco, 1948), 53.

44 See AHT Robb-Smith, 'Osler's Brain,' OL *Newsletter* 60 (Feb. 89); William Feindel,
    'Osler's Brain Again,' OL *Newsletter* 64 (June 1990); Alvin Rodin and Jack Key,
    'Osler's Brain and Related Mental Matters,' *Persisting Osler*, 303–12; correspondence
    in Osler Brain file, Mutter Medical Museum, College of Physicians of Philadelphia,
    and interview with the director of the Museum, Gretchen Worden.

Acknowledgments

In this as in all my work I owe more than can be said to Elizabeth Bliss. We have made our lives together for almost four decades and keep no chloroform handy.

Most of this book was written during two years when I was released from undergraduate teaching as the holder of an I.W. Killam Research Fellowship administered by the Canada Council. I am deeply indebted to the University of Toronto for its substantial contribution to the Killam arrangements, and particularly to the Faculty of Medicine and former Dean Arnold Aberman for accommodating me in its History of Medicine Program. Grants-in-aid from the Hannah Institute for the History of Medicine, which is funded by Associated Medical Services, underwrote many of my direct research expenses. Without all this assistance the project would have taken many more years to complete.

Before leaving Canada to become the historian of St Mary's Hospital, London, my former student Elsbeth Heaman did heroic research preparing and organizing my files of Osleriana. Her enthusiasm for the project was extraordinarily helpful, as were her later incisive comments on the manuscript. I am also indebted for spot research help to Ed Benoit in Montreal and Shelley McKellar in Toronto.

While this was not in any way an official or sanctioned biography, I received only enthusiasm and cooperation from members of the Osler and Francis families whom I approached, most notably Eve Osler Hampson and Marian Francis Kelen. The Curators of the Osler Library for the History of Medicine at McGill University oversee a wonderful institution; the hospitality, help, good advice, patience, and much else that I received from the staff of the Osler Library – including June Schachter, Wayne LeBel, Pam Miller, and former Osler librarian, Professor Faith Wallis – were exemplary. The Osler Library is one of the best history of medicine libraries in the world; it welcomes private support through the Friends of the Osler Library, a very good cause for those who wish to perpetuate Osler's memory. All of the research material and manuscripts generated in this project will go to the Osler Library.

I was made welcome in every library and archive I visited, as well as by telephone, fax, and e-mail at institutions I may never see. Nancy McCall and her staff at the Chesney Archives of the Johns Hopkins Medical Institutions were particularly helpful, as were Charles Greifenstein and the staff at the Library of the College of Physicians of Philadelphia and Gretchen Worden of the Mütter Museum. The Huntington Library in Pasadena is an unusually wonderful place to work; so, of course, is Oxford's Bodleian Library. The archive of the Osler Club of London, located in its Club Room at the Royal College of Physicians of London, was uniquely charming; Yale University Library's policy of making the Harvey Cushing Papers available on microfilm made their use uniquely convenient. Thanks for hospitality, help, and often quite extensive service to the staff of the Archives of the Province of Ontario, the Thomas Fisher Rare Book Library of the University of Toronto, McGill University's Archives, the Sophia Smith Collection at the Nielson Library of Smith College, the Eisenhower Library of Johns Hopkins University, the Library of the Medical and Chirurgical Faculty of Maryland, the Cushing-Whitney Medical History Library of Yale University, the Hamilton (Ontario) Academy of Medicine, the Dundas (Ontario) Public Library, the American Philosophical Society Library (Philadelphia), Philadelphia City Archives, Thomas Jefferson University Archives, the University of Pennsylvania Archives, the Rare Books Division of the University of Pennsylvania Library, the Countway Medical Library of Medicine of Harvard University, the Woodward Biomedical Library of the University of British Columbia, the Phleger Room of the Health Sciences Library of the University of California at San Francisco, the Library of the Royal College of Surgeons of England, the Library of the Royal College of Physicians of London, the Bernard Becker Medical Library of the Washington University School of Medicine, the South Caroliniana Library of the University of South Carolina (Columbia), Trinity University Library (San Antonio, Texas), the Eskind Biomedical Library of Vanderbilt University Medical Center, the New York Public Library, and Trinity College School library (Port Hope, Ontario).

Gerry Hallowell of the University of Toronto Press and Jeff House of Oxford University Press saw the potential in this project and shepherded it to completion. I received useful suggestions about improving the manuscript from my publishers' anonymous readers, and detailed, invaluable comment from Drs Charles S. Bryan and W. Bruce Fye, as well as from Elizabeth Bliss – three eagle-eyed and erudite critics. Drs Jeremiah A. Barondess and John Dirks gave me special help and insight into Osler's last illness. Carlotta Lemieux is an amazing copy editor. The shortcomings of the text are solely my responsibility. Special thanks to Drs Arthur Gryfe, Andrew Baines, and Lynn Russell for making it possible for me to observe autopsies and outstanding teachers of medicine, and to the outstanding teachers I observed, Drs Herbert Ho Ping-Kong and Michael Hutcheon.

For help with research, leads, documents, arrangements, contacts, interviews, and everything else that went into a very complex project, thanks to Dr Donald Bates, Dr John Carson, Andrea Clark, Jim and Jennifer Connor, Sue O'Reilly Davis, Muriel Howard Douglas, Mrs Jane Farrar, Katherine I. Ferguson, Dr Palmer H. Futcher, Dr Charles M. Godfrey, Dr Richard L. Golden, Dr George T. Harrell, Marian Hebb, Dr David B. Hogan, Tom

Horrocks, Susan Kelen, Dr Harold M. Malkin, Professor A. E. Malloch, Donald Matthews, Sandra McRae, Dr Victor A. McKusick, Dr Jock Murray, Dr Earl F. Nation, Carol Nash, Dr Richard T. O'Kell, Michael Osler, Violet Andras Peard, Felicity Pope, Dr Charles G. Roland, Dr Jesse Roth, Dr Alex Sakula, Dr Clark Sawin, Eric and Lois Sinclair, Edward Shorter, Dr Marvin Stone, Dr John D. Stobo, Philip Teigen, Sylvia Van Kirk, Lord (John) Walton of Detchant, Dr Leonard Weistrop, William Westfall, Alan Wilkinson, Dr Charles F. Wooley, and other colleagues, associates, and friends in the American Osler Society and the Toronto Medical Historical Club. Thanks and apologies to those whom I have inadvertently neglected to mention.

Illustration Credits

Alan Mason Chesney Medical Archives of the Johns Hopkins Medical Institutions: Johns Hopkins Hospital, c. 1892; The Women's Committee; *The Four Doctors* by John Singer Sargent; Franklin P. Mall; Harvey Cushing; Lewellys Barker; 'The Saint' by Max Brödel

Dr. Palmer Futcher: Donkey riding

Journal of the American Medical Association, **1901**: An 'Observation' Class

National Library of Medicine, Bethesda, Md: Osler, 1919, B20151

Osler Library of the History of Medicine, McGill University: William Osler; Featherstone Lake Osler; Ellen Pickton Osler; The Rectory; Ellen Osler and her 'Tecumseth Cabbages'; William Osler as prefect; Jennette Osler; Marian Osler Francis; Osler's mentors: W.A. Johnson, James Bovell, and Palmer Howard; Osler at McGill; instructing in the Blockley Dead House; Osler, pathologist; writing *The Principles and Practice of Medicine*; Grace Revere Osler and her trophy husband; Inspection, palpation, auscultation, contemplation; 'Open Arms'; the Oslers in Oxford; the children's doctor; cavorting on a beach; Sir William Osler, age 63; Father and son, peace; Father and son, war; W.W. Francis

Index

Also by Michael Bliss

Medical History

The Discovery of Insulin

Banting: A Biography

Plague: A Story of Smallpox in Montreal

Canadian History

Right Honourable Men: The Descent of Canadian Politics
from Macdonald to Mulroney

Northern Enterprise: Five Centuries of Canadian Business

A Canadian Millionaire: The Life and Business Times
of Sir Joseph Flavelle

A Living Profit: Studies in the Social History
of Canadian Business, 1883–1911